AF383059

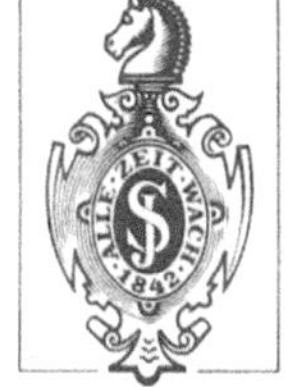

P.C. Leung (Ed.)

Current Practice of Fracture Treatment

New Concepts and Common Problems

With 248 Figures and 10 Tables

Springer-Verlag

Berlin Heidelberg New York London Paris
Tokyo Hong Kong Barcelona Budapest

Prof. P.C. Leung
Department of Orthopaedics & Traumatology
Faculty of Medicine
The Chinese University of Hong Kong
Prince of Wales Hospital
Shatin, N.T., Hong Kong

ISBN-13: 978-3-642-78605-1   e-ISBN-13: 978-3-642-78603-7
DOI: 10.1007/978-3-642-78603-7

Library of Congress Cataloging-in-Publication Data. Current practice of fracture treatment: new concepts and common problems / P.C. Leung, ed. p. cm. Includes bibliographical references and index. ISBN 0-387-57367-4 (U.S.) 1. Fractures — Treatment. I. Leung, Ping-Chung, 1941–RD101.C893 1994 617.1'5 — dc20 94-2609 CIP

24/3130 – 5 4 3 2 1 0 – Printed on acid-free paper

Foreword

This book, under the skillful editorship of Prof. P.C. Leung, will be a very welcome addition to the libraries of many postgraduates, junior orthopaedic surgeons and trauma surgeons, who have the responsibility of not only practicing a high standard of fracture care but also for keeping up to date. Indeed, one of the chapter titles contained the word "contemporary" which can be defined as "occurring at the same moment of time."

The numerous authors, all expert in their particular fields, have tackled interestingly and written succinctly on the perspectives, the controversies, dilemmas and problems as well as the emerging science of biomechanics in fracture repair and fixation and microvascular surgery.

In the "contemporary" world of trauma on the roads, in the work place and on the battle fields, fracture treatment still remains the raison d' etre for the majority of surgeons both in training and in practice. This book will be of help to many.

Oxford   ROBERT B. DUTHIE

Notes from the Editor

Many books have been written on fracture management. Large volumes giving comprehensive accounts of all types of fractures are available for reference purposes, and special fractures sometimes arouse so much interest and controversy that short monographs are specially written to offer an answer to the problem. This volume is a medium-sized reference, dealing with commonly occurring and yet difficult problems. It is particularly designed as an aid for those colleagues who are required to deal with fracture problems every day.

Such physicians may have easy access to large, comprehensive volumes of fracture management in the hospital library; however, they need to familiarize themselves thoroughly with useful options of treatment for commonly occurring, difficult fractures. All the details of concept and procedures involved in treating these common fractures which need to be learned are available in this volume. The book can be used as a check list to ensure that the right choice of treatment is made.

With this in mind, the book starts by supplying the basic principles of fracture fixation and biomechanical principles which provide the scientific background for making a wise choice. The subsequent chapters discuss popular methods of internal fixation, including intramedullary nailing and the use of external fixations. Plating and screwing are not discussed separately since this method of fixation is becoming less popular and few recent advances are known currently.

Compound fractures are everyday problems, and the principles of their management and practical solutions deserve separate discussion. The value of microsurgical techniques has been underestimated by orthopaedic experts and the indications, choices and procedures have been put into proper perspective.

Following basic principles and special topic discussions, the book turns to practical problem-solving areas, namely the hand, wrist, elbow, shoulder, hip, knee, ankle and foot, and spine and special problems in children. These are mainly juxta-articular regions which are known to produce severe functional disturbances after injuries. The recent developments in treatment concept, options and procedures have brought about remarkable improvements in the functional outcome, and so options and tricks to bring about better results have been offered.

This book is a practical guide for the treatment of commonly occurring, difficult fractures. Orthopaedic surgeons will find sufficient basic information and principles to back up their choices of treatment.

Contents

1 General Perspectives on Fracture Management
   P.C. Leung 1

2 Biomechanics of Fracture Repair and Fracture Fixation
   E.Y.S. Chao and H.T. Aro 9

3 Contemporary Applications of External Fixation in Fracture
   Treatment
   S. Nayagam and J.B. Jupiter 59

4 Current Use of the Intramedullary Nail
   D. Pennig 119

5 Problems in Compound Fractures
   N.P. Suedkamp and H. Tscherne 167

6 Microvascular Reconstruction in Limb Trauma
   L.K. Hung 187

7 Problems in Children's Fractures
   J.C.Y. Cheng 218

8 Hand Fractures: Controversies and Dilemmas
   L.K. Hung and P.C. Leung 248

9 Fractures of the Distal Radius and Ulna
   K.S. Leung and P.C. Leung 308

10 Problems in Elbow Fractures
    W.Y. Shen and J.C.Y. Cheng 327

11 Problems in Shoulder Fractures
    S.Y.C. Hsu 354

12 Fractures Around the Hip
    K.S. Leung 373

13 Problem Fractures Around the Knee
    K.M. Chan 399

14 Fractures Around the Ankles and Foot
    K.S. Leung 419

15 Problems in Spinal Fractures
    S.Y. Lee 440

Subject Index 471

List of Contributors

ARO, H.T., Biomechanics Laboratory, Department of Orthopaedics, Johns Hopkins University, 720 Rutland Ave, Baltimore, MD 21205, USA

CHAN, K.M., Department of Orthopaedics & Traumatology, The Chinese University of Hong Kong, Prince of Wales Hospital, Shatin, N.T., Hong Kong

CHAO, E.Y.S., Biomechanics Research Laboratory, Department of Orthopaedics, Johns Hopkins University, 5601 Loch Raven Blvd 4th Fl, Baltimore, MD 21239, USA

CHENG, J.C.Y., Department of Orthopaedics & Traumatology, The Chinese University of Hong Kong, Prince of Wales Hospital, Shatin, N.T., Hong Kong

HSU, S.Y.C., Consultant Orthopaedic Surgeon, Department of Orthopaedics & Traumatology, Team A, Princess Margaret Hospital, Kowloon, Hong Kong

HUNG, L.K., Department of Orthopaedics & Traumatology, The Chinese University of Hong Kong, Prince of Wales Hospital, Shatin, N.T., Hong Kong

JUPITER, J., Orthopaedic Trauma Service, Massachusetts General Hospital, Harvard Medical School, Ambulatory Care Center, Boston, MA 02114, USA

LEE, S.Y., Hong Kong Society for Rehabilitation, Margaret Trench Medical Rehabilitation Centre, Rehab Path, Kwun Tong, Kowloon, Hong Kong

LEUNG, K.S., Department of Orthopaedics & Traumatology, The Chinese University of Hong Kong, Prince of Wales Hospital, Shatin, N.T., Hong Kong

LEUNG, P.C., Department of Orthopaedics & Traumatology, The Chinese University of Hong Kong, Prince of Wales Hospital, Shatin, N.T., Hong Kong

NAYAGAM, S., 14, Wensley Drive, Withington, Manchester, M203DD, England

PENNIG, D., Abteilung für Trauma-, Hand- und Wiederherstellungs chirurgie, St. Vinzenz-Klinik, Westfälische-Wilhelms-Univcr sität, Merheimer Straße 221–223, D-50733 Köln, Germany

SHEN, W.Y., Consultant Orthopaedic Surgeon, Department of Orthopaedics & Traumatology, Team 1, Queen Elizabeth Hospital, Kowloon, Hong Kong
SUEDKAMP, N.P., Medizinische Hochschule Hannover, Unfallchirurgische Klinik, Konstanty-Gutschow-Straße 8, D-30625 Hannover, Germany
TSCHERNE, H., Medizinische Hochschule Hannover, Unfallchirurgische Klinik, Konstanty-Gutschow-Straße 8, D-30625 Hannover, Germany

1 General Perspectives on Fracture Management

P.C. Leung

Introduction

The treatment of fracture has a history perhaps as long as that of fairly institutionalized human civilization itself. In fact, this is only to be expected, since injuries resulting from work and daily activities are particularly common in upright walking human beings. Both the human posture and the extremely varied demands of work and recreation make human limbs and the supporting skeleton especially vulnerable to injuries and particularly to fractures. Our ancestors knew long ago that fractures heal spontaneously, albeit slowly, and they attempted to splint them in order to relieve pain, while leaving nature to heal the injuries. Resting and immobilization for a painful limb were also practised, although this is perhaps instinctive.

As early as the first century AD the Chinese began to develop their system of fracture fixation, and historical records are available from that period on (Fig. 1). In China a comprehensive system of fracture treatment, including a manual of reduction techniques and other adjunctive measures, was established during the Chin Dynasty (fourth century) by a Taoist monk called Gue Hung. This manual formed the basis of all later books and commentaries on the management of fractures and dislocations (Fig. 2).

The following review of the history of fracture treatment adds an important aspect not only by illustrating the cultural heritage but also by enabling us to take a paramedic's view of the development of fracture management. Because of my own personal background I am in a better position to review historical trends in the Orient – China and Japan – and therefore concentrate on fracture treatment in the Far East rather than on that in early Roman and Egyptian civilizations. Chinese civilization shows a very strong heritage in the treatment of bone and joint diseases. If modern theories and practices were not derived purely from intuition and brilliant innovation, they must have drawn inspiration from such earlier endeavours.

History of Fracture Treatment in the Far East

Curative arts comprised a very strong element in ancient Chinese culture, particularly in the area of bones and joints. A review of the available

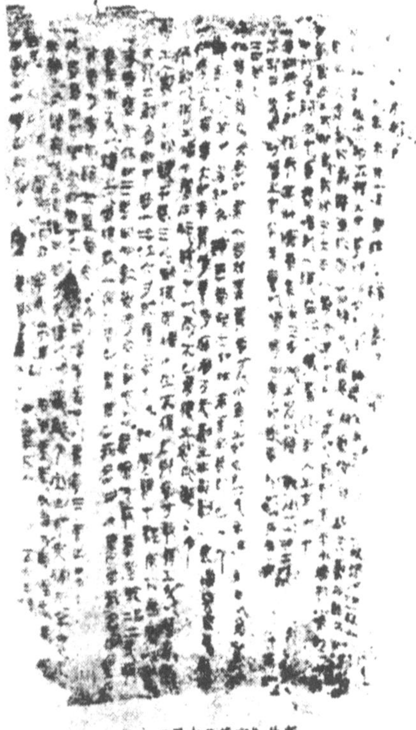

Fig. 1. Ancient manuscript on the treatment of fracture (around the first century)

literature confirms that up to the middle of the nineteenth century, Chinese bone setters possessed a genuine command of the treatment of fractures and dislocations. Their Japanese counterparts learned these arts from the Chinese, refering to their writings and applying their techniques.

The earliest record of the surgical treatment of bone disease describes a mighty warrior in the second century who was shot in the arm with a putatively poisoned arrow. The legendary surgeon cut open the warrior's arm, removed the arrow and curetted the affected bone. Whether the affected bone was suffering as the result of actual poison or of simple infection remains a matter of speculation. According to the story, the warrior was engaged in a game of chess with an aide while the surgeon-physician used a knife to curette his poisoned bone. His apparent serenity during the operation suggests that the curettage procedure may have been carried out under some form of local anaesthesia.

A century later (in the year 250) a healer of joint pains wrote a book on the use of acupuncture in the treatment of joint pain. Less than a century after this the first volume on the technique of reducing fractures and dislocations appeared. The author, a Taoist, was probably the greatest bone setter who ever lived. He worked out the basic procedures for closed

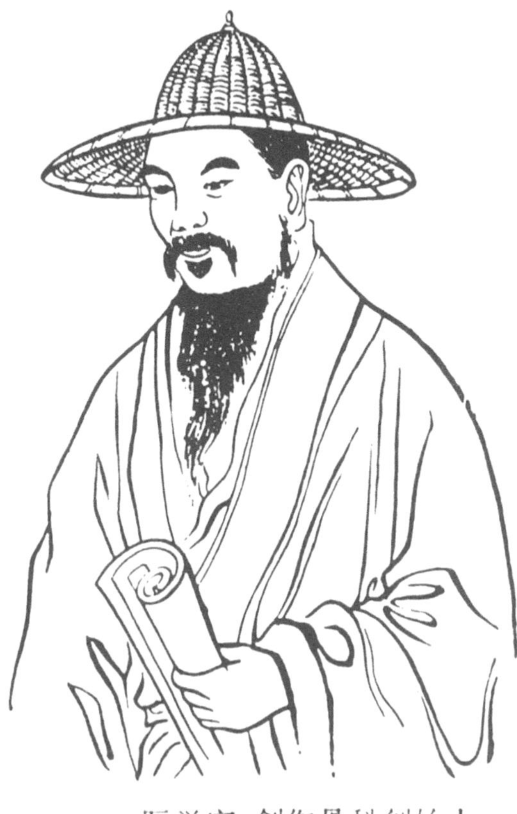

Fig. 2. Gue Hung, Taoist monk who described fractures and dislocations in great detail. His manual on their treatment challenges many modern methods

reduction, and in terms of modern concepts these are by no means out of date even today. Such classical accounts of fracture treatment and other aspects of bone problems certainly indicate that fracture treatment in China enjoyed a very early development, much earlier in fact than that in Western culture.

Since the Tang Dynasty (618–907) many other important writings on fracture treatment have appeared. The first account of the treatment of osteomyelitis dates from 1189; the procedure involved the removal of dead bone and curettage of apparently healthy bones. During these centuries, Japanese healers followed in the footsteps of the Chinese, and their writings reflected the Chinese experience. During the Yüan Dynasty (1280–1386) Li Chongnam worked out an approach for the treatment of fractured spine using the methods of traction and extension.

In 1578, during the Ming Dynasty (1368–1644), an important manual on the use of herbal plants was produced by a physician called Li Xichun. This manual contained a full description of herbs used for the healing of fractures and joint pains. Around this time, in the seventeenth century, while Oriental healers were still concentrating on the treatment of traumatic conditions, Western researchers such as Fabricius Hildanus (1560–1634) described in detail the conditions of scoliosis and Framis Glisson (1597–1677) described distraction treatment for spinal deformities.

In the period of the Ching Dynasty (1644–1911) all areas of Chinese culture enjoyed thorough scholastic review and analysis of past works. As old concepts were analysed, new ideas came to be elaborated. China at this time was quite isolated from the rest of the world, as Western science and technology was developing with a logic of direct deduction and didactics. The work of John Hunter (1728–1798) on the pathology of bone, including fractures and infections, was unknown to the Orient throughout the nineteenth century. The first orthopaedic hospital – the Royal Orthopaedic Hospital – was founded in England in 1837 by a physician-surgeon called Little, while Chinese healers were still busy collecting traditional methods for the management of bone and joint disorders. Monks living in the monasteries on mountains in China were great contributors to the art of bone setting, and an herbalist by the name of Jiang, in the middle of the Ching Dynasty, made a trip to the mountains to visit exponents of the various schools of bone setting and compiled a book on the basis of his experiences to give a comprehensive account of what he had discovered.

Surgery in the West took great strides as anaesthesia was developed in the nineteenth century (1846), and the aseptic technique was introduced by Lister in 1867. Japan began to adopt a much more open stance to the outside world, and important books on surgery were introduced and translated into Japanese as early as 1851. From then on, important publications were translated continuously. In China the first translated book on surgery was entitled *The First Line of Practice of Surgery in the West*, by Benjamin Hobson. This book was published in Shanghai in 1857, after which further works were not identified. Japanese interest was very much committed to the area of military medicine, which was best developed in Prussia in the middle of the nineteenth century. All the important manuals and books on military medicine at this time were translated into Japanese. During the Meiji era (1867–1912), more active programmes for the adoption of Western science and technology were implemented. Starting with techniques for bandaging and splinting fractures and later developing into basic orthopaedic areas, however, the written work produced in this period was not particularly illuminating.

The leading role of the West in the field of orthopaedic surgery was evidenced, finally, by the initiation of orthopaedic journals (*Revue d' Orthopaedie* in 1890, *Zeitschrift für Orthopädische Chirurgie* in 1892, *Journal of Bone and Joint Surgery* in 1919). Japan established her Surgical Association in 1898, which began publication of its journal the following year.

Orthopaedic surgery experienced another breakthrough when Röntgen invented an X-ray machine to examine the human body, making possible more direct observation and analysis based on the study of X-ray shadows. Since then it has become clear that further developments in the treatment of fractures must rely on the Western approach. The traditional methods of healing have made great contributions in the past, but these have limitations. The traditional methods of treatment, however, should not be seen as being of merely historical interest. It remains the task of modern researchers to reexamine the technical procedures and other means of treatment that have been applied in the past (such as herbal medicine) and to extract from these effective components that may further enrich more modern therapeutic modalities.

Principles of Fracture Treatment

All viable tissues possess the power of healing after damage. One should not assume that because bone is a rigid, hard tissue, it heals with more difficulty. As a matter of fact, the metabolic activities of bone are so active that the speed of catabolic and anabolic changes in bony tissues is faster than that in any other tissue in the body other than blood. Bone healing after injury is therefore guaranteed as long as the environmental circumstances are in order. It is said that the stimulating factor for bone healing is injury itself. Indeed, anthropologists who studied gibbons living in the forests found that a large percentage of them showed evidence of healed fractures. Although different degrees of deformities are found, fractures in the upper limbs always healed. Lower limb fractures likewise healed except when they occurred in the femoral neck region. One may therefore conclude that even without treatment nature heals fractures under most circumstances.

Management of human fractures therefore began with reducing and realigning the displaced fracture ends and protecting the reduced and re-aligned ends by external splintage, first in the form of wooden sticks and later with plaster of paris casts. Nature was the proven healer.

Casting brought with it, however, the unwanted result of joint stiffness in the adjacent joints. A method for overcoming this problem was to free the joints by functional braces. Skin-tight application of the braces produced sufficient support to the reduced fractures to protect the fracture ends from motion while the adjacent joints were mobilized. This was an impressive development of external splintage for suitable fractures, namely fractures of diaphyseal regions. Unfortunately, fractures of other sites and of more complicated nature could not be treated by functional bracing.

Open operative treatment was originally used only for the open type of fracture or when there were complications such as nerve and vascular damage or infection. Screws, plates and other implants were designed for fixing such fractures. It must be noted, however, that screws and plates did not heal fractures; only nature (normal physiological healing power) healed fractures.

The Swiss group that studied fracture healing (AO) contributed substantially to the conceptualization of open treatment for fractures. These researchers worked on the biomechanics of fracture fixation, metallurgy of implants and atraumatic techniques for approaching fractures. The same group also introduced the concept of fracture healing without callus (primary bone healing) as the optimum method of fracture healing. The upshot of this concept for the management of fractures is, of course, that virtually all fractures should be treated by open reduction and rigid internal fixation, i.e. applying compression to fracture ends to achieve "primary non-callus forming bone healing".

While fixing with open techniques and fracture end compression produce remarkable radiological pictures, it was soon discovered that healing without callus produces a weak union which relies on implant strength. "Primary bone healing" may therefore, after all, not be wholly desirable. Healing, whether enhanced by closed or open technique, may proceed best with both internal and external callus formation. This cannot be achieved by applying internal fixation with such rigidity as to allow virtually no motion at the fracture site. A compromise may therefore provide the ideal situation: a means of internal fixation that maintains perfect alignment of the fracture ends while allowing minor degrees of movement at the fracture site to stimulate external callus formation. On the basis of this concept, intramedullary nails and "semi-rigid" implants, for example, of carbon substance, were introduced.

This history of attempts to manage the healing of bone fractures underscores the fact that nothing has yet replaced nature as *the* effective healer in bone healing. Management concepts that did not respect this fact, for example, those completely proscribing joint motion, led to healing that was often imperfect.

What then are the effects of open management and internal fixation? Should they not be dropped as treatment methods, leaving us to rely on natural healing alone? Apart from such complications as open wounds or vascular and nerve damage, open treatment does have a definite place. Fractures should heal with maximal functional recovery. Functional recovery is of course adversely affected by deformities, joint stiffness and intra-articular derangements. Although open management may slow bone healing, in many instances it is the only means of producing perfect reduction, preventing deformities, maintaining articular integrity and allowing immediate joint motion. Special techniques such as bone grafting and special implant fixation likewise require open management.

The apparent controversies are in fact more understandable when one recalls the basic factors governing fracture fixation: reduction, immobilization and rehabilitation. All current procedures in fracture treatment concentrate on perfect reduction followed by temporary rigid fixation or semi-rigid fixation. The former requires the early introduction of controlled motion while the latter depends more on metallurgic inventions. External fixators with telescoping bars are claimed to supply rigid fixation while at the same time allowing axial movement. Although experimental models have failed to demonstrate successfully the real mechanical effects of "dynamization", clinically a timely release of the rigidity given by the external fixator (which is still being used as effective means of immobilization) does give better radiological results of callus formation or consolidation. This of course has been a clinical observation, and the principle of so-called "release of rigidity" has been arbitrarily applied: the timing has been arbitrary and the stress allowed has been arbitrary.

While accepting that perfect and early functional recovery often requires operative treatment and internal fixation, the temptation to over-operate is dangerous. More stress should therefore be put on the identification of fracture types that heal safely without complications. Such fractures should not require operative treatment. Are there such fractures? Apart from minor fractures without displacement, all diaphyseal fractures of spiral nature have such large areas of fracture contact and healing is more or less guaranteed.

Difficult Areas

It is equally important for the surgeon to recognize the difficult areas that are not able to enjoy natural healing to the same extent as others. There are three situations which inevitably present problems for fracture healing, namely, when fragments do not stay together, when blood supply is deficient, and when wide bone gaps exist.

When a fracture occurs, there may be comminutions, and yet the fragments tend to stay together because of periosteal linkages and soft tissue tension around the fracture, unless it is an open type of fracture in which soft tissue losses are extensive. Healing can therefore be expected to be problematic in this type of compound fracture. When comminution occurs in an intra-articular fracture, the fragments float apart due to the lack of soft tissue tension around the fracture; intra-articular fractures therefore often present problems of healing.

The blood supply to a fracture site relies on the original blood flow to the fragments and the surrounding vasculature. Disruption of the blood supply to the fracture fragments is often compensated by a soft tissue environment of rich blood flow. Nevertheless, when soft tissue damage is so severe that bone coverage is hardly attained, revascularization faces a problem. John Charnley remarked that "It is not so much the methods of osteosynthesis but the vascularity of the surrounding tissues that affects the outcome of the fracture healing." Unique anatomical regions may be responsible for the selective disruption of blood flow to a fracture site and hence jeopardize its healing or subsequent well-being. Well-known examples of segmental ischaemia leading to necrosis include the femoral head in femoral neck fracture, proximal segment of the scaphoid in scaphoid fracture and dome of the talus in fracture of the talus.

Fractures often create gaps at the fracture sites. Small gaps are easily bridged spontaneously. Those wider than 0.5 cm require a lengthy period even when conditions are favourable. Early clinical and radiological assessment is important so that problems of healing in situations of comminution can be predicted. Early cancellous grafting is then indicated to obtain better results of union. Failing this, healing will be unduly delayed.

Conclusion

Efforts over the past centuries in the treatment of fracture have been directed towards the facilitation of union and the preservation of function. The achievements based on biomechanical considerations have been remarkable. We are now good at keeping a fracture reduced and in an environment of reasonable stress to allow healing to occur. In other words, the mechanical factors that affect fracture healing can now be controlled and even utilized to stimulate callus formation. Each individual surgeon must assess the force transmission across any difficult fracture and estimate during the treatment planning the bending, rotatory and axial loads that are likely to be exerted on the fracture site, so that the best means of immobilization may be instituted. The biomechanical control on most fractures should be positively controllable.

There are other equally important factors which are not easily controlled. Firstly, the nature of the fracture itself is predetermined, and degree of displacement and comminution affect the outcome of the healing. Secondly, the patient's general well-being and associated bone pathology (e.g. osteopenia or other more serious disorders) could have an adverse influence on fracture healing. This type of host-dependent consideration, unfortunately, is not widely considered by junior surgeons, and this very often causes complications.

Future advances in the treatment of fractures may lie in promoting the host's ability to heal. This could, perhaps, take the form of promoting fracture site circulation, and promoting callus formation by using humoral factors.

2 Biomechanics of Fracture Repair and Fracture Fixation

E.Y.S. Chao and H.T. Aro

Introduction

Knowledge of the basic biomechanical principles is essential throughout the care and management of patients with long-bone fractures. This starts from the evaluation of fracture mechanism and extends to the phase of treatment when the structural strength of the healed bone is evaluated after removal of the fixation device.

Selection of the fixation method is multifactorial. Factors such as the patient's age, the affected bone, the existence of multitrauma, the severity of local soft-tissue injury, and others, including the personal preference and clinical experience of the surgeon, are involved in the selection process. Most importantly, the selection of fixation rigidity determines the mode of bone healing. Hence, the mechanism of bone fracture healing chosen should dictate the further course of patient care.

Fracture healing results in reconstitution of the original bony structure and material properties. The healing involves a number of important developmental processes which can be regarded as temporary reversal to embryonic state. The mechanisms controlling the repair processes of fractures are the most fundamental in biology, involving the molecular stimulus that prompts the cells at the fracture site to alter their normal rate of growth and the stimuli which recruit cells outside the fractured bone to participate in the healing processes.

Understanding the basic events in bone healing is a prerequisite for the successful outcome of fracture treatment, regardless of the method of immobilization to be utilized. The need for deep insight into the bone healing mechanisms will be even more important in the future development of mechanical, physical, or biological stimuli in fracture healing modulation. It is also well known that different types of tissue may form or remodel under a specific stress or loading condition (Fig. 1). However, many of such generalized mechanophysiological concepts are unproven under in vivo animal models. These considerations open up the possibilities to manipulate specific tissue formation in many orthopedic reconstructive procedures, including bone fracture healing management.

Orthopedic surgeons are faced with increasing numbers of fixation devices and treatment alternatives in fracture management. Biomaterial

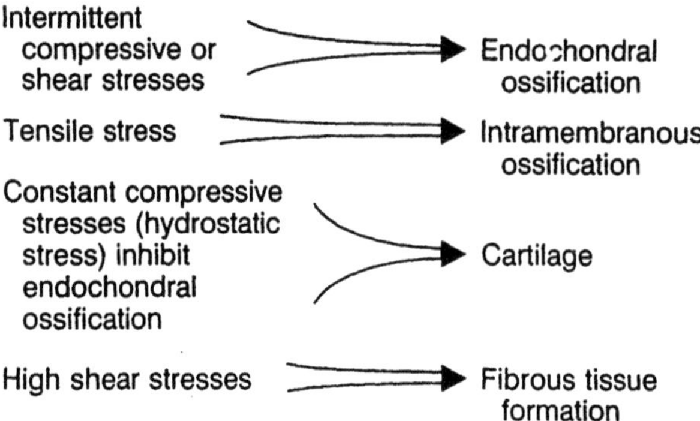

Fig. 1. Hypothetical mechanisms between mechanical stresses and connective tissue formation

technology is offering solutions to the many problems related to the use of conventional metal implants in fracture fixation. The successful clinical application of the new methods, however, requires a good knowledge of the biomechanics of these devices, the biological demands of the healing process, and the ability to manipulate tissue formation using either mechanical, physical, or biological stimuli.

Each of the well-established fixation methods (rigid compression plating; reamed intramedullary nailing, with or without interlocking of the fracture fragments; and external fixation) has advantages and disadvantages as well as special biomechanical characteristics. Vast clinical experience combined with the data produced from theoretical and experimental studies have described many of the problems related to the biomechanics of these fracture fixation devices. These findings have, in many cases, resulted in the improved design of the devices, with a more reliable clinical result. Because of the inherent differences, one method may have a preferred advantage in certain fracture cases over another, and there is general agreement on the indications and contraindications for each method. Proper surgical technique must be utilized, however, to ensure the desired biomechanical outcome of the fixation and to avoid additional tissue trauma and devascularization at the fracture site.

Current treatment results of long-bone fractures are generally rated from good to excellent, even in high-grade open fractures. Modern guidelines for intra-articular fracture management, including anatomical reduction of the fragments and rigid internal fixation, have produced satisfactory results even under rather difficult situations. Only in certain types of long-bone fractures, especially those involving the tibia, are there treatment problems that require special attention. Operative management of fractures presents the risk of infection which could result in the development of chronic osteomyelitis or even in amputation. Undoubtedly, many noninfectious complications originate from incomplete evaluation of the biomechanical characteristics of the fracture type and the inherent biomechanical limitations and physiological disadvantages of the selected fixation method. The purpose of this chapter is to give an overview of fracture mechanics of long bones and the healing mechanisms of diaphyseal fractures under stable and unstable mechanical conditions, with special emphasis on the comparison of fracture fixation and bone healing characteristics related to the use of rigid compression plates, intramedullary nails, and external fixators.

Fracture Mechanism of Long Bones

Fractures can be classified in terms of the factors characterizing the force having caused the fracture. Fractures caused by direct forces can be subclassified according to the magnitude and area distribution of the force as well as according to the rate at which the force acted on the bone. Soft-tissue injury and fracture comminution are especially related to the loading rate. Trauma energy is dependent upon the second power of loading rate, and this energy is released when a bone fractures. Thus, high-velocity gunshot wounds result in considerably more soft-tissue damage and bone comminution than low-velocity gunshot wounds as a result of the application of a greater, more rapidly loaded force. The destructive effect of high-velocity bullets is even increased if the impact area (bullet dimension) is decreased.

Fractures due to indirect forces are produced by a force acting at a distance from the fracture site. When a long bone is loaded, each section of the bone is subject to both normal and shear stress (Fig. 2). When these stresses exceed the limit of the bone according to certain failure criteria, the bone fractures. Different loads generate different normal and shear stresses

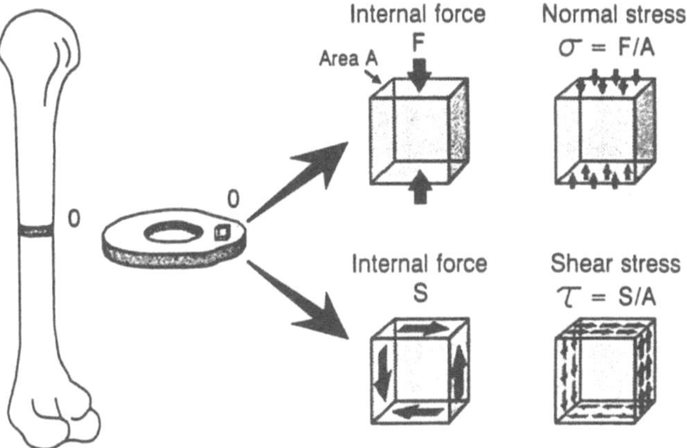

Fig. 2. Normal and shear stresses in a long bone under internal and external loading

along different orientation planes within the bone. Judging the morphology of fracture lines, it is possible to estimate the type of indirect injury mechanism (Fig. 3).

In general, depending upon material strength, certain combinations of the three principal stress planes (maximum tensile stress, maximum compressive stress, and maximum shear stress) dictate the fracture plane and when and how the material will fail. Cortical bone as a material is generally weak in tensile and shear, particularly along the longitudinal plane. Hence, cortical bone is not regarded as an isotropic material since its strength is directionally dependent, which also influences bone fracture failure under external loads.

The failure patterns of long bones follow basic rules. Under bending, the convex side is under tension and the concave side under compression. Since bone is more susceptible to failure in tension than in compression, the tension (convex) side fails first. Tension failure then occurs progressively across the bone, creating a transverse fracture without comminution. Occasionally, the cortex under compression breaks due to shear stress before the tension failure progresses all the way across the bone; comminution on the compression side occurs which often creates a single "butterfly" fragment or multiple fragments. Under torsion injury, there is always a certain bending moment which prevents the propagation of an endless spiral fracture line. The 45° fracture line (theoretically) is a result of maximum tensile stress acting at a 45° plane. Shear stress may cause small longitudinal cracks on the spiral fracture line. Under experimental conditions, an average fracture angle of a spiral fracture is approximately 30° of the longitudinal axis, and combined axial loading has little effect on the torsional properties of whole bone [84].

The susceptibility of a bone to fracture under a single injury is related to its energy-absorbing capacity and modulus of elasticity. The loading rate of

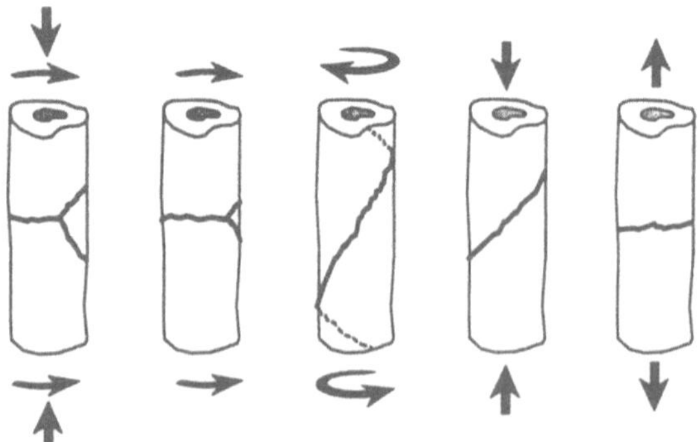

Fig. 3. Typical long-bone fracture morphology corresponding to the type of external load applied to the long bone. The fracture pattern may vary depending upon the magnitude of the composite loading mode involved

bone affects its energy-absorption capacity. Bone undergoing rapid loading absorbs more energy than when loaded at a slower rate [78]. However, there appears to occur a decline in energy absorbed at very high loading rates [84]. The energy absorbed by the bone during loading is released when the bone fractures. This phenomenon helps to explain why injuries with rapid loading involving higher velocities dissipate greater energy and result in greater fracture comminution and displacement. The clinical estimation of fracture energy is of great value. Long-bone shaft fractures resulting from high-energy injuries have a higher rate of bone healing complications than fractures of low-energy injuries. This difference has been explained by the severity of soft-tissue injury associated with high-energy injuries. Experimental studies [115] have demonstrated the retarding effect of muscle damage on bone healing.

Clinically, it is well known that spiral and oblique tibial fractures tend to heal faster than some transverse fractures. This difference in the inherent healing rate has been commonly related to as the difference in the amount of soft-tissue destruction, that is, in the difference in injury mechanism and fracture energy [47]. Another variable is the increased surface area of fracture ends in oblique/spiral fractures. The following in vitro experiment was designed to explore the possible difference in fracture energy under transverse and spiral failure of a loaded bone. Using eight pairs of canine tibiae, one bone of each pair was loaded to failure under torsion, while the contralateral side was loaded to failure under bending. The loading rate was slow and similar between the two loading modes. Load-displacement curves were recorded (Fig. 4) and analyzed for the stiffness (the initial slope of the

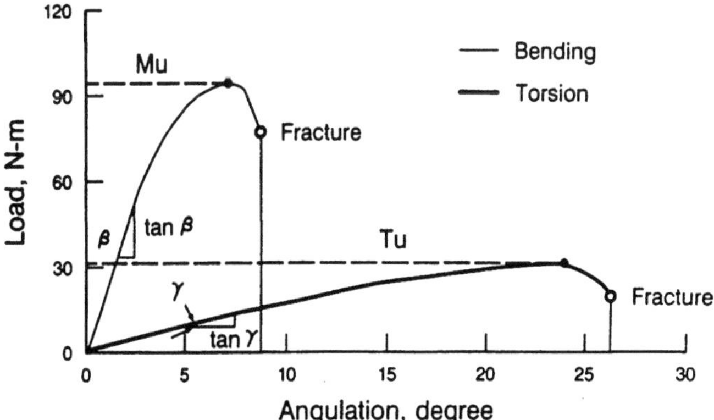

Fig. 4. A comparison of the load and angular deformity curve for canine tibiae under three-point bending and torsional load. Although the total energy to failure under torsion is approximately equal to that produced under bending, the ultimate load to failure for torsion (T_u) was substantially lower than the optimal load to failure through bending (M_u). Such difference in failure load may affect the degree of soft tissue and periosteum damage after bone fracture

load-displacement curve), maximum load at failure, deformation at failure, and the energy absorption at failure (the area of the load-displacement curve). Bending loading resulted in a transverse fracture, usually with some comminution on the compression side. Torsion loading caused a spiral fracture. Analysis of the load-displacement curves showed no statistically significant difference in the amount of energy absorption at failure. However, the maximum load to failure was about three times greater on the side of transverse failure. This difference was due to the different stiffness properties of the bone under torsion and bending. Under torsion, the bone exhibited relatively low stiffness and, on average, 23° of deformation before failure. During bending, the bone was relatively stiff and underwent, on average, only 8° of angulation before failure. In this experiment, the force needed to produce a transverse bending fracture was approximately three times greater than that required to produce a spiral fracture. This finding corroborates clinical experience of the injury mechanisms. Interestingly, the experiment did not suggest any difference in the amount of energy released when a bone develops a transverse or spiral fracture. However, the larger load under bending failure may cause the surrounding soft tissues and periosteum to sustain more damage and thus affect bone fracture healing potential.

The susceptibility of bone to fracture under fluctuating forces (or stresses) is related to its crystal structure and collagen orientation, which reflects the viscoelastic properties of the bone. Cortical bone is vulnerable to both tensile and compressive fluctuating stresses. Under each cycle of loading, a small amount of strain energy may be lost through microcracks along the cement lines. Fatigue load under certain strain rates can cause progressive accumulation of microdamage in cortical bone. When such a process is prolonged, bone may eventually fail through fracture crack propagation. Although bone has rather poor fatigue resistance in vitro, it is a living tissue and can undertake a repair process simultaneously. Periosteal callus and new bone formation near the microcracks can arrest crack propagation by reducing the high stresses at the tip of the crack. However, for this repair process to be effective, a relatively low level of stress must be applied and maintained on the bone.

Biological and Biomechanical Characteristics of Fracture Callus

Biological Processes of Fracture Healing

Fracture repair follows the principles which govern embryonic and fetal development of the skeleton and its physiological remodeling and functional adaptation [97,100]. A fractured bone has lost its mechanical integrity and continuity. The unique feature of fracture healing is restoration of the original tissue structure with mechanical properties equal to those before fracture. Injured skin, muscle, and tendon are unable to copy such a real regeneration process after injury but rather heal with permanent scar tissue. Factors that influence fracture healing are both systemic and local:

Systemic
    Age
    Hormones
    Functional activity
    Nerve functions
    Nutrition
Local
    Degree of local trauma
    Vascular injury
    Type of bone affected
    Degree of bone loss
    Degree of immobilization
    Infection
    Local pathological conditions

Fracture healing can be considered a series of phases occurring in sequence and also overlapping to a certain extent. The process can be divided into at least three distinct stages, those of inflammation, reparation, and remodeling [30]. Bone reacts to fracture within a few hours in uniform periosteal cell activity, and the initial cellular reaction is considered a very fundamental response of bone to any injury (so-called primary callus response) [71].

The inflammation phase may be most critical for the reparative phase of fracture healing, similar to that in soft-tissue wounds. If serious impairment of the inflammation phase occurs, tissue healing is compromised [53]. The inflammation phase includes activation of the cellular mechanisms necessary for the subsequent repair and also the processes protecting the healing tissue from infection. In brief, injury is translated to the waves of chemical messengers, such as kinins, complement factors, histamine, serotonin, prostanoids, and leukotrienes. The coagulation cascade contributes fibrin and fibrinopeptides. These together mediate the inflammatory reaction by causing vasodilation, migration, and chemoattraction, thus initiating the next step in repair. Platelets also assist, but, in addition, they contribute growth factors which initiate angiogenesis and mesenchymal cell proliferation. Upon reaching the injured tissue, the granulocytes ingest and destroy bacteria but do not contribute to repair. Macrophages and, to a lesser extent, lymphocytes aid in the destruction of bacteria but also stimulate repair by releasing angiogenesis factor(s) and other cell growth factors [53].

During the reparative phase, the pattern of fracture healing is highly susceptible to mechanical factors, that is, to the amount of interfragmentary motion. The natural histological course of fracture healing (without immobilization), described in detail by Ham [43] starts with interfragmentary stabilization by periosteal and endosteal callus formation. The process restores continuity, and bone union occurs by intramembranous and endo-chondral ossification. Avascular and necrotic areas of fracture ends are substituted by haversian remodeling. Malalignment of fragments may be corrected to a certain extent by remodeling of the fracture site and by functional adaptation, particularly in children or adolescents with remaining bone growth potential. Fracture remodeling generally does not correct torsional deformities.

At the inflammatory stage of healing, external callus tissue consists of primitive-looking mesenchymal cells, particularly granulation-tissue fibro-blasts, macrophages, and blood vessels. At this stage of healing, callus tissue shows the highest content of procollagen mRNA for type III collagen [75]. The origin of periosteal callus cells is still controversial, but, undoubtedly, the cambium layer of the periosteum plays an important role as a source of cells with both osteogenic and chondrogenic potential. The blood vessels of periosteal callus are entirely new, or almost so, and originate from sur-rounding extraskeletal tissues (muscles) [40] and from the medullary cavity [89]. It is not known whether invading vascular endothelial cells have osteogenic or chondrogenic potential. Angiogenesis, i.e., the growth of new capillaries, involves migration and proliferation of endothelial cells, and the process can be stimulated by so-called angiogenetic growth factors [7,39]. A hypoxic tissue gradient seems to be essential for the maintenance of angio-genesis in a healing tissue. Angiogenesis may be controlled by macrophages which produce angiogenic factors under hypoxic conditions [62]. Fracture callus [16,48] as well as the medullary cavity during external callus formation [3] show low tissue oxygen tension.

The induction and proliferation of undifferentiated periosteal callus tissue is the first critical step in fracture healing by external callus. Formation of such callus is suppressed by rigid immobilization. Excessive fracture motion is equally harmful. Its formation depends upon several humoral fac-tors. Most importantly, the induction and proliferation periods of periosteal callus are finite.

During the next phase, primitive callus tissue shows a very rapid chondrogenic transformation. The appearance of cartilage cells is reflected by the high levels of type II collagen mRNA. It has not been determined whether the cells with the condrogenic potential are derived from specific periosteal prechondrogenic cells or represent chondrocytes differentiated from primitive mesenchymal cells through signals created by the environ-ment. The size of early external callus ("soft callus") corresponds to that of cartilaginous callus as well as to that of the final bony callus. In addition, the DNA content, as an indicator of cell number, does not change during the maturation process.

The next critical step in obtaining union of a fracture is the establish-ment of an intact bony bridge between the fragments, and since this involves the joining of hard tissue, it follows that the whole system must become immobile at least momentarily [24]. At this stage of healing, an inefficient fracture immobilization by flexible stainless steel or plastic intramedullary rods [4,17] or by plates with low axial bending and torsional stiffnesses [119], as well as the presence of excessive fracture gap with no inherent fracture instability [74], may cause a pending hypertrophic nonunion because of the persistence of fibrous tissue or fibrous transformation of osteogenic callus tissue between the frontiers of bridging external callus. It seems that there is a narrow threshold for permissible interfragmentary motion, and the use of fixation flexibility as a method of callus stimulation at this stage would be difficult when the fracture healing pathway has already become committed to certain biological and mechanical conditions.

The osteoblastic activity, in conjunction with evaluation of osteoclastic activity, can also be quantitated using a histomorphometric technique developed for the evaluation of metabolic bone diseases from iliac crest bone biopsies [49,72]. Using this method, a recent study [5] showed that the osteoclastic number, measured per the woven new bone surface length, reaches the maximum value at an early stage of endochondral ossification, suggesting that there is a close coupling phenomenon between osteoblasts and osteoclasts in fracture callus.

During the ossification process of external callus, the total amount of calcium per unit volume of callus shows approximately a fourfold increase, hydroxyproline (an indicator of total collagen content) a twofold increase, and the breaking strength of the callus in tensile test a threefold increase (Fig. 5) [2]. The time-related changes in the amounts of the chemical callus components (total nitrogen, hydroxyproline, and minerals) are similar to those in

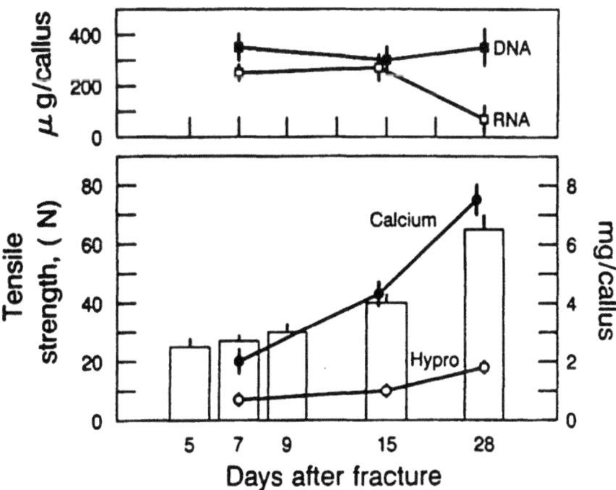

Fig. 5. Time-related change in nucleic acid in terms of DNA and mRNA (*above*), calcium, and hydroxyproline contents and the mechanical strength (*below*) of fracture callus as a function of healing time (rat tibia model, $n = 6$). *Vertical bars* (*below*), failure load of the callus in tensile test

breaking strength of the callus in tensile test. However, the chemical parameters of callus production are not correlated with the strength at any time period of healing [80]. Radiographic size of external callus is a poor predictor of fracture strength [79] and does not indicate at a given healing time the amount of chemical components in the fracture callus [4]. The restoration of fracture strength and stiffness seems to be related to the amount of new bone connecting the fracture fragments (measured from the failure plane in the tensile test) and less to the overall amount of uniting callus [11].

Biomechanical Properties of Fracture Callus

The structural properties of a healing fracture are dependent on the material properties of the uniting callus. To determine the material properties of callus tissue, uniform fracture callus specimens were loaded under axial compression using a circular indentor at a low deformation rate [5]. Callus tissue deformation, calculated from the impression of the indentor during loading, was continuously recorded with the applied load, and the modified Brinell's hardness value was calculated.

The results showed that the staged differentiation and mineralization of fracture callus have a profound influence on its compressive behavior (Fig. 6). Because mineralization is a major determinant of the mechanical behavior of fracture callus, we also examined the correlation between the mechanical properties of the callus tissue and its mineral content. A trochar-type indentor was used to obtain a full-length biopsy of the callus tissue, which was tested mechanically. The tissue sample with a known preloading volume was analyzed for calcium content. The results showed a close correlation ($r = 0.830$, $p < 0.001$) between the hardness of the fracture callus and its calcium content.

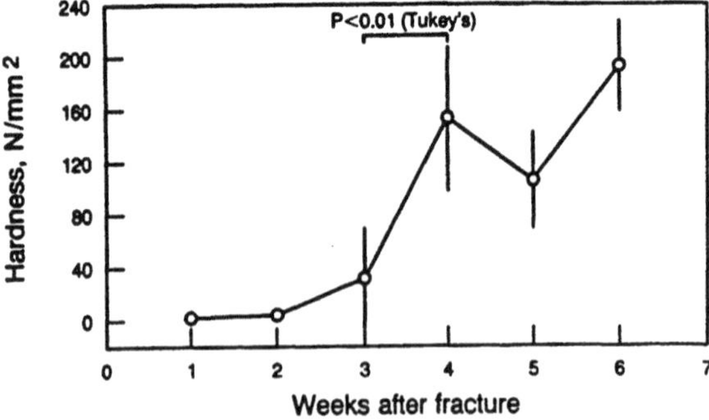

Fig. 6. Time-related change in callus hardness after initial bone fracture (rat tibia model). The increasing hardness with time reflects the differentiation of callus tissue to woven bone (1–4 weeks) and subsequent bone remodeling (4–6 weeks)

Once the external bony bridge has been established between the fracture fragments, provided that adequate mechanical protection is given, the other processes such as the formation of medullary callus and reconstruction of cortical bone can be expected to follow [71]. The medullary osteoblasts differentiate directly from undifferentiated osteogenic cells (stromal cells of the medullary cavity). This process is slow compared with periosteal activity. It is enhanced by adequate blood supply.

Looking at the whole period of fracture healing, four biomechanical stages can be defined:

Stage I: The bone fails through the original fracture site with a low-stiffness, rubbery pattern.

Stage II: The bone fails through the original fracture site with a high-stiffness, hard tissue pattern.

Stage III: The bone fails partially through the original fracture site and partially through the previously intact bone with a high-stiffness, hard-tissue pattern.

Stage IV: The site of failure is not related to the original fracture site and occurs with a high-stiffness pattern.

These stages correlate with the progressive increase in average torque and energy absorption to failure as healing progresses and also with the average healing time [114]. The distinct change from a low-stiffness, rubbery quality (Stage I) to a hard-tissue type of resiliency (Stage II) occurs during a rather short period of time. The same phenomenon is observed in indentation testing of fracture callus between 3 and 4 weeks (Fig. 6). This change is sometimes evident also in clinical practice during conservative treatment of a fracture.

Basic Mechanisms of Bone Fracture Union and Remodeling

In the 1960s it was discovered that rigid compression plating of an osteotomy inhibits callus formation and bone ends unit directly by haversian remodeling in contact areas (so-called "contact healing") and noncontact areas (so-called "gap healing") [98]. Subsequently, fracture healing was divided into two patterns, primary bone healing and secondary (spontaneous) fracture healing. Spontaneous fracture healing (healing with periosteal and endosteal callus formation; Fig. 7) was considered "secondary" mainly because, initially, an intermediate fibrous tissue or fibrocartilage is formed between the fracture fragments and is replaced only subsequently by new bone [97].

The ultimate structural goal of fracture healing is reconstruction of the original cortical bone. Due to the damage to bone and surrounding soft tissue during trauma, the cortical ends at the fracture site are avascular and necrotic during the initial stages of healing. This inevitable vascular compromise does not prevent the avascular fracture ends from playing an important biomechanical role and serving as the mechanical supportive elements

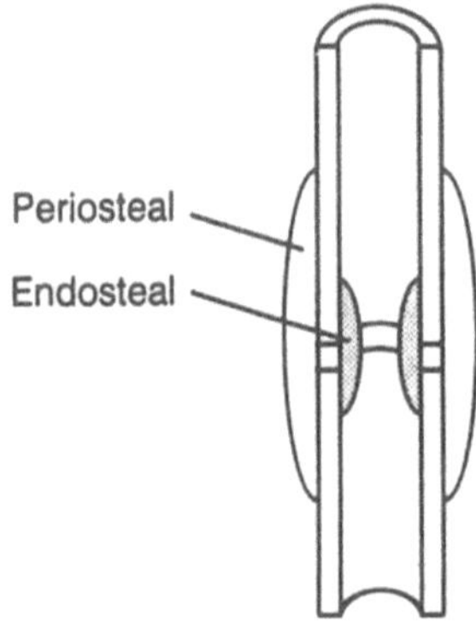

Fig. 7. Schematic diagram illustrating the non-osteonal bone healing mechanism with abundant periosteal callus and a small amount of endosteal callus without osteon formation across the fracture gap. The union of the fracture relies on maturation and remodeling of the periosteal osseous tissue with extensive remodeling processes of the fracture ends

for any fixation device. Haversian remodeling has two main functions: (a) the revascularization of necrotic fracture ends and (b) reconstitution of the intercortical union. There are three requirements for the haversian remodeling across the fracture site: (a) exact reduction (axial alignment), (b) stable fixation, and (c) sufficient blood supply.

The growth of secondary osteons starts in the dog in the second month after fracture and later in man [97]. This means that there is always a lag period before the activation of haversian remodeling during fracture healing. The factors which initiate the dramatic increase in secondary osteons in healing fractures and influence the direction of their growth are not known. It has been postulated that the activation of haversian remodeling is related to the tissue damage (avascular necrosis) at the fracture site. Static pre-loading, studied with compression plates in intact and osteotomized bones [50,68,104] does not seem to influence the rate of osteonal remodeling. Fracture fragments which are deprived of their vascular supply for too long a period of time fail to be remodeled for years [97]. This important observation clearly shows that the signal for the growth of secondary osteons after fracture is time limited, confirming the theory of biochemical induction of haversian remodeling.

The growth of secondary osteons from one fracture fragment to another does not necessarily require intimate contact of fracture fragments. Even after perfect reduction and compression plating there are incongruencies at the fracture site which result in small gaps intermitten with contact areas or even contact points. These gap regions are filled, within weeks after fracture with no lag period, by direct lamellar or woven new bone formation (appositional bone formation) [97]. The woven bone formed within the gap acts as a spacer but does not "unite" the fracture ends. The boundary between the new bone and the original cortex is the weak link of the union process at this stage of healing [5]. Secondary osteons use the gap tissue as a scaffold to grow from one fragment to another. Although this is the crucial step for the final union, the growth of secondary osteons results, paradoxically, in a transitory compulsory reduction of cortical bone density. The gap new bone also shows a similar "porotic change" as a part of the union process with the fragments [5].

In any form of fracture fixation, bone fragments under load experience a certain amount of relative motion which, by unknown mechanisms, determines the morphological features of fracture repair. Perren [81] proposed an hypothesis (so-called "interfragmentary strain hypothesis") which refines the notion that the tissue response is affected by the local mechanical environment. This theory is not entirely consistent with the experimental results produced in the validation studies [26]. The interfragmentary strain is defined as the ratio of the relative displacement of fracture ends versus the initial gap width (Fig. 8). Interfragmentary strain is believed to govern the type of tissue that forms between the fracture fragments. According to the theory, a balance between the local interfragmentary strain and the mechanical characteristics of the callus tissue is the determining factor in the course of both primary bone healing and spontaneous fracture healing. Fracture healing results in a gradual decrease in interfragmentary motion. Different tissues can sustain different maximum tensile strains before failure. Granulation tissue can tolerate 100% of strain, while fibrous tissue and cartilage tolerate appreciably lesser amounts of strain. Compact bone can resist only 2% of strain. Thus, the fracture gap tissue transformation can be assumed to prepare the fracture mechanical and biological environment for solid bone union (Fig. 9). The time-related changes in the compression behavior of

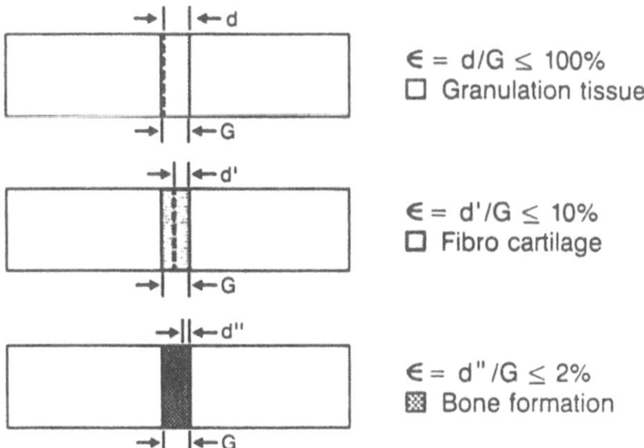

Fig. 8. The concept of interfragmentary strain theory as reflected by the type of tissue formation as a function of the magnitude of the strain occurring in the tissue located in the fracture gap. The strain (ε) is defined as the ratio of the fragment relative motion (*d, d', d"*) and the original gap (*G*) between the bone fragments. Fracture healing results in a gradual decrease of interfragmentary motion (*d, d', d"*). Different tissues can sustain different maximum tensile strains before failure

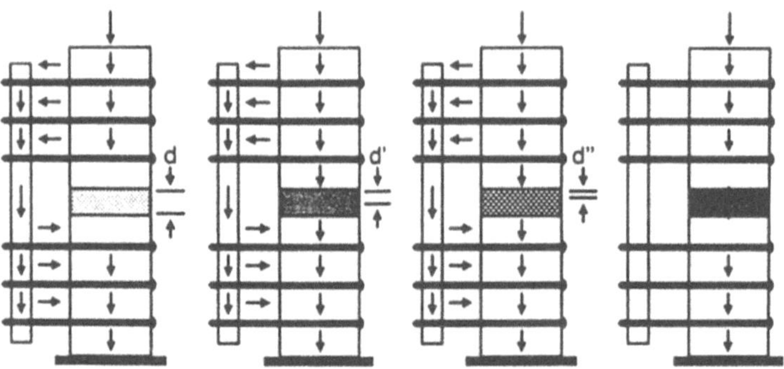

Fig. 9. Adaptation of the interfragmentary strain theory to explain fracture healing under external fixation. When the fracture gap tissue has a low modulus, bone stress passes mainly through the fixation pins and the side bar, bypassing the fracture gap. As the fracture callus begins to mature, more bone stress passes through the fracture site, thereby releasing the load passing through the external fixation side bars

external callus (Fig. 6) appears to support this theory although its deformation under load does not fit the interfragmentary strain definition.

It is important to realize that interfragmentary strain is inversely proportional to the fracture gap size. When the fracture gap is small, even slight interfragmentary motion can increase the strain to the extent that the granulation tissue may not be able to form. To circumvent this situation, small sections of bone near the fracture gap may undergo resorption, thus making the fracture gap larger and reducing the overall strain. This important biological response is histologically evident in gap healing areas of fractures treated by rigid external fixation (Fig. 10) [6].

The original interfragmentary strain theory considered only longitudinal strains associated with the applied interfragmentary strain. Analytical three-dimensional analyses [31] have revealed that interfragmentary motion applied to a plate/bone/gap system results in a complex gap deformation and multidirectional principal strains. However, the interface between the fracture fragment ends and the gap tissue represents a critical plane of high distortion containing maximum principal strain magnitudes and severe endosteal to periosteal strain gradients. With bone resorption and callus formation, the largest strain reductions (up to 50%) occur in these gaps, confirming the original hypothesis.

During the past few years several experimental studies of external fixation with controlled mechanical conditions of osteotomy healing [1,6,44,116] have suggested that there are many combinations of the healing processes. Also clinical experience has indicated that "callus free healing" after dynamic compression plating is not a rule. A recent report of the AO/ASIF group,

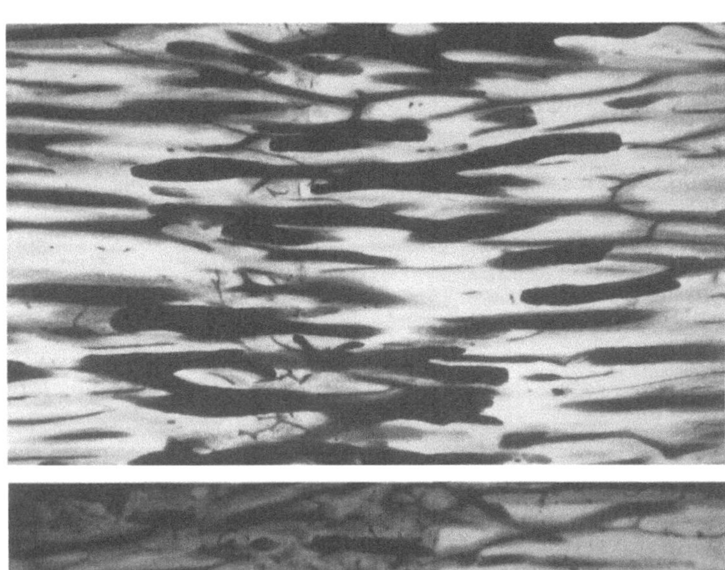

a

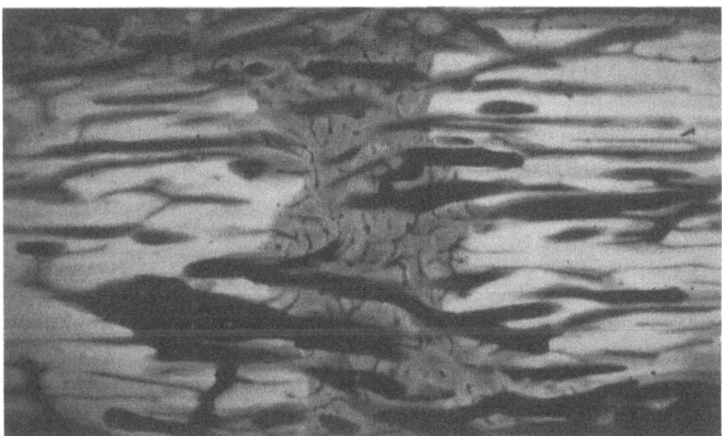

b

Fig. 10a,b. The histological appearance of bone fracture repair under rigid external fixation with constant fracture gap (a) or with dynamic compressive loading (b). Newly formed woven bone has a transverse orientation while the dynamized side is dominated by direct osteon migration. The rough edge at the cortical ends in the gap side represents bone resorption

which popularized the concept of primary bone healing, reported that only 37% of patients in a clinical study showed primary bone union (no radiographic callus) in tibial fractures treated by dynamic compression plate [99].

Therefore, a modified bone union classification was considered in place of the oversimplified terms "primary bone healing" and "secondary bone healing:"

Nonosteonal bone union (Fig. 7)
Osteonal bone union (Fig. 11)
    Primary bone healing

Primary contact healing
Primary gap healing
Secondary bone healing
Secondary contact healing
Secondary gap healing

The modified classification emphasizes the mechanism of cortical reconstruction (osteonal versus nonosteonal union). In addition, the classification includes the fact that contact healing can occur with or without external callus, and that the gap healing mechanism can be achieved when the fracture ends are not in intimate contact (Fig. 11). The gap healing mechanism also can occur with or without external callus formation [5]. The term of primary bone union was originally a radiographic definition, while the lack of external callus formation and the gradual disappearance of the narrow fracture line served as the main criteria [97]. This clinically accepted terminology was maintained in the modified classification. Accordingly, secondary bone union means a healing mechanism of substantial radiographic external callus formation. The histological criteria for the gap healing mechanism were (a) the formation of lamellar bone in the fracture gap with perpendicular orientation of collagen to the bone axis and (b) the growth of secondary osteons through this lamellar bone from one fragment to another. Nonosteonal bone union includes all the healing patterns which do not exhibit the direct growth of osteons across the fracture site. The conditions for nonosteonal bone union may include: (a) axial malalignment, (b) excessive fracture gap, or (c) unstable fixation in the presence of axial alignment. The critical gap size is not completely known but seems to be within the limit of 1 mm, as previously suggested [97].

The biomechanical basis for the modified classification is the crucial role of cortical reconstruction to retain the ultimate bone union strength. Cortical reconstruction is the best radiological indicator of bone union strength [79]. The strength of bone union seems to be related to the number of osteons crossing the union site [25]. However, it is still unproven whether osteonal reconstruction shortens the time to the return of normal bone strength and stiffness compared with nonosteonal cortical reconstruction. On the other hand, a recent study [6] showed that there is no obvious difference in the time needed for the return of normal bone strength and stiffness between the primary and secondary healing mechanisms of osteonal bone repair. However, during early stages of fracture healing, the formation of external callus is mechanically sound to cover the lag period before the activation of haversian remodeling during osteonal bone repair, indicating the benefits of secondary, osteonal bone healing. Static compression of bone fragments is not a prequisite of contact healing. Dynamic compression of bone fragments (obtained by axial dynamization of external fixation without jeopardizing the torsional and bending rigidity of fixation) results in contact healing with periosteal callus formation [6].

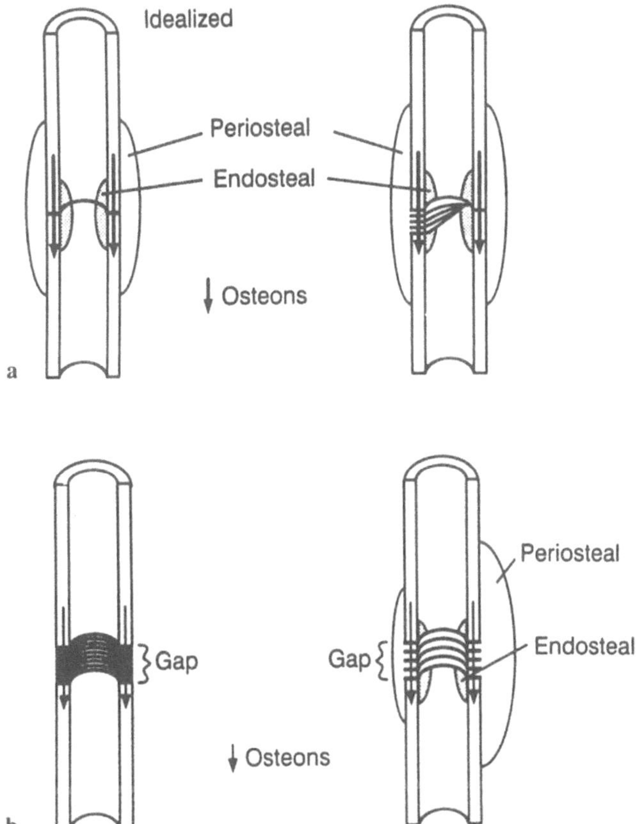

Fig. 11. a Schematic diagrams illustrating the secondary contact healing mechanism. This bone-healing pattern is characterized by periosteal callus formation and direct cortical reconstruction by secondary osteons. Even under contact healing (*right*) there are small gaps located asymmetrically around the circumference of the bone cortex. Thus, contact healing does not imply that the entire cortex undergoes the contact healing mechanism. Primary contact healing (not shown) is characterized by equivalent direct cortical reconstruction but without substantial periosteal new bone formation. **b** Schematic diagram illustrating primary (*left*) and secondary (*right*) gap healing mechanisms under rigid external fixation. The primary healing mechanism does not show substantial radiographic external callus formation. *Arrows*, intracortical secondary osteons bridging direction across the fracture gap. Formation of periosteal callus under rigid external fixation is related to high axial compression through weight bearing

The challenge of biomechanical research on fracture healing is to improve the biomechanics of fracture fixation so that, after satisfactory reduction, a fracture can heal through the secondary bone union mechanism. This goal seems to be relevant for the improvement of both plate fixation [119] and external fixation methods [20]. This question is less critical in intramedullary nailing. Reamed intramedullary nailing results in axial alignment of the bone fragments while permitting axial dynamic compaction, and thus the nailed fracture heals with external callus followed by osteonal reconstruction of the cortex.

Mechanical Properties of Internal and External Fixation Devices

In evaluation of the effects of fixation rigidity on fracture healing processes and in the comparison of different fixation devices used for fracture management, it is important to use quantitative parameters for the expression of fixation rigidity. The understanding of the basic definitions of structural rigidity or stiffness of bone fragment fixation is also essential in evaluation of the factors which determine the biomechanical properties of a fixation method. Such knowledge is clinically important not only during the application of each fixation method but also when one must consider and evaluate the consequences of many variables and options available in the fixation techniques. The need of this knowledge is especially crucial in external fixation, where many types of frames as well as the numerous different fixation configurations are available.

The structural rigidity (or stiffness) of a fixation device can be determined in vitro using a universal mechanical testing machine. The device is applied, using the recommended application technique, to an osteotomized cadaver or synthetic bone. The bone ends of the device-bone system are then loaded under axial compression, bending in two planes, and in torsion. During each mode of loading, the load versus deformation curve is recorded and subsequently analyzed to define the three basic stiffness parameters: axial, bending (flexural), and torsional stiffness. In each load-deformation curve, the slope of the linear portion of the curve is defined as the fixation rigidity or stiffness (Fig. 12).

Using this type of testing procedure of device-bone systems, it is possible to compare the fixation stiffnesses of different types of fixation. In an experimental study (Williams et al. 1988, unpublished data), plate fixation, intramedullary nailing, and external fixation apparatus of two different configurations were compared. The study used osteotomized cadaver canine tibiae, and the stiffness of each fixation device was expressed as a percentage of the intact bone stiffness. As shown in Fig. 13, the stiffness values of the different fixation methods were mismatched. The plated bones behaved as intact bones under the different loading conditions. The stiffness properties of the external fixators with full pins or half pins were different in magnitude, but they followed a similar pattern. Osteotomies stabilized by fluted intramedullary rods showed, compared with other devices, low bending and torsional stiffnesses. In this experiment, bone ends were in contact during loading. Therefore, the measured distraction stiffness values in this particular experiment describe the inherent axial stiffness of each method in the absence of fracture contact.

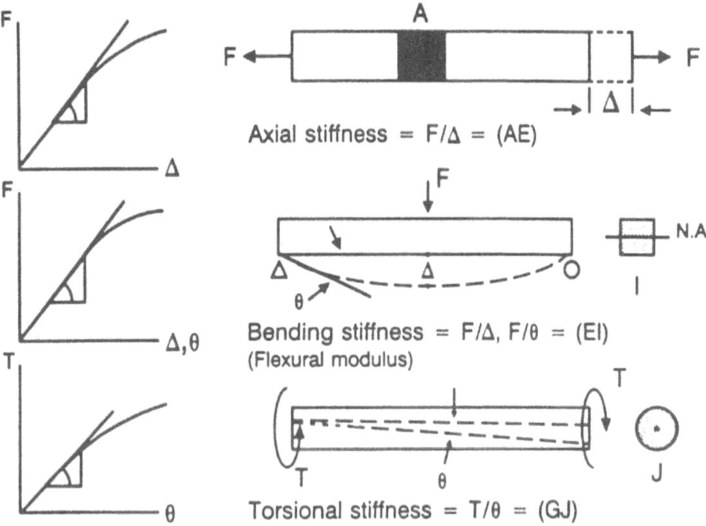

Fig. 12. Using the load deformation curve for each loading mode, the slope of the linear portion of the curve defines the structural rigidity or stiffness property of the intact bone or the bone fragments fixed with either internal or external fixation devices

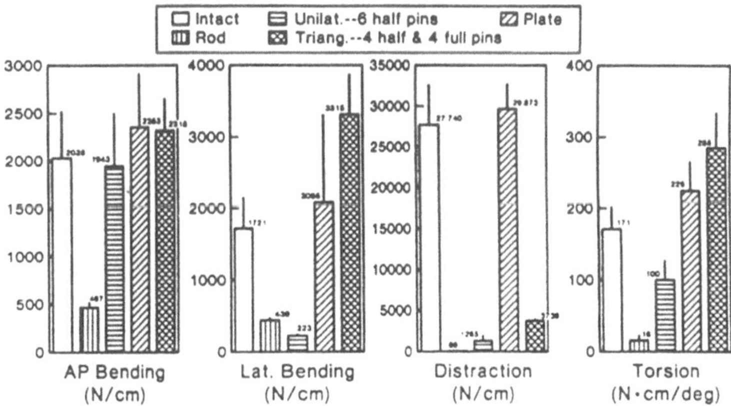

Fig. 13. Rigidity comparison between different fixation methods using dog tibiae as the in vitro model. All fixation stiffness values are compared with those of intact bone. To eliminate the fracture site effect, only distraction is included in the axial loading mode

Mechanical Performance of External Fixation

As is evident, the axial stiffness of external fixation tends to be low. The axial stiffness of most frames and pin configurations (using simulated clinical dimensions) varies between 2000–4000 N/cm [14,21,33,70], which means partial weight bearing (about 20 kg) causes 0.5–1.0 mm axial cyclic movement of fracture fragments if the fracture ends are not in contact. This biomechanical characteristic of external fixation emphasizes the importance of considering the effects of weight bearing together not only with the frame and pin configuration used but also with the modes of fracture reduction. Using in vitro standard testing conditions, it is possible to determine how the mode of fracture reduction (contact with or without compression versus neutralization) and the type of fracture (stable versus unstable) affects the stability of a fixation method. In an experimental study, paired canine tibiae were used. One bone of each pair was osteotomized and fixed with a unilateral external fixator. Osteotomy was performed transversely in five pairs of bones (a model of stable fracture), while an oblique osteotomy (45°) was performed in the other five pairs of bones. The rigidity of fixation provided by the fixator was compared with the contralateral intact bone. The osteotomized bone was loaded in contact mode of fixation (osteotomy ends in contact) as well as in the presence of fracture gap. The results showed that simulated stable fractures (transverse osteotomies) fixed in the contact bone behave as contralateral intact bones in all loaded bones except in anteroposterior bending. On the other hand, the unstable versus stable fracture type as well as the contact mode versus the gap mode of fixation showed the main difference in axial stability. These findings emphasize that the axial rigidity of the bone-fixator system is crucially dependent on the type of fracture and the modes of reduction.

During the past few years there has been increasing interest in circular external fixation configurations, especially for certain reconstructive and limb-lenthening procedures. These devices generally use four pairs of crossed Küntscher wires (diameter of approximately 2 mm or less) that are held under high tension by screws on circular or semicircular frames. The wires can be oriented at different angles across the bone, and tension in the pins provides fixation rigidity. Mechanical comparison of one of the fixator types [70] shows low overall fixation stiffness and especially in the axial direction when compared with the standard Hoffmann-Vidal quadrilateral frame. As expected, the bending stiffness of the frame was independent of the loading direction. Consequently, the device showed a high anteroposterior bending stiffness, which is usually low in unilateral and bilateral noncircular configurations. The rigidity of the circular frame device with K-wires is dependent on wire tension, wire group separation on either side of the fracture, and ring diameter. This type of fixator also exhibits a nonlinear stiffness behavior mainly due to the large deflection of the thin wires [37]. A disadvantage of this type fixation, aside from the complexity of the frame and its application, is the possible sliding action of the bone fragment over the wires during functional loading. The use of threaded wires can eliminate such motion, but the threads may significantly weaken the strength of the wire as it must sustain extremely high tension due to pretension plus loading.

The stiffness of a bone-plate system can be duplicated in a bone-external fixator system if closed reduction (contact of fracture surfaces) can be achieved. The major factors determining external fixation rigidity are the fouowing: (a) increased pin diameter, (b) increased pin number, (c) decreased side bar separation, (d) decreased pin separation, and (e) increased pin group separation. These variables have different effects on the axial, bending, and torsional stiffness, and varying these key parameters is possible to achieve a desired fracture stability. In general, bilateral configurations (using full pins) show 50% higher overall rigidity than unilateral configurations (using half pins). However, unilateral external fixators with increased pin diameter [21] or with one-plane or two-plane frame geometries [9] can provide stiffness characteristics comparable to bilateral configurations. Knowledge of the mechanical performance of external fixators is essential if one is considering adjusting (decreasing or increasing) the stiffness of external fixation as a means to manipulate bone healing progress.

In the clinical situation, the overall rigidity of a fixation system is dependent not only on the frame used and on the pin configuration. A theoretical model can be used to predict the mechanical performance standard unilateral or bilateral fixators under any combination of pin and frame parameters [22,51]. In evaluation of the amount of interfragmentary motion and, thereby, the mode of fracture healing, equally important factors are the type of fracture, the accuracy of reduction, the amount of physiological loading, and the performance of pin-bone interface. Such principle should be noted in the use of different types of fracture fixation devices.

Clinical experience [32,41] as well as both three-dimensional and two-dimensional finite element analyses [22,51,52] have clearly indicated biomechanical and other factors which are involved in the pathogenesis of pin loosening and subsequent infection. The results of recent animal experimental studies [5,85] have corroborated and also expanded the theoretical predictions. This knowledge has aided efforts to improve the design of fixators and fixation pins, and, clinically, it gives measure to prevent pin tract complications.

Biomechanically, there are four distinct factors to improve the performance of pin-bone interface: pin geometry and thread design, bone thread preparation, pin insertion technique, and pin/bone stress. There seems to be a race between the gradually increasing load carrying capacity of a healing bone and failure of the pin-bone interface. Under various loading modes, pins are primarily subjected to bending. In unstable fractures, the bone stress at the pin tract can approach a very high level, which may create localized yielding failure. Such stresses can be reduced by increasing the bending rigidity of the pin (high-modulus pin material, large pin diameter), reducing the side-bar separation, and applying a full-pin configuration. Half pins generate high stress primarily at the entry cortex. Stress-related pin-bone failures of half pins occur mainly at the entry cortex. According to analytical studies, the location of maximum stress within a pin group varies according to the loading mode. To avoid high pin-bone interface stresses, weight bearing should be avoided in fractures without cortical contact. Axial dynamization of an external fixator, on the other hand, restores the cortical contact in stable fractures and thus decreases the pin/bone stresses. Undoubtedly, the surgical pin insertion technique must also play a very important role for the uneventful performance of the pin-bone interface. If the pin insertion technique is inadequate (such as eccentric location of the pins, thermal necrosis of the bone tissue due to the use of a power drill), the loosening of the applied pin can be predicted. The measurement of pin insertion torque, at least with the use of tapered fixation pins, seems to be a good indicator if the applied pin is eccentrically (through one cortex) in the bone.

Mechanical Performance of Compression Plate Fixation

The importance of accurate reduction of fracture fragments and the secure permanent contact of fracture fragments is a general principle in fracture management. The goal of bringing the entire fracture surfaces into contact and compressing the fracture surface by a fixation device is based on the widely known principles of rigid compression plating. The biomechanical principles of rigid compression plating, according to Hayes [45] and Perren and Cordey [82] are as follows:

Plate positioning: The plate should be applied such that acting forces tend to close the fracture site (applying the plate to the convex or tensile surface of the bone).

Interfragmentary compression: Fixation should produce a sufficiently high amount of compression to counter tension and shear forces under functional load. The plate is applied under tension which, in turn, compresses the plated bone segment axially. Applied interfragmentary compression increases the rigidity of the plate-bone system.

Prebending of plate: A plate which is contoured to fit the bone surface exactly produces eccentric compression; the cortex beneath the plate is compressed, and the opposite cortex opens. Asymmetric compression is especially inefficient in stabilizing against torque. Use of prebent plates results in more uniform compressive contact stresses across the fracture site. Only small bending angles are required in prebending, and too much prebending should be avoided because of plastic plate shaping.

Plate screws: With plate screws, used to fix the implant to bone, the full metal thread contacts a full bone thread. It is important to use screws close to the fracture site to reduce unsupported length.

Lag screw compression fixation: A screw may also be used to compress fracture surfaces as a lag screw. The principle of a lag screw is that a partially threaded screw, shaft screw, or a partially-threaded bone-hole, gliding hole, permits interfragmentary compression. Lag screw compression fixation, protected by a neutralization plate, is efficient and most powerful, because a screw placed perpendicularly to the fracture surface results in a high normal component of force.

These principles were developed to improve the rigidity of plate fixation, i.e. to prevent the micromotion of fracture fragments which results in fracture end resorption [81]. Fracture end resorption jeopardizes the rigidity of plate fixation. Under external fixation or intramedullary nailing, the fracture end resorption may be less harmful. Under intramedullary fixation, the bone fragments can be brought together under functional load. On the other hand, external fixation is the only form of fracture fixation which allows the change in fixation rigidity at different phases of fracture management. Hence, the fracture end resorptive gap during external fixation can be reduced by readjusting the device, for example, through axial dynamization (relaxation of the axial constraint) in stable fracture types or merely by improving the apposition of the fracture fragments in less stable fracture types.

Interfragmentary compression means any type of constant, static compression exerted across the surfaces of fracture fragments. Two basic principles of action of the interfragmentary compression are preload and friction between the plate and the bone cortex and between the bone fragment surfaces. Preloading means creating compression which prevents any separation of the fracture surfaces as long as the amount of preload is greater than the functional load (bending or distraction) which tends to separate the fragments. Friction prevents axial sliding under distraction and tangential displacement under shear or torsion.

Interfragmentary compression can be achieved using so-called dynamic compression plates. These plates have a self-compression action, permitting horizontal gliding and inclination of the plate screw which can be used as a lag screw, also maintaining a congruent fit between the spherical undersurface of the screw and the cylindrical portion of the screw hole. The static compression obtained with these plates is not constant but decreases as a function of time; however, it seems to be present until far beyond the time of bone union [83]. Therefore, when compression plating is to be used, established surgical techniques must be followed judiciously.

An undesirable consequence of the use of rigid compression plates is postunion osteopenia, which means porotic transformation of the cortex beneath the plate with a net decrease in bone mass and with impaired mechanical properties of the healed bone. This phenomenon has been described in every detail in experimental studies [12,104,109,110,119]. This phenomonon, with the lack of callus healing, has been related to the occurrence of refractures after plate removal. Most investigators believe that the structural change is secondary to the overprotection of the underlying bone from normal stresses ("stress protection"). Experimental studies have offered three potential solutions (reviewed by Woo et al. [119]), to overcome these disadvantages: (a) continue to use rigid plates but modify the timing of plate removal, (b) the use of biologically degradable materials for internal fixation plates, and (c) the use of a fracture fixation system of reduced rigidity. The main problem of nonrigid systems is that such fixation may fail to ensure the main goal of treatment, i.e., union of the fracture. Woo et al. [119] proposed, based on theoretical analyses, bench tests, and animal experiments, that a change in the design of the plate would offer the optimal healing mechanism. Their biomechanical rationale for improved plate design is:

The plate is subjected to dynamic bending and torsional loads in the early phase of bone healing because of the discontinuity of bone (the neutral axis of the plate-bone system is along the plate itself, assuming that the plate is the only load transmitting structure).

Therefore, the plate should have adequate flexural and torsional rigidities so that the motion of the fractured ends can be limited to an appropriate degree to facilitate the union of fracture with external callus but without bone angulation or implant failure.

As healing progresses and the bone ends unite, the bone itself becomes a load-transmitting structure, and subsequently the neutral axis of the plate-bone system shifts toward the bone and the plate is subjected to tensile or compressive loads.

In these late phases of bone union and remodeling, the axial stiffness of the plate must be sufficiently low so that the underlying bone is permitted to share a higher portion of the physiological stresses needed to facilitate normal bone remodeling.

Their main argument is that the axial stiffness of a rigid stainless plate is several times that of an intact bone. The improved plate design seeks to lower the axial stiffness of the plate to the level of the underlying bone so that the bone and plate can deform in unison. However, bone fragment displacement at the fracture site is always nonuniform under plate fixation, regardless of its stiffness property. The ability to compress bone ends uniformly under loading can be achieved only through intramedullary nailing or external fixation with dynamization.

The prevalence of postunion osteopenia in plated human fractures is unknown. There is also some controversey about the mechanism causing postunion osteopenia. In animal studies comparatively large plates are often applied to small bones, and the amount of stress protection has been out of proportion [28]. The concept that cortical transformation under the plate is related to the "stress protection" includes an assumption that the applied rigid plate is firmly attached to the underlying bone still months or even years after surgery. Recently Cordey and Perren [27] suggested that the limit of frictional transmission between a plate and bone may be reached under certain loading conditions, resulting in plate loosening, followed by bone resorption, and cortical thinning under the plate. At present, there are no data to show how rigidly a plate is fixed to a human bone, for example, 2 years after plating. Experimental studies [54] have shown low removal torques of screws in plated bones after 16–32 weeks, suggesting that plates are not firmly pressed on bones after a certain time period. Using a quantitative bone densitometry, Schwyzer et al. [99] performed computed tomography of human tibiae after fracture plate removal (about 18 months after plating of a fracture). The bone density of the fracture site was reduced by an average of 8%, which was not considered to increase the risk of refracture. The average bone loss was offset by an increase in the total area of the bone. An interesting finding was that fractures that healed without external callus did not show such geometric change in the presence of reduced density. These results emphasize that further studies must be carried out to correlate the pattern of bone healing and the incidence of refracture.

Mechanical and Biological Characteristics of Intramedullary Nails

In 1940 Küntscher introduced the closed intramedullary nailing technique of the femur and, in 1950, added reaming of the medullary canal to improve the contact between the nail and the cortical wall for better stability of the fixation [64]. Reaming allows the placement of a large nail that resists bending, thus allowing early mobilization of the limb without plaster support. At present there is increasing agreement that Küntscher's method, supplemented with interlocking design, is the treatment of choice for essentially all closed fractures of the femur located between the lesser trochanter and femoral condyles, regardless of the fracture pattern or degree of comminution [118]. The use of reamed nailing in fresh tibial fractures is more controversial. Devascularization of the inner cortex, a consequence of reaming [89], is risky in high-energy tibial fractures with compromised soft tissue coverage and periosteal blood supply. Acute nailing of open fractures of the tibia with intramedullary reaming is generally contraindicated [23]. Recent experimental studies of using the microsphere technique have confirmed that intramedullary nailing (Sampson rod following graduated reaming) damages the perfusion of cortical bone at the fracture site during the early phases of fracture healing (4 h–14 days), but that by 90 days this effect is overcome by collaterization of blood vessels to the endosteal cortex [106].

Intramedullary nailing has some favorable biomechanical features. A proper nailing technique, including the correct point of pin insertion and prevention of eccentric reaming of the medullary cavity [117], places the neutral axis of the nail-bone structure at the center of the bone itself. Axial alignment, a natural consequence of the introduction of a fitted medullary nail after reaming, restores the load-bearing capacity of a bone with a fracture in the isthmus region of the shaft, allowing protected early weight bearing. Plate fixation, after perfect reduction, also restores such an anatomical condition but does not allow weight bearing until partial bone union since the neutral axis of the plate-bone system is along the plate, and dynamic forces may result in fatigue breakage of the plate or the screws under bending or torsion.

The intramedullary fixation is based mainly on elastic three-point contact in a longitudinal direction, and reaming prepares a cylindric channel of uniform diameter for a firm fit of the nail. Outside the isthmus region the medullary cavity is large, and conventional Küntscher nailing does not generally provide sufficient rotational stability in proximal and distal fractures. In addition, in comminuted fractures a regular nail does not prevent axial telescoping and hence may cause fracture collapse and loss in reduction. To overcome these biomechanical difficulties the interlocking intramedullary nail concept was introduced. The interlocking feature of intramedullary nails has widened the indications of intramedullary fixation (Fig. 14).

The biomechanical characteristics of interlocking nailing are different from those of the conventional closed Küntscher nailing [59,61], and functional rehabilitation must be adjusted to complement the unique biomechanical characteristics of the nailing technique. Following insertion of threaded bolts on both sides of the fracture (so-called static interlocking

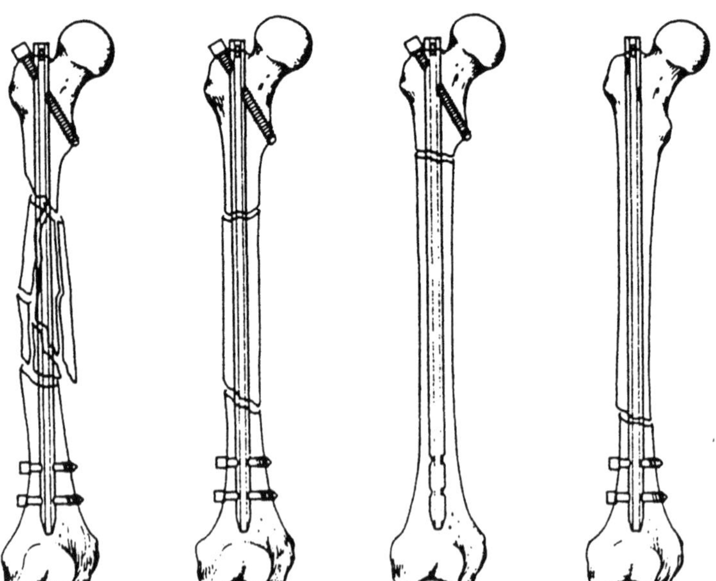

Fig. 14. Common fracture types amenable by interlocking intramedullary nailing using either proximal or distal, or both, interlocking features

nailing), forces are transmitted from the intact bone tube proximally via the bolts through the nail which span the fracture site and back to the intact cortical bone anchored distally by the transverse locking bolts. This type of fixation, without cortical contact, does not allow immediate weight bearing [59] because of the risk of nail fatigue failure. Interlocking nails can be used also to stabilize transverse and short oblique fractures above and below the isthmus, using the bolts to lock the smaller fracture fragment (so-called dynamic interlocking nailing). The principle of static interlocking nailing originally included the procedure of dynamization (removal of proximal or distal bolts) to allow unrestricted dynamic axial compression of the fracture site after initial union. Increasing clinical experience has not uniformly shown the need for such a procedure during uncomplicated bone healing, but it may be useful in fractures with signs of delayed healing. The latter findings emphasize that the intrameduallry nail is a load-sharing device during the early stages of fracture healing and, after the reconstruction of cortical continuity, bone remodeling takes place, even under the static interlocking mode. In this respect, external fixation seems to be capable of duplicating the beneficial biomechanical characteristics of intramedullary nailing. After cortical union (Fig. 9), an externally fixed bone is subjected to physiological dynamic loads necessary for structural maturation and does not seem to develop stress-protection osteopenia during osteotomy union [5].

Fractures of the subtrochanteric region of the femur represent a difficult biomechanical problem in trauma surgery. The subtrochanteric region is an area of high stresses due to bending moments and compressive forces. Fixation systems for fractures in this region are exposed to high stresses, even without ambulation. Flexion and extension of the hip, even while in bed, can produce forces at the femoral head as large as 2.5–3 times body weight, while slow walking can result in hip forces of up to 4.9 times body weight [92]. Comminution of subtrochanteric fractures can further increase the stress applied to the implant because a comminuted bone cannot act as a load shearing part of the fixation system. Tencer et al. [108] made a comparative study to evaluate the stabilization of simulated subtrochanteric fractures by different intramedullary and plate fixation implants (Fig. 15). They measured the torsional and bending stiffnesses of the implant-bone systems and compared these stiffness values with intact bone values. They also determined the maximum load carrying capacity (failure load) of each device in combined bending and compression, a simulation of the action of weight bearing. All the intramedullary devices (including two types of interlocking nails, Zickel nail and multiple Enders pins) showed low torsional stiffness (maximum of 5% of control intact femur) while the plate-bone systems (blade plate or compression hip screw) had higher torsional stiffness (about 50% of intact bone). In bending, all devices except Enders pins were about 80% as stiff as intact femora. As shown in Fig. 15, an interlocking nail system provides the highest failure loads under simulated

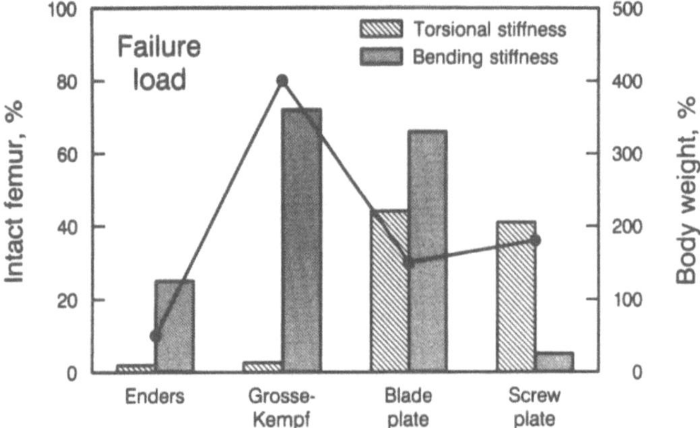

Fig. 15. Comparison of intramedullary and plate fixation devices in fixation of unstable subtrochanteric fractures of the femur. The bending stiffness (*bars*, percentage of intact femur) and the failure load (*dots connected by lines*, percentage of intact femur and percentage of body weight) is highest for the Grosse-Kempf interlocking nail

weight bearing (between 300% and 400% of body weight). It should be emphasized that this study did not include fatigue testing of the bone-device system, which usually is the clinical course of implant failure in subtrochanteric fractures.

Recent clinical experience [13,36,103] has indicated a high success rate in the treatment of subtrochanteric fractures of the femur by the use of interlocking nails. These results indicate that although the interlocking designs prevent relative rotation between the nail and the cortex, they do not change the inherent low torsional stiffness of the nail itself. This feature, in the case of intramedullary fixation, does not seem to be detrimental to bone healing results. However, improvements in nail designs (elimination of posterior slot) have been made to improve torsional rigidity of the device [59,107]. Such change may be efficacious since the slotted section provides the essential flexibility needed for the nail to follow the medullary cavity, while the combination of the slot and the cover-leaf profile (of the original Küntscher nail) aids in fixation between the implant and bone. It should be emphasized that a low torsional stiffness of a device is not synonymous to torsional instability of the fixation system which reflects uncontrolled motion between the nail and bone.

Biomechanical Characteristics of Fracture Healing Under Internal and External Fixation

In order to explore the possibility of using mechanical stimuli of a certain type to modulate fracture union, it is essential that the normal healing characteristics under different fixation methods are well understood. Therefore a series of experiments was carried out for this purpose. Since only external fixation can provide active control of fixation rigidity and fracture gap mechanical environment, such mode of immobilization was selected as the primary model. The experiments were carried out using the same experimental setup (canine tibial shaft osteotomy) to eliminate other variables such as the extent of soft-tissue injury, the variation of fracture surface, the accuracy of reduction, and the type of fracture configuration, which may influence bone healing.

The purpose of these experiments was not to show the superiority of any particular device or a fixation mode over another. Instead, the experiments were designed to demonstrate the model of healing expected by each type of fixation rigidity under standardized, uncompromised healing conditions. Under clinical fracture healing conditions, the fixation rigidity and the type of fixation are among other variables influencing the outcome of the treatment. The use of intra-animal comparison in statistical analysis also minimizes the many interanimal variables, such as individual differences in functional activity and loading magnitude. It must be emphasized that the studies of external fixation do not represent only the healing modes provided by external fixators. External fixation, allowing controlled adjustment of fixation rigidity, is an important experimental tool to study the mechanical factors influencing fracture healing, and the data can be used not only to speculate as to possible mechanical factors to enhance the fracture union process but also to improve the designs of other fixation devices.

Plate Fixation Versus Intramedullary Fixation

The effects of compression plating (eight-hole dynamic compression plates) and intramedullary nailing after reaming (fluted Sampson rod) on the vascular supply of the canine tibial osteotomy site and on the rate and quality of osteotomy union were studied [87]. A total of 45 adult, mongrel dogs were used in this experiment to establish the fracture model. The animals were killed at 1, 14, 42, 90 and 120 days to show the time-related changes in osteotomy-site blood flow (measured by strontium clearance) and in the morphology and mechanical properties of the osteotomies. The results showed that blood flow reaches higher levels and remains elevated longer in osteotomies that are fixed with a rod than in those fixed with a plate (Fig. 16). Rod-fixed osteotomies healed by periosteal callus, whereas plate fixed osteotomies showed predominantely endosteal callus formation (Fig. 17). There were no significant differences in bone porosity between the fixation methods. The plated osteotomies displayed higher torsional stiffness values than rod-fixed osteotomies at 90 days ($p < 0.005$), but this difference was no longer apparent at 120 days. Maximum torque values of the plated osteotomies were significantly higher at 90 days ($p < 0.01$), but this difference also disappeared by 120 days.

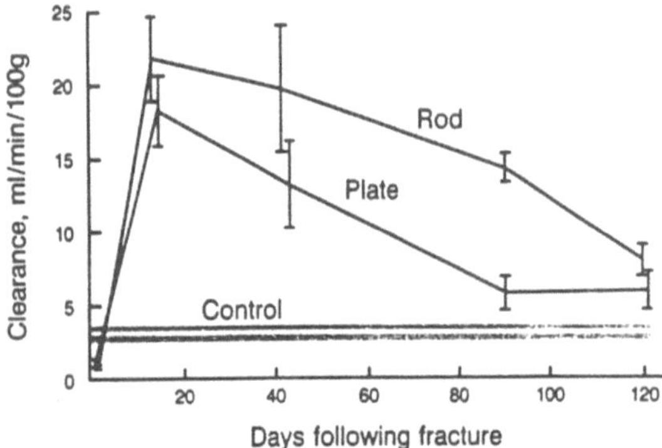

Fig. 16. Fracture-site bone blood flow measured by strontium clearance in plate-versus rod-fixed animal model as compared to the intact control at different time periods

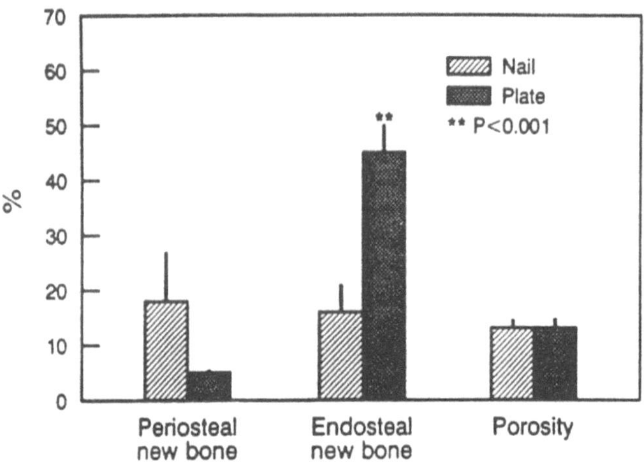

Fig. 17. Comparison of new bone formation and porosity between intramedullary nailing and compression plate fixation (canine tibial osteotomy model). Significantly higher endosteal new bone formation occurred on the plated side. Intramedullary nail fixation produced greater periosteal new bone formation

It is evident that bone union occurs through different mechanisms after intramedullary rod fixation and plate fixation. Interestingly, rigid plate fixation improved the recovery of mechanical properties at the early phases of healing, although the rigidity of plate fixation inhibited periosteal callus formation. The time needed for the return of normal strength and stiffness was, however, the same between the two methods, indicating that the end result of the different healing patterns was biomechanically indifferent.

Plate Fixation Versus External Fixation

The bone osteotomy union characteristics between compression plating (eight-hole prebent dynamic compression plates) and unilateral external fixation (Sukhtian-Hughes design) were compared [66]. The fixator was applied using six stainless steel Schanz screws, 4 mm in diameter. In vitro mechanical testing showed that the plate-bone system was significantly more rigid than the external fixator-bone system in all testing modes except in lateral bending, where the external fixator was more rigid. In vivo study showed that the use of both methods led to osteotomy union by 120 days. However, the maximum torque and stiffness of the plated osteotomies were significantly higher than those of the external fixator side ($p < 0.05$ and $p < 0.01$, respectively). Histologically, there was more porosity ($p < 0.05$) on the external fixator side compared to paired osteotomies treated with compression plates (Fig. 18). The external fixator side also had significantly less intracortical new bone ($p < 0.01$). Increased bone turnover on the fixator side was accompanied by increased blood flow, ($p < 0.05$, compared with the plated side).

This was the first demonstration that external fixation can achieve bone osteotomy union under experimental conditions. It is well demonstrated that the rigidity of fixation is an important factor in early bone healing, not the type of device used. Less rigid external fixation has been shown to increase bone resorption and decrease intracortical bone formation compared with rigid compression plating. This study, as well as the study of Rand et al.

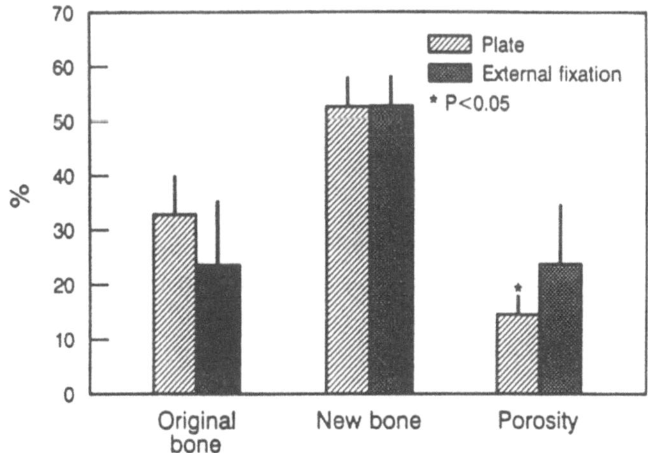

Fig. 18. The relative amounts of original cortical bone, new bone, and porosity between the plated side and the external fixation side in a midtibial canine osteotomy model. The porosity in the external fixation side was greater compared to the compression plated side. This finding may reflect the higher fracture site movement and nonosteonal bone healing mechanics under the less rigid external fixation

[87], did not show in the canine tibia porotic transformation of the cortical bone beneath a rigid plate, suggesting that such a phenomenon must be a late effect.

Four-Pin Versus Six-Pin Unilateral External Fixation

Wu et al. [120] compared the healing pattern of osteotomies fixed with more rigid (six half pins) and less rigid (four half pins) unilateral external fixator configurations. The Sukhtian-Hughes model fixator was used, and the pins were 4-mm stainless steel Schanz screws. In vitro testing showed that the axial, torsional, and lateral bending stiffness of the four-pin configuration was about 70% that of the six-pin configuration. The anteroposterior bending stiffness in the four-pin side was only 50% of the six-pin side. In vivo study showed increased periosteal callus formation in the four-pin side, based on the planimetry of sequential radiographs. At 120 days the osteotomies treated by the two configurations did not show significant differences in the maximum torque to failure or in stiffness. Histologically, the four-pin side showed increased porosity of the osteotomy area ($p < 0.05$, compared with the six-pin side; Fig. 19). The incidence of pin loosening was significantly higher in the four-pin side than in the six-pin side.

This experiment confirmed that less rigid external fixation results in enhanced periosteal callus formation but, at the same time, increases bone porosity without any beneficial effects on the mechanical recovery. This study also showed that the low initial stiffness of external fixation carries the potential to pin-bone interface problems.

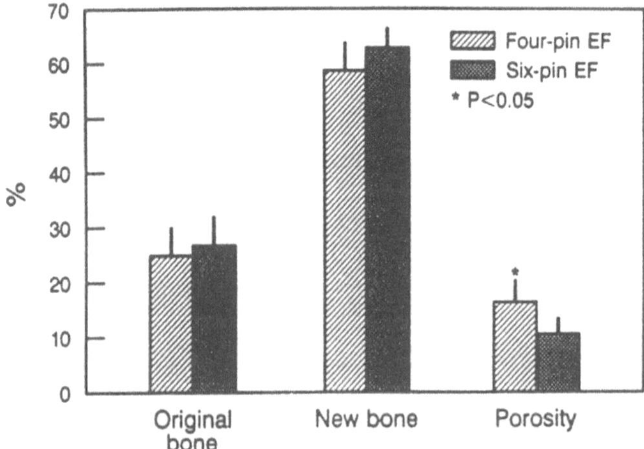

Fig. 19. New bone formation and bone porosity comparison in four-pin (less rigid) versus six-pin (more rigid) unilateral external fixation configuration (canine tibial osteotomy model). The intracortical porosity was significantly greater in the less stiff four-pin external fixator side

Compression Versus No Compression Under External Fixation

Hart et al. [44] focused on examining the effects of constant compression on osteotomy healing. The static compression of 80 N was applied across the tibial osteotomy site by the Sukhtian-Hughes unilateral external fixator. The contralateral side was treated with the same fixator, but the osteotomy ends were not in intimate contact (osteotomy gap 20 µm). The fixator was applied using a six-pin configuration (4.5-mm custom-made, titanium, self-tapping pins). In vitro study showed that the static compression of osteotomy ends increased the rigidity of fixation, especially in lateral bending and torsion. All the osteotomies were healed at 90 days. No statistical differences were observed between the paired osteotomies in mechanical testing or in histological analysis (Fig. 20). The osteotomy-site blood flow did not show any significant differences. On both sides, periosteal new bone formation was less in the mediolateral plane than in the anteroposterior plane, which seemed to correlate inversely with the amount of bending stiffness of the unilateral external fixator. Some of the osteotomies, regardless of the mode of fixation, showed haversian remodeling across the osteotomy site through a contact or gap type of healing mechanism.

This study showed that compression, applied through an external fixation system, increases the rigidity of fixation. Relative to the rigidity of the intact tibia, this increase was small, and no significant biological or biomechanical benefits were observed for the bone union process. Therefore, static compression does not seem to enhance healing when adequate rigidity and small fracture gap are maintained by the fixator system.

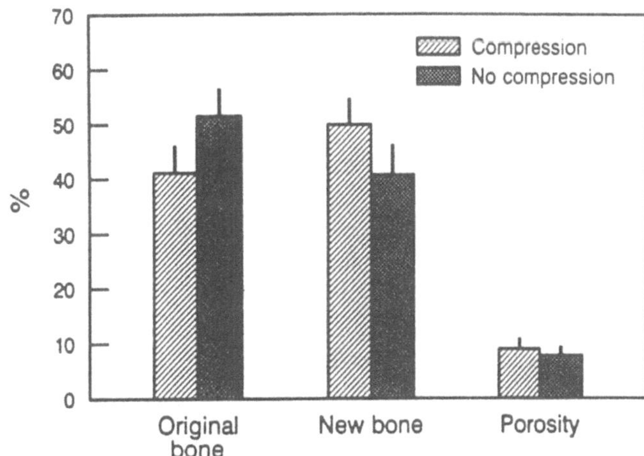

Fig. 20. Static compression did not change new bone formation or porosity at the osteotomy site under external fixation (canine tibial model)

Unilateral Versus Bilateral Two-Plane External Fixation

The study of Williams et al. [116] was designed to compare bilateral, two-plane external fixation to unilateral external fixation. The two-plane fixator included two transfixation full pins and two half pins above and below the site of osteotomy. The unilateral fixator was the Sukhtian-Hughes fixator with six titanium half pins. In vitro testing showed that the bilateral, two-plane configuration significantly improves the torsional stiffness as well as the bending stiffness in the plane perpendicular to the plane of half pins of the unilateral fixation. In the animal study the bilateral two-plane configuration induced less periosteal callus formation, and the in vivo measurement of osteotomy stiffness (at 4, 6, and 9 weeks using an instrumented device) showed higher values on this side compared with those on the unilateral fixation side. The ratio of static versus dynamic bone scan activity, serving as an indicator of bone turnover, was increased at the early stages of osteotomy healing on the side of unilateral external fixation. Histologically at 13 weeks, the bilateral two-plane fixation side showed cortical reconstruction more frequently by haversian remodeling across the osteotomy site. The porosity of the osteotomy site was also lower on the side of bilateral fixation ($p < 0.05$; Fig. 21). Torsional testing showed that the osteotomies fixed with the more rigid bilateral two-plane fixation are stiffer ($p < 0.025$) than those fixed with unilateral fixation, but no statistical difference was observed in the maximum torque to failure.

Therefore, higher rigidity external fixation with small or no gap results in osteotomy healing with less callus formation and stiffer union during the

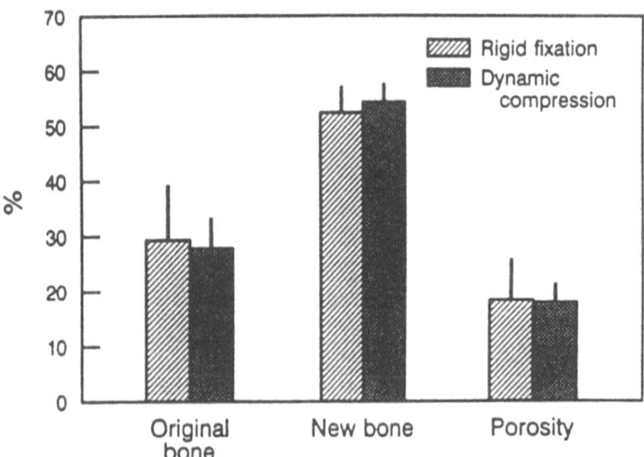

Fig. 21. Comparison of new bone formation and bone porosity between the bilateral full-pin plus half-pin fixation configuration and the unilateral half-pin external fixator. Porosity was significantly higher in the less rigid unilateral external fixator

healing process. The results agree with the previous experimental data on internal and external fixation, indicating that the healing pattern of a bone osteotomy can be augmented by the rigidity of fixation.

Constant Rigid Versus Dynamic Compression Under External Fixation

A well-controlled experiment was designed to study the effects of dynamic, axial compression on bone healing after an initial, short period (2 weeks) of a neutralization mode of rigid fixation [5]. The control side was treated by the same unilateral external fixator (Orthofix) but maintained in the neutralization mode (gap 800 µm) throughout the healing process. The half pins with a tapered threaded portion had a shank diameter of 6 mm. In vitro studies showed that the introduction of axial dynamization did not alter the fixation rigidity under either torsion or bending, while axial compressive load was transmitted through the bone. In the rigidly fixed side, axial load of less than 200 N was insufficient to close the osteotomy gap. In vivo, dynamization reduced the osteotomy gap and induced contact healing with periosteal callus formation (secondary contact healing, Fig. 11). Nondynamized, rigidly fixed bones healed through a gap healing mechanism with or without external callus (primary gap healing or secondary gap healing) while the distribution of external callus was nonuniform around the osteotomy site. The paired comparison of the control and dynamized osteotomies showed no statistical differences in the total quantity of external callus. At 90 days both sides showed a high rate of cortical reconstruction through haversian remodeling, and no differences were observed in the histological composition of new bone formation and bone porosity (Fig. 22) or in

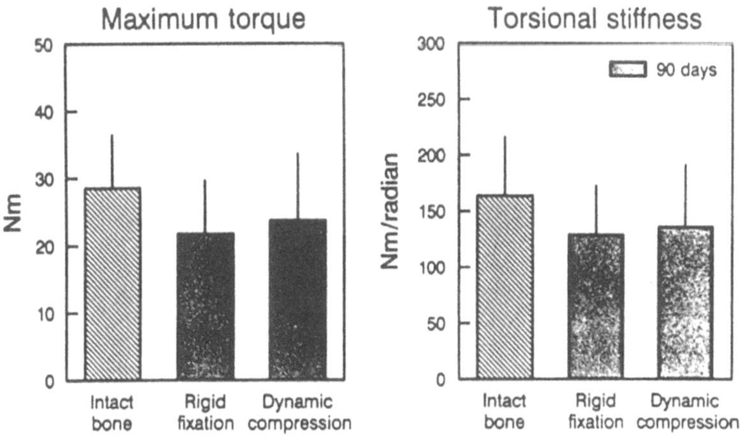

Fig. 22. Comparison of rigid external fixation under neutralization and dynamic compression modes. No significant differences were found in new bone formation or bone porosity

osteotomy-site blood flow and bone scan activity at this postunion stage. Intracortical porosity was low on both sides, with minimal endosteal new bone formation. The torsional strength and stiffness of the healed tibiae were not significantly different from those of intact tibiae (Fig. 23). The dynamization decreased pin loosening, measured by pin removal torque, among pins closest to the osteotomy site. The overall clinical, radiographic, and biomechanical performance of the tapered pin appeared to be good, with well-formed new bone within the pin thread space. Such pin tract behavior may be related to the thread design in the tapered pin since no tapping is necessary to create the threads in the bone.

This study showed that the axial readjustment of external fixation rigidity during the bone healing process can facilitate contact osteonal bone healing. The results of the rigidly fixed control side showed that rigid external fixation may prevent periosteal callus formation. The fast mechanical healing of the bones, compared with the previous studies of external fixation, demonstrated the efficiency of osteonal bone healing and the stability of the fixation used in this experiment. Undoubtedly, the tapered pin design with increased shank diameter plays an important role in this achievement. Furthermore, the experiment confirmed the theoretical prediction that rigid external fixation does not cause postunion osteopenia, dissimilar to rigid plate fixation. The dynamization manuever, relying on the ability of the bone to transmit axial load, appears to reduce pin bending load and, subsequently, the risk of pin-bone interface failure.

These experimental results seem to suggest that the rigidity of fixation is an important factor governing not only whether the fracture heals but also

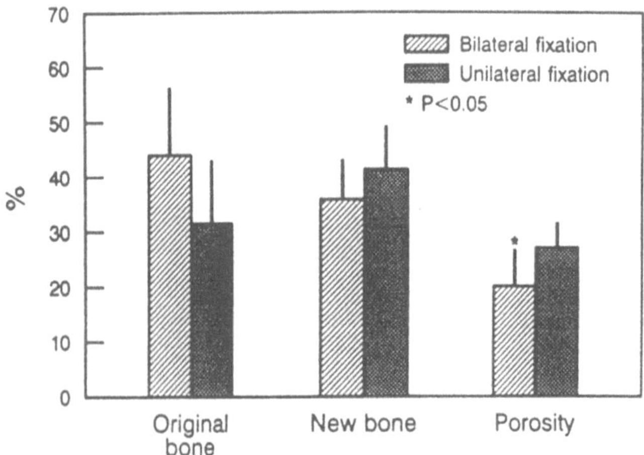

Fig. 23. The maximum torque to failure of the bone union site and the torsional stiffness of the healed tibia after 90 days were found to be similar to intact bone strength and stiffness. There was no difference between the rigidly fixed and dynamized sides of the experimental model

the mechanism through which bone union takes place. The biological and biomechanical pathways to osseous union can be attenuated by changing the rigidity of fixation during the treatment course. It has been well established that internal or external fracture fixation devices as dictated by their biomechanical characteristic can lead to the same final end result of fracture union but through slightly different biological processes. Plate fixation favors endosteal healing, while intramedullary fixation and less rigid external fixation encourage periosteal healing. Rigid external fixation prevents periosteal callus formation and thus relies on osteonal cortical reconstruction with minimal endosteal healing. Axially dynamized external fixation facilitates secondary contact healing, i.e. direct cortical reconstruction with periosteal new bone formation. Fluctuating stress induced by unstable fixation and the associated fracture gap movement is an important contributing factor in pin loosening. Careful pin insertion technique, increased pin diameter, improved pin geometry and thread design, the load carrying capacity of the healing fracture, and the magnitude of loading under external fixation are other involving factors in the prevention of pin loosening and pin tract infection.

Finally, it remains unknown whether mechanical stimuli significantly improve the normal fracture healing process, or whether abnormal or delayed union can be enhanced by such external factors. The existing data strongly support such assumption, and future studies should be encouraged to verify this exciting contention. The following section outlines various possibilities to modulate or attenuate bone union.

Bone Fracture Healing Enhancement

Present attempts to enhance bone healing processes can be divided into three categories: biological, electromagnetic, and mechanical stimulations.

Biological Factors

Fracture healing is a cascade of cellular and biochemical events, and a biological enhancement in one step can expect to result in stimulation of the whole healing process. There are several requirements for well-balanced healing and remodeling processes of bone, which include: an available pool of precursors for each type of cell involved, proper stimulants for bone cell differentiation, mechanisms for positioning and distribution of the specialized osteogenic cells, and coordinated mechanisms for their activation and synthesis. The numerous biological factors which theoretically can be used in the enhancement of the cascade events include:

- Pool of osteogenic cells
- Osteogenic cell division and proliferation

- Cell recruitment and cell attachment
- Angiogenesis
- Cell differentiation
- Cell metabolism for matrix production
- Osteoblast-osteoclast interaction during bone remodeling

Precursor elements, for example, can be increased by local bone marrow injections [42] and probably by improved cell attachment [113]. The control of macrophage functions [62] and the production of other chemoattractant substances for endothelial cells [39] may help to promote angiogenesis and cell proliferation. Transforming growth factors as well as bone-derived osteoinductive growth factors also seem to be involved in the control of tissue repair. Transforming growth factors are a heterogeneous family of polypeptides that can induce nonneoplastic cells to express a transformed phenotype. Indeed, they are found in many tissues, both neoplastic and nonneoplastic, including platelets; they may also have a role in wound healing [90].

Recently, two cartilage-inducing factors similar to other bone-derived growth factors [88,111] capable of eliciting intramuscular biological response that has all the elements of endochondral ossification, were identified as the two types of transforming growth factor-β (β_1 and β_2) [101,102]. Studies using cloned cDNA probes [75] can be focused in the future to detect expression of growth factor/proto-oncogene mRNAs during various stages of callus formation in order to better understand the regulation of cell division, metabolism, and differentiation during fracture repair. In the near future, with the development of recombinant DNA technology, it will be possible to verify the production of natural growth factors in healing bones and thereby open the chance to control the target processes by manufacturing growth factors.

Electromagnetic Factors

Bone can transduce mechanical deformations into electrical potentials. Methods of electrically stimulating bone repair include: implanted electrodes, induction coupling, capactitive coupling, which corresponding to piezoelectric effect, streaming potential effect, and endogenic bioelectric effect respectively. This effect may be related to the piezoelectric properties of bone matrix. Another strong hypothesis is that streaming potentials could be produced in bone as a result of the flow of fluid through the solid matrix when bone is deformed. Bone tissue also exhibits endogenous ionic currents (bioelectric potentials) after injury which are due to the functions of living cells (reviewed by [65]). Wolff's law – the very architecture of bone being a response to the mechanical demands placed on it – has been explained as a self-regulating feedback mechanism in which the appearance of stresses and strains in the bone modifies the electrical evironment of the bone cells in such a way as to modify their behavior [8].

Electrical stimulation of fracture healing has this strong bioelectric background. The method seems to be an alternative treatment modality of fracture nonunions, in some cases of delayed unions, for example, in scaphoideum, and congenital pseudoarthroses. The three most commonly used modalities for electrical stimulation involve currents that are delivered internally by means of implanted electrodes or externally by mounted devices that inductively (time-varying magnetic field) or capacitively (time-varying electric field) couple currents to the appropriate site. Unfortunately, the basic mechanisms by which these different types of electrical stimulation work remain one of the most complex issues in the entire problem of bone fracture repair. One clinically important fact is that the type of tissue between the ununited bone fragments seems to be crucial in predicting the treatment response. On the other hand, the clinical results will always be open to question until randomized, double-blind trials are performed.

Mechanical Factors

According to Wolff's law, mechanical loading elicits an osteogenic response in the loaded bone structure. Studies by Rubin and Lanyon [91] have shown that compressive loading results in osteogenic response in an isolated bone segment, and the response is related to the tissue strain during loading. Controlled weight bearing under functional braces has a positive effect on healing of tibial fractures [96]. The mechanism of action of such a treatment is probably related not only to the introduction of compressive forces but also to other biological and physical factors.

The clinical experience favors the advantages of early functional loading. This concept of axial stimulation of osteogenesis has been adopted in external fixation which has the unique feature to allow a controlled adjustment of fixation rigidity during the progress of fracture healing. The three basic alternatives during external fixation to attempt axial stimulation of osteogenesis are:

Passive dynamization: Load transmission through fracture site due to pin bending under weight bearing (rigid side bar). Removal of additional sidebar or pins results in proportional reduction of axial, torsional, and bending stiffness.

Active axial dynamization: Load transmission through fracture site under weight bearing without pin bending (telescoping side bar). Relaxation of the axial constraint in the fixator does not affect the torsional or bending stability of the fixation.

Controlled axial micromovement: Load transmission through fracture site using controlled force/displacement actuator (telescoping side bar).

The rigidity of external fixation can be gradually decreased by reviewing pins or side bars as the healing progresses. Such a maneuver not only decreases axial stiffness, but the corresponding torsional and bending stiffness are also affected. Use of the telescoping mechanism in the side bar to allow dynamic compression of fracture fragments is advantageous since the original bending and torsional rigidity is maintained. However, the proper timing to introduce dynamic compression in different types of fracture is still unknown and must be carefully established in order to benefit fully from such a treatment modality, which is available only in external fixation. The controlled axial micromotion by the displacement actuator has been applied in a clinical trial of tibial fractures [60]. The regimen includes a treatment of controlled micromotion for 30 min per day, starting 1–3 weeks after injury and continuing until partial weight bearing is permitted. Although such treatment appears to be novel and attractive, careful clinical and basic science investigations must be performed so that the optimal treatment environment and time period can be established to cope with the widely varying fracture conditions.

It is important to realize that numerous factors, both local and systemic, have been reported to stimulate bone healing under experimental fracture healing conditions. Recently, ultrasound [73] and factor XIII [25] have been found to be beneficial for bone repair. However, at the present time, we have no pharmacological or other agents available for clinical use to stimulate normal fracture healing. After an intensive review of literature, Brighton [15] concluded that none of the studies involving the manipulation of biomechanical factors could show that the experimental fracture is able to reach the healed state more rapidly than the control fracture. The only exception seems to be functional weight bearing [95], which was also proven to be useful and clinically reproducible. Brighton emphasized that many factors may improve mechanical properties in the early and midphase of fracture healing, but the fractures do not heal in a shorter period of time. The normal biological response suggests that uncomplicated fracture healing repairs at a rate that is near optimal. Enhancement of fracture healing is possible and desirable only when the normal healing rate is significantly compromised.

Noninvasive Assessment of Fracture Healing

There is a definite need for noninvasive, quantitative techniques to assess the progress of fracture healing and remodeling. A reliable noninvasive method, more sensitive and accurate than conventional radiography, would be extremely valuable for both experimental studies and management of clinical fracture cases. If validated, such methods would allow earlier prediction of delayed unions, allowing timely intervention or alteration in treatment of such cases. Noninvasive quantitative measurement of bone mass and density would be of great value in prediction of the risk of refracture, especially after plate removal. In external fixation of fractures, noninvasive methods are needed to determine when to vary fixation rigidity.

At present, other promising methods include computed tomography, photon densitometry, and magnetic resonance imaging. Ultrasonic high-resolution computed tomography [121] is a new, noninvasive imaging modality which may be helpful in assessment of very early stages of fracture healing. Vibration methods [29] and ultrasonic velocity measurement [38] have also been employed in assessment of mechanical properties of healing fractures, but no definitive conclusions can be drawn.

Dynamic bone scans (using ^{99m}Tc-labeled methylene diphosphonate), as an indicator of blood flow [77], and static bone scans have been used in evaluation of osteotomy-site blood flow and bone matrix production in experimental studies [6,116] and clinically in prediction of the outcome of fracture treatment [105]. However, the specificity and sensitivity of the quantitative radionucleotide imaging needs further investigation.

External fixation provides an opportunity nonivasively to assess the bioemchanical progress of fracture healing. Strain gages can be attached to the fixator frame, and bending deformations can be measured as a function of healing time [18]. Similar healing curves of tibial farctures have been generated by removal of the side bars of the Hoffmann fixator and measuring the relative pin motion in response to an applied bending moment [55]. In experimental studies the increasing rigidity of the osteotomy site has been quantitated by measuring (with the side bar of an external fixator in place) the displacement of transfixing pins in response to axial tensile loads [56] or by measuring osteotomy-site strain in response to distraction of the osteotomy site [116]. In these methods, the state of pin-bone interface remains an unknown source of error.

Noninvasive methods for measurement of bone mass and density, such as single- and dual-photon absorptiometry as well as computed tomgraphy have been applied mostly for assessment of metabolic bone diseases, particularly osteoporosis. Each of these methods has advantages, disadvantages, and specific indications [69]. In common, they seem to be accurate in indirect measurement of bone mineral content, which might be very valuable in evaluation of fracture area mineralization and postunion remodeling processes. Compressive strength and modulus of trabecular bone are closely related to its apparent density, and the hardness of fracture callus is related to its mineral content. In a recent study, a high-resolution single-photon densitometry technique [5] proved to be most promising to quantitate the mineral density of fracture callus. The noninvasively measured local mineral density in fracture callus correlated highly with the hardness of the callus, indicating that this method may serve as a good predictor of fracture strength.

Musculoskeletal applications of magnetic resonance imaging are expanding rapidly. It has several features which make it superior to computed tomography in many situations [10]. Quantitative magnetic resonance imaging has already been applied in experimental fracture healing studies [67] to quantitate signal activity in external callus and in cortical bone areas at the fracture site. The correlation of in vivo signal activity with invasive test data on tissue properties validates the potential of magnetic resonance imaging as a noninvasive indicator of tissue quality during normal fracture healing and in pending nonunions. Magnetic resonance imaging spectroscopy, which is still an experimental tool, has also been used to monitor local pH changes during fracture repair [76], but further research is required before its true merit can be fully appreciated.

Summary and Concluding Remarks

Bone fracture management and the related clinical and basic sciences have always been regarded as the fundamental disciplines in orthopedics and traumatology. In the wake of the dramatic achievement of artificial joint replacement, the emphasis of basic research on bone fracture biomechanics and physiology has experienced a temporary setback. Fortunately, the new knowledge, unique experimental tools, and research methodology introduced and perfected by scientists and bioengineers working in the field of prosthetic joint development have all been adopted in bone fracture research. Consequently, the amount of progress achieved recently in the basic understanding of bone fracture repair and remodeling has surpassed any of our previous investigatory periods.

The physiology and biomechanics of bone fracture union is one of the most widely studied subjects in orthopedic surgery. Although much has been written and discussed, many fundamental issues still remain controversial and poorly understood. One of the possible reasons for such deficiency may be related to the heavy clinical influence of basic research. Frequently, scientific inquires have been stimulated by the introduction of a new treatment modality or device. Very few well-conceptualized hypotheses and systematic investigations have been able to pace the advances of the field. Furthermore, well-developed techniques or devices for specific applications have all too often tended to overexpand their indications, even at the risk of contradicting the orginal working principles. These potential pitfalls must be carefully avoided to ensure the quality and originality of research in the field of bone fracture repair.

Each bone fracture fixation method, either internal or external, has its specific advantages and disadvantages according to its original development concept and specific indications. No single method or device can be so universal as to be applicable for every fracture type and location. It is therefore logical to select the best treatment modality and fixation device according to the lesion and clinical conditions of the patient. Once the method of fixation has been selected, a thorough knowledge of its biomechanical function and biological response is required to optimize its effectiveness, since each method or fixation device bears its own bone fracture healing mechanism through characteristic clinical responses. It would be unreasonable to change the treatment modality in midcourse, as each fixation or immobilization method requires a specific biological environment which may not exist after the initial time period has elasped.

This chapter documents the fact that bone fracture union can follow any one of many combinations of pathways to the final stage. The choice of healing mechanism should be based on many factors, including the treating surgeon's expertise and experience. It would be wrong to assume that a certain method which appears easier requires less technical demand. Many clinical factors such as the patient's expectations, compliance to treatment, degree of tolerance, and socioeconomic considerations are likely to play an important role in the selection of fixation method. A biological system appears to have a high level of tolerance and adaptability to even the most adverse conditions. If the fundamental biomechanical and biological principles for any fracture fixation modality are well understood and carefully applied in patient management, it would be hard to believe that successful bony union will not occur.

Compression plate fixation may have potential drawbacks, such as stress shielding bone osteopenia and refracture after plate removal, but its advantages in many special circumstances appear to outweight these considerations. Redesigning the plate geometry or material composition to minimize its axial stiffness would appear ineffective and contradictory to the underlying principle of compression plate fixation. On the other hand, lack of torsional rigidity in intramedullary nail fixation should not be regarded as an intrinsic deficiency of such method since the functional principle of intramedullary nailing is to promote axial compaction of the bone ends at the fracture site. Increasing torsional rigidity of the nail (fluted cross-section) or fixation (interlocking feature) may reduce the axial stimulation characteristics inherent in such method of fracture fixation. Therefore, in changing the structural properties of any internal fixation devices, the benefits to be gained may be overshadowed by the loss of certain fundamental functional principles upon which the original fixation concept was based.

Although the uncertainty that exists among some surgeons concerning the use of external fixation for fracture treatment is due mainly to the fear of pin tract infection and fracture nonunion, much of the clinical experience and basic science research results have proven the reverse. Many of the potential benefits of external fixation, such as dynamization and the change of fixation stiffness, are not yet fully appreciated. Additional research and well-organized clinical trials must be performed. Pin tract problems can be controlled, but the surgeon utilizing such a device must be familiar with the techniques and clinical care of the patients. One common mistake is to assume that external fixators, especially those of the simpler unilateral configuration, are easy to use and do not require learning or mastering the surgical techniques until the time of application. On the other hand, external fixation also has its limitations and unavoidable shortcomings from a clinical

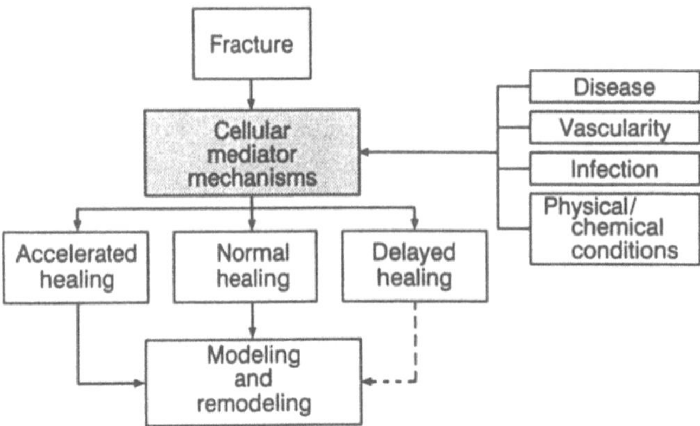

Fig. 24. Proposed regulatory mechanisms for bone fracture healing and remodeling

point of view. It would be a disservice to the external fixation technique if one overextended its indications in certain patients with specific clinical conditions which may be more amenable to another form of treatment.

Finally, the importance of balancing between the biomechanical properties and the biological behavior of different fracture fixation methods has been demonstrated. Understanding this knowledge and the application techniques associated with each fixation modality is the prerequisite to selecting the optimal treatment for each patient and the involved pathological and clinical conditions. Some of the basic knowledge related to both internal and external fixation is still unknown. This should provide the impetus for surgeons, bioengineers, and medical scientists to continue collaborative basic and applied research with carefully formulated hypotheses as well as organized specific aims. Furthermore, recognizing the proper cell mediator and the physical means to stimulate these cellular elements, the bone fracture healing process may be modulated, regardless of the fixation technique (Fig. 24). The end result of such effort should not be limited by establishing proper guidelines of fracture management under each method of fixation. A better understanding of how bone repairs itself under variable conditions and environment can help the future development of noninvasive fracture healing monitoring techniques and identify bone union enhancing and inhibiting factors.

References

1. Aalto K, Holmström T, Karaharju E, Joukainen J, Paavolainen P, Slätis P (1987) Fracture repair during external fixation. Torsion tests of rabbit osteotomies. Acta Orthop Scand 58:66–70
2. Aro H (1985) Fracture healing in the rat tibio-fibular bone with special reference to the effects of denervation. Thesis, University of Turku
3. Aro H, Eerola E, Aho AJ, Niinikoski J (1984) Tissue oxygen tension in externally stabilized tibial fractures in rabbits during normal healing and infection. J Surg Res 37:202–207
4. Aro H, Eerola E, Aho AJ (1985) Determination of callus quantity in 4-week-old fractures of the rat tibia. J Orthop Res 3:101–108
5. Aro H, Wippermann B, Hodgson S, Wahner H, Lewallen D, Chao E (1988) Noninvasive monitoring of fracture callus mineralization using high-resolution single-photon absorptiometry. Transactions of the 34th Annual Meeting of the Orthopaedic Research Society, Febr 1–4, Atlanta, p 415
6. Aro H, Kelly PJ, Lewallen DG, Chao EYS (1988) Comparison of the effects of dynamization and constant rigid fixation on rate and quality of bone osteotomy union in external fixation. Transactions of the 34th Annual Meeting of the Orthopaedic Research Society, Febr 1–4, Atlanta, p 303
7. Banda MJ, Knighton DR, Hunt TK, Werb Z (1982) Isolation of a nonmitogenic angiogenesis factor from wound fluid. Proc Natl Acad Sci USA 79:7773–7777
8. Bassett CAL (1971) Biophysical principles affecting bone structure. In: Bourne GH (ed) The Biochemistry and physiology of bone, vol 3. Academic, New York, pp 1–76
9. Behrens F, Johnson WD, Koch TW, Kovacevic N (1983) Bending stiffness of unilateral and bilateral fixator frames. Clin Orthop 178:103–110
10. Berquist TH (ed) (1987) Magnetic resonance of the musculoskeletal system. Raven, New York
11. Black J, Perdigon P, Brown N, Pollack SR (1984) Stiffness and strength of fracture callus. Relative rates of mechanical maturation as evaluated by a uniaxial tensile test. Clin Orthop 182:278–288
12. Bradley GW, McKenna GB, Dunn HK, Daniels AU, Statton WO (1979) Effects of flexural rigidity of plates on bone healing. J Bone Joint Surg [Am] 61:866–872
13. Brien W, Wiss DA, Peter K, Merritt PO (1987) Subtrochanteric fractures of the femur: treatment with locked medullary nails. Proceedings of the 54th Annual Meeting of the American Academy of Orthopaedics Surgeons, San Fransisco, p 121
14. Briggs BT, Chao EYS (1982) The mechanical performance of the standard Hoffmann-Vidal external fixation apparatus. J Bone Joint Surg [Am] 64:566–573
15. Brighton CT (1984) Principles of fracture healing. Instr Course Lect 33:60–82
16. Brighton CT, Krebs AG (1972) Oxygen tension of healing fractures in the rabbit. J Bone Joint Surg [Am] 54:323–332
17. Brown SA, Gillet NA, Broaddus TW (1984) Biomechanics of fracture fixation by plastic rods with transverse screws. In: Perren SM, Schneider E (eds) Biomechanics: current interdisciplinary research. Nijhoff, Dordrecht, pp 475–480
18. Burny FL (1979) Strain gage measurement of fracture healing. In: Brooker AF, Edwards CC (eds) External fixation – the current state of the art. Williams and Wilkins, Baltimore, pp 371–382
19. Chao EYS (1976) Principles of orthopedic biomechanics. Biomechanics Laboratory, Department of Orthopedics, Mayo Clinic/Mayo Foundation, Rochester
20. Chao EYS (1983) Fissazione externa e guardigione delle fratture: proprietà biomeccaniche di strumenti diversi. In: Ricciardi L (ed) Attulita in traumatologia. Gaggi, Bologna, pp 191–206

21. Chao EYS, Hein TJ (1988) Mechanical performance of standard Orthofix external fixator. Orthopedics 11:1057–1069
22. Chao EYS, Kasman RA, An KN (1982) Rigidity and stress analyses of external fracture fixation devices – a theoretical apporach. J Biomech 15(12):971–983
23. Chapman MW (1986) The role of intramedullary fixation in open fractures. Clin Orthop 212:26–34
24. Charnley J (1970) The closed treatment of common fractures. Livingstone, Edinburgh
25. Claes L, Burri C, Gerngross H, Mutschler W (1985) Bone healing stimulated by plasma factor XIII. Osteotomy experiments in sheep. Acta Orthop Scand 56:57–62
26. Claes L, Wilke JH, Kemper F (1987) Interfragmentary strain and bone healing – an experimental study. Proceedings of the International Society for Fracture Repair, Aug 31–Sept 2, Helsinki, Stockholm, pp 64–65
27. Cordey J, Perren SM (1986) Limits of plate on bone friction in internal fixation of fractures. Proceedings of the 5th Meeting of the European Society of Biomechanics, September, Berlin, p 102
28. Cordey J, Perren SM, Steinemann S (1986) Parametric analysis of the strain distribution in bone after plating. Proceedings of the 5th Meeting of the European Society of Biomechanics, September, Berlin, p 103
29. Cornelissen M, Mulier M, Sleeckx E, Van der Perre G (1987) Dynamic behaviour of healing bones. Proceedings of the International Society for Fracture Repair, Aug 31–Sept 2, Helsinki, Stockholm, pp 72–73
30. Cruess RL, Dumont J (1975) Fracture healing. Can J Surg 18(5):403–413
31. DiGioia AM, Cheal EJ, Hayes WC, Perren SM (1987) Biomechanics of bone resorption, callus formation and medullary pressurization in healing plated fractures. Transaction of the 33rd Annual Meeting of the Orthopaedic Research Society, San Francisco, p 100
32. Edwards CC (1983) Staged reconstruction of complex open tibial fractues using Hoffmann external fixation. Clin Orthop 178:130–161
33. Finlay JB, Moroz TK, Rorabeck CH, Davey JD, Bourne RB (1987) Stability of ten configurations of the Hoffmann external-fixation frame. J Bone Joint Surg [Am] 69:734–744
34. Frankel VH, Burstein AH (1970) Orthopaedic biomechanics. Lea and Febiger, Philadelphia
35. Frankel VH, Nordin M (1980) Basic biomechanics of the skeletal system. Lea and Febiger, Philadelphia
36. Garbarino JL, Brumback RJ, Poka A, Burgess AR (1987) Closed interlocking nailing of subtrochanteric fractures. Proceedings of the 54th Annual Meeting of the American Academy of Orthopaedics Surgeons, San Fransisco, p 121
37. Gasser B, Wyder D, Schneider E (1987) The stiffness behaviour of the circular, wire-based frame in contrast to conventional external fixators. Proceedings of the International Society for Fracture Repair, Aug 31–Sept 2, Helskinki, Stockholm, pp 95–96
38. Gerlanc M, Haddad D, Hyatt GW, Langloh JT, Hilaire PS (1975) Ultrasonic study of normal and fractured bone. Clin Orthop 111:175–180
39. Glaser BM, D'Amore PA, Seppa H, Seppa S, Schiffmann E (1980) Adult tissues contain chemoattractants for vascular endothelial cells. Nature 288:483–484
40. Göthman L (1961) Vascular reactions in experimental fractures. Microangiographic and radioisotope studies. Acta Chir Scand 284 [Suppl]
41. Green SA (1981) Complications of external skeletal fixation: causes, prevention and treatment. Thomas, Springfield
42. Guse R, Lippiello L, Connolly J (1988) Percutaneously injected marrow augments osteosynthesis in a rabbit delayed union mode. Transactions of the 34th Annual Meeting of the Orthopaedic Research Society, Febr 1–4, Atlanta, p 556

43. Ham AW (1930) A histological study of the early phases of bone repair. J Bone
    Joint Surg 12:827–844
44. Hart MB, Wu J-J, Chao EYS, Kelly PJ (1985) External skeletal fixation of
    canine tibial osteotomies. Compression compared with no compression. J Bone
    Joint Surg [Am] 67:598–605
45. Hayes WC (1980) Basic biomechanics of compression plate fixation. In: Uhthoff
    HK (ed) Current concepts of internal fixation of fractures. Springer, Berlin
    Heidelberg New York, pp 49–62
46. Hayes WE, Snyder BD (1981) Toward a quantitative formulation of Wolff's
    law in trabecular bone. In: Cowin SC (ed) Mechanical properties of bone.
    ASME, New York, pp 43–68 (AMD, vol 45)
47. Heppenstall RB (1980) Fractures of the tibia and fibula. In: Heppenstall RB
    (ed) Fracture treatment and healing. Saunders, Philadelphia, pp 777–802
48. Heppenstall RB, Grislis G, Hunt TK (1975) Tissue gas tensions and oxygen
    consumption in healing bone defects. Clin Orthop 106:357–365
49. Hodgson SF (1986) Skeletal remodeling and renal osteodystrophy. Semin
    Nephrol 6(1):42–55
50. Holmström T, Paavolainen P, Slätis P, Karaharju E (1986) Effect on compres-
    sion on fracture healing. Plate fixation studied in rabbits. Acta Orthop Scand
    57:368–372
51. Huiskes R, Chao EYS (1986) Guidelines for external fixation frame rigidity and
    stresses. J Orthop Res 4:68–75
52. Huiskes R, Chao EYS, Crippen TE (1985) Parametric analyses of pin-bone
    stresses in external fracture fixation devices. J Orthop Res 3:341–349
53. Hunt TK (1984) Can repair processes be stimulated by modulators (cell growth
    factors, angiogenetic factors, ect.) without adversely affecting normal processes?
    J Trauma 24(9):S39–S46
54. Hutzschenreuter P, Brummer H (1980) Screw design and stability. In: Uhthoff
    HK (ed) Current concepts of internal fixation of fractures. Springer, Berlin
    Heidelberg New York, pp 244–250
55. Jörgensen TE (1979) A simple method of assessing fracture healing. In: Brooker
    AF, Edwards CC (eds) External fixation – the current state of the art. Williams
    and Wilkins, Baltimore, pp 383–392
56. Kaplan SJ, Hayes WC, Mudan P, Lelli JL, White AA (1985) Monitoring the
    healing of a tibial osteotomy in the rabbit treated with external fixation. J
    Orthop Res 3:325–330
57. Kelly PJ (1983) Pathways of transport in bone. In: Geiger SR (ed) Peripheral
    circulation and organ blood flow. American Physiological Society, Bethesda,
    pp 371–396 (Handbook of physiology, vol 3: The cardiovascular system,
    part 1)
58. Kelly PJ, An K-N, Chao EYS, Rand JA (1985) Fracture healing: biomechanical,
    fluid dynamic, and electrical considerations. In: Peck WA (ed) Bone and
    mineral research, vol 3. Elsevier, Amsterdam, pp 295–319
59. Kempf I, Karger C, Willinger R, Francois JM, Cornet A, Renault D, Bonnel F
    (1984) Locked intramedullary nailing – improvement of mechanical properties.
    In: Perren SM, Schneider E (eds) Biomechanics: current interdisciplinary
    research. Nijhoff, Dordrecht, pp 487–492
60. Kenwright J, Goodship AE, Kelly DJ, Newman JH, Harris JD, Richardson JB,
    Evans M, Spriggins AJ, Burrough SJ, Rowley DI (1986) Effect of controlled
    axial micromotion on healing of tibial fractures. Lancet 2:1185–1187
61. Klemm KW, Borner M (1986) Interlocking nailing of complex fractures of the
    femur and tibia. Clin Orthop 212:89–100
62. Knighton DR, Hunt TK, Scheuenstuhl H, Halliday BJ, Werb Z, Banda MJ
    (1983) Oxygen tension regulates the expression of angiogenesis factor by
    macrophages. Science 221:1283–1285
63. Kopman CR, Boskey AL, Lane JM, Pita JC, Eaton B (1987) Biochemical
    characterization of fracture callus proteoglycans. J Orthop Res 5:7–13

64. Küntscher G (1965) Intramedullary surgical technique and its place in orthopaedic surgery. My present concept. J Bone Joint Surg [Am] 47:809–818
65. Lavine LS, Grodzinsky AJ (1987) Electrical stimulation of bone repair. J Bone Joint Surg [Am] 69:626–630
66. Lewallen DG, Chao EYS, Kasman RA, Kelly PJ (1984) Comparison of the effects of compression plates and external fixators on early bone healing. J Bone Joint Surg [Am] 66:1084–1091
67. Lewallen DG, Aro HT, Chao EYS, Bergquist TH, Kelly PJ (1988) Noninvasive evaluation of bone healing using quantitative MRI imaging. Transactions of the 34th Annual Meeting of the Orthopaedic Research Society, Febr 1–4, Atlanta, p 409
68. Matter P, Brennwald J, Perren SM (1974) Biologische Reaktion des Knochens auf Osteosyntheseplatten. Helv Chir Acta 12 [Suppl]:1–44
69. Mazess RB (1983) The noninvasive measurement of skeletal mass. In: Peck WA (ed) Bone and mineral research. Annual 1. Excerpta Medica, Amsterdam, pp 223–279
70. McCoy TM, Chao EYS, Kasman RA (1983) Comparison of mechanical performance in four types of external fixators. Clin Orthop 180:23–33
71. McKibbin B (1978) The biology of fracture healing in long bones. J Bone Joint Surg [Br] 60:150–162
72. Meunier PJ (1983) Histomorphometry of the skeleton. In: Peck WA (ed) Bone and mineral research. Annual 1. Excerpta Medica, Amsterdam, pp 191–222
73. Mont MA, Pilla A, Tenreiro RA, Kaufman JJ, Sadeh A, Campos-Marquetti A, Burstein AH, Siffert RS (1987) The effects of ultrasonic stimulation on fresh fracture repair in rabbits. Transaction of the 33rd Annual Meeting of the Orthopaedic Research Society, San Fransisco, p 97
74. Müller J, Schenk R, Willenegger H (1968) Experimentelle Untersuchungen über die Entstehung reaktiver Pseudarthrosen am Hunderadius. Helv Chir Acta 1/2:301–308
75. Multimäki P, Aro H, Vuorio E (1987) Differential expression of fibrillar collagen genes during callus formation. Biochem Biophys Res Commun 142(2): 536–541
76. Newman RJ, Francis MJO, Duthrie RB (1987) Nuclear magnetic resonance studies of experimentally induced delayed fracture union. Clin Orthop 216: 253–261
77. Nutton RW, Fitzgerald RH Jr, Kelly PJ (1985) Early dynamic bone-imaging as an indicator of osseous blood flow and factors affecting the uptake of $^{99\,m}$Tc hydroxymethylene diphosphonate in healing bone. J Bone Joint Surg [Am] 67:763–770
78. Panjabi MM, White AA, Southwick WO (1973) Mechanical properties of bone as a function of rate of deformation. J Bone Joint Surg [Am] 55(2):322–330
79. Panjabi MM, Walter SD, Karuda M, White AA, Lawson JP (1985) Correlations of radiographic analysis of healing fractures with strength: a statistical analysis of experimental osteotomies. J Orthop Res 3:212–218
80. Penttinen R (1972) Biochemical studies on fracture healing in the rat with special reference to the oxygen supply. Acta Chir Scand Suppl 432 [Suppl]
81. Perren SM (1979) Physical and biological aspects of fracture healing with special reference to internal fixation. Clin Orthop 138:175–196
82. Perren SM, Cordey J (1980) Mechanics of interfragmentary compression by plates and screws. In: Uhthoff HK (ed) Current concepts of internal fixation of fractures. Springer, Berlin Heidelberg New York, pp 184–191
83. Perren SM, Huggler A, Russenberger M, Straumann F, Muller ME, Allgöwer M (1969) A method of measuring the change in compression applied to living cortical bone. Acta Orthop Scand Suppl 125:7
84. Peterson DL, Skraba JS, Moran JM, Greenwald AS (1984) Fracture of long bones: rate effects under singular and combined loading states. J Orthop Res 1:244–250

85. Pettine KA, Kelly PJ, Chao EYS, Huiskes R (1986) Histologic and bio-mechanical analysis of unilateral external fixator pin-bone interface. Proceedings of the 32nd Annual Meeting of the Orthopaedic Research Society, New Orleans, p 472
86. Posner AS (1985) The mineral of bone. Clin Orthop 200:87–99
87. Rand JA, An KN, Chao EY, Kelly PJ (1981) A comparison of the effect of open intramedullary nailing and compression-plate fixation on fracture site blood flow and fracture union. J Bone Joint Surg [Am] 63:427–442
88. Reddi AH (1981) Cell biology and biochemistry of endochondral bone development collagen. Clin Orthop 1:209–226
89. Rhinelander RW (1972) Circulation of bone. In: Bourne GH (ed) The biochemistry and physiology of bone, vol 2. Academic, New York, pp 1–77
90. Roberts AB, Frolik CA, Anzano MA, Sporn MB (1983) Transforming growth factors in neoplastic and nonneoplastic tissues. Fed Proc 42:2621–2626
91. Rubin CT, Lanyon LE (1987) Osteoregulatory nature of mechanical stimuli: functions as a determinant for adaptive remodeling in bone. J Orthop Res 5:300–310
92. Rydell NW (1966) Forces acting on the femoral head prosthesis: a study on strain gauge supplied prostheses in living persons. Acta Orthop Scand 88 [Suppl]
93. Sandberg M, Vuorio E (1987) Localization of mRNAs for fibrillar collagens in developing human skeletal tissues by in situ hydridization. J Cell Biol 104: 1077–1084
94. Sandberg M, Aro H, Multimäki P, Aho H, Vuorio E (1988) In situ localization of collagen production by chondrocytes and osteoblasts in fracture callus tissue. J Bone Joint Surg [Am] 71A:69–77
95. Sarmiento A, Schaeffer JF, Beckerman L, Latta LL, Enis JE (1977) Fracture healing in rat femora as affected by functional weight-bearing. J Bone Joint Surg [Am] 59:369–375
96. Sarmiento A, Sobol PA, Hoy AL, Ross SDK, Racette WL, Tarr RR (1984) Prefabricated functional braces for the treatment of fractures of the tibial diaphysis. J Bone Joint Surg [Am] 66:1328–1339
97. Schenk RK (1986) Histophysiology of bone remodeling and bone repair. In: Lin OCC, Chao EYS (eds) Perspectives on biomaterials. Elsevier, Amsterdam, pp 75–94
98. Schenk RK, Willenegger H (1963) Zum histologischen Bild der sogeinannten Primärheilung der Knochenkompakta nach expermentellen Osteotomien am Hund. Experientia 19:593
99. Schwyzer HK, Cordey J, Brun S, Matter P, Perren SM (1984) Bone loss after internal fixation using plates, determination in humans using computed tomograpy. In: Perren SM, Schneider E (eds) Biomechanics: current interdisciplinary research. Nijhoff, Dordrecht, pp 191–195
100. Sevitt S (1981) Bone repair and fracture healing in man. Churchill Livingstone, Edinburgh
101. Seyedin SM, Thompson AY, Bentz H, Rosen DM, McPerson JM, Conti A, Siegel NR, Galluppi GR, Piez KA (1986) Cartilage-inducing factor-A. Apparent identity to transforming growth factor-beta. J Biol Chem 261:5693–5695
102. Seyedin SM, Segarini PR, Rosen DM, Thompson AY, Bentz H, Graycar J (1987) Cartilage-inducing factor-B is a unique protein structurally and functionally related to transforming growth factor-beta. J Biol Chem 262:1946–1949
103. Shifflett MW, Bray TJ (1987) Subtrochanteric fractures treated by Zickel and Grosse-Kempf nailing. Proceedings of the 54th Annual Meeting of the American Academy of Orthopaedics Surgeons, San Francisco, p 121
104. Slätis P, Karaharju E, Holmström T, Ahonen J, Paavolainen P (1978) Structural changes in intact tubular bone after application of rigid plates with or without compression. J Bone Joint Surg [Am] 60:516–522

105. Smith MA, Jones EA, Strachan RK, Nicoll JJ, Best JJK, Tothill P, Hughes SPF (1987) Prediction of fracture healing in the tibia by quantitative radionucleotide imaging. J Bone Joint Surg [Br] 69:441–447
106. Smith SR, Bronk JT, Kelly PJ (1987) Effect of fracture fixation on blood flow. Proceedings of the International Society for Fracture Repair, Aug 31–Sept 2, Helsinki, Stockholm, p 69
107. Taylor JC, Russell TA, LaVelle DG, Calandruccio RA (1987) Clinical results of 100 femoral shaft fractures treated with the Russell-Taylor interlocking nail system. Proceedings of the 54th Annual Meeting of American Academy of Orthopaedics Surgeons, San Francisco, p 155
108. Tencer AF, Johnson KD, Johnston DWC, Gill K (1984) A biomechanical comparison of various methods of stabilization of subtrochanteric fractures of the femur. J Orthop Res 2:297–305
109. Uhthoff HK, Dubuc FL (1971) Bone structure changes in the dog under rigid internal fixation. Clin Orthop 81:165–170
110. Uhthoff HK, Finnegan M (1983) The effects of metal plates on post-traumatic remodeling and bone mass. J Bone Joint Surg [Br] 65:66–71
111. Urist MR (1983) The origin of cartilage: investigations in quest of chondrogenic DNA. In: Hall BK (ed) Cartilage, vol 2. Academic, New York, pp 1–85
112. Urist MR, Mikulski A, Lietze A (1979) Solubilized and insolubilized bone morphogenetic protein. Proc Natl Acad Sci USA 76:1828–1832
113. Weiss RE, Reddi AH (1981) Role of fibronection in collagenous matrix-induced mesenchymal cell proliferation and differentiation in vivo. Exp Cell Res 133: 247–254
114. White AA III, Panjabi MM, Southwick WO (1977) The four biomechanical stages of fracture repair. J Bone Joint Surg [Am] 59:188–192
115. Whiteside LA, Lesker PA (1978) The effects of extraperiosteal and subperiosteal dissection. II. On fracture healing. J Bone Joint Surg [Am] 60:26–30
116. Williams EA, Rand JA, An KN, Chao EYS, Kelly PJ (1987) The early healing of tibial osteotomies stabilized by one-plane or two-plane external fixation. J Bone Joint Surg [Am] 69:355–365
117. Winquist RA, Hansen ST, Clawson DK (1984) Closed intramedullary nailing of femoral fractures. J Bone Joint Surg [Am] 66:529–539
118. Wiss DA (1986) Editorial comment. Clin Orthop 212:2–3
119. Woo SLY, Lothringer KS, Akeson WH, Coutts RD, Woo YK, Simon BR, Gomez MA (1984) Less rigid internal fixation plates: historical perspectives and new concepts. J Orthop Res 1:431–449
120. Wu JJ, Shyr HS, Chao EYS, Kelly PJ (1984) Comparison of osteotomy healing under external fixation devices with different stiffness characteristics. J Bone Joint Surg [Am] 66:1258–1264
121. Ylitalo J, Greenleaf JF (1987) Correction method for speed variations in high-resolution ultrasound reflection mode CT imaging. Ultrasonic Technology 55–62

3 Contemporary Applications of External Fixation in Fracture Treatment

S. Nayagam and J.B. Jupiter

Introduction

Fracture care at the close of the twentieth century has evolved into an area of specialisation for the orthopaedic surgeon. In its evolution over the past 30 years we have seen the role of non-operative treatment better defined, the advancement of internal fixation techniques and materials, a better understanding of the limb as a complete functional unit and subsequently an appreciation that fractures always involve damage to the soft-tissue envelope. In this era we have also witnessed the development of the external fixator from an option in the care of severe open fractures to a versatile instrument in the arena of trauma care.

Historical Perspective

The first recorded use of an external fixator to restore and maintain alignment of fracture fragments was by Malgaigne in 1843 (cited in [20]). The application of his *griffe metallique* (metal claw; Fig. 1), initially used as a stabiliser of external splints, was modified by Rigaud to perforate the skin and obtain direct contact with the fracture fragments [158]. This was probably the first use of an external device in conjunction with percutaneous points, forming an assembly which maintained fracture reduction [51]. In the nineteenth century Keetley in the United Kingdom [110] and Parkhill in the United States [147] were also responsible for designs which enabled the control of fracture alignment. Both designs incorporated the introduction of pins or screws into fracture fragments and an external linkage assembly. At the turn of this century, Lambotte recorded the use of his external fixator (Fig. 2) on fractures of both long and short tubular bones [119]. His unilateral frame design was later joined by biplanar and multiplanar frame designs in the 1930s by Cuendet and Hoffmann [59,95] (Fig. 3).

The initial response to the external fixator from the surgical fellowship was poor, partly a consequence of variable results and a reported high rate of complications [5,84]. A rapid phase of development soon followed reports of successful use in compression arthrodesis by Charnley in 1953 [43], and later in diaphyseal non-unions by Judet [106] and Müller [141]. The use of the external fixator was extended into trauma as an alternative to skeletal

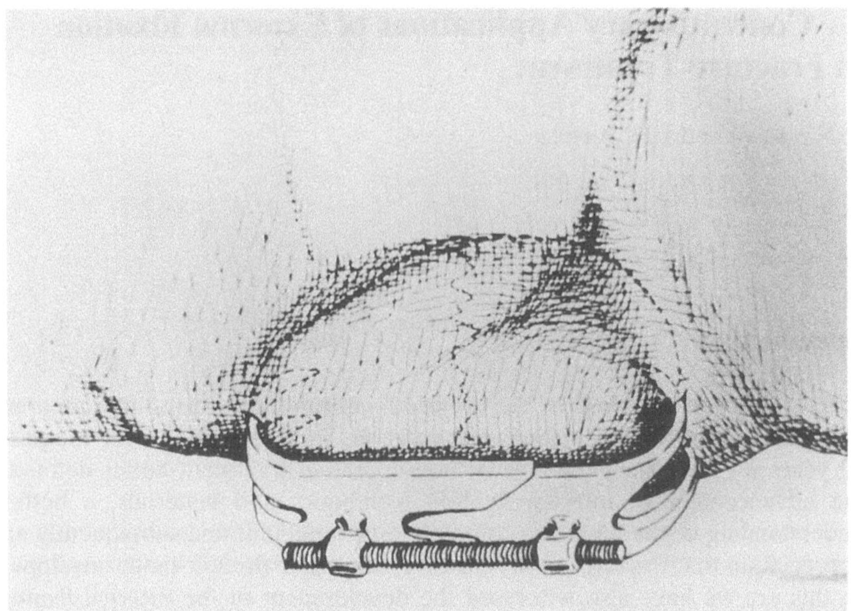

Fig. 1. Malgaigne's *griffe metallique* was the first recorded use of external fixation

traction in the immediate care and stabilisation of open fractures. Internal fixation techniques carried a significant infection rate with more severe open injuries, and functional bracing was inadequate for the highly complex extremity injuries that were being seen with increasing frequency. Our present understanding of the mechanical principles and frame configurations behind effective and appropriate use of the external fixator derives from the enthusiastic efforts of a small number of surgeons. This coupled with technological advancements in design has provided a foundation on which fracture care with external fixation can be developed.

Principles

The external fixator is a modular frame affixed to bone through percutaneously inserted pins and wires. Its modularity allows adjustment both at the time of application and subsequently. Unlike internal fixation, mechanical control and stabilisation of the bony elements at the site of injury is achieved without additional damage to the vital soft-tissue envelope. Access to wounds is accomplished with the fixator in situ, allowing soft-tissue and neurovascular repair in the presence of stable bony supports. In most situations it is possible to utilise the fixator in a configuration which permits the movement of adjacent joints.

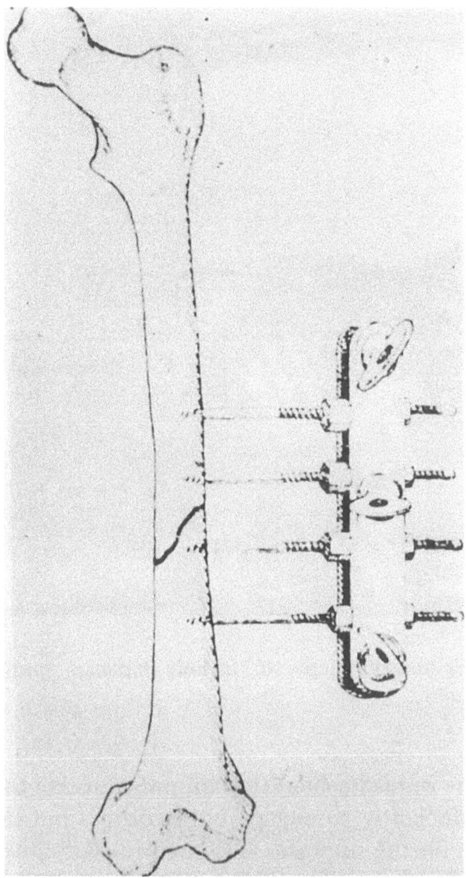

Fig. 2. Lambotte at the turn of the twentieth century developed and applied numerous forms of external fixation in a unilateral frame design

The Device

Although several designs of external fixator are available, the components are similar. The elements of the device are pins, clamps, rods and frames.

Pins

Pins provide the link between the bone fragments and the external assembly. Most pins are inserted percutaneously or via stab incisions. Some pins are threaded to varying lengths; some possess fluted tips to obviate predrilling. Three basic types exist (Fig. 4): (a) transfixion pins are inserted through skin

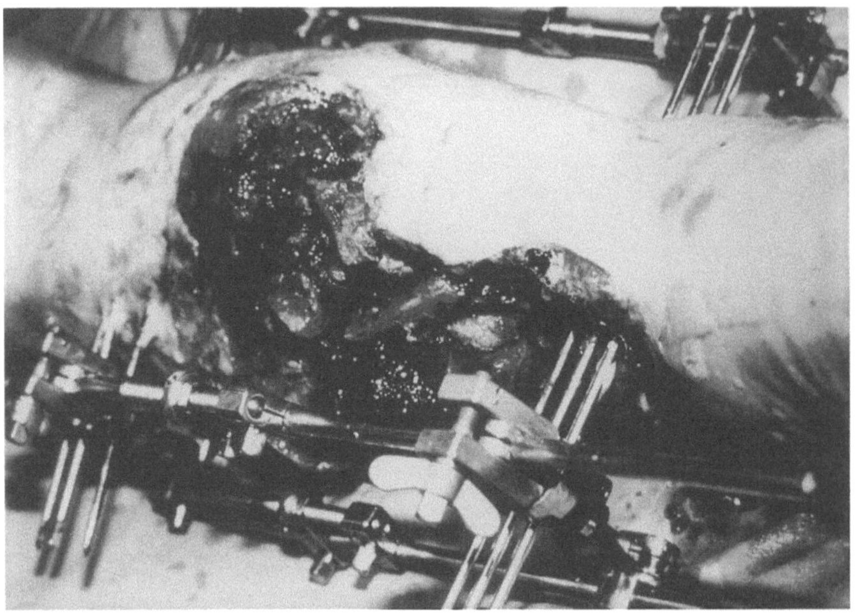

Fig. 3. Hoffman extended Lambotte's developments to include biplanar frame designs

and bone to exit through skin on the opposite side; (b) half pins traverse the diameter of the bone fragment sufficiently to engage both cortices but do not pierce the soft-tissue envelope on the opposite side; and (c) Kirschner wires are of a much smaller diameter than either of the others but are also transfixion pins penetrating the soft-tissue envelope on two sides [14,15] – these are often used as tensioned wires in conjunction with ring fixators.

Pin Number and Placement

The bone-pin interface remains the weakest link in the external fixator [39,173], especially in cancellous bone. A poor interface has been associated with failure of the external fixator system as well as a higher incidence of soft-tissue and bone infection [91]. The interface is the point of maximal stress concentration of the bone-fixator assembly during normal and maximal loading [29,40]. This weak link can be minimised by increasing the number of pins in each bone fragment and ensuring that the pins are placed as far apart as possible within each fragment. A minimum of two pins should be used for each major bone fragment, usually inserted into the same plane [29]. The addition of a third pin, in the plane with least resistance to deformation, does improve rigidity, but further additional pins contribute little to the overall stability [35].

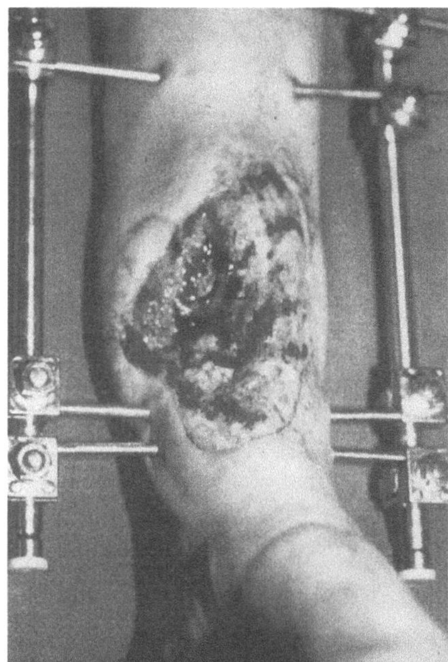 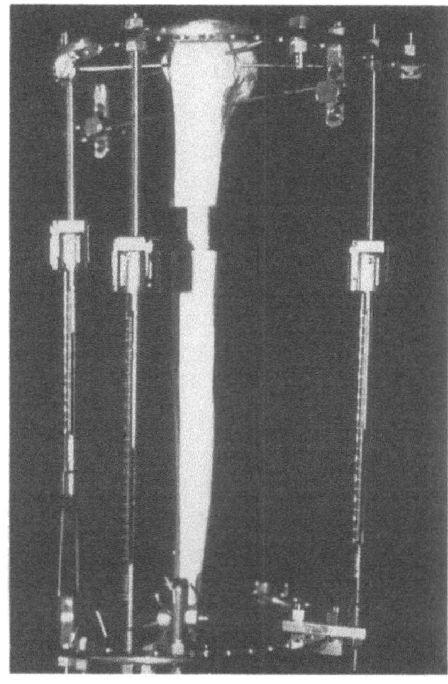

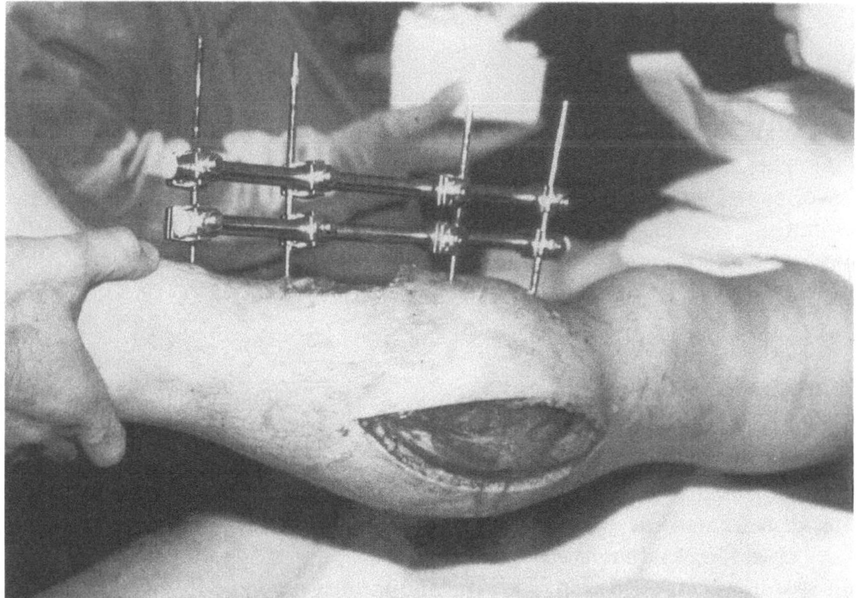

Fig. 4a–c. External fixation frames are based upon pins linking the frame to the bone. **a** Transfixion pins extend through both sides of the soft-tissue envelope. **b** Half pins engage both cortices of bone but only one side of the soft tissue. **c** Flexible wires penetrate both sides of the soft tissue and bone and are tensioned as they are attached to ring

Pin Holding Strength

Some studies have emphasized the importance of the bone-pin interface by investigating the parameters which affect pin holding power. In vitro studies on the holding power of screws as tested by their pull-out strengths are limited owing to other stresses that are present in real-life models [170]. Although the maximum holding power of a pin depends on the shear strength of the material into which it is inserted [99], this does not acknowledge the changes that occur at the bone-pin interface after insertion, especially if the insertion was traumatic to the surrounding tissue.

Despite the limitations of assessing holding power by a tensile stress mode, research has provided data on improvements in pin design and application. Pull-out strength has been related to the interference [7], which is expressed as: (major diameter − pilot hole diameter)/(major diameter − minor diameter). However, selection of the largest diameter pin as a means of maximising interference [91,174] must be reconciled with the risk of iatrogenic fracture. A maximum of 20%–30% of the bone diameter is recommended to minimise this potential problem [13,36]. Alternatively, decreasing the minor diameter has an inversely proportional effect on the torsional strength [6].

Thermal Necrosis

The influence of thermal necrosis on the bone-pin interface, as induced by pin insertion, has been evaluated. High temperatures are generated in the immediate vicinity which may be associated with failure of pin-holding power as the necrotic bone is resorbed. Predrilling is an effective method of minimising temperature elevation [127]. Conversely, there is no difference between pretapping or the use of self-tapping pins [170].

Preloading

With earlier pin designs adjacent pins were preloaded by bending adjacent pins either towards or away from each other. This utilised the compressive strength of the bone fragment held by the pins and created high local contact pressures at the bone-pin interface [189]. Prestressing prevented lateral movement of the bone fragment on the pin; in addition to greater stability to the external fixator assembly, it had a positive impact on lessening pin loosening and infection. This technique of preloading by bending is now succeeded by radial preloading, which is more effective [21,100]. The core diameter of most present pins exceeds the pilot hole diameter by approximately 0.2 mm; this difference has been found to provide excellent purchase without disrupting the surrounding cortex [142].

In summary, an accurate understanding of the multiple factors which influence the integrity of the pin-bone interface will guide the surgeon to good planning decisions for pin choice and placement. The issue of good pin anchorage is paramount when the external fixator is used in neutralisation or lengthening modes; it is here that stresses in loading are not shared by the frame and bone fragments but are transferred entirely through the frame, with the maximum stress concentration at the bone-pin interface. The interface thus becomes a potential site of loosening and subsequent infection.

Clamps

Clamps are the connecting elements between pins and the rods or rings (Fig. 5). There are various degrees of complexity incorporated into these devices, with the more complicated ones accomodating a greater degree of variation in the relative pin-rod or pin-ring position. The connectors associated

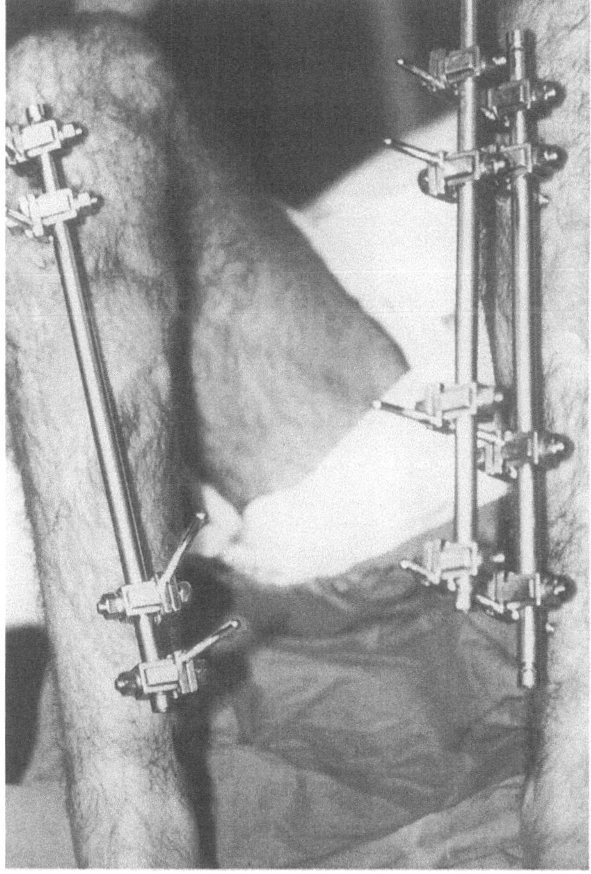

Fig. 5. Pins are connected to rods by individual clamps in half-frame or unilateral external fixation constructs

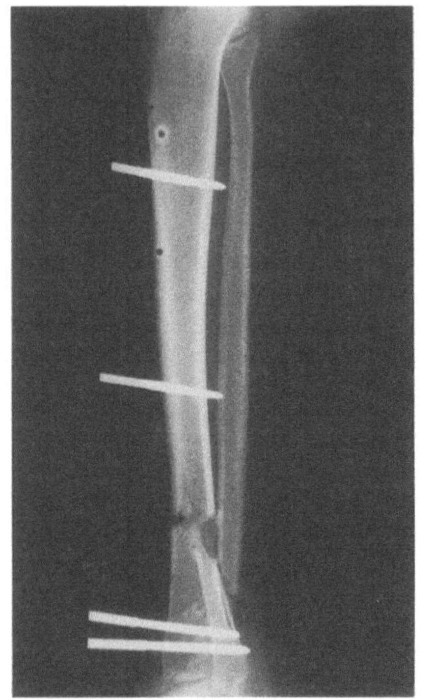

a

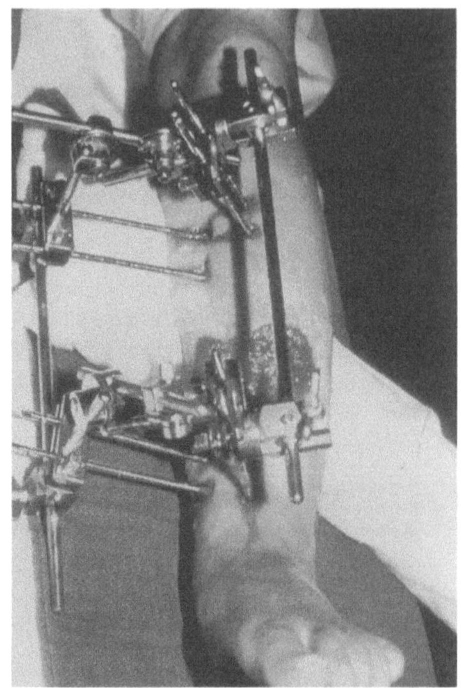

b

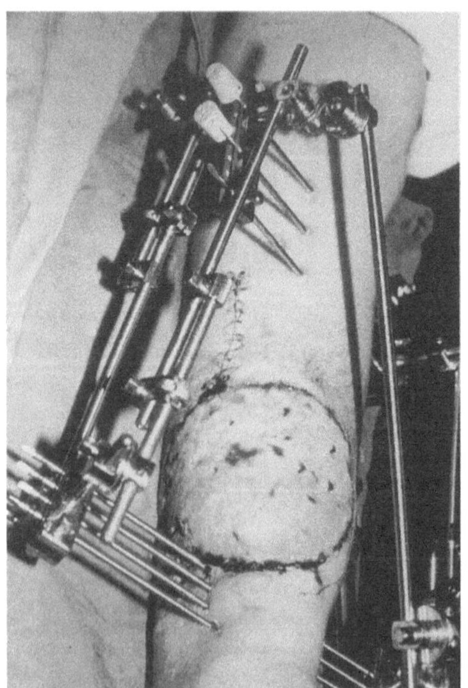

c

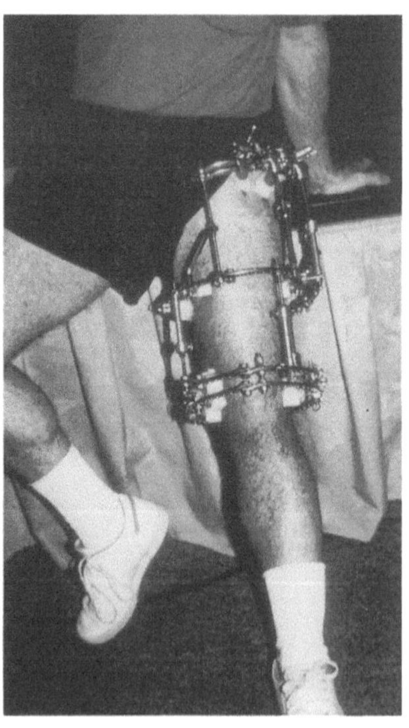

d

with ring fixators allow for tensioning of the wires; this property is essential to the ring fixator as it provides translational stability but allows axial micromotion.

Some authors [15,35] have reserved the term "clamp" to devices that hold two or more parallel aligned pins and connect them to a rod, usually via a universal joint. The other forms of connections are distinguished and named by the two components of the external fixator assembly that are connected, for example, single pin-rod joints, pin-ring joints and ring-rod joints. This allows for a more accurate nomenclature of the connecting device.

The performance of the clamp has been linked to pin movement at the bone-pin interface. The use of pins with larger diameter and their symmetrical placement within a multiple-pin clamp provides the best pin fixation strength [7]. It has been shown that the rigidity of external fixation is increased by applying either the single pin-rod joint or the multiple-pin clamp close to bone [29].

Rods

Together with pins, rings and clamps, rods constitute the external fixator assembly. The rod is the connecting component across the fracture site. More recent designs have incorporated modularity, with rod-to-rod articulations or central telescopic elements which facilitate alignment or length adjustments, respectively. The trend towards increasing modularity has provided an improved versatility to the external fixator. This advance will have to be balanced with the apparent greater freedom for error in pin placement that modularity may give; assessment of future results with such designs must consider this possibility.

Frames

There are four primary frame configurations (Fig. 6): unilateral-uniplanar, unilateral-biplanar, bilateral-uniplanar and bilateral-biplanar.

The Bilateral Frame

The use of tranfixion pins with a bilateral frame configuration has been recommended by Weber [189]; the symmetrical stress transfer and greater stability of this arrangement make this a better choice when the frame is used in the absence of bony fragment contact, as in neutralisation or

Fig. 6a–d. External fixation frames can be constructed in a number of basic designs. **a** Unilateral-uniplanar frame. **b** Unilateral-biplanar frame. **c** Bilateral-uniplanar. **d** Bilateral-multiplanar lengthening mode. The bilateral frame is, however, disadvantaged by interfering with the contralateral leg, making walking difficult. Some authors have questioned the safety in using transfixion pins; several reports of neurovascular injury or muscle and tendon transfixion have led to a more recent popularity of the unilateral frame [84,114,155].

Earlier designs of unilateral-uniplanar frames were not rigid enough for unstable fractures. Axial loading forces were partially transformed into shear and pivotal bending, resulting in non-union and soft-tissue problems. This lead to the initial popularity of the bilateral frame, as noted above.

A Case for the Unilateral Frame

The recognised deficiencies in early unilateral frames led to improvements in design, manufacture and methods of application of the half-frame – in particular, the techniques described earlier for maximising the pin-bone interface, attaching a double rod to the same pins, or using the unilateral-biplanar configuration.

Several authors have demonstrated that bending moments in the AP plane are greater than in the transverse plane when the externally fixated lower limb is elevated and the ankle allowed to perform active exercises; furthermore, this ratio of anteroposterior to transverse bending moments changes little in partial or full weight bearing [28,173]. In response to this information it has been shown that for the tibia, the unilateral frame applied in double plane configuration is clinically and mechanically the most effective at neutralising these moments. A double-bar anterior unilateral frame provides almost comparable qualities. More recent designs with 6-mm-diameter pins and stiffer components have provided unilateral-uniplanar devices that are suitable for even the most complex fractures [62]. The mechanical performance of these newer fixators coupled with a better understanding of the application techniques, have led some authors to conclude that the unilateral-uniplanar configuration is suitable for over 80% of fractures requiring external fixation [18].

Multiplanar Frames

The multiplanar configurations usually comprise transfixion wires or half pins attached to ring or arc frames [73,86]. Interconnecting rods link the frames to constitute an external fixator assembly. The stated advantages of a multiplanar frame include the ability to neutralise effectively bending moments in more than two planes. Furthermore, control or readjustment is possible in one selected plane after completion of the frame assembly. This is accomplished without the need to disassemble the frame or lose control of fracture alignment in other planes [73,104]. Most modular uniplanar devices allow for readjustments after fixator application but require adjustments in all planes to be made simultaneously.

Fixation Modes

The fixation mode refers to the function of the external fixator in relation to bone fragments. The intrinsic stability of the assembly reflects the capability of the chosen fixator type and configuration to resist displacing moments. This resistance may be accomplished by the fixator assembly alone or as a collective stability by the fixator and bone fragments.

There are three main fixation modes: compression, neutralisation and distraction.

Compression Mode

When axial compression is applied across the fracture site through the external fixator, the bone and fixator form a collective assembly which together provide intrinsic stability to the system (Fig. 7). For the fracture fragments to impart a contribution to the overall stability, there must therefore be interfragmental contact through compression; in theory, only tranverse fractures would be suitable for this compression as other fracture configurations (spiral, oblique, comminuted types or major bone loss) may displace with axial loading. With these other fracture types it is still possible to achieve compression in the absence of interfragmental contact by the following methods.

Shortening. Bony stability can be restored at the expense of a mild degree of shortening. Oblique fractures can be wedged together by back-cutting; this involves cutting a wedge into one fragment and fitting the apex of the other into this [35]. Squaring off the apices of spiral or oblique fracture ends also allows axial loading across the fragments.

Interpositional Graft. Cortico-cancellous graft would be more suitable to pressures of axial loading; an iliac crest graft can appropriately bridge a defect created by a sparing resection of the area of comminution.

Adjunctive Internal Fixation. The use of interfragmentary lag screws with spiral or oblique fractures may produce sufficient stability between the fracture fragments to allow axial compression from the external fixator. However, the external fixator acts principally as a neutraliser to bending moments. This approach must be balanced with the added soft-tissue dissection that inevitably results from internal fixation methods; there are also reports that union is delayed after adjunctive internal fixation [37].

Transverse Compression. The use of fixator pins close to and on either side of a short oblique fracture allows for transverse compression; this is achieved if tension or compression is applied to the pins in the coronal plane. Such an assembly is feasible only with bilateral or multiplanar frame configurations.

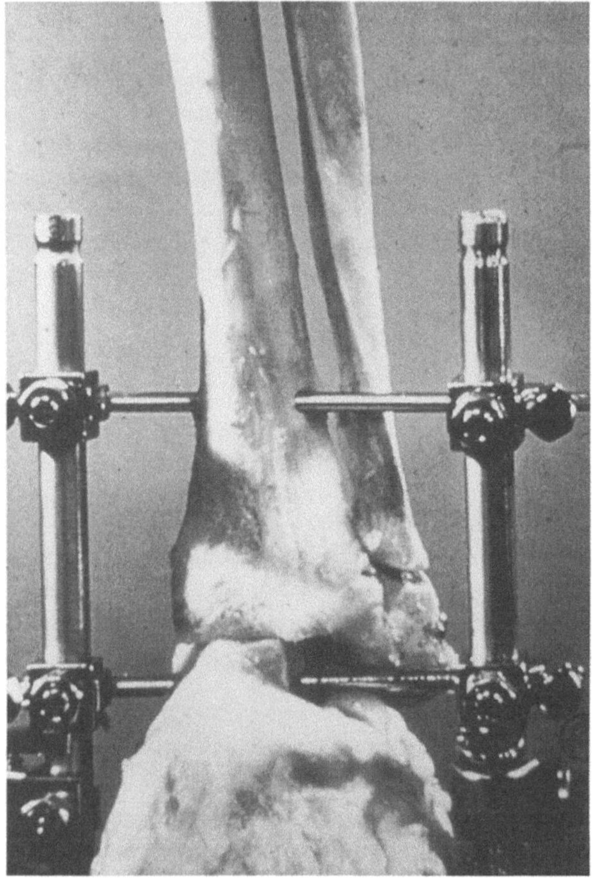

Fig. 7. External skeletal fixation used in a compression mode achieving some axial compression

The aim of these techniques is to allow the external fixator frame to be applied in compression mode. This in turn maintains positive interfragmental pressure under conditions of cyclical loading, an environment that encourages stability and the remodelling of early fixation callus.

Dynamisation

Although constructing an external fixator assembly in compression mode allows for axial loading through the fracture fragments, there is stress shielding to a variable degree. The unilateral frame configuration is a two-pillar system with asymmetrical loads through the external fixator and bone. Initially it is favourable to have most of the loads taken through the external pillar. This minimises the risk of loss of reduction. As soft-tissue and bone healing consolidates, the progressive increase in axial force transmission through the fracture site appears to encourage bone formation and callus remodelling. Stress shielding by the external fixator assembly as this stage would be counterproductive. A decrease in this stress shielding can be achieved through dynamisation.

Dynamisation is accomplished through a gradual build-down of the frame or via the release of an axial sliding mechanism; the choice of method depends on the type of fixator. The rationale in frame build-down is a stepwise reduction in frame stability, with protection against sagittal bending moments maintained. This allows a progressive increase in axial load through the fracture while preserving alignment. The sequence of build-down for modular or simple rod fixators is as follows:

1. Converting a complex frame configuration to a unilateral-uniplanar system, usually choosing the plane which provides maximum resistance to sagittal bending moments (for the tibia, this is the anterior plane).
2. Reducing a double-rod system to single.
3. Increasing the bone-rod distance (this significantly alters the resistance to frontal and torsional bending moments while minimally affecting control in the sagittal plane).
4. Loosening the central pin-rod articulations to increase sagittal pin movement.
5. (Crosswise slackening of pin-rod articulations to allow longitudinal sliding of the rods; this step may be performed on a double-rod unilateral-uniplanar system if step 2 is omitted).

Some newer unilateral-uniplanar fixators accomplish dynamisation though gradual loosening of a locking cam which controls axial sliding. The timing of dynamisation is often left to when the patient is capable of full weight bearing through the frame. It is usually at this stage that fracture consolidation is sufficiently advanced to commence a reduction in stress shielding. Interestingly, recent evidence suggests that the application of axial micromovement, with defined characteristics and for very short periods, within 2 weeks of fracture enhances healing [113].

Neutralisation Mode

The use of the external fixator in compression mode may not be feasible in extensive bone loss or comminution, despite the methods described above. The external fixator, however, would still be an appropriate choice for skeletal stabilisation in view of the considerable soft tissue injury that accompanies fractures of these types. It restores alignment and limb length; this is the neutralisation mode (Fig. 8).

In this fixation mode the fracture fragments are often not in contact, with reliance on stability and stress transfer entirely on the external fixator frame. Demands on the frame are therefore inversely proportional to the

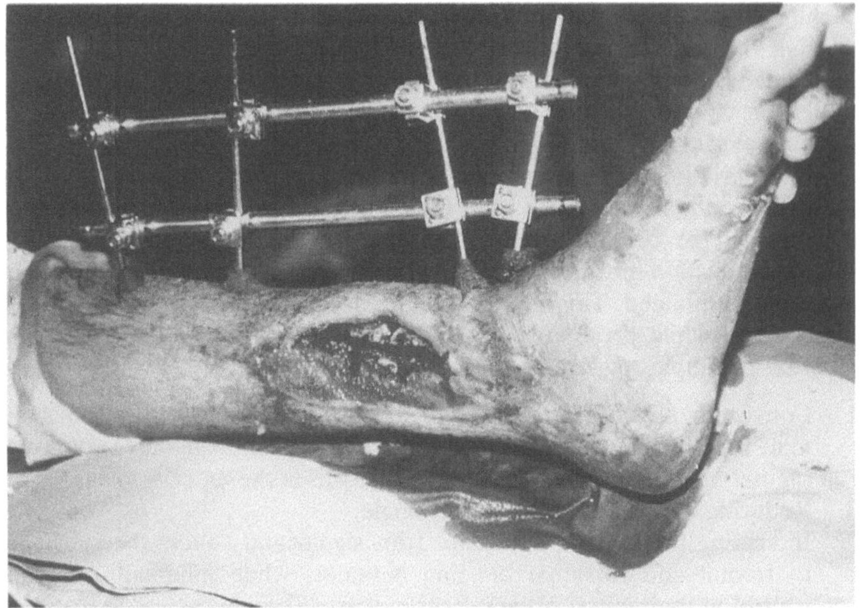

Fig. 8. External fixation used in a neutralization mode often requires bony reconstruction with autogenous bone grafts

stability provided by the fracture configuration [35]. It also follows that particular attention to details of maximising the bone-pin interface and rigidity of the frame is required.

Use of the external fixator in neutralisation mode usually requires a secondary procedure for fracture healing. This is frequently autogenous bone grafting, performed when healing of soft tissues allows surgical intervention and support of non-vascularised graft.

Secondary Procedures

The case for secondary operative stabilisation after initial treatment with the external fixator is controversial. This problem arises when delayed union, malunion or non-union occurs in a fracture stabilised by the fixator. The major concern is sepsis if internal fixation techniques are used in a surgical field potentially contaminated through external fixator pins.

The present recommendation of delayed secondary operative stabilisation is with an interim period, usually of 8–10 days, following pin removal. It is based on the presumption that superficial infection from pin sites will resolve in this period. Use of antibiotics in the interim period and for the secondary procedure is also encouraged [3]. Some promising results have been achieved using unreamed intramedullary nails or plate osteosynthesis under antibiotic cover [70]. Despite this it has also been reported that a high incidence of complications follows secondary internal fixation after initial stabilisation with an external fixator. These complications often relate to deep sepsis, the incidence reportedly 44% in one series [109,129,132]. The results reflect the heterogeneous group of injuries in these studies, most of which were severe and contributed to the incidence of complications. It is difficult to isolate the influence of prior use of the external fixator from the severity of the injury or the method of internal fixation on the outcome. Well-controlled trials in this area of trauma management are needed to provide answers to the timing of secondary operative stabilisation, the method of internal fixation and the concurrent use of antibiotics.

Distraction Mode

Although the application of the external fixator in compression mode would provide stability through interfragmental pressure, this is not always feasible for all fracture types. In contrast, distraction through the external fixator can be used as a method of fracture reduction (Fig. 9). This technique of ligamentotaxis is helpful in periarticular fractures when the fragments still possess joint capsule or ligament attachments. In this mode of fixation the fixator is not used as a definitive form of fracture stabilisation. Further additional procedures are needed to augment the frame – commonly, internal fixation and bone-grafting.

Bone Healing with the External Fixator

Union in fractures treated with the external fixator has been observed with and without the formation of intervening callus; however, primary bone healing is seen less frequently. Despite the use of the external fixator in compression mode, the stability and compression at the interfragmentary interface is insufficient for either gap or contact healing to occur.

The vascularity of the fragments are important determinants of the type of bone healing. External fixators are often used for fractures associated with a marked degree of soft-tissue injury; the hypovascularity of bone fragments from such severe injuries also makes primary bone healing unlikely.

Bone healing with the external fixator is therefore usually secondary bone healing with callus formation. However, there are differences when compared to secondary healing by cast methods of treatment. The amount of medullary osteogenesis in externally fixed fractures is greater; this arises from the rapid reestablishment of an intramedullary blood supply in the presence of stable fixation. Rigid fixation has been shown to enhance the intramedullary blood supply. In contrast, the periosteal reaction is significantly more pronounced with cast-treated fractures. Medullary osteogenesis in this method of treatment is delayed owing to the extended resorption of

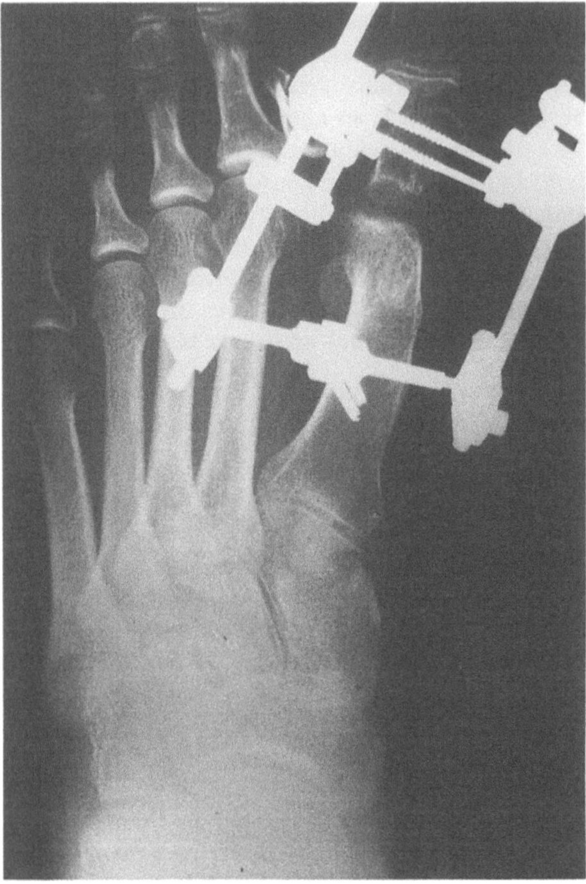

Fig. 9. External fixation used in a distraction mode applying distraction on the fracture fragments through their soft-tissue attachments

fracture haematoma and continued presence of an inflammatory exudate; there is late in-growth of new vessels.

Open Fractures

Open fractures remain a formidable challenge to the orthopaedic surgeon's skill. Historically, the significance of open fractures shows a recognition of the severity of the injury and its known association with a poor, often fatal outlook. The techniques of fracture splinting that were widely practised earlier were used with varying success, but more severe open injuries brought such a grave prognosis that amputation was frequently the immediate treatment.

Until the turn of this century, the treatment of open fractures by primary amputation was a reflection of the limited ability for limb salvage. Attempts at salvage were often fatal; the few successes documented from that period were notable for splintage of the injured limb and open wound treatment. The evolution of surgical techniques in soft-tissue management and the advance of antiseptic, and later aseptic methods ushered in prospects of limb salvage for open fractures.

Influence of Soft-Tissue Damage

The arrival of the external fixator in the management of open fractures provided an alternative to skeletal traction and casting techniques. The current role of the external fixator in the management of fractures is related to the extent of soft-tissue damage; its unique advantages are valuable in severe cases, irrespective of whether skin has been breached [145].

Initial classifications of open fractures were unanimous in demonstrating the effect of injury severity on prognosis. Gustilo's classification of open fractures of long bones included an assessment of laceration size and extent of soft-tissue damage [88]. The importance of soft-tissue integrity is emphasised by current proposals for its evaluation in closed fractures.

Simpler classification systems, although possessing the merit of easy recall, allow the presence of heterogeneous examples within a single category; this questions the validity of results of studies based on these systems. The extent of a skin laceration often does not reflect the degree of underlying soft-tissue contusion or neurovascular injury. As a principal objective in managing these severe fractures is union without sepsis, it has become clear that the size of the portal of wound contamination is not as critical as the viability of the underlying tissue [12,68]. The state of soft-tissue viability reflects the capacity of tissue to respond to residual bacterial contamination after surgical débridement.

The AO Classification

A more recent classification proposed by the ASIF group combines their comprehensive classification of fractures with a soft-tissue grading system that includes separate categories for closed and open fractures. It incorporates individual evaluation of muscle, tendon and neurovascular injury [142]. Admittedly more complex, this system gives credence to the damage inflicted upon the elements of the soft tissue envelope, and links this to the fracture configuration. The nature of the fracture, for example, segmental and complex types, often emphasizes the injury to the surrounding soft tissue and therefore cannot be excluded from a comprehensive classification.

Fracture Types

Current indications for use of the external fixator have been developed through retrospective and prospective evaluations in different fracture types.

A treatise of this subject would be incomplete if results of using the external fixator were not measured against other methods of management that provided a comparable outcome. The indications below are considered according to fracture site.

Tibia: Diaphyseal Fractures

The tibial diaphyseal fracture is widely acknowledged as the commonest diaphyseal fracture [80]. Application of an external fixator to this injury begins with an understanding of the fracture and its associated soft-tissue damage.

There is a wide spectrum of severity in this fracture group. The subcutaneous nature of the anteromedial border of this bone increases the likelihood of open injuries. Severe damage to the soft-tissue envelope is not restricted to open fractures; it can be evident in closed injuries. As there are strong proponents to each of several available treatment options, constructing a universal treatment algorithm for the tibial diaphyseal fracture becomes difficult.

Priorities

The surgeon's immediate responsibility is to assess the need for emergency surgery in an injury that is limb threatening. There are three principal criteria that require evaluation:

- An adequate blood supply to the limb, distal to the fracture, as evidenced by palpable pulses, good capillary refill and skin warmth.
- A compartment syndrome; awareness of its possible occurrence in all types of tibial shaft fractures coupled to repeated assessments for the presence of symptoms and signs lessens the risk of a delayed or missed diagnosis. Measurement of intracompartmental pressures are confirmatory.
- An open fracture increases the likelihood of severe damage to the soft-tissue envelope and potential wound contamination. Evidence to support the significance of bacterial contamination from the hospital environment [89,148] has emphasised the need for prompt wound coverage with a sterile dressing. Some trauma units use Polaroid photographs taken of the wound on arrival at the emergency unit followed by prompt coverage; this minimises the period of wound exposure outside an operating-room environment.

Indications

The unique advantages of the external fixator for skeletal stabilisation with a minimum of additional soft-tissue injury in its application provides the orthopaedic surgeon with an instrument suited to dealing with fractures with a large component of soft-tissue damage. The treatment methods of closed tibial shaft fractures have advocates for casting, functional bracing, plating and intramedullary nailing techniques. As the degree of soft-tissue injury increases, its influence on the prognosis rises. This can reveal limitations in techniques which require additional soft-tissue dissection to accomplish fracture stabilisation or fixation.

The external fixator has a definite role in managing tibial shaft fractures with the following groups (AO types) of soft-tissue injury:

IO2, IO3, IO4: These refer to open injuries varying from wounds larger than 1 cm with contused edges to extensive open degloving and skin loss (IO2 and IO3 grades parallel Gustilo and Anderson's types II and III).

MT3, MT4, MT5: With reference to the muscular and tendinous elements, these grades encompass muscle injury in multiple compartments, extensive contusion, muscle defects and compartment syndrome.

NV3, NV4, NV5: Vascular damage, localised or segmental with combined neural damage, demands prompt identification of the nature and site of injury; external fixation allows rapid skeletal stabilisation with minimal interference to efforts at repair of the vascular injury.

If Gustilo's [88] classification is used, the above categories of soft-tissue injury would include types II and IIIA–IIIC.

These indications are based on the extent of soft-tissue damage; the underlying fracture configuration may be variable, but comminuted and segmental fractures serve to emphasise the degree of soft-tissue injury.

The principle of minimal interference with the soft-tissue envelope applies to closed injuries that have severe contusion or crush. Tscherne's classification has been adopted by the AO group [142,145]; injuries of classes IC2 and IC3 would also be candidates for external fixation, especially if associated with complex fracture patterns [186].

Technique

Soft Tissue. Management of the soft-tissue envelope is a priority. The essentials of soft-tissue management include a thorough inspection of the extent of damage, débridement of devitalised tissue coupled with removal of all particulate foreign matter, followed by pulsatile irrigation with copious amounts of isotonic solution (Fig. 10). This can be achieved only if adequate access to the soft-tissue envelope is gained. Often this involves surgical extension of the wound; as fracture stabilisation requires preoperative planning, so does wound extension. Care is taken not to create flaps of devitalised skin whilst keeping the incision as close to an extensile approach. Concurrent use of intravenous antibiotics for prophylaxis against wound infections is adjunctive to débridement and irrigation; the type of antibiotic depends on the likely contaminating agent and results of wound cultures taken on arrival at the emergency unit and at post-débridement [148].

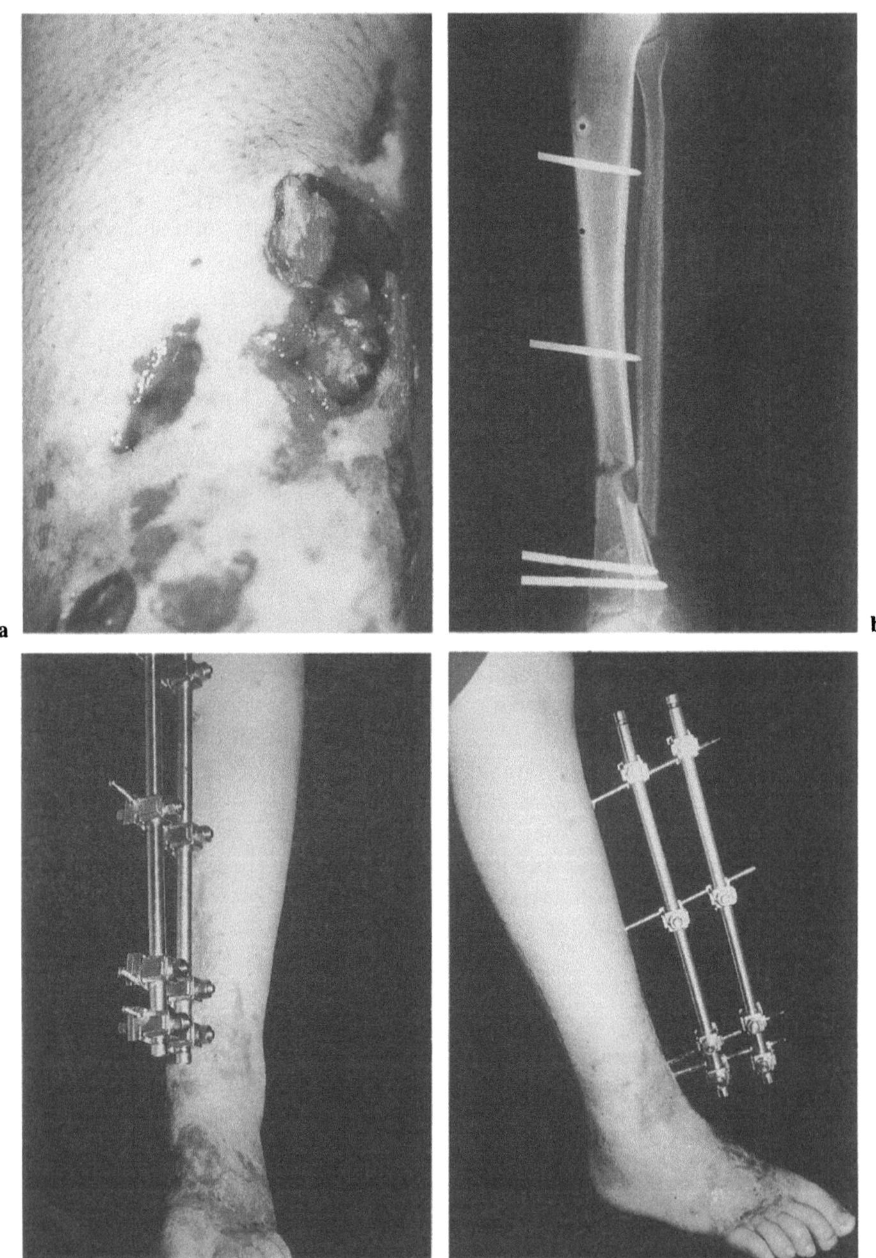

Fig. 10a–h. A 20-year-old woman with an open tibial diaphyseal fracture from high-energy trauma. **a** Extensive soft-tissue disruption is evident. **b** The X-ray reveals a complex diaphyseal fracture pattern. **c,d** Following initial débridement, a unilateral

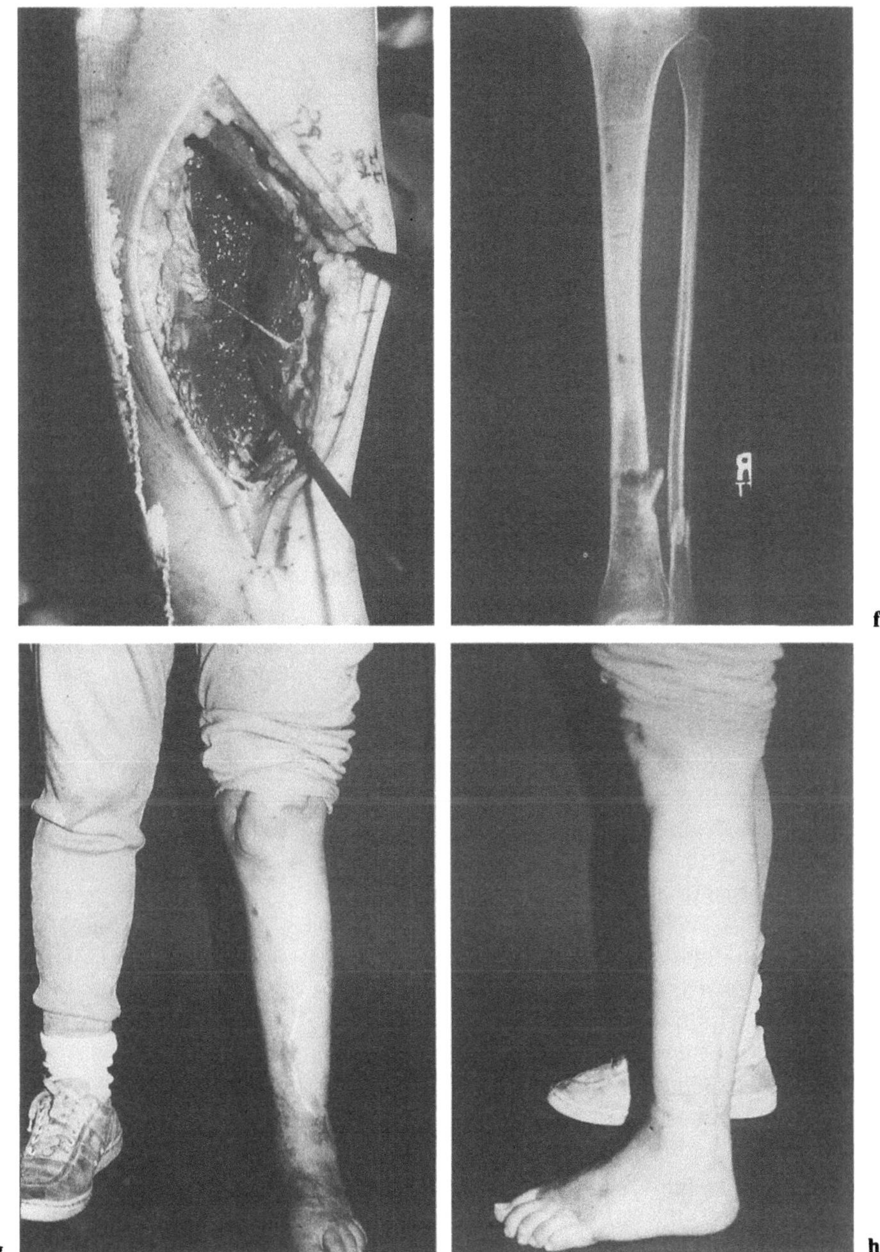

external fixation frame is applied with the fracture held out to length. **e** Once the soft-tissue envelope has been restored, cancellous iliac crest bone graft is placed posteriorly. **f–h** Fracture union occurred while still in the external fixator

Fracture Stabilisation. Use of the external fixator on diaphyseal fractures of the tibia requires knowledge of "safe corridors" [14–16,18] and preoperative planning. This reduces iatrogenic injury from improper pin placement and produces a frame assembly that will achieve optimal stabilisation but still allows access for soft-tissue procedures at a later time.

In the tibia proximal to the tibial tubercle, pin insertion is safe in an arc which subtends 220° from the tibiofibular joint to the posteromedial edge of the subcutaneous border. The area occupied by the patellar tendon is obviously excluded. Distal to this area and up to the junction of middle and distal thirds of the tibial shaft, this safe corridor reduces to a 140° arc. Pin insertion here should be kept inside an arc from the posteromedial border of the subcutaneous surface to just lateral to the anteromedial edge. In the distal third of the tibia this safe corridor is decreased further by encroachment from the lateral side by musculotendinous units of the anterior and lateral compartments. When fractures of the distal third of the tibial diaphysis involve damage to the soft-tissue envelope around the ankle, insertion of pins into the metatarsals is helpful; these are conveniently inserted into the first or second metatarsals and aid in supporting the ankle in neutral position.

Assembly

Pin insertion techniques should follow guidelines stated above. Care should be paid to minimise soft-tissue damage and limit thermal necrosis of bone, yet maximise the strength of the bone-pin interface. If the pin design used does not incorporate radial preloading, this should be accomplished on attaching pins to the external fixator. Construction of the external fixator assembly depends on the type of fixator available; most are simple tubular designs and as such suffice for over 80% of fractures if used in a double anterior bar configuration [18]. Occasionally, delta frame (unilateral-biplanar) configurations are required; pin placement follows the same guidelines and are located within the same "safe corridors".

With most tubular fixators, application involves initial provisional reduction of the fracture and placement of the first pin in a main fragment, preferably to one end of the tibia. The fracture is then reduced formally, and an assembled tube with the necessary number of clamps, as determined by preoperative planning, is attached to the first pin. The next pin is inserted at the opposite end of the tibia with the clamp usually acting as placement and drill guide. Reduction is then maintained if the tube is tightened to proximal and distal pins. Additional pins and tubes can be added after this stage to enhance the rigidity of the overall frame assembly.

Modular tubular fixators have helped considerably in making application of an external fixator "user-friendly". Fracture reduction can be postponed to after applying pins and short tubular rods to the main fragments; reduction is achieved with these rods assisting in manipulation of the fragments. The rods are finally interconnected through rod-rod clamps, often with an additional interlinking tube; tightening the rod-rod clamps maintains reduction.

Aftercare

There are four main points of after care in fractures treated with the external fixator:

Pin Care. Pin sites should be cleaned daily with normal saline or an antiseptic agent. The screw portions immediately adjacent to skin should also be cleaned and the area covered with sterile gauze; some surgeons prefer to impregnate this light covering with an antibacterial agent such as povidone iodine. Any evidence of skin tenting around pin sites should be released promptly by extending the incision under local anaesthesia. Although some serous exudation can be tolerated, obvious inflammation or infection may require local or systemic antibiotic treatment. Occasionally removal of the problematic screw remains the only option, with replacement at an alternative site.

Fracture Alignment. Appropriate follow-up includes serial checks by X-ray. Initially this should be weekly; any minor losses in alignment can be corrected easily in the first 2–3 weeks owing to the plasticity of early callus.

Dynamisation. Certain fracture types, for example, transverse fractures, permit a degree of weight bearing early after external fixation owing to the inherent collective stability of the bone and fixator. A greater proportion of fractures require some evidence of consolidation, often the radiological presence of callus, before the stress-shielding effect of a rigid external fixator assembly is reduced. The time for dynamisation, which should ideally allow axial loading without sacrifice of control of bending or torsional moments at the fracture site, therefore depends on the factors which influence the speed of fracture and soft-tissue healing. Clinically dynamisation is commenced when the patient is capable of full weight bearing comfortably through the frame.

Joint Movement. Most external fixators for tibial shaft fractures can be applied without crossing a joint. This allows physical therapy for active and active-assisted range of movement exercises to the knee and ankle joints. Modern unilateral fixators have avoided transfixing pins of bilateral frames, which were responsible for tethering muscles and compromising ankle function.

Comparative Results

Charnley, in the preface to the third edition of his classic treatise on the closed treatment of fractures, noted many fractures of the tibia for which conservative treatment is not adequate by itself. He found many cases of redisplacement after what was initially a satisfactory reduction [44]. Nevertheless, union rates of 90%–97.5% have been reported with closed treatment, when coupled to a programme of early weight bearing [154,166,168]. Achieving a good outcome with this method of treatment requires patient selection. It is best suited to closed, low-velocity injuries with stable fracture patterns and minimal shortening; with these criteria, it is possible to limit malalignment of more than 10° to about 4% [154,166].

Intramedullary nailing of tibial shaft fractures has been used with impressive success. Union rates of 88%–98% have been reported using reamed and unreamed nails [124,154]. Interlocking intramedullary nails have expanded the application of this method of fixation from the added torsional control provided. However, some reports of infection rates as high as 20% [117] with type IO1 and IO2 fractures have cautioned against universal adoption of this treatment choice. The unreamed interlocked nail has provided a method of fracture fixation with minimal interruption of the endosteal blood supply and injury to the soft-tissue envelope; recent studies have shown results comparable to the external fixator without problems of pin tract sepsis or loosening [97,165]. It is a formidable option in the management of open tibial shaft fractures, in particular open injuries of types IO1 and IO2.

In open tibial fractures of greater severity, there is new evidence to support use of the unreamed interlocked intramedullary nail [57,165,187]. Similar infection rates to the external fixator have been reported, with a lower incidence of malunion. Although classed as type IIIB (Gustilo et al.), the classification system used in these studies was sufficiently broad to encompass heterogeneous examples within each category. Fractures that had better results of union and lower infection rates did not involve bone loss; as most studies of external fixation of open type IIIB fractures have involved injuries with bone loss and crushing, a meaningful comparison is difficult. The unreamed intramedullary nail may become the treatment method of choice for open fractures of type IIIB (AO type IO3), but the present data are new, and critical comparison to older published results of external fixation in these situations may not be valid. In addition, use of the unreamed intramedullary nail for severe open fractures may need a transient form of fracture stabilisation; this frequently is os calcis skeletal traction, enabling repeated débridements or delayed coverage to be performed for the soft-tissue injury. External fixation possesses the advantage of definitive and immediate fracture stabilisation with easy repeated access for surgery to the soft tissue envelope. A structured protocol for limb salvage in severe open injuries is often accomplished most easily with the external fixator

[30,45,66]. It is for these reasons the external fixator remains an instrument of choice in open fractures type IO3 or higher.

Tibia: Metaphyseal Fractures

Tibial Plateau and Plafond

Short metaphyseal fragments or articular fractures present specific problems in assembly of the external fixator. This is due largely to the size of fracture fragments involved; placement of half pins is often multiplanar to afford suitable purchase on the fragment. An alternative strategy is construction of the fixator across the joint involved. Although contraditory to the principle of early movement in periarticular fractures, joint mobility is preserved if the period of external fixation is restricted [169].

Fractures of the tibial plateau and plafond have also been amenable to fixation with combined internal and external techniques. This is in sharp distinction to diaphyseal fractures, where problems with delayed union, non-union and sepsis are prevalent if combination techniques are used [85].

Indications

The indications for use of an external fixator in metaphyseal and periarticular fractures of the tibia are as follows:

- Open fractures of type IO3 or greater. Severe open metaphyseal fractures necessitate the same protocol of soft-tissue management as do diaphyseal fractures. Approximately 1%–3% of tibial plateau fractures are open [96]; external fixation provides either temporary or definitive stabilisation of joints in the presence of serious soft tissue or ligamentous injury. Closed ankle and pilon fractures associated with major soft tissue disruption frequently swell and require judicious timing for surgery. The external fixator provides a means of stabilisation, with a distraction force to maintain reduction if necessary, until resolution of soft-tissue oedema allows operative intervention.
- In polytrauma, external fixation across a joint provides a better mode of rapid temporary fracture stabilisation compared to skeletal traction. With external fixation, the patient can avoid prolonged periods in the supine position; cast treatment is a suitable alternative although length control over time is poorer [169].
- The external fixator can also be used to bridge a joint for prophylaxis of joint contractures or deformities. This mode of use is temporary, with later definitive fracture stabilisation allowing removal of the fixator and commencement of active joint movement.

Technique

Most modular tubular fixators possess tibial epiphyseal clamps which allow attachment of pins inserted in the tibial epiphyseal and metaphyseal areas. The wide safe corridor for pin insertion in the proximal tibia (220°) enables multiple pin insertion in the transverse plane; this provides adequate control of short metaphyseal fragments and secure fixation to the diaphysis (Fig. 11). Assembly of a transverse epiphyseal clamp to a sagittal anterior rod produces a modified two-plane unilateral fixator which is suited to these metaphyseal fractures.

The wide safe corridor in the proximal tibia has been utilised by certain types of external fixator for definitive treatment of tibial plateau injuries. Half pins are inserted into the larger metaphyseal fragments and can number

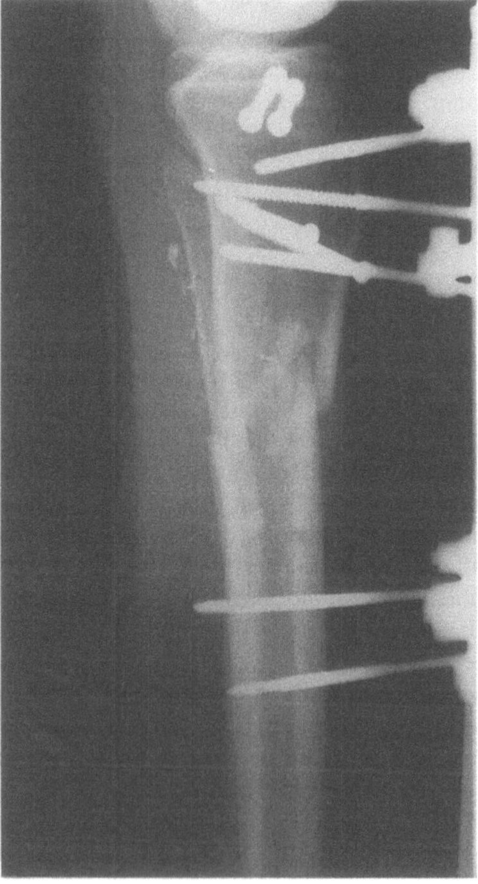

Fig. 11. A complex proximal tibial fracture is stabilized with a modular external fixation frame using half pins in the metaphyseal segment

five or more. These pins are clamped using a special transverse epiphyseal fixator bar; each pin is held within a universal joint which allows pin movement in a 30° arc in any direction, permitting manipulation of the fragments held by the pins prior to tightening of the clamps. Such a facility enables condylar fracture fragments to be reduced with greater accuracy before final assembly of the fixator. Although an approximate closed reduction is a prerequisite of this technique, the entire process can be performed under radiological control, thereby minimising further soft-tissue dissection. Use of a fixator in this mode avoids crossing the knee. Care should be taken with epiphyseal pins not to transfix collateral ligaments, the iliotibial band or pes anserinus as this would effectively restrict any beneficial joint movement. Ranging the knee through a full arc of movement after placement of epiphyseal pins helps ensure that this problem is avoided [142].

Circular external fixators using tensioned Kirschner wires are an alternative (Fig. 12). Ilizarov's multiplanar fixator was initially used for fracture management; olive-tipped wires used as directional wires allow manipulation of displaced fracture fragments into place. A distinct advantage of this technique is the ability to control small epiphyseal fragments and apply a combination of axial and lateral compression through the fixator assembly. The size of wires (1.5–1.8 mm diameter) and multiplanar use allow reduction and stabilisation of tibial metaphyseal and epiphyseal fractures without spanning the adjacent joint. In contrast, modular tubular fixators are often unable to achieve this control in either unilateral or bilateral configurations without bridging the joint; however, modular tubular fixators allow better access for soft-tissue management.

External Fixation Across a Joint: The Tibial Plateau

This can be accomplished using fixators based on half pins, transfixation pins or tensioned wires. Pin placement demands careful consideration of the different safe corridors in the femur and tibia together with individual characteristics of the injury; in addition, access for prospective internal fixation must be regarded. With half pins, lateral tibial and lateral femoral insertion avoids compromising a mid-line approach to the tibia should internal fixation be considered when soft-tissue healing is appropriate. Anterior tibial and femoral pin placement is less satisfactory.

Although more common in compression arthrodesis, transfixation pins can also be used. The type of frame assembly may differ among Charnley, Hoffmann, and Roger Anderson devices; however, the pins are similarly inserted in a mediolateral plane. Use of external fixator pins through large muscle masses in the thigh or lateral aspect of the tibia requires detailed attention to minimise damage to the soft-tissue sleeve during pin insertion. As the indications for using an external fixator across a joint are few and usually for temporary stabilisation, pin tract problems are resolved on disassembly of the fixator.

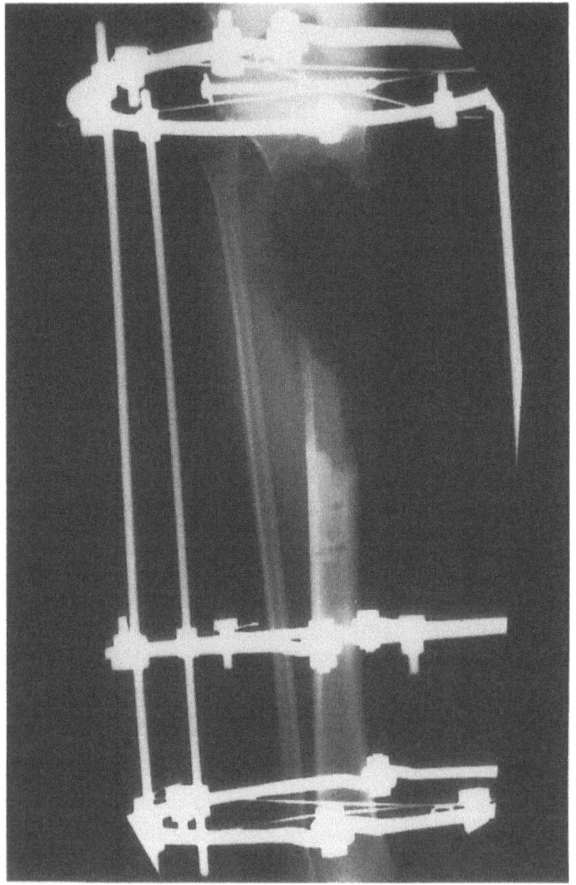

Fig. 12. A circular frame using tensioned thin wires is extremely effective for complex proximal tibial metaphyseal fractures

External Fixation Across a Joint: The Tibial Plafond

External fixation across the ankle joint presents less of a dilemma; modular tubular fixators can easily be assembled over half pins inserted anteriorly into the distal tibial diaphysis and into the first and fifth metatarsals (Fig. 13). An alternative arrangement involves connecting an anterior tibial bar to a transfixation calcaneal pin. Whichever technique is selected, it is important to ensure the ankle is maintained in approximately 5°–10° of dorsiflexion to avert problems with development of an equinus contracture [18].

The use of an external fixator across a joint contravenes a principle fundamental to present-day orthopaedics; joint fractures are best managed by accurate reduction, stabilisation and early movement. Bridging a joint with an external fixator deletes movement at the joint. However, the indi-

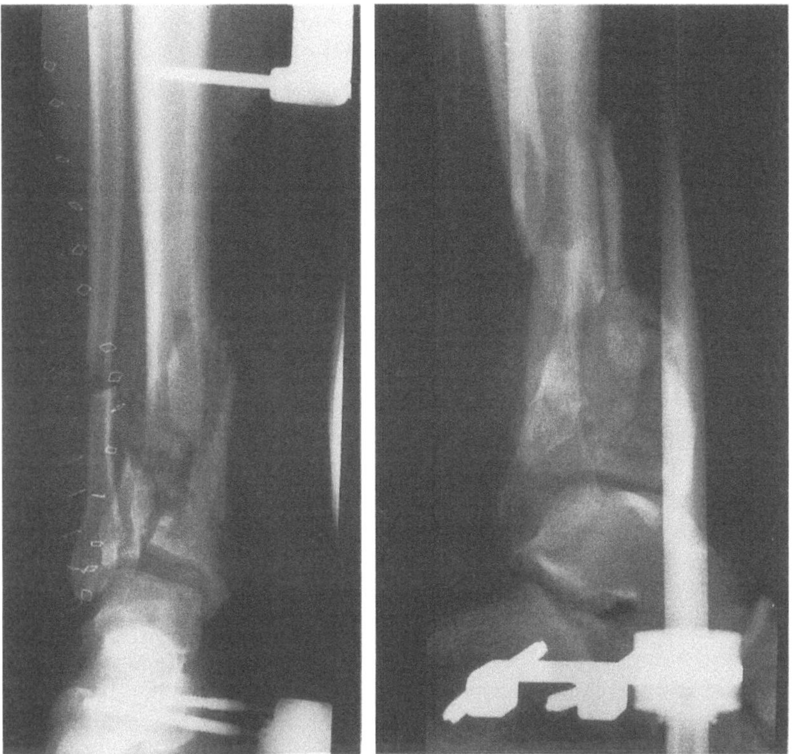

Fig. 13a,b. A complex tibial plafond fracture with extensive soft-tissue damage is stabilized with an external fixation frame. Once the soft-tissue has been restored, limited external fixation of the articular fragments is done

cations described earlier refer to injuries that involve such soft-tissue damage that open procedures would jeopardise the soft-tissue sleeve further. Temporary use of the external fixator in these situations can thus be ratified. It is encouraging to note that a surprisingly good range of movement is attainable even after 4 weeks of immobilisation [169].

Finally, techniques involving a combination of internal and external fixation are suitable to fractures in these areas. This contrasts to results achieved when such combined techniques are used for diaphyseal fractures; there is strong evidence here for a increased incidence of delayed and non-union unless additional procedures (bone grafting, removal of the fixator and support through functional bracing, etc.) are included in later stages of management. Combined internal and external fixation in metaphyseal fractures of the tibia is successful in providing the collective advantages of accuracy of reduction and rigid stabilisation without extensive soft-tissue dissection. Good results with open type VI (Schatzker) tibial plateau fractures have been achieved with lateral plate internal fixation and a medial half pin external fixator for neutralisation [157].

Femur

The unique strength and deep soft-tissue sleeve of the femur imparts certain qualities with respect to fractures of the femur. With the possible exception of fractures in children, fractures of the shaft of femur are the result of high-energy injuries. This type of trauma occurs most frequently in young male adults; several epidemiological studies confirm this [81,92]. Interestingly, the incidence of femoral shaft fractures in the elderly is rising [140].

Diaphyseal fractures of the femur are suited to stabilisation by the external fixator; whether this option is appropriate depends on other qualities of the fracture. There is little question to the merits of prompt stabilisation of femoral shaft fractures; the restoration of anatomical and functional integrity to the injured limb have been shown to benefit the patient beyond the boundaries of fracture healing [24,79,105,160,171]. This rapid skeletal stabilisation achieved through surgical means avoids periods of prolonged recumbency associated with closed methods of treatment, in particular, traction.

Fractures of the femoral shaft in adults are consistently the result of high-energy trauma; this is a refection of the strength of the bone and deep soft-tissue sleeve. Open injuries are comparatively common as a consequence of this high-energy impact, although lower grades of open injuries comprise a greater number. The open femoral fracture denotes the severity of the causative injury and extent of resultant soft-tissue damage; immediate surgical débridement with pulsatile lavage is required to reduce high infection rates associated with operative management of these injuries.

Intramedullary nailing has become a superior technique for treating closed femoral shaft fractures [103,193]; comminution and extent within the diaphysis determines the choice of locking and non-locking types of nail [31,32]. Despite initial reservations [42], this technique has been extended to IO1 and IO2 open-shaft fractures where excellent results have been achieved when combined with early thorough débridement and lavage prior to nailing [33,122].

The primal role of débridement and pulsed lavage in all open injuries has been established. With remarkable achievements by the intramedullary nail, work at present has centred on extending its application to open fractures of type IO3 or higher; the advent of unreamed nails has further increased prospects of establishing this technique in open fractures. Prior to this, external fixation or closed techniques were the principal methods used. Comparative studies demonstrate a 7%–8% delayed union with the external fixator, coupled to pin tract problems (7%–17%) and loss of movement at the knee (28%–45%) [11,143]. De Bastiani's work with the dynamic axial fixator (Orthofix) reported an 87% union rate with open fractures of the femur, with overall infection at 0.3% [62]. The rate of significant deficits in knee range of movement was 2.3%.

With more severe injuries, the influence of soft-tissue and bony damage on outcome may exceed that of the method of fracture stabilisation. Comparative studies on the use of either the intramedullary nail or external fixator for IO3 or IO4 fractures are pending; preliminary impressions suggest similar union and infection rates. This impressive achievement of the intramedullary nail in open femoral shaft fractures has restricted indications for use of the external fixator. Choosing the external fixator as a method of femoral fracture stabilisation must be justified after a careful balance of the advantages and drawbacks. Present indications for the external fixator in femoral shaft fractures are therefore:

- Open femoral shaft fractures of grade IO3 or greater
- Femoral shaft fractures with an associated vascular injury [156]
- Temporary stabilisation in patients with multiple trauma. In selecting the external fixator for this role, secondary fixation with intramedullary nails may be compromised; there has been an associated high incidence of osteomyelitis [42,143].

Technique

Pin insertion for the femoral shaft requires a clear understanding of regional cross-sectional anatomy. Transfixation pins in the proximal two-thirds are unsafe. If anteroposterior pins are used, half pins are necessary to avoid damage to the sciatic nerve. The thick soft-tissue sleeve dictates use of generous skin incisions to allow predrilling of the bony cortex with minimal trauma to this sleeve.

Lateral to medial half pins are safest for femoral shaft fractures. Anteroposterior pin placement is a second choice owing to the attendant quadriceps transfixing problems. Selection of pin placement may, however, be decided by the site and size of the wound. Pin insertion technique is the same as for the tibia, with attention paid to soft-tissue protection, predrilling and manual preloading if the pin design does not incorporate radial preloading (Fig. 14). Preliminary reductions are important with attention to alignment in sagittal, coronal and axial planes. This is especially so with non-modular fixators which possess little allowance for realignment after assembly of the fixator. After assembly of the external fixator, the hip and knee joints must be ranged to determine whether further releasing incisions in skin and fascia lata are required to accommodate this movement.

The double lateral bar configuration or newer single large modular fixators (e.g. dynamic axial fixator) provide sufficient rigidity for femoral shaft fractures. This maximal rigidity is important in the initial stages where the fracture configuration cannot contribute towards a collective bone-frame stability. Fracture stabilisation also confers a biological environment that

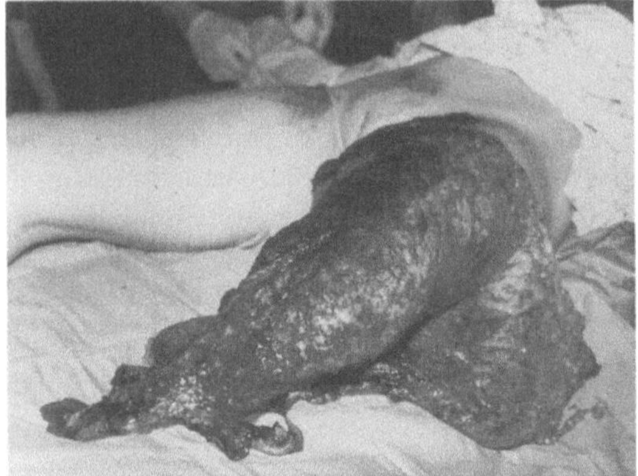

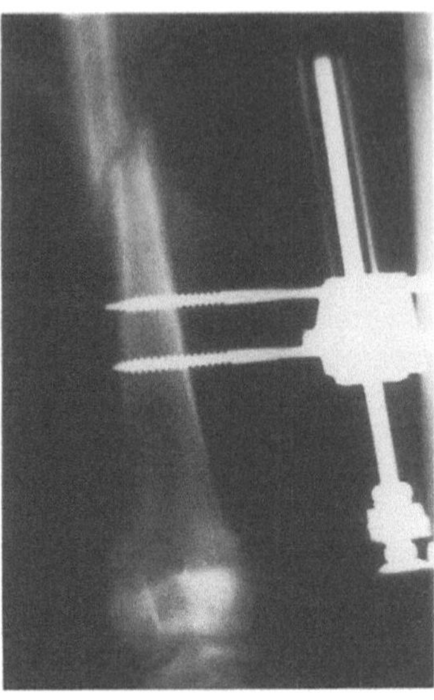

Fig. 14a–e. A 13-year-old girl suffered a mutilating injury to her lower extremity. a The extent of the injury included a traumatic amputation of the lower leg, a femoral shaft fracture, and extensive soft-tissue degloving leaving an exposed knee joint and denuded proximal tibial shaft. b Following débridement, the femur was stabilized with a unilateral Wagner external fixator. c A free flap was created from the amputated lower limb and used to provide immediate coverage of the knee and preserve a functional below knee amputation level. d,e The femoral fracture healed while in the external fixator, and a functional knee joint was preserved

supports soft-tissue healing. Dynamisation is commenced upon radiological detection of callus at the fracture site; this can be started earlier if the fracture pattern is stable.

Secondary reamed intramedullary nailing is inadvisable if external fixation was the initial mode of fracture stabilisation; functional bracing or casting are safer alternatives. This recommendation stems largely from a reported high incidence of osteomyelitis [42,109,129,132,143], presumed to arise from preceding pin tract infections. The criteria for safe secondary intramedullary nailing have yet to be established, although current guidelines advise a delay between removal of pins and nailing, with concomitant antibiotic prophylaxis [3,70]. Use of the unreamed interlocking nail may alter the incidence of this complication, but definitive evidence is still pending.

Comparative Results

It is important to recognise that in most published series, femoral fractures that were treated with the external fixator were often the most severe open

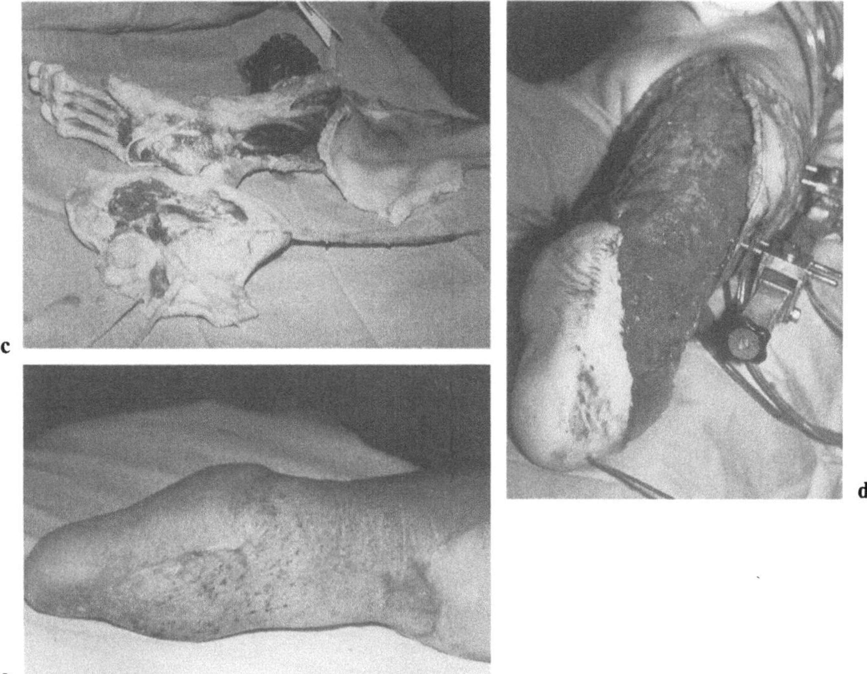

Fig. 14c–e.

injuries. Comparative studies on the intramedullary nail and external fixator for type IIIB and IIIC [89] are forthcoming. It is likely that the severity of injury in these classification groups exert a much greater influence on outcome than the mode of fracture stabilisation. De Bastiani's impressive results with the dynamic axial fixator highlights the capability of a well-designed external fixator in the field of both closed and open femoral fractures [62].

Initial enthusiasm for plating femoral fractures was led by the aim to restore bony anatomy and allow early ambulation and joint movement. Analyses of results for closed femoral shaft fractures show union rates of approximately 90%–95% [126,164] coupled to infection rates of 5%–15% [144,164,178], with implant or fixation failure at 5%–10% [1,126,164]. Application of this technique to open fractures results in unacceptably high infection rates [10,25,161,162]. Despite a change in strategy from anatomical reduction and rigid compression to indirect reduction, minimal soft-tissue stripping and long fracture-spanning plates, this mode of fixation remains applicable mainly to closed femoral fractures.

Intramedullary nailing has emerged as the fixation mode of choice for most femoral shaft fractures. Union rates of 98%–99% with infection rates less than 1% [23,47,193] in closed injuries have been reported. Better results are achieved for open femoral fracture types I, II and IIIA with the intramedullary nail than with the external fixator [3,60]. Although Chapman [41] suggested delayed nailing of types I and II fractures as a means of avoiding subsequent infection, a principal objective of early definitive fracture stabilisation is sacrificed. Infection rates of 2%–6% can be achieved with immediate nailing when performed with appropriate surgical wound management and antibiotic prophylaxis [33,122,181]; this is not dissimilar to the incidence of infection with delayed intramedullary nailing.

De Bastiani's results with the dynamic axial fixator for open femoral fractures remain singularly impressive [62]. Most reported series have a much higher incidence of sepsis, delayed union, malunion and loss of knee movement. Although it would reasonable to attribute the differences to the type of external fixator used, studies are needed to determine whether results comparable to these are reproducible using modern fixators on a similar protocol. Until similar results are again reported, use of the external fixator must remain with severely contaminated type IIIB and type IIIC open femoral fractures.

Pelvic Ring Disruptions

The evolution of treatment principles in pelvic fractures was facilitated by the emergence of accurate classification systems. Prior to the advent of radiographic imaging, management guidelines were based on characteristics that were determined from history and physical examination; it was difficult to differentiate instability arising from ligamentous injury, fracture or both.

In the latter half of this century, Peltier [150], Pennal et al. [151], Tile [182–185] and Young [196,197] have contributed significantly to an understanding of the pathogenesis of pelvic ring disruptions. The accuracy of these classification systems have enabled most pelvic fractures to be categorised and the associated instability inferred. The relationship of certain fracture patterns to visceral, vascular, head and thoracic damage has also been verified [63]).

Stability in the pelvic ring depends on each hemipelvis retaining the ability to resist rotational, anteroposterior and cephalocaudal displacing moments; the integrity of ligamentous and bony elements involved in the sacroiliac and symphyseal joints underlie this ability. An understanding of the anatomical relationships and mechanistic classifications is the key to management of these injuries.

Mechanism of Injury

Pelvic fractures result from either high- or low-energy impacts. The latter group of injuries often leave the integrity of the pelvic ring undisturbed; these include solitary fractures of the iliac wing, pubic rami and transverse fractures of the sacrum and coccyx. These fractures are stable (Tile type A [183]).

Motor vehicle accidents remain a main source of high-energy trauma to the pelvis [63]. These injuries have been grouped according to the mode of damage; Young [196,197] has classed injuries arising from lateral compression, anteroposterior compression and vertical shear modes. Each class within a particular group is a grade of severity and instability within the group. Tile's classification centres on the direction of potential instability that results from the bony and ligamentous injury; there are groups for stable injuries, rotationally unstable injuries, and rotationally and vertically unstable injuries [182].

Diagnosis

A distinction between high- and low-energy trauma together with the possible mechanism of injury can be made from history taking. This information contributes to an overall clinical picture from which a management plan is derived. In assessing the high-energy group, a full physical examination is essential owing to the 60%–80% incidence of associated musculoskeletal injuries [131]. Certain fracture classes also have a higher risk of accompanying intra-abdominal, thoracic and head injuries [63]. With the pelvis, inspection for deformity, leg length inequality, perineal bruising and haematomas, areas of contusion or poor skin viability, and the presence of blood at the urogenital and gastrointestinal orifices should be systematic. A gap in the symphysis pubis should be sought, in addition to testing for rotational and vertical stability. This assessment of stability, if performed at a later stage, can be aided by X-ray or fluoroscopic screening and a general anaesthetic. If the testing is performed in the emergency room this is done preferably when haemodynamic stability is obtained; forceful rotational or axial loading moments on an unstable pelvic injury may aggravate haemorrhage [34].

The anteroposterior radiograph of the pelvis is part of the initial series of X-ray images, including supine chest and lateral cervical spine views, that is essential in assessing the victim of multiple blunt trauma [78]. Inlet and outlet views are complementary to the initial anteroposterior radiograph; they enable better identification of sacroiliac widening, sacral fractures, and posterior displacements of the hemipelvis which suggest a vertical shear mechanism [182]. Computed tomography has provided a means for accurate confirmation of the category of the pelvic injury; in addition, in both axial scanning mode and three-dimensional reconstructions, it is invaluable in assessing acetabular and pelvic anatomy prior to reconstructive surgery.

Pelvic Ring Disruptions and the External Fixator

In high-energy pelvic injuries the external fixator is used either acutely or as a delayed means of stabilisation. It can function as either temporary, definitive or adjunctive means of fixation.

Almost all frame configurations for pelvic injury are based anteriorly; it follows that the fixator substitutes for mechanical stability that is lost principally in the anterior pelvis. Some degree of posterior instability can be moderately overcome by frame configurations of the trapezoidal [176] or rectangular types [183] or through the use of transiliac pins with anterior and posterior pelvic frames [137]; however, the latter poses numerous problems with nursing aftercare.

These limitations of the external fixator therefore define a group of pelvic injuries that are most suited to this technique of stabilisation:

- Anteroposterior compression injuries with diastasis of the symphysis and tearing of the anterior sacroiliac, sacrotuberous and sacrospinous ligaments; the posterior sacroiliac and iliolumbar ligaments remain intact. These injuries correspond to Young's APC-II and APC-III fracture patterns, and to Tile's types B1.2 and B1.3.
- Lateral compression injuries with a contralateral anterior ring (pubic ramus or symphyseal) fracture and an ipsilateral posterior iliac wing fracture; these injuries, although stable to axial loading (vertical stresses) are internally able to rotate in the manner of a bucket handle, with resultant proximal displacement of the hip joint and leg length inequality. These are LC-II fractures or type B2.2.
- In spite of limitations in stabilising injuries which involve loss of the posterior bony-ligamentous hinge, the external fixator can be used as an adjunctive form of stabilisation if posterior internal fixation is performed. It would therefore be indicated together with posterior internal fixation in vertical shear injuries (VS or type C). This combined technique betters symphyseal plating and external fixation [182] for injuries with posterior instability from a superior resistance to vertical loads.

Haemorrhage and Pelvic Fracture

Haemorrhage is the most serious complication from a pelvic fracture [58,65,71]. It arises most commonly from injury to the presacral venous plexus, although bleeding from the fracture surface, small local vessels and larger named vessels may be responsible [112].

Haemorrhage is responsible for hypotension in the multiply injured patient 95% of the time [34]. Severe haemorrhage is more likely in pelvic injuries which result in a shearing force across vessels of the posterior pelvic wall. Injuries such as the APC-II, APC-III, LC-III and VS patterns have been associated with severe retroperitoneal haemorrhage [63].

The external fixator is one of the most effective means of bleeding control in pelvic trauma. It reduces bleeding from open cancellous surfaces through compression and establishes a tamponade effect on haemorrhage by maintaining a fixed pelvic volume. Stabilisation of severe pelvic injuries minimises the risk of clot displacement and subsequent repeat haemorrhage;

in addition, it facilitates care and pain management in the acute phase [111,192].

Use of the external fixator as an aid to resuscitation requires careful evaluation with regard to the likely source of bleeding. Haemorrhage from large named vessels are unlikely to be controlled with application of the external fixator; differences in lower limb pulses should alert the surgeon to the possibility of major vessel injury and a need for urgent laparotomy. Similarly, a positive peritoneal lavage in a haemodynamically unstable patient requires general surgical attention for the cause; the external fixator can be applied after laparotomy with pelvic packing if retroperitoneal bleeding is significant. In patients with a positive peritoneal lavage but who are haemodynamically stable, a case for application of the external fixator prior to laparotomy can be made [112]; a possibility of loss of tamponade at laparotomy should be considered.

The external fixator should be applied urgently in the patient with poor haemodynamic control, a negative peritoneal lavage and the presence of equal lower limb pulses. This clinical situation strongly suggests haemorrhage from the presacral venous plexus or a sacral fracture; reduction and stabilisation by the external fixator achieves tamponade of haemorrhage, in particular with the type of injuries outlined earlier. The effect of external fixation on other types of pelvic injuries (e.g. LC-I, LC-II) may be less pronounced. Failure to control haemorrhage despite this should indicate a need for urgent angiography, with possible embolisation [135].

Technique

When used in resuscitation, application of the external fixator can be accomplished in less than 30 min. Early use of the fixator is also indicated in the presence of local wound problems which will postpone internal fixation methods for stabilisation. Acute application is performed preferably within 4 h of injury; establishing a stable pelvic ring facilitates treatment of other visceral injuries [63].

The method of fixator assembly is similar irrespective of whether external fixation is definitive, temporary or adjunctive stabilisation. Technical aspects of pin insertion remain the same as for other fractures; frame configurations, however, differ. It was noted above that anteriorly placed fixator frames are insufficient to control sacroiliac instability that arises from loss of the posterior bony-ligamentous hinge [182]. In these cases the external fixator should be used initially with traction; traction is later substituted with posterior fixation. Anterior symphyseal plating combined with a trapezoidal frame moderately stabilises APC-III and VS injuries, but the overall stability is inferior to posterior internal fixation combined with an external fixator [182] (Fig. 15).

There are three sites of pin insertion: iliac crest, between the anterior iliac spines, and transiliac. With all sites, direct visualisation of the portion

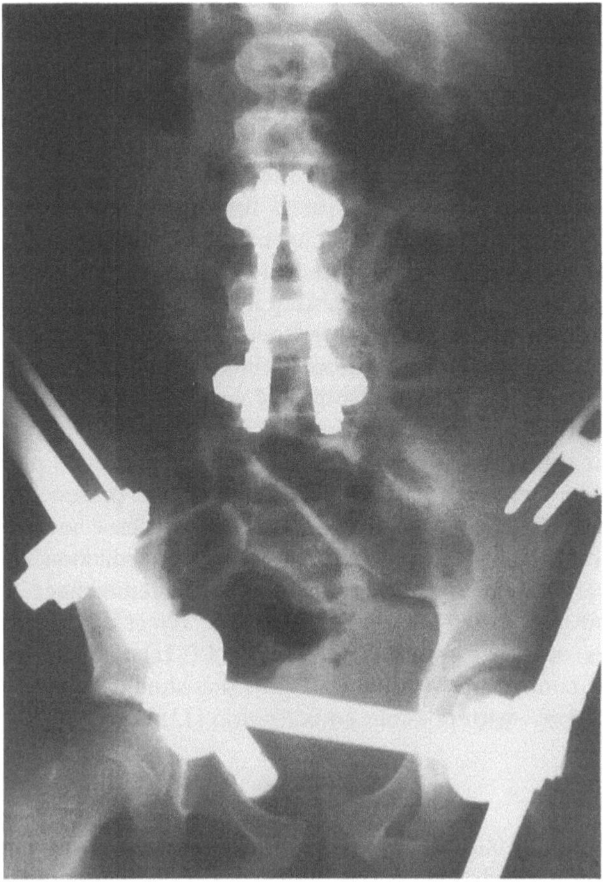

Fig. 15. A complex open-book pelvic fracture associated with intrapelvic bleeding and spinal trauma was successfully stabilized with an anteriorly placed external fixator. The bleeding stopped immediately following application of the pelvic frame

of the ilium prior to insertion is safer than percutaneous techniques. Skin incisions for pin insertion should account for the change in position of the pelvis on reduction; this often requires the addition of releasing incisions around pin sites. This potential problem may be averted by placing skin incisions after preliminary manual reduction.

Iliac Crest. Placing an incision over the palpable crest is less flexible to adjustments; a curved incision extending medially towards the umbilicus is less affected by skin tenting at the pin sites when the pelvis is reduced. Kirschner wires against either the outer and inner tables of the iliac wing provide an alignment check to the plane of insertion. Drilling the outer cortex of the iliac crest aids insertion of the pin by hand. The plane of the iliac wing and the obliquity of the pelvis to the operating table must be borne in mind during pin insertion. Pins of 5- to 6-mm diameter are preferable for use on pelvic fixators. The first pin is inserted just behind the anterior superior iliac spine, directed parallel to the plane of the iliac wing and towards the sacroiliac joint; subsequent pins are placed posterior to the first with 1 cm between pins [182]. Some fixator assemblies enable subsequent pins to be inserted through a clamp which is positioned over the first pin.

Anterior Insertion. The incision is started over the anterior crest and extended distally and medially, inferior to but in line with the ilioinguinal ligament. Sartorius and rectus femoris are reflected from their origins with care to avoid damage to the lateral cutaneous nerve of the thigh. Direct visualisation of the thin crest between the superior and inferior anterior iliac spines is important. The pin is again inserted by hand from anterior to posterior; use of X-ray guidance may help avoid penetration of the hip joint [176]. This position of pin placement is useful when the iliac crest is underdeveloped, as in children, or when wounds exclude use of the usual crest placement.

Transiliac Insertion. Described by Mears in 1980 [137], transiliac insertion involves use of a jig which is placed over the anterior inferior iliac spine, with the posterior superior iliac spine as exit point. The frame assembly which utilises transiliac pins was designed to overcome limitations of anterior frames in providing posterior stability. A circumferential assembly is constructed from anterior and posterior frames linked to these transiliac pins; however, the system has technical difficulties with assembly and nursing aftercare.

Frame Configurations

Various configurations have been described, but it is important for the surgeon to familiarise himself with the assembly of one or two configurations that can be applied swiftly when used to control haemorrhage. The simplest connection between two groups of iliac pins is a single transverse rod. This configuration is hampered by poor abdominal clearance and poor flexibility for adjustments. Two shorter rods forming an apex over the abdomen overcomes both disadvantages. This arrangement is quick to assemble and is the configuration of choice when used as part of initial resuscitation.

Selection of a frame configuration for definitive or adjunctive management depends on the nature of pelvic instability. The simple double-bar arrangement described above stabilises type B1.2 injuries adequately. Injuries with greater anterior diastasis (type B1.3), loss of the posterior bony-ligamentous hinge (type C), or unstable lateral compression injuries (type B2.2) require more complex configurations.

Trapezoidal [176], rectangular [182] and double-cluster [137] configurations have been described; some provide a modicum of posterior support. The trapezoidal frame is assembled anteriorly over a cluster of three pins in each iliac crest. The middle transverse bars, when approximated, provide compression over the posterior parts of the pelvis. The rectangular frame configuration is assembled in the coronal plane, again anchored to the pelvis through three iliac crest pins on each side. In contrast, the double-cluster assembly attaches to the pelvis through pins inserted in the crest and anteriorly; two rectangular frames are assembled based on the anterior and crista pins respectively. Cross-linking the rectangular frames can increase the rigidity of the overall construct. However, when assessed biomechanically, none of the above configurations prove adequate on their own to sufficiently stabilise vertical shear and type B1.3 pelvic disruptions [182]. The circumferential frame with transiliac pins as described by Mears is an exception, but difficulties in its application and aftercare have been highlighted. Posterior internal fixation was found to increase sacroiliac stability as much as four to five times; reliance on anterior external fixator frame configurations alone for such injuries is therefore not recommended.

Open Pelvic Injuries

The severity of trauma that results in an open pelvic fracture also produces a higher associated mortality and morbidity. There are four mechanisms that cause an open pelvic fracture: severe open-book injuries which tear the perineum; high-energy crush injuries; severe lateral compression injuries, notably the type B2.1 pattern with a tilt of the fractured rami into the perineum; and direct laceration from the impacting structure which causes the pelvic injury. The majority of these severe injuries require acute pelvic stabilisation with external fixation. A simple crossed anterior bar configuration or the antishock pelvic clamp as described by Ganz [76] would be appropriate. Open pelvic fractures are often associated with urogenital and gastrointestinal injuries. For the orthopaedic surgeon, the nature of these injuries are important in the management of the fracture. Faecal contamination precludes internal fixation if the wounds are in close proximity to the proposed site of surgery. All wounds require débridement and irrigation; the presence of faecal contamination may necessitate diversion of the faecal stream by colostomy, in addition to distal bowel wash-outs and broad-spectrum antibiotic cover [128]. External fixation may be a necessity even if only moderate stability is provided; minimal lag screw fixation with external fixation may be a better compromise for minimally contaminated wounds [112].

Comparative Results

Controlled trials of external fixation over other methods of treatment in pelvic fractures are few [94,175,183,192]. Non-operative treatment which includes the use of slings, spical casts and MAST trousers impose restricted mobility; optimal pulmonary ventilation is affected by virtue of delayed mobilisation. With spica casts and MAST trousers, care of lower extremity wounds is also potentially compromised [34].

Double plating of a symphyseal diastasis is biomechanically superior to any of the external fixator frame configurations described above [182]. This factor has prompted some surgeons to recommend internal fixation of such injuries if a concurrent laparotomy is performed acutely for associated intraperitoneal injuries [34]. However, the speed at which an external fixator can be applied and the relative simplicity of the procedure still support this technique of stabilisation for the acute stages. The additional stability from double anterior plating, if required, can be carried out at a later stage.

The limitations of most anterior external fixator configurations in providing posterior stability has been discussed. Posterior internal fixation, usually through transverse transiliac bars or lag screw fixation across the sacroiliac joint, provides much better stability. This form of fixation can be combined with external fixation to produce an overall assembly that is sufficiently stable for type C and type B1.3 injuries.

In summary the external fixator should be used acutely in pelvic ring disruptions with retroperitoneal haemorrhage. Its application as a definitive form of pelvic stabilisation must take into account its limitations in providing stability when the posterior bony-ligamentous hinge is lost; it is therefore probably best suited as a solitary form of stabilisation for types B1.2 and B2.2 injuries only.

Radius: Distal Fractures

Closed reduction and casting remain a widely practised mode of treatment for fractures of the distal radius. the assumption of a universally good result through conservative treatment, as first proposed by Colles [50], has, however, been questioned [82]. His assertion of a poor correlation between residual deformity and functional ability is verified only in the elderly population, where life-style demands and loading expectations of the injured wrist are substantially lower.

This injury is the commonest fracture; it comprised nearly 75% of all forearm fractures in Alffram's epidemiological survey in Sweden [2]. Recognition of the importance of articular anatomy and its congruence at both radiocarpal and radioulnar joints was emphasised by Frykman in 1967 [75]. Further studies have established radial length, radial inclination and dorsal or volar angulation as important prognostic criteria. A link between the severity of injury and the incidence of displacement after reduction has focused attention on alternative modes of treatment [52,190].

Classification

The challenge to conservative methods as a successful universal treatment for fractures of the distal radius arose when several classification systems allowed the study of outcome on different fracture grades; high-energy fractures, with marked displacement and joint involvement, produced poor results when treated by closed means. This finding is common for younger individuals [27,108,115], in whom functional demands of the wrist are significantly greater than the older population described earlier. Although several classification systems exist, that proposed by McMurtry and Jupiter highlights the importance that anatomy, local and patient-related factors have in forming a clinical composite that is fundamental in establishing the "personality" of the fracture [133]. A distinction between intra-articular and extra-articular fractures is made; the former, a subclassification is based on the number of main fragments which show a displacement greater than 1–2 mm. Local factors which have a direct influence on obtaining and maintaining a reduction, namely comminution, bone quality, energy of the injury and degree of displacement, are also included. These aspects are considered with the patient's age, handedness, occupation, life-style, loading expectations and compliance to a proposed treatment regime. This tripartite classification avoids the use of dogmatic treatment protocols based solely on anatomical features; such protocols lose the ability of selecting a treatment mode that achieves a functional outcome that best serves the individual.

Clinical examination and radiographic imaging, which may include standard and trispiral tomograms, establish the character of the fracture. Radial length, radial inclination and dorsal/volar angulation can be determined. Poor function is more likely if dorsal angulation is greater than 20°, radial shortening beyond 5 mm and joint line incongruence more than 2 mm [133].

Indications

Stable extra-articular fractures are successfully treated with manipulation and casting; however, the issue of long- versus short-arm casting has not been resolved. Distal radio-ulnar joint alignment has also emerged as a critical factor; malalignment can result in significant functional deficits, which are not uniformly resolved through distal ulnar resections. This factor has generated protagonists for long-arm bracing in neutral rotation or in full supination. Despite the different approaches, these fractures often unite without complications.

An unstable distal radius fracture is one with comminution, intra-articular involvement, or avulsions of either radial or ulnar styloid processes. Comminution often results in loss of cortical support despite an adequate reduction [38,82,190]; casting as a means to maintain reduction often fails to neutralise the tendency of these fractures to shorten. Adjunctive techniques to casting, such as percutaneous Kirschner wiring, are used to overcome this problem. Several techniques of pinning have been described; from Clancey's crossed and transverse wires [46] and Rayhack's multiple pins from the radial styloid to the ulnar cortex [107] and Kapandji's intrafocal technique. These techniques succeed in maintaining reduction after manipulation but are less effective in higher energy, complex fractures. Control of fracture alignment and bone length in such injuries is difficult without ligamentotaxis; this can be accomplished through use of the external fixator.

External fixation of fractures of the distal radius is indicated for unstable, high-energy injuries. Specifically these are comminuted, intra-articular fractures of two or more parts (McMurtry and Jupiter [133]), Frykman [75] type III or higher, or type II, IVA and IVB (Universal [77]). Open fractures are also appropriate for external fixation.

The significant advantages of the external fixator have been confirmed in the results of several prospective studies [98,102,116,120,121]. Distraction applied through the external fixator achieves significantly better control of radial length than casting [54,98]; this has resulted in a lower incidence of remanipulation and a better functional outcome [98,116]. However, prolonged distraction has resulted in wrist stiffness. This potential problem has led this technique to be combined with one of the following:

Percutaneous pinning. Using any of the techniques mentioned earlier, this method enables direct control over intra-articular fragments.

Autogenous bone grafting. This can be performed as a primary procedure at the time of application of the external fixator or delayed for 2–3 weeks. Primary autogenous grafting has been shown to increase the rigidity of fixation by four times [120]. Early removal of the external fixator at 3 weeks, followed by functional bracing, avoids wrist stiffness [120,121]. The grafted cancellous bone prevents late collapse at the fracture site after discontinuation of ligamentotaxis.

Dynamic external fixators. To overcome stiffness with prolonged distraction, these external fixators enable early wrist movement but maintain ligamentotaxis.

Specific Fractures

Two-Part Intra-articular Fractures. Where the second part consists of a volar or dorsal fragment that carries the carpus with it in its displacement (Barton's or reverse Barton's), buttress plating through either an anterior or dorsal approach affords excellent stability for this unstable, high-energy injury. The die punch injury, which is either a two- or three-part intra-articular injury, is perhaps more appropriately treated with external fixation. Distraction through the external fixator provides preliminary reduction; the lunate fossa is then approached dorsally through the third and fourth extensor compartments. Reduction is finalised by direct elevation of the fragment, with primary cancellous grafting to metaphyseal defects if these are created. Transverse Kirschner wiring augments fixation and enables early removal of the fixator for functional bracing.

Three-Part Intra-articular Fractures. The external fixator, used in conjunction with percutaneous Kirschner wiring, is the treatment method of choice. After preliminary application of the fixator in distraction mode, the main fracture fragments are held reduced with a transverse and an oblique Kirschner wire. Occasionally direct manipulation of the lateral fragment (lunate fossa) is required; this is carried out through an approach between the third and fourth extensor compartments as described above [72].

Four-Part Intra-articular Fractures. The ability to maintain reduction through ligamentotaxis becomes vital in fractures of increasing complexity. Here the lunate fossa is split coronally into two fragments; external fixation is similarly used in distraction prior to direct manipulation of the individual fracture fragments. The radial styloid fragment is often fixed first to provide a scaffold onto which the lunate fossa fragments can be held [133]. This can be achieved with use of interfragmentary lag screws or Kirschner wiring. The volar fragment of the lunate fossa often requires open reduction through an anterior approach and fixation by Kirschner wiring or buttress plating [72,139]. Such injuries, which have a large component of soft-tissue damage and are also subjected to surgical dissection, are best combined with primary autogenous bone grafting.

Intra-articular Fractures with Five or More Parts. The principles involved in these severe injuries are as for the four-part intra-articular fracture. The aim of restoring articular anatomy [9,27,115,139] must be weighed against possible damage inflicted by open reduction and adjunctive internal fixation. Delayed open reduction and fixation often provides the necessary allowance for resolution of soft-tissue swelling. The external fixator therefore enables a provisional reduction to be maintained whilst allowing recovery of the soft-tissue envelope. It can subsequently be used in conjunction with internal fixation techniques to restore and maintain articular anatomy and fracture alignment.

Technique

Strict attention to detail forms the basis of use of the external fixator for fractures of the distal radius. The application technique is similar for the variety of fracture types for which it is indicated.

Applying the external fixator is made easier if distraction can be maintained during its assembly. Use of traction through wire or raffia finger traps, with countertraction at the upper arm, enables this. Some modular external fixator systmes allow attachment of a distractor for the same effect.

After suitable skin preparation and draping, the pin insertion sites over the distal third of the radius and second metacarpal are located with the aid of an image intensifier and marked. Two pins in the radius and second metacarpal suffice. An improved bone-pin interface is obtained if the pins are angled at 60° to the cortical surface; as such each pair of pins subtend an angle of 60° (Fig. 16).

A limited open approach enables safer pin placement without the risk of transfixing nerve or tendon. This is particularly important in the radius, where the superficial branch of the radial nerve and tendons of extensor pollicis brevis and abductor pollicis longus are at risk. Pin insertion into the second metacarpal should be carried out with the metacarpophalangeal joint flexed and the thumb held in abduction; this places the intrinsics out at maximum length and similarly holds out the first dorsal interosseous muscle. The use of 4-mm pins through the cortices of the second and third metacarpal bases (six cortices) has been shown to provide an optimal biomechanical configuration without compromising the interosseous muscles of the second intrinsic compartment [172]. Although both metacarpal pins are inclined at 60° to each other, they should also lie at 45° to the plane of the palm to avoid interference with thumb adduction. Use of soft tissue guards and predrilling is recommended.

The degree of fine adjustment allowed after assembly of the frame depends on the external fixator system used; final reduction is confirmed by radiographs, and the clamps holding the connecting rod between metacarpal and radial pins are tightened. Aftercare includes physical therapy to encourage hand movements and pronation/supination. Pin site care should be demonstrated to the patient.

Dynamic external fixators differ in that alignment of the hinge of the fixator to the screw axis of the wrist is important [134,195]. The proximal capitate has been identified as the centre of the screw axis; precise positioning can be achieved only if an accurate fracture reduction is performed prior to application of the external fixator [48]. Early experience with dynamic external fixators showed a loss of reduction if wrist extension was allowed early in fractures with dorsal comminution. Flexion is therefore encouraged early but extension limited until 2–3 weeks following the injury [49].

Dynamic external fixators with distal pin placement into the distal fragment of the fracture allow early wrist movement as the joint is not spanned by the fixator. Such an application of the external fixator is restricted to distal fragments at least 6 mm in length and is contraindicated in fractures with marked comminution or intra-articular involvement [138]. The potential early recovery of wrist movement is offset by a higher incidence of pin tract infection secondary to increased skin motion over pin sites; this may be overcome by earlier conversion at 3 weeks to functional bracing [120,121].

Comparative Results

A successful result in fractures of the distal radius is a composite of normal articular anatomy, good grip strength, range of movement, endurance and

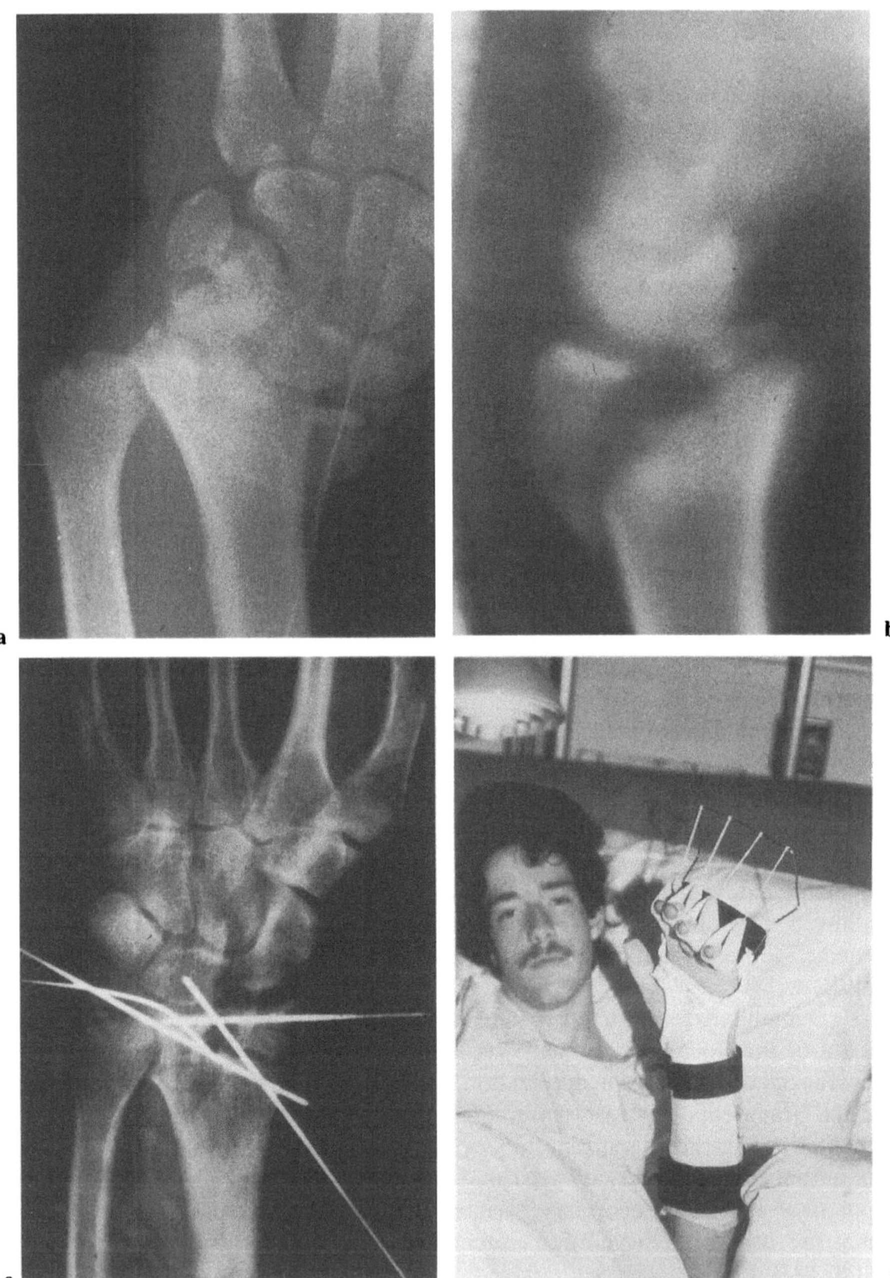

Fig. 16a–h. A complex distal radius fracture in a young adult. **a,b** Anteroposterior and lateral X-rays reveal the extensive disruption of the articular surface. **c** The fracture was treated by open reduction through a dorsal and volar approach. Skeletal fixation was with Kirschner wires. Axial length was maintained by an external

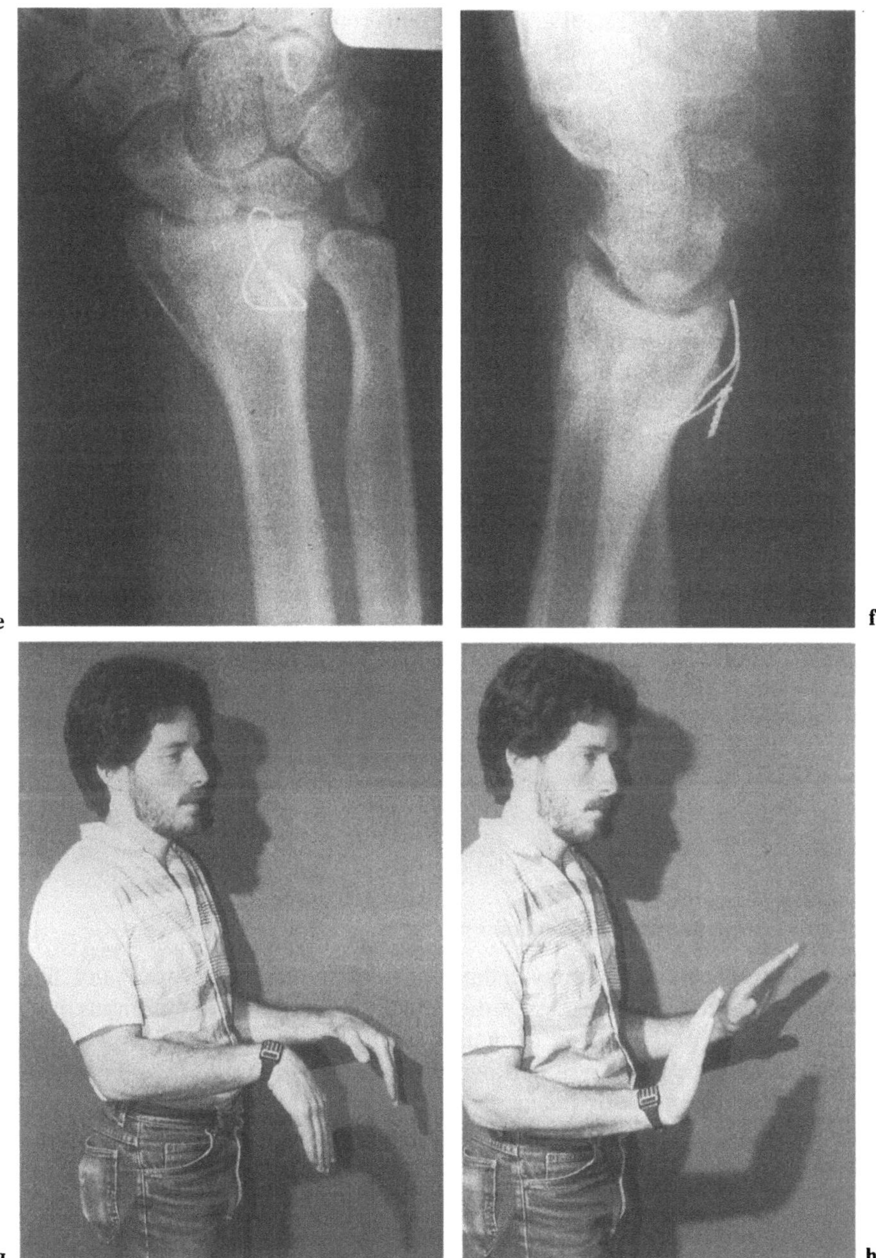

fixation frame. **d** The frame permitted rehabilitation of the hand beginning on the first post-operative day. **e,f** The fracture healed, and at 5-year follow-up the patient was functional. **g,h** At 5-year follow-up, some radiocarpal joint space narrowing is evident although non-progressive fine dexterity. These factors probably deliver the best functional outcome, but individual weighting of the component parts has yet to be determined.

Severe, comminuted distal radius fractures in young adults require accurate restoration of articular anatomy. Open reduction and internal fixation techniques achieve this aim at the expense of additional soft-tissue dissection; used in adjunct to the external fixator, this soft-tissue injury can be minimised. At a mean follow-up of 5 years, Bradway et al. [27] found an 81% good or excellent anatomical rating in patients with displaced, intra-articular fractures treated by open reduction and internal fixation. Similar studies report 83%–93% good to excellent results on anatomical scoring [67,98,101] and 76%–89% [98,116] on functional scoring with external fixation. This does not vindicate external fixation over open techniques but highlights the capabilities of external fixation in restoring and maintaining articular anatomy through ligamentotaxis. Fernandez and Geissler [72] have emphasised the need for combining these techniques in more severe injuries. Comparative studies of plaster casting and external fixation for these injuries have also unanimously demonstrated the significantly better results with external fixation in young adults [98,116].

The presumption of a good functional outcome despite deformity in young adults with fractures of the distal radius is therefore unsupported. Several studies have affirmed a relationship between articular anatomy and function [9,27,72,82,98,115,139,152]. Stable, extra-articular fractures are, however, amenable to closed reduction and casting, with good results [4,177]. This method of treatment can be extended to most fractures of the distal radius in the elderly, where for reasons outlined above, a successful result often depends more on early hand and wrist rehabilitation than restoration of articular anatomy [64,130,136,163].

Hand: Metacarpal and Phalangeal Fractures

The hand represents a finely balanced combination of osseous and ligamentous support on which extrinsic and intrinsic musculo-tendinous units interact; this affords a blend of unique qualities and functional capabilities, including dexterity, strength and precision. Injury to any of the elements of this composite alters this balance, which then manifests as functional loss. The close relationships between structures in the hand also exist on a physiological level; the extensive dysfunction witnessed in reflex sympathetic dystrophy emphasises the need for normal structural and functional integrity in all the elements.

Experience in managing fractures of the tubular skeleton of the hand has stressed the importance of early functional rehabilitation. Swanson has cautioned against overzealous treatment which too often results in stiffness [180]. The goals in treating these fractures have been elucidated and include [107]: (a) restoration of articular congruity, (b) reduction of malrotation or angulation, (c) maintenance of reduction with minimal surgical intervention, and (d) prompt mobilisation.

The majority of fractures involving the tubular skeleton of the hand can be managed non-operatively; a fundamental decision lies in selecting those injuries for which this mode of treatment is successful and those for operative intervention. Two important criteria that assist in this decision are the degree of displacement and potential fracture instability. With displaced metacarpal and phalangeal fractures, the criteria for acceptable alignment are [153]: (a) 10° of angulation in the saggital or coronal plane for diaphyseal fractures, 20° being acceptable for metaphyseal fractures; (b) at least 50% of fracture overlap; and (c) an absence of any rotational deformity.

The potential for displacement or instability can also be determined from the site and fracture pattern [153]. Those that are unstable include: rotated spiral fractures, comminuted and severely displaced fractures, multiple fractures, displaced articular fractures, subcondylar proximal phalanx fractures, and base of middle phalanx fractures. Displaced fractures can be reduced either by closed means or surgically; the options available for maintaining reduction differ with the reduction method employed. With closed reduction, further fracture support can be effected through functional bracing, percutaneous Kirschner wiring or external fixation.

Functional bracing is suitable for fractures that are inherently stable; the extensor hood is stretched over a flexed metacarpo-phalangeal joint, acting as a tension band to the palmar cortex of either metacarpal or phalangeal fracture [56]. Although suitable for fractures that are transverse or short oblique, regular radiographic and clinical follow-up is vital to ensure that reduction is maintained with this method.

Percutaneous Kirschner wiring, when applied after closed reduction, satisfies the aim of stabilisation with minimal surgical intervention. To many, it is the standard for the fixation of hand fractures [19,83]. Despite the versatility of Kirschner wiring, wires do loosen and often require additional fracture support [188] if early hand mobilisation is to be achieved. It is also used in conjunction with open reduction techniques, where it may be combined with tension band or intraosseous wiring [87,123], screw or plate fixation [93] to stabilise severely comminuted fractures. These internal fixation methods are often sufficiently stable to permit early hand rehabilitation without any further external support, thereby offsetting any disadvantage from the additional soft-tissue dissection that is required for their insertion.

The mini-external fixator in fractures of the hand provides a means of fracture stabilisation of sufficient rigidity to allow early hand rehabilitation. Its application is often accomplished with little further damage to the soft-tissue sleeve. More recent designs of the mini-external fixator permit adjustments to fracture alignment post-operatively [159]. In one series, fracture union was accomplished in an average of 6 weeks, with a 10% pin sepsis complication rate [159]; there were no non-unions or osteomyelitis. Most modern mini-fixators have adopted application principles that were derived from their larger relations; this does not detract the pioneering work by Henri Jaquet in popularising this mini-fixator for fractures of the hand. The culmination of a fracture stabilisation method that allows early hand rehabilitation, and yet minimises additional soft-tissue dissection when applied, is evidenced by the success of this device in open hand fractures [74]. This achievement has extended the role of the mini-external fixator beyond complex open injuries; there is now an increasing list of indications for which external fixation is appropriate. The general indications for external fixation for fractures of the hand are [107]: highly comminuted fractures, fractures with severe soft-tissue injury, open fractures, infected fractures, fractures with bone loss, complex fracture dislocations of the proximal interphalangeal joint, and maintenance of the first web space.

Technique

Several mini-external fixator systems are available; most are based on 1.5- and 2.0-mm pins. Differences refer mainly to ease of application and the feasibility of post-assembly alterations in fracture alignment.

The pins are of two types: transfixing and half pins. Pin insertion is aided by pin placement guides which usually double in function as drill guides; they also ensure that pairs of pins inserted are parallel. The site of pin application depends on the location and pattern of the fracture. With diaphyseal fractures, locating pins on either side of the fracture line avoids spanning a joint. However, this is occasionally not viable for highly comminuted or periarticular fractures.

The pins are inserted under direct vision; they are placed to lie in the coronal plane at the lateral edges of the extensor hood or just dorsal to the mid-axial line. Transfixing pins, by necessity, must be placed in the coronal plane across the longitudinal axis of the bone. This plane of insertion avoids impinging the gliding surfaces of extensor and flexor mechanisms. Assembly of pin holders, swivel clamps, articulated couplings and connecting rods depends on the frame configuration needed; for most cases unilateral half frames suffice for half pins, bilateral frames for transfixing pins, and occasionally a triangulated mini-frame. The additional swivel clamps greatly assists post-assembly alterations in fracture alignment.

Specific Indications in Metacarpal Fractures

Comminuted First and Fifth Carpo-metacarpal Fracture Dislocations. Although simpler epibasal and two-part (Bennett's and reverse Bennett's) fracture dislocations are successfully treated by traction and percutaneous Kirschner wire fixation, the higher energy three-part or comminuted injuries often benefit from distraction through a mini-external fixator in adjunct to a limited open reduction [61,107]. Distraction is accomplished between pins in the metacarpal and either the hamate or trapezium. In severe comminution, cancellous grafting of metaphyseal defects created after elevation of fracture fragments aids in supporting the reconstructed articular anatomy. Supplemental internal fixation by Kirschner wiring may be needed. Ligamentotaxis is maintained through the external fixator for 4 weeks after which sufficient support from early callus permits use of a thumb spica for a further 2 weeks [107]. With first carpo-metacarpal fracture dislocations associated with a large soft-tissue injury component, maintenance of the first web space is important to avert subsequent contracture. The external fixator can be assembled in the manner of a delta frame; pins in the first and second metacarpals are cross-linked to achieve this [74].

Metacarpal Shaft Fractures. External fixation is indicated for fractures with severe comminution where internal fixation methods would be difficult [74]. Primary restoration of skeletal length through external fixation allows later reconstructive procedures to the bony component of the injury; prompt management of the soft-tissue envelope is facilitated with the external fixator, which seldom impedes access. On achieving a clean, well-vascularized bed, autogenous bone graft can be introduced. Further definitive fixation, which may be a combination of internal and external fixation, should then allow mobilisation to commence [74]. Distraction-fixation is also indicated in the primary treatment of metacarpal bone loss [149]. Its success depends on a staged protocol of management which includes reconstructive procedures to the bony and soft-tissue elements combined to a continual programme of rehabilitation. Although distraction-fixation can similarly be accomplished through intermetacarpal Kirschner wires, the external fixator provides greater latitude of adjustment post-operatively.

Diaphyseal Fractures of the Proximal Phalanx. With the phalanges, dimensions of the tubular skeleton and its surrounding soft-tissue sleeve impose a restriction on the size of internal implants used if the functional integrity of the gliding surfaces is to be preserved. Internal fixation techniques employing interfragmentary screws, Kirschner wires or tension band wiring are of adequately low profile. With higher degrees of comminution, external fixation offers a method to realign through ligamentotaxis, with little additional trauma to the vascularity and integrity of the soft-tissue sleeve. Application of the fixator is technically less demanding and permits early hand rehabilitation [22]. Attention to detail is vital to the success of the technique; Freeland [74] has cautioned on the possibility of delayed union, collapse and subsequent deformity in such comminuted injuries that do not have the additional support of primary cancellous bone grafting.

Comminuted Articular Fractures. In some comminuted periarticular fractures, definition of articular anatomy is poor without an approximate reduction through distraction; application of the external fixator in this mode facilitates an improved anatomical appraisal of the articular damage. In addition, surgical restoration is aided by distraction; a gradual reassembly of the fragments on a template of the opposing articular surface is followed by cancellous grafting to the metaphyseal defects that result from fragment elevation. Often the difficulty lies in stabilising the reassembled puzzle; fixation may require a combination of techniques, such as interfragmentary screws, wiring or 1.5-mm condylar plates in adjunct to external fixation. When used in this manner, the external fixator may be removed at 3–4 weeks if sufficient radiological evidence is present to document healing progress at the fracture site; attempts at hand rehabilitation can start with the support of functional finger bracing. The extent of comminution in some severe periarticular fractures frustrates attempts at providing anatomical reconstruction of sufficient stability for early rehabilitation to commence. Even so, the approximate restoration of articular congruity through distraction fixation serves to preserve length and alignment in anticipation of severe joint limitation or ankylosis, facilitating a later task of arthrodesis or arthroplasty. If the external fixator is constructed to span only the involved joint, mobilisation of adjacent joints assists in achieving a functional result that is optimal for the severity of the injury involved [74].

Mini-external Fixation: A Comparison

Prospective studies comparing mini-external fixation to the other, longer established methods of fracture stabilisation in the hand are pending. Several authors have documented the success of this appliance in managing severe hand fractures [22,74,107,149,159]; a substantial credit must lie in the ability for establishing stable fixation with minimal surgical dissection, and the early restitution of functional activity. It is possible that problems concerning pin tract sepsis and loosening are fewer with mini-external fixation as the loads and bending moments are of a totally different magnitude compared to external fixation of weight-bearing bones. Certainly, the incidence of these complications is low for the severity of the injuries involved [8,74]. Although much of the performance and characteristics of external fixation have been derived from studies on the tibia, the tubular skeleton of the hand may eventually prove to be the ideal site for external fixation owing to its good vascularity, slim soft-tissue sleeve, and lower bone-pin interface stresses.

References

1. Akeson WH, Woo SLY, Rutherford L, Coutts RD, Gonsalves M, Amiel D (1976) The effects of rigidity of internal fixation plates on long bone remodelling. Acta Orthop Scand 47:241–249
2. Alffram PA, Göran CHB (1962) Epidemiology of fractures of the forearm. J Bone Joint Surg [Am] 44:105–114
3. Alonzo J, Geissler W, Hughes JL (1989) External fixation of femoral fractures: indications and limitations. Clin Orthop 241:83–88

4. Altissimi M, Antenucci R, Fiacca C, Mancini GB (1986) Long-term results of conservative treatment of fractures of the distal radius. Clin Orthop 206:202–210
5. Anderson R (1934) An automatic method of treatment for fractures of the tibia and fibula. Surg Gynaecol Obstet 58:6–39
6. Ansell BH, Scales JT (1968) A study of some factors which affect the strength of screws and their insertion and holding power in bone. J Biomech 1:279
7. Aro HT, Hein TJ, Chao EYS (1989) Mechanical performance of pin clamps in external fixators. Clin Orthop 248:246–253
8. Asche G (1989) Hand. In: Coombs R, Green S, Sarminento A (eds) External fixation and functional bracing. Orthotext, London, pp 161–166
9. Axelrod TJ, McMurtry RY (1990) Open reduction and internal fixation of comminuted intraarticular fractures of the distal radius. J Hand Surg [Am] 15:1–11
10. Bach AW, Hansen ST (1989) Plate versus external fixation in severe open tibial shaft fractures. Clin Orthop 241:89–94
11. Barquet A, Silva R, Massaferro J, Dubra A (1988) The AO tubular external fixator in the treatment of open fractures and infected non-unions of the shaft of the femur. Injury 19:415–420
12. Bauer GCH, Edwards P, Widmark PH (1962) Shaft fractures of the tibia: etiology of poor results in a consecutive series of 173 fractures. Acta Chir Scand 124:386–395
13. Bechtol CO, Lepper H Jr (1956) Fundamental studies in the design of metal screws for internal fixation on bone. J Bone Joint Surg [Am] 38:1385
14. Behrens F (1989) General theory and principles of external fixation. Clin Orthop 241:15
15. Behrens F (1989) A primer of fixator devices and configurations. Clin Orthop 245:5–14
16. Behrens F (1989) General theory and principles of external fixation. Clin Orthop 241:15–23
17. Behrens F, Johnson WD (1989) Unilateral external fixation: methods to increase or reduce frame stiffness. Clin Orthop 241:48
18. Behrens F, Searls K (1986) External fixation of the tibia. J Bone Joint Surg [Br] 68(2):246–254
19. Belsky MR, Eaton RG, Lane LB (1984) Closed reduction and internal fixation of proximal phalangeal fractures. J Hand Surg [Am] 9: 725–729
20. Bérenger Féraud LJB (1867) De l'emploi de la pointe de Malgaigne dans les fractures. Rev Ther Med Chir 15:228–232, 256–262
21. Biliouris T, Schneider E, Rahn BA, Gasser B, Perren SM (1989) The effect of radial pre-load on the implant-bone interface: a cadaveric study. J Orthop Trauma 3:323–332
22. Bilos ZJ, Eskestrand T (1979) External fixator use in comminuted gunshot fractures of the proximal phalanx. J Hand Surg 4:357–359
23. Böhler J (1968) Closed intramedullary nailing of the femur. Clin Orthop 60:51–67
24. Bone LB, Johnson KD, Weigelt J, Scheinberg R (1989) Early versus delayed stabilisation of femoral fractures: a prospective randomised study. J Bone Joint Surg [Am] 71:336–340
25. Böstman O, Varjonen L, Vainionpää S (1989) Incidence of local complications after intramedullary nailing and after plate fixation of femoral shaft fractures. J Trauma 29:639–645
26. Bower WH (1988) The distal radio-ulnar joint. In: Green DP (ed) Operative hand surgery, 2nd edn. Lippincott, Philadelphia, pp 939–989.
27. Bradway J, Amadio PC, Cooney WP (1989) Open reduction and internal fixation of displaced, comminuted intra-articular fractures of the distal end of the radius. J Bone Joint Surg [Am] 71:839–847
28. Bresler B, Frankel JP (1950) The forces and moments in the leg during level walking. Trans Am Soc Mech Eng 72:27

29. Briggs BT, Chao EY (1982) The mechanical performance of the standard Hoffmann-Vidal external fixation apparatus. J Bone Joint Surg [Am] 64:566
30. Brumback RJ (1992) Open tibial fractures: current orthopaedic management. Instr Course Lect 41:101–117
31. Brumback RJ, Reilly JP, Poka A (1988) Intramedullary nailing of femoral shaft fractures. I. Decision-making errors with interlocking fixation. J Bone Joint Surg [Am] 70:1441–1452
32. Brumback RJ, Uwagie-Ero S, Lakatos RP (1988) Intramedullary nailing of femoral shaft fractures. II. Fracture healing with static interlocking fixation. J Bone Joint Surg [Am] 70:1453–1462
33. Brumback RJ, Ellison PS, Poka A (1989) Intramedullary nailing of open fractures of the femoral shaft. J Bone Joint Surg [Am] 71:1324–1330
34. Burgess AR (1991) Fractures of the pelvis. In: Rockwood CA, Green DP, Buchholz RW (eds) Fractures in adults, 3rd edn. Lippincott, Philadelphia, pp 1399–1442
35. Burgess AR, Poka A, Browner BD, First KR (1992) Principles of external fixation. In: Browner BD, Jupiter JB, Levine AM, Trafton PG (eds) Skeletal trauma, vol 1. Saunders, Philadelphia, pp 231–242
36. Burnstein AH, Currey J, Frankel VH, Heiple KG, Lunseth P, Vessely JC (1972) Bone strength – the effect of screw holes. J Bone Joint Surg [Am] 54:1143
37. Burny F, Donkerwolcke M, Saric O (1982) Elastic external fixation of tibial fractures: influence of associated internal fixation. In: Uhthoff HK (ed) Current concepts of external fixation of fractures. Springer, Berlin Heidelberg New York, pp 159–167
38. Carrozzella J, Stern PJ (1988) Treatment of comminuted distal radius fractures with pins and plaster. Hand Clin 4:391–397
39. Chao EY, Malleuge JK (1981) Pin bone interface stresses in the application of external fixation and traction devices. Orthop Trans 5:259
40. Chao EY, Kasman RA, An KN (1982) Rigidity and stress analysis of external fixation devices – a theoretical approach. J Biomech 15:971
41. Chapman MW (1986) The role of intramedullary fixation in open fractures. Clin Orthop 212:26–34
42. Chapman MW, Mahoney M (1979) The role of early internal fixation in the management of open fractures. Clin Orthop 138:120
43. Charnley J (1953) Compression arthrodesis. E. and S. Livinstone, Edinburgh
44. Charnley J (1961) The closed treatment of common fractures, 3rd edn. Churchill Livingstone, Edinburgh
45. Cierny G, Byrd HS, Jones RE (1983) Primary versus delayed soft tissue coverage for severe open tibial fractures: a comparison of results. Clin Orthop 178:54–63
46. Clancey GJ (1984) Percutaneous Kirschner wire fixation of Colles' fractures. J Bone Joint Surg [Am] 66:1008–1014
47. Clawson DK, Smith RF, Hansen ST (1971) Closed intramedullary nailing of the femur. J Bone Joint Surg [Am] 53:681–692
48. Clyburn TA (1989) The wrist. In: Commbs R, Green S, Sarmiento A (eds) External fixation and functional bracing. Orthotext, London, pp 167–171
49. Clyburn TA (1987) Dynamic external fixation for comminuted intraarticular fractures of the distal end of the radius. J Bone Joint Surg [Am] 69:248–254
50. Colles A (1814) On the fracture of the carpal extremity of the radius. Edinb Med Surg J 10:182–186
51. Colton CL (1992) The history of fracture treatment. In: Browner BD, Jupiter JB, Levine AM, Traftion PG (eds) Skeletal trauma, vol 1. Saunders, Philadelphia, pp 3–30
52. Cooney WP, Linscheid RL, Dobyns JH (1979) External pin fixation for unstable Colle's fractures. J Bone Joint Surg [Am] 61:840–845

53. Cooney WP, Dobyns JH, Linsheid RL (1980) Complications of Colles' fractures. J Bone Joint Surg [Am] 62:613–619
54. Conney WP, Linscheid RL, Dobyns JH (1991) Fractures and dislocations of the wrist. In: Rockwood CA, Green DP, Buchholz RW (eds) Fractures in adults, 3rd edn. Lippincott, Philadelphia, pp 563–678
55. Coonrad R, Goldner JL (1968) A study of the pathological findings and treatment in soft tissue injury of the thumb metacarpo-phalangeal joint. J Bone Joint Surg [Am] 50:439–451
56. Coonrad R, Pohlman M (1969) Impacted fractures in the proximal portion of the proximal phalanx of the finger. J Bone Joint Surg [Am] 57:1291–1296
57. Court-Brown C (1991) Grade IIIB open tibia fracture – the Edinburgh experience of intramedullary nailing. 5th Edinburgh Trauma Symposium, Edinburgh
58. Cryer HM, Miller FB, Evers BM, Rouben LR, Seligson DL (1988) Pelvic fracture classification: correlation with haemorrhage. J Trauma 28:973–980
59. Cuendet S (1936) Procédé de réduction des fractures de la diaphyse des deux os de l'avant-bras à l'aide de l'appareil à broches jumeliées. Livre jubilaire Albin Lambotte. Vromant, Brussels
60. Dabezies EJ, D'Ambrosia, Shoji H (1984) Fractures of the femoral shaft treated by external fixation with the Wagner device. J Bone Joint Surg [Am] 66:360–364
61. Dammisse IG, Lloyd GJ (1979) Injuries to the fifth carpometacarpal region. Can J Surg 22:240–244
62. De Bastiani G, Aldegheri R, Renzi-Brivio L (1986) Dynamic axial fixation. A rational alternative for the external fixation of fractures. Int Orthop 10(2):95–99
63. Delal SA, Burgess AR, Siegel JH, Young JW, Brumback RJ, Poka A, Dunham CM, Gens D, Bathon H (1989) Pelvic fracture in multiple trauma: classification by mechanism is key to pattern of organ injury, resuscitative requirements and outcome. J Trauma 29:981–1002
64. Dias JJ, Wray CC, Jones JM, Gregg PJ (1987) The value of early mobilisation in the treatment of Colle's fractures. J Bone Joint Surg [Br] 69:463–467
65. Dove AF, Poon WS, Weston PAM (1982) Haemorrhage from pelvic fractures: dangers and treatments. Injury 13:375–381
66. Edwards CC, Shelton SC, Browner BD, Weigel MC (1988) Severe open tibial fractures: results treating 202 injuries with external fixation. Clin Orthop 230: 98–115
67. Edwards GS (1991) Intra-articular fractures of the distal part of the radius treated with the small AO external fixator. J Bone Joint Surg [Am] 73: 1241–1250
68. Edwards P (1965) Fracture of the shaft of the tibia: 492 consecutive cases in adults: importance of soft tissue injury. Acta Orthop Scand Suppl 76:1–83
69. Ellis H (1958) The speed of healing after fracture of the tibial shaft. J Bone Joint Surg [Br] 40:42–46
70. Etter C, Burri C, Claes L, Kinzl L, Raible M (1983) Treatment by external fixation of open fractures associated with severe soft tissue damage of the leg. Clin Orthop 178:80–88
71. Evers BM, Cryer HM, Miller FB (1989) Pelvic fracture haemorrhage: priorities in management. Arch Surg 124:422–424
72. Fernandez DL, Geissler WB (1991) Treatment of displaced articular fractures of the radius. J Hand Surg [Am] 16(3):375–384
73. Fischer DA (1983) Skeletal stabilization with a multiplane external fixation device: design rationale and preliminary clinical experience. Clin Orthop 180: 50–62
74. Freeland AE (1987) External fixation for skeletal stabilisation of severe open fractures of the hand. Clin Orthop 214:93–100
75. Frykman G (1967) Fracture of the distal radius including sequelae – shoulder hand finger syndrome, disturbance in the distal radio-ulnar joint and impair-

ment of nerve function. A clinical and experimental study. Acta Orthop Scand Suppl 108:1–155
76. Ganz R, Krushell RJ, Jakob RP, Küffer J (1991) The antishock pelvic clamp. Clin Orthop 267:71–78
77. Gartland JJ, Werley CW (1951) Evaluation of healed Colles' fractures. J Bone Joint Surg [Am] 33:895–907
78. Gillott A, Rhodes M, Lucke J (1988) Utility of routine pelvic X-ray during blunt trauma resuscitation. J Trauma 28:1570–1574
79. Goris RJA, Gimbrere JSF, van Niekerk JLM (1982) Early osteosynthesis and prophylactic mechanical ventilation in the multitrauma patient. J Trauma 22:895–903
80. Grazier KL, Holbrook TL, Kelsey JL, Stauffer RN (1984) Frequency of occurrence, impact and cost of selected musculoskeletal conditions in the United States. American Academy of Orthopaedic Surgeons, Chicago, pp 73–135
81. Grazier KL, Holbrook TL, Kelsey JL, Stauffer RN (1984) The frequency of occurrence, impact, and cost of musculoskeletal conditions in the United States. American Academy of Orthopaedic Surgeons, Chicago
82. Green DP (1975) Pins and plaster treatment of comminuted fractures of the distal end of the radius. J Bone Joint Surg [Am] 57:304–310
83. Green DP, Anderson JR (1973) Closed reduction and percutaneous pin fixation of fractured phalanges. J Bone Joint Surg [Am] 55:1651–1654
84. Green SA (1981) Complications of external skeletal fixation. Charles, Springfield
85. Green SA (1989) Combined internal and external fixation. In: Green S, Coombs R, Sarmiento A (eds) External fixation and functional bracing. Orthotext, London, pp 233–237
86. Green SA (1992) The Ilizarov method. In: Browner BD, Jupiter JB, Levine AM, Trafton PG (eds) Skeletal trauma, vol 1. Saunders, Philadelphia, pp 543–570
87. Greene TL, Noellert RC, Belsole RJ (1987) Treatment of unstable metacarpal and phalangeal fractures with tension band wiring techniques. Clin Orthop 214:78–84
88. Gustilo RB, Anderson JT (1976) Prevention of infection in the treatment of one thousand and twenty five open fractures of long bones; retrospective and prospective analyses. J Bone Joint Surg [Am] 58(4):453–458
89. Gustilo RB, Merkow RL, Templeman D (1990) Current concepts review: the management of open fractures. J Bone Joint Surg [Am] 72:299–303
90. Gylling SF, Ward RE, Holcroft JW (1985) Immediate external fixation of unstable pelvic fractures. Am J Surg 150(6):721–724
91. Halsey D, Braden Fleming MS, Pope MH, Krag M, Kristiansen T (1992) External fixator pin design. Clin Orthop 278:305–312
92. Hedlund R, Lindgren U (1986) Epidemiology of diaphyseal femoral fracture. Acta Orthop Scand 57:423–427
93. Heim U, Pfeiffer KM (1988) Internal fixation of small fractures, 3rd edn. Springer, Berlin Heidelberg New York
94. Henderson RC (1988) The long term results of non-operatively treated major pelvic disruptions. J Orthop Trauma 3(1):41–47
95. Hoffmann R (1938) Rotules à os pour la réduction dirigée, non sangalante, des fractures (ostéotaxis). Helv Med Acta 6:844–850
96. Hohl M (1991) Fractures of the tibial plateau. In: Rockwood CA, Green DP, Bucholz RW (eds) Fractures in adults, vol 2, 3rd edn. Lippincott, Philadelphia, pp 1725–1761
97. Holbrook JL, Swiontkowski MF, Sanders R (1989) Treatment of open fractures of the tibial shaft: ender nailing versus external fixation: a randomised, prospective comparison. J Bone Joint Surg [Am] 71:1231–1238
98. Howard PW, Stewart HD, Hind RE, Burke FD (1989) External fixation or plaster for severely displaced comminuted Colles' fractures? J Bone Joint Surg [Br] 71:68–73

99. Hughes AN, Jordan BA (1969) The mechanical properties of surgical boen screws and some aspects of insertion practice. Injury 4:25
100. Hyldahl C, Pearson S, Tepic S, Perren SM (1988) Induction and prevention of pin loosening in external fixators in the sheep tibia. Orthop Trans 12:378
101. Jakim I, Pieterse HS, Sweet MBE (1991) External fixation for intra-articular fractures of the distal radius. J Bone Joint Surg [Br] 73:302–306
102. Jenkins NH, Jones DG, Johnson SR, Mintowt-Czyz WT (1987) External fixation of Colles' fractures: an anatomical study. J Bone Joint Surg [Br] 69:207–211
103. Johnson KD (1992) Femoral shaft fractures. In: Browner BD, Jupiter JB, Levine AM, Trafton PG (eds) Skeletal trauma, vol 2. Saunders, Philadelphia, pp 1525–1641
104. Johnson WD, Fischer DA (1983) Skeletal stabilisation with a multiplane external fixation device: biomechanical evaluation and finite element model. Clin Orthop 180:34–43
105. Johnson KD, Cadambi A, Seibert GB (1985) Incidence of adult respiratory distress syndrome in patients with multiple musculoskeletal injuries: effect of early operative stabilisation of fractures. J Trauma 25:375–384
106. Judet R, Judet J, Roy-Camille R (1958) La vascularisation des pseudoarthoses des os longs d'après une étude clinique et expérimentale. Rev Chir Orthop 44:5
107. Jupiter JB, Belsky MR (1992) Fractures and dislocations of the hand. In: Browner BD, Jupiter JB, Levine AM, Trafton PG (eds) Skeletal trauma, vol 2. Saunders, Philadelphia, pp 925–1024
108. Jupiter JB, Masem M (1988) Reconstruction of post-traumatic deformity of the distal radius and ulna. Hand Clin 4:377–390
109. Karlstrom G, Olerud S (1983) External fixation of severe open tibial fractures with Hoffmann frame. Clin Orthop 180:69–77
110. Keetley CB (1893) On the prevention of shortening and other forms of malunion after fracture, by the use of metal pins passed into the fragments subcutaneously. Lancet 137–139
111. Kellam JF (1989) The role of external fixation in pelvic disruptions. Clin Orthop 241:66–82
112. Kellam JF, Browner BD (1992) Fractures of the pelvic ring. In: Browner BD, Jupiter JB, Levine AM, Trafton PG (eds) Skeletal trauma, vol 1. Saunders, Philaedlphia, pp 849–897
113. Kenwright J, Goodship AE (1989) Controlled mechanical stimulation in the treatment of tibial fractures. Clin Orthop 241:36–47
114. Kimmel RB (1982) Results of treatment using the Hoffmann external fixator for fracture of the tibial diaphysis. J Trauma 22:960–965
115. Knirk JL, Jupiter JB (1986) Intraarticular fractures of the distal end of the radius in young adults. J Bone Joint Surg [Am] 68:647–659
116. Kongsholm J, Olerud C (1989) Plaster cast versus external fixation for unstable intraarticular Colles' fractures. Clin Orthop 241:57–65
117. Koval KJ, Clapper MF, Brumback RJ (1991) Complications of reamed intramedullary nailing of the tibia. J Orthop Trauma 5:184–189
118. Kristiansen T, Fleming B, Neale G, Reinecke S, Pope MH (1987) Comparative study of fracture gap motion in external fixation. Clin Biomech 2:191
119. Lambotte A (1913) Chirurgie opératoire des fractures. Masson, Paris
120. Leung KS, Shen WY, Leung PC, Kinninmonth AWG, Chang JCW, Chan GPY (1989) Ligamentotaxis and bone grafting for comminuted fractures of the distal radius. J Bone Joint Surg [Br] 71:838–842
121. Leung KS, Shen WY, Tsang HK, Chiu KH, Leung PC, Hung LK (1990) An effective treatment of comminuted fractures of the distal radius. J Hand Surg [Am] 15(1):11–17
122. Lhowe DW, Hansen ST (1988) Immediate nailing of open fractures of the femoral shaft. J Bone Joint Surg [Am] 70:812–820

123. Lister G (1978) Intraosseous wiring of the digital skeleton. J Hand Surg 3:427–435
124. Lottes JO (1954) Blind nailing technique for insertion of the triflange medullary nail. JAMA 155:1039–1042
125. Lynch AC, Lipscomb PR (1963) The carpal tunnel syndrome and Colles' fractures. JAMA 185:363–366
126. Magerl F, Wyss A, Brunner C, Binder W (1979) Plate osteosynthesis of femoral shaft fractures in adults: a follow-up study. Clin Orthop 138:62–73
127. Matthews LS, Green CA, Goldstein SA (1984) The thermal effects of skeletal fixation – pin insertion in bone. J Bone Joint Surg [Am] 66(7):1077–1083
128. Maull KI, Sachatello CR, Ernst CB (1977) The deep perineal laceration – an injury frequently associated with open pelvic fractures: a need for aggressive surgical management. J Trauma 17:685–696
129. Maurer DJ, Merkow RL, Gustilo RB (1989) Infection after intramedullary nailing of severe open tibial fractures initially treated with external fixation. J Bone Joint Surg [Am] 71:835–838
130. McAuliffe TB, Hilliar KM, Coates CJ, Grange WJ (1987) Early mobilisation of Colles' fractures: a prospective trial. J Bone Joint Surg [Br] 69:727–729
131. McCoy GF, Johnstone RA, Kenwright K (1989) Biomechanical aspects of pelvic and hip injuries in road traffic accidents. J Orthop Trauma 3(2):118–123
132. McGraw JM, Lim EVA (1988) Treatment of open tibial shaft fractures. J Bone Joint Surg [Am] 70(6):900–911
133. McMurtry RY, Jupiter JB (1992) Fractures of the distal radius. In: Browner BD, Jupiter JB, Levine AM, Trafton PG (eds) Skeletal trauma, vol 2. Saunders, Philadelphia, pp 1063–1094
134. McMurtry RY, Youm Y, Flatt AE, Gillespie TE (1978) Kinematics of the wrist. II. Clinical application. J bone Joint Surg [Am] 60:955–961
135. McMurty RY, Walton D, Dickinson D (1980) Pelvic disruption in the polytraumatised patient: a management protocol. Clin Orthop 151:22–30
136. McQueen MM, MacLaren A, Chalmers J (1986) The value of remanipulating Colles' fractures. J Bone Joint Surg [Br] 68:232–233
137. Mears DC, Fu FH (1980) Modern concepts of external fixation of the pelvis. Clin Orthop 151:65–72
138. Meléndez EM, Mehne DK, Posner MA (1989) Treatment of unstable Colles' fractures with a new radius mini-fixator. J Hand Surg [Am] 14(5):807–811
139. Melone CP (1984) Articular fractures of the distal radius. Orthop Clin North Am 15:217–236
140. Moran CG, Gibson MJ, Cross AT (1990) Intramedullary locking nails for femoral shaft fractures in elderly patients. J Bone Joint Surg [Br] 72:19–22
141. Müller ME (1965) Treatment of non-unions by compression. Clin Orthop 43:83
142. Müller ME, Allgöwer M, Schneider R, Willenegger H (1992) Manual of internal fixations, 3rd edn. Springer, Berlin Heidelberg New York
143. Murphy CP, d'Ambrosia RD, Dabezies EJ (1988) Complex femur fractures: treatment with the Wagner external fixation device or the Grosse-Kempf interlocking nail. J Trauma 28:1553–1561
144. O'Beirne J, O'Connell RJ, White JM, Flynn M (1986) Fractures of the femur treated by femoral plating using the anterolateral approach. Injury 17:387–390
145. Oestern HJ, Tscherne H (1984) Pathophysiology and classification of soft tissue injuries associated with fractures. In: Tscherne H, Gotzen L (eds) Fractures with soft tissue injuries. Springer, Berlin Heidelberg New York
146. Overgarrd S, Solgaard S (1989) Osteoarthritis after Colles' fracture. Orthopaedics 12:413–416
147. Parkhill C (1897) A new apparatus for the fixation of bones after resection and in fractures with a tendency to displacement. Trans Am Surg Assoc 15:251–256
148. Patzakis MJ, Wilkins J, Moore TM (1983) Use of antibiotics in open tibial fractures. Clin Orthop 178:31–35

149. Peimer CA, Smith RJ, Leffert RD (1981) Distraction-fixation in the primary treatment of metacarpal bone loss. J Hand Surg 6(2):111–124
150. Peltier LF (1958) Joseph Francois Malgaine and Malgaine's fracture. Surgery 44:777–784
151. Pennal GF, Tile M, Waddell JP, Garside H (1980) Pelvic disruption: assessment and classification. Clin Orthop 151:12–21
152. Porter M, Stockley I (1987) Fractures of the distal radius. Intermediate and end results in relation to radiologic parameters. Clin Orthop 220:241–251
153. Pun WK, Chow SP, Luk KDK (1989) A prospective study on 284 digital fractures of the hand. J Hand Surg [Am] 14:474–481
154. Puno RM, Teynor JT, Nagano J, Gustilo RB (1986) Critical analysis of results of treatment of 201 tibial shaft fractures. Clin Orthop 212:113–121
155. Raimbeau G, Chevalier JM, Raguin J (1979) Les risques vasculaires du fixateur en cadre à la jambe. Rev Chir Orthop 65 Suppl 11:77–82
156. Rich NM, Metz CW, Hutton JE Jr (1971) Internal vs. external fixation of fractures with concomitant vascular injuries. J Trauma 11:463
157. Ries MD, Meinhard BP (1990) Medial external fixation with lateral plate internal fixation in metaphyseal tibia fractures; a report of eight cases associated with severe soft tissue injury. Clin Orthopa 256:215–223
158. Rigaud C (1850) Des vis métalliques enforcées dans le tissue des os pour le traitement de certaines fractures. Rev Med Chir Paris 8:113–114
159. Riggs SA Jr, Cooney WP (1983) External fixation of complex hand and wrist fractures. J Trauma 23:332–336
160. Riska EB, von Bonsdorff H, Hakkinen S (1977) Primary operative fixation of long bone fractures in patients with multiple injuries. J Trauma 17:111–121
161. Rittmann WW, Schibli M, Matter P, Allgower M (1979) Open fractures; long term results in 200 consecutive cases. Clin Orthop 138:132–140
162. Roberts JB (1977) Management of fracture and fracture complications of the femoral shaft using the ASIF compression plate. J Trauma 17:20–28
163. Roumen RMH, Hesp WLEM, Bruggink EDM (1991) Unstable Colles' fractures in elderly patients: a randomised trial of external fixation for redisplacement. J Bone Joint Surg [Br] 73:307–311
164. Ruedi T, Luscher N (1979) Results after internal fixation of comminuted fractures of the femoral shaft with DC plates. Clin Orthop 138:74
165. Santoro V, Henley M, Bernischke S (1990) Prospective comparison of unreamed interlocking IM nails versus half-pin external fixation in open tibial fractures. 6th Annual Meeting of the Orthopaedic Trauma Association, Nov 7–10, Toronto
166. Sarmiento A (1974) Functional bracing of tibial fractures. Clin Orthop 105:202–219
167. Sarmiento A, Pratt GW, Berry NC, Sinclair WF (1975) Colles' fractures: functional bracing in supination. J Bone Joint Surg [Am] 57:311–317
168. Sarmiento A, Gersten LM, Sobol PA, Shankwiler JA, Vangness CT (1989) Tibial shaft fractures treated with functional braces. J Bone Joint Surg [Br] 71:602–609
169. Schatzker J (1992) Tibial plateau fracture. In: Browner BD, Jupiter JB, Levine AM, Trafton PG (eds) Skeletal trauma, vol 2. Saunders, Philadelphia, pp 1745–1769
170. Schatzker J, Sanderson R, Murnaghan JP (1975) The holding power of orthopaedic screws in vivo. Clin Orthop 108:115–126
171. Seibel R, LaDuca J, Hassett JM (1985) Blunt multiple trauma(ISS-36), femur traction and the pulmonary failure septic rate. Ann Surg 202:283–295
172. Seitz WH, Froimson AI, Brooks DB, Postak PD, Parker RD, LaPorte JM, Greenwald AS (1990) Biomechanical analysis of pin placement and pin size for external fixation of distal radius fractures. Clin Orthop 251:207–212
173. Seligson D, Pope MH (1982) Concepts in external fixation. Grune and Stratton, New York

174. Seligson D, Donald GD, Stanwyck TS, Pope MH (1984) Consideration of pin diameter and insertion technique for external fixation in diaphyseal bone. Acta Orthop Belg 50:441
175. Semba RT, Yakusawa K, Gustilo RB (1983) Critical analysis of results of 53 Malgaine fractures of the pelvis. J Trauma 23(6):535–537
176. Slätis P, Karaharju EO (1975) External fixation of the pelvic girdle with a trapezoid compression frame. Injury 7:53–56
177. Smaill GB (1965) Long term follow-up of Colles' fracture. J Bone Joint Surg [Br] 47:80–85
178. Sprenger TF (1983) Fractures of the shaft of the femur treated with a single AO plate. South Med J 76:471–474
179. Stein AH (1962) The relation of median nerve compression to Sudek's syndrome. Surg Gynaecol Obstet 115:713–720
180. Swanson AB (1970) Fractures involving digits of the hand. Orthop Clin North Am 1:261–274
181. Templeman D, Sweeney C, Chapman MW (1990) Critical analysis of the management of open femur fractures at two regional trauma centres. Orthop Trans 14:675
182. Tile M (1984) Fractures of the pelvis and acetabulum. Williams and Williams, Baltimore
183. Tile M (1988) Pelvic ring fractures: should they be fixed? J Bone Joint Surg [Br] 70:1–12
184. Tile M (1991) Fractures of the acetabulum. In: Rockwood CA, Green DP, Bucholz RW (eds) Fractures in adults, 3rd edn. Lippincott, Philadelphia
185. Tile M, Pennal GF (1980) Pelvic disruption: principles of management. Clin Orthop 151:56–64
186. Trafton PG (1988) Closed unstable fractures of the tibia. Clin Orthop 230: 58–67
187. Tscherne H (1991) Open tibia fracture – IIIB: the Hanover experience. 5th Edinburgh Trauma Symposium, Edinburgh
188. Vanik RK, Weber RC, Matloub HS (1984) The comparative strengths of internal fixation techniques. J Hand Surg [Am] 9:216–221
189. Weber BG, Magerl F (1985) The external fixator. Springer, Berlin Heidelberg New York
190. Weber ER (1987) A rational approach for the recognition and treatment of Colles' fractures. Hand Clin 3:13–21
191. Weber SC, Szabo RM (1986) Severely comminuted distal radius fracture as an unsolved problem: complications associated with external fixation and pins and plaster techniques. J Hand Surg [Am] 11:157–165
192. Wild JJ, Hansen GW, Tullos HS (1982) Unstable fractures of the pelvis treated by external fixation. J Bone Joint Surg [Am] 64:1010–1020
193. Winquist RA, Hansen ST Jr, Clawson DK (1984) Closed intramedullary nailing of femoral fractures: a report of 520 cases. J Bone Joint Surg [Am] 66:529–539
194. Wu JJ, Shyr HS, Chao EYS, Kelly PJ (1984) Comparison of osteotomy healing under external fixation devices with different stiffness characteristics. J Bone Joint Surg [Am] 66(8):1258–1264
195. Youm Y, McMurtry RY, Flatt AE, Gillespie TE (1978) Kinematics of the wrist. I. An experimental study of radial-ulnar deviation and flexion-extension. J Bone Joint Surg [Am] 60:423–431
196. Young JWR, Burgess AR, Brumback RJ, Poka A (1986) Lateral compression fractures of the pelvis: the importance of plain radiographs in the diagnosis and surgical management. Skeletal Radiol 15:103–109
197. Young JWR, Burgess AR, Brumback RJ, Poka A (1986) Pelvic fractures: value of plain radiography in early assessment and management. Radiology 160: 445–451

4 Current Use of the Intramedullary Nail

D. Pennig

History

In 1968 Küntscher patented an "intramedullary nail for the treatment of comminuted fractures, with its insertion apparatus". Küntscher's original drawings are presented in Fig. 1. Figure 1b illustrates the proximal locking principle, for which Küntscher described a cannulated screw and a nail-mounted targetting device for the distal screw, and Fig. 1c shows the distal locking screw in place and a comminuted fracture being stabilized with the intramedullary nail. According to his description, Küntscher's main reason for designing this novel device was that the current practice of open reduction and internal fixation using metal plates required a major surgical intervention [36,78] and impaired the blood supply of the fracture fragments [52,79]. With his invention Küntscher wanted to provide an internal intramedullary fixation with a surgical intervention that is minor and distant from the fracture site.

This first locking nail was called a "detensor" and was based on the straight cloverleaf design which Küntscher used successfully for the treatment of femoral fractures [45]. Küntscher had realized that the unlocked nail could be used safely only for a noncomminuted midshaft fracture whereas proximal, distal and comminuted midshaft fractures could not. In Küntscher's opinion, reaming of the nail is necessary to permit the insertion of a nail of sufficient size and to allow the patient ambulation and early weight bearing [45].

After Küntscher's death in 1972, Klemm and Schellmann [44] in Frankfurt and later Grosse and Kempf [30,41,42] in Strasbourg enlarged on Küntscher's ideas, and with two different manufacturers they created implants that have been used successfully for more than 20 years. Compared to Küntscher's original design there were two major changes introduced by Klemm and Schellmann and by Grosse and Kempf: the proximal locking screw was inserted obliquely rather than transversely, and the nail was curved to accomodate an average curvature of the femur rather than being straight as in the original [37]. Based on these initial models in the 1980s other locking nails with similar features have since become available.

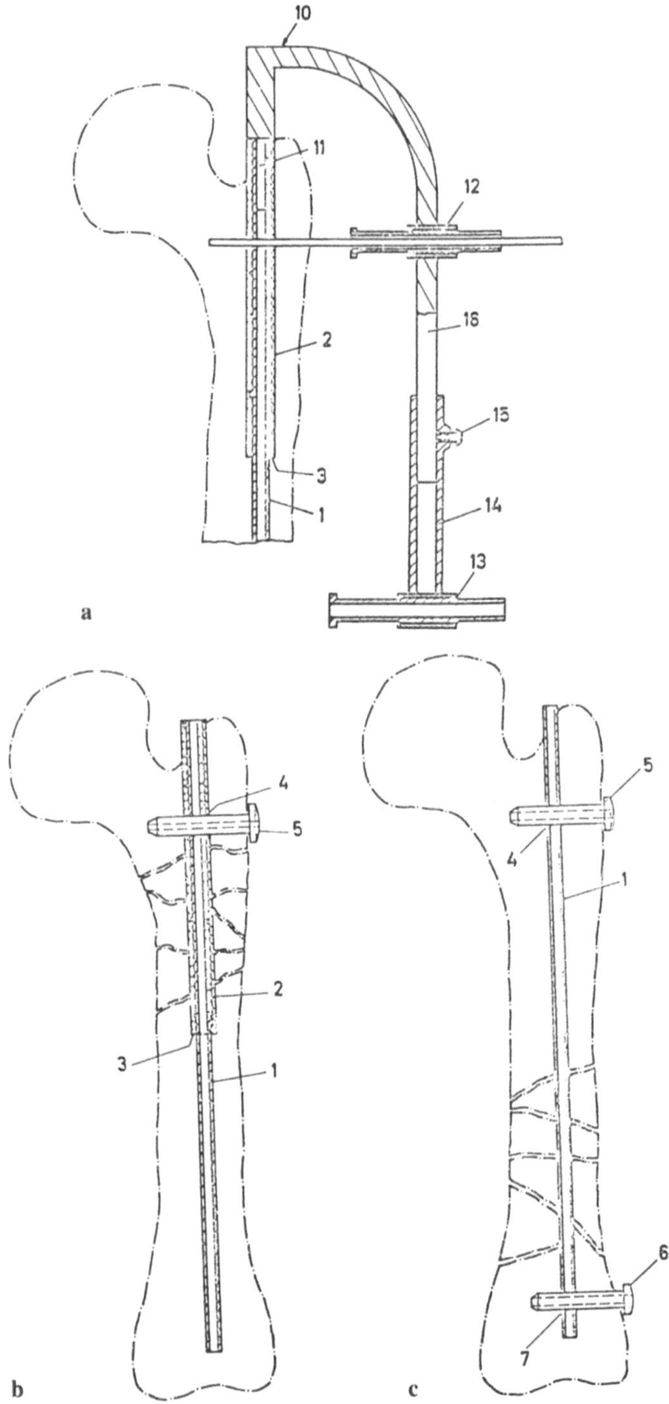

a

b

c

Principles of Locked Nailing

In locked nailing the nail acts as an intramedullary fixator [38]. Stabilization of the fracture is not achieved by elastic deformation of the nail and tight fit in the fractured disphysis (isthmus) but by insertion of locking screws proximal and distal to the fracture [13,14]. Nail locking above and below the fracture is referred to as static nailing and insertion of the proximal and/or distal locking screw as dynamic nailing [13,14]. In the latter the locking screws nearest the fracture line are inserted. This should be used, if at all, only in stable fractures in which shortening due to the full contact of the fragments is impossible. Most surgeons today, however, use locked nailing of fresh fractures in the static mode [16,17].

The term dynamization refers to the removal of the locking screw(s) farthest from the fracture line. After the locking nail became available, this was carried out routinely, but recent studies have shown that routine dynamization of femoral fractures is not justified [17]. Similar findings have been reported for the tibia [1,23]. Dynamization does seem to be necessary, however, in those cases in which locked nailing in the static mode has caused distraction, or when there is an obvious delay in union with little callus formation [28]. The decision whether dynamization or exchange nailing will best lead to consolidation requires individual assessment of the situation and its course [17]. In nonunion, especially in the tibia, the value of dynamization has not been assessed, and we recommend dynamic nailing for stable situations [14]. If dynamization is to be carried out at 12–16 weeks, one must assess the potential of the fracture to shorten [16]. If there is any inherent risk of shortening, dynamization should be postponed.

Reamed and Unreamed Nailing

Intramedullary nailing originally used an unreamed procedure. Initially, Küntscher [45] did not have flexible reamers, but he then welcomed their arrival enthusiastically. The unreamed insertion of a nail allowed the use of only small-diameter implants. Bending and failure of the nail were the logical consequences in some cases [45]. Therefore Küntscher decided for a reaming procedure to allow the implantation of nails of larger diameter and to extend the indication for his type of nailing. In reaming, the medullary canal part of the endosteum is taken out, and fragments of it are pushed into the fracture gap. Experiments with these reamer products have shown that they act as a cell source providing osteoblasts [14,59].

Fig. 1a–c. Drawings from Küntscher's original patent file. **a** Design of a locking nail with nail-mounted jig for distal locking. **b** Proximal locking with a cannulated screw. **c** A comminuted fracture with both proximal and distal locking screws in place

There has been some controversy regarding the tibial blood supply following nailing [43]. After a fracture the intramedullary nutrient artery is disrupted [12], and the periosteal blood supply with its segmental arteries still exists down to the fracture line [45]. The contention that the endosteal blood supply through the nutrient artery is less traumatized by unreamed than by reamed nailing has not been verified in the clinical situation. Using labelled microspheres, it has been shown that the periosteal blood supply is most important [25,49,59], and that the role of the nutrient artery in earlier studies [67,77] may have been exaggerated. The periosteal blood supply reserve in these experiments compensated for the loss of the medullary blood supply [73]. With unreamed nailing the advantage of early loading of the fracture site and thereby weight bearing and recovery of the limb function is not ensured. There is no question but that excessive reaming with thinning of the cortices should be avoided. On the other hand, it is not only the alignment of the fracture but also the capacity of the implant to accept weight bearing that permits restoration of normal function.

The use of unreamed nails in open fractures of the tibia is currently under investigation, and due to the lack of prospective randomized trials no firm recommendation can be made. Two recent investigations allow comparison of unreamed locked nailing and the standard reamed nailing procedure. Court-Brown et al. [24] reported a series of 41 type II and III open tibial fractures (classified according to Gustilo) in which 27 were of type IIIa or IIIb. The incidence of infection in these fractures was 7.4% and all were nailed using a reaming procedure for the Grosse-Kempf locking nail. Results of a similar study by Whittle et al. [82] on the use of the Russell-Taylor unreamed locking nail showed an average time to union of 28 weeks and an infection rate of 12% in 36 type IIIa and IIIb fractures. In the former study 14 fractures were of type IIIa and 13 of type IIIb while in the latter there were 22 type IIIa and 12 type IIIb fractures. It is worth noting that during the period of the Whittle et al. [82] study only about 20% of the total number of compound tibial fractures were treated by unreamed nailing. Both institutions have documented their familiarity with locked nailing in previous publications [22,82].

Since the main objective in the use of unreamed nailing is the avoidance of infection, the unreamed technique seems to have a disadvantage compared to the standard procedure using a reamed locking nail. In addition to the unreamed locking nail, a patella tendon bearing cast must be used for 4 weeks after the operation. This obviously is not necessary with the reamed locking nail. Considering the present financial constraints in most countries, it does not seem justified to add the unreamed locking nail to the necessary equipment in trauma departments since no advantage has been demonstrated for it, and unreamed tibial fractures show an even higher infection rate.

The reamed nails studied are cannulated, and in case of breakage the distal nail end may be removed using this cannula. After breakage of the material with solid-section nails, however, removal in the tibia and especially in the femur can be expected to be hazardous.

At present, reasonable reaming to fit a nail of sufficiently large diameter for the femur and tibia seems an attractive solution: in the femur nails generally of 12 or 13 mm and in the tibia those of 11 mm. Larger medullary canals, however, may accommodate nails of larger diameters.

Technical Aspects of Locked Nailing

Fracture Reduction

Femur

In the femur the recommended position for traction is the supine [22,30,80]. For multiple-trauma victims this position is safer and allows easy access by the anaesthesiologist [15,85]. This also facilitates positioning of the image intensifier and handling of the instruments for distal locking. Most authors therefore recommend the patient be on his back rather than in the lateral decubitus position, which was used in most of Küntscher's original nailings.

Reduction starts with correct insertion of the Steinmann pin in the condyles. The Steinmann pin, with a centrally threaded portion, is inserted from the medial to the lateral site just above the condylar roof. Obviously, the more distal the fracture the more critical this position is. In distal fractures of the femur it is therefore recommended to insert the 5-mm Steinmann pin with the assistance of an image intensifier. In the coronal plane the Steinmann pin is placed in line with the diaphysis of the femur. It should be connected securely to the traction table. To avoid the Steinmann pin slipping out the clamps may have grooves to increase friction. The traction must be counteracted by a central pole against which the patient is pulled. This pole must be covered with suitable material to avoid compression injury to the pudendal nerve [22]. The patient's trunk is bent towards the uninjured site and secured with a support. This allows easy instrumentation of the trochanteric insertion point [30].

The reduction itself is carried out on the traction table and under control of an image intensifier. It is crucial to achieve reduction in both planes before beginning the operation (Fig. 2). In delayed procedures it may be difficult to reach this position [5,9], and nailing should therefore be carried out as early as possible, especially in fermoral fractures associated with head injuries [14,39,47,64,83,84]. In proximal femoral fractures the usual anterior displacement of the proximal fragment can make reduction difficult in the lateral plane, but the axis should be aligned in the anteroposterior plane prior to surgery. Rotation must be controlled carefully, and if the lesser trochanter is fully visible, the distal fragment is rotated outwards appropriately to avoid a rotational deformity. Most com-

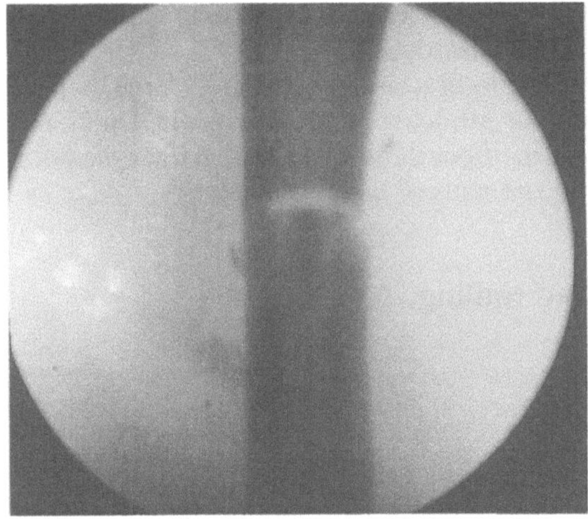

Fig. 2. Intraoperative image of an anatomical reduction prior to guide wire insertion. Femoral shaft fracture

monly the tibia is rotated outwards by about 10°–15°, creating an external rotation of the distal femoral fragment.

With all screws at the traction table tightened securely, the patient's leg is washed circumferentially from above the iliac crest down to the knee. Disposable drapes with a slot are ideal for draping, but these should be sturdy enough to avoid penetration by the Steinmann pin. If there is any doubt, the Steinmann pin ends should be either trimmed or covered with a sterile cloth to avoid compromising sterility. Two slotted drapes are necessary, and the first is placed just above the Steinmann pin. No space should be wasted, especially in distal fractures, to allow free access to the lateral aspect of the femur for the locking procedure. The second slotted drape is applied from above with the tip of the slot, centred on the anterior superior iliac spine. An incision drape should be used, and after application of this drape a horizontal drape is attached to the posterior aspect of the thigh to provide a barrier when an image intensifer is used to screen the lateral aspect of the femur.

Tibia

In the tibia one can use either the traction shoe or in very distal fractures a Steinmann pin through the os calcis [22]. The knee is flexed to about 90°, and the distal femur supported by a leg rest. It is important to leave the popliteal fossa free since the support may press the neurovascular structures against the bone, thereby making them particularly vulnerable to injury when drilling is carried out for the anteroposterior locking screw. When using the traction shoe, this should never extend above the medial malleolus. As an alternative to the traction shoe, the plate of this shoe can be used, with the foot appropriately padded and fixed with adhesive tape 5 cm in width. This fixation must be secure but should not hinder perfusion of the foot. If there is any doubt, it is certainly safer to use an os calcis traction pin [22,30].

Reduction is carried out with the assistance of an image intensifier and is usually more straightforward than in the femur. In cases of an intact fibula, however, reduction may be more difficult. Again, it is emphasized that anatomical positioning of the fragments prior to surgery is crucial for a successful procedure. Before washing the skin one must check that ample space is available for the distal locking screws inserted from the medial side. Again, two slotted drapes should be used, one coming distally from the anterior aspect of the ankle joint and the second entering from above the upper pole of the patella. The rest of the draping is as in the femur.

Humerus

In the humerus no traction device is used. The shoulder should be supported by a sandbag which leaves free access for the image intensifier to provide an unobscured image of the proximal humerus. The trunk of the patient is elevated about 30° and the humerus flexed by about 10°–15° in the shoulder joint. Traction and reduction in nailing procedures of the humerus are carried out manually. The shoulder and arm are washed from the medioclavicular region down to the midshaft of the forearm. A small drape is used to wrap the forearm, and a slotted drape is used from the medioclavicular region down to the axilla. An incision drape is used, but no barrier is necessary [72].

Guide Wire Insertion

Femur

The medullary canal of the femur is opened at the piriform fossa with a pointed awl. The anticurvature of the femur must be considered as well as a possible displacement of the short femoral fragment in a proximal femoral fracture [30]. If in doubt, an image intensifier check is carried out to verify the correct position. The pointed awl should be inserted to a depth of about 2.5–3 cm, and after withdrawing it the guide wire is inserted. The diameter is 4 mm, and the ideal length of the femoral guide wire is 1 m, which is particularly helpful in very distal fractures. If shorter guide wires are used, withdrawal of the reamers causes the entire extraosseous portion of the guide wire to disappear in the reamer and to be removed involuntarily from the distal femoral fragment. The tip of the guide wire should be armed with an olive and be bent by about 25°. This has proven helpful when the entry point of the distal fragment is sought [22].

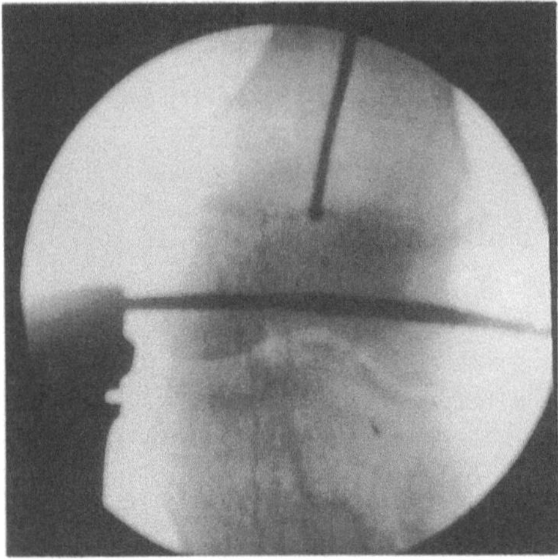

Fig. 3. Correct positioning of the guide wire in a distal femoral fracture. Note the very distal position of the transverse Steinmann traction pin

The guide wire is inserted down the proximal fragment under image intensifier control and is pushed into the distal fragment. If this is difficult, the correct positioning of fragments in the anteroposterior and lateral views must be verified. With the assistance of a short Küntscher nail introduced into a short proximal fragment this can be manipulated until reduction is carried out. If necessary, the fragments are be pushed into place manually while the guide wire is inserted. Particularly in segmental fractured feeding the guide wire into the distal fragment can be difficult. It may be helpful temporarily to stabilize the proximal of the two fracture lines with a small-diameter nail, and a further attempt to insert the guide wire into the distal fragment can then be made. The guide wire should then be pushed down, and the condyles should be displayed on the image intensifier screen. The correct point of the guide wire distally is just above the condylar roof (Fig. 3). Any positioning of the guide wire to the medial or lateral side results in valgus or varus positioning of the nail. This is particularly crucial in distal fractures in which the medullary canal is so wide that misplacement of the nail can easily occur.

Tibia

In the tibia the patellar ligament should be split after a longitudinal incision, and the medullary canal is opened just below the tibial plateau. Especially in osteoporotic bone care must be taken not to penetrate the posterior cortex with the pointed awl or the guide wire. A slightly shorter guide wire (0.8 m) may be used, and the insertion to the distal fragment follows the technique described for the femur. In the tibia the ankle joint must be displayed clearly in the image intensifier, and the tip of the guide wire should sit in the subchondral bone just above the centre of the talus.

Humerus

In the humerus all current techniques employ a deltoid-splitting approach with a longitudinal incision of the rotator cuff. Just medial to the greater tubercle the medullary canal is opened, and care is taken to avoid a crushing injury to the cuff. Reduction is carried out manually, and the guide wire inserted into the distal fragment. This guide wire can be 0.6 m in length and the olive should sit just above the fossa olecrani. The correct positioning of the guide wire is always verified in both planes.

Reaming

A soft-tissue protector must be fastened securely prior to reaming. A variety of reamers are available, but we prefer the type that cuts both at the tip and at the side of the reamer head. The procedure begins with an 8- or 9-mm reamer depending on the width of the medullary canal. In older patients 1-mm steps can be taken but in younger patients 0.5-mm increments. We routinely ream 1 mm more than the selected nail size, and in general we prefer nails of smaller diameter unless the skeleton can easily accommodate a larger implant. If there is a significant curvature, especially in the femur, reaming should be 1.5 or 2 mm more than the selected nail size. It is important always to ream the full length of the medullary canal to direct the nail down into the cancellous metaphyseal bone. Undue pressure must be avoided while reaming.

If the reamer head becomes stuck, it can be taken out with the assistance of the olive at the tip of the guide wire [81]. This helps to withdraw the reamer when the guide wire is held with forceps, against which gentle taps with a hammer are carried out. In segmental fractures of the tibia care is taken that the segment does not rotate [81]. Increments of 0.5 mm in reaming are therefore mandatory. In a free-floating segment it may be helpful to hold it with a pair of forceps to avoid rotation of the fragment, which invariably impairs vascularization [81]. Especially in nailing of atrophic nonunions the reamer products should be harvested and may be inserted at the end of the reaming process into the nonunion site with the aid of a nasogastric tube. This provides excellent bone graft and, in our experience, promotes callus formation [13].

Nail Insertion

Prior to nail insertion the correct length of the required nail must be measured. The direct method consists of using a ruler to measure the length from the supracondylar area to the greater trochanter in the femur and the length from the supramalleolar region to the tibial tuberosity. In the humerus the position at which the guide wire ends can be taken as the reference point for measuring. Alternatively, the length of the guide wire can be established beforehand and the section of the guide wire outside the bone measured, thereby allowing calculation of the nail length.

The correct alignment of the fracture must be checked again before nail insertion. Reaming is carried out with a 4-mm guide wire for nail insertion, but this can be replaced by a 5-mm nail insertion wire [30]. For this, a sufficiently long polyethylene tube is pushed over the first guide wire. The two guide wires are now exchanged, and nail insertion may begin. Most nailing systems provide a handle that guides the nail down the medullary canal and also allows hammering on it. A 500-g mallet may be used to drive the nail down with gentle taps. No undue force must be used, and in the femur care is to be taken not to insert the nail pushing too hard against the medial cortex in the subtrochanteric region. This may lead to additional fractures or cracking of the bone [16,22,81]. In the tibia a particularly vulnerable area is the posterior cortex, which especially in osteoporotic bone is rather fragile. If the point of entry is too far laterally, the medial cortex is in danger and, conversely, if too far medially the lateral cortex. If the nail does not progress despite gentle driving taps, it is safer to remove the nail and to ream 0.5–1 mm more.

If a fracture occurs during nail insertion, the nail should always be locked statically [16,81]. Weight bearing may have to be delayed depending on the site and the severity of the problem. With the exception of the humerus the nail should be long enough to pass down to the metaphyseal bone and should not significantly exceed the greater trochanter and, for the tibia, not beyond the tibial tuberosity. In the later case the patient invariably complains of knee pain, and constant irritation may be the consequence.

Hammering during nail insertion may loosen the guide wire, which has been anchored in the subchondral bone and force it upwards. One must be aware of this problem and avoid it by an assistant holding the guide wire firmly down and pushing it forward in the medullary canal. If this is not closely observed, the nail especially in the femur may end up in a valgus position with the tip of the nail sitting in the medial condyle.

Proximal Locking

All currently available locking nail systems allow proximal locking with a nail-mounted template. There is no clinical evidence that more than one locking screw should be used, but in osteoporotic bone single locking may present a problem [56]. This extends the working length of the nail if the locking screws are sited in the trochanteric region and do not reach below the lesser trochanter. Holes in the nail create a mechanical weakness, and the highest forces occur in the area of the nail just below the lesser trochanter [37]. Therefore an oblique locking screw or locking screws above or at the level of the lesser trochanter seem to be more reasonable (Fig. 4). With the proximal locking in this position, in principle all fractures below the lesser trochanter can be nailed as long as it is intact. In systems with a smooth proximal nail hole the screw is engaged in the cancellous bone and finds anchorage in the medial cortex at the end of the femoral neck. In some

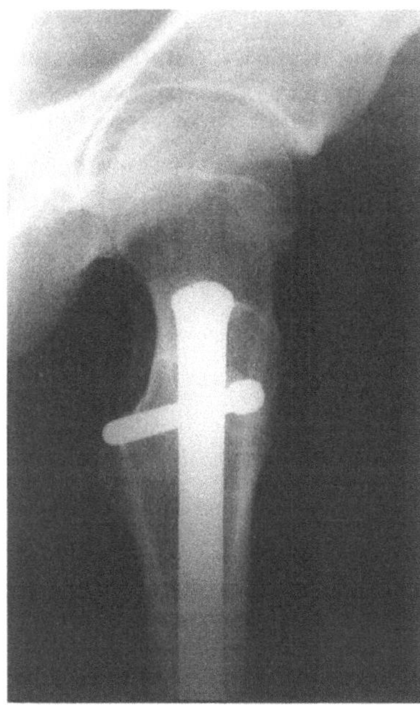

Fig. 4. Correct positioning of a femoral locking nail (lateral view). Note the posterior position of the proximal locking screw due to nail rotation

nails the hole is threaded, and an appropriate locking screw must be used [30]. In any case, the correct alignment of nail and template must be tested prior to nail insertion [81]. This allows identification of a deformed template that may have been abused during previous operations. The locking screw length should be sufficient to pass the inner cortex of the calar.

Distal Locking

Distal locking is seen by some surgeons as the Achilles tendon of the locking nail concept. To circumvent the insertion of distal locking screws some nail systems (e.g. that of Brooker and Wills) have used flanges which extrude from the nail after an inner metal rod pushes them out. In midshaft fractures these flanges theoretically provide sufficient rotational stability, but in distal fractures and in osteoporotic bone problems are evident. Also during nail removal the flanges may not retract and may lead to considerable problems [22].

Most currently available systems use two distal locking screws to provide rotational stability and avoid shortening. Despite several attempts to design a nail-mounted device the free-hand technique for insertion of the screws seems the most popular. The nail-mounted insertion jig is not effective since the nail usually rotates and deforms during insertion [22]. An early solution to distal locking that was elegant but cumbersome proposed mounting the jig on the image intensifier [41]. This allows distal screw insertion without any radiation to the surgeon's hands; however, this is time consuming and requires considerable expertise with the adjustment. The radiographer must be trained and familiar with the technique to perform the necessary steps without significant delay [22].

The use of hand-held pointed awls is extremely popular, but there is considerable risk of involuntary radiation to the hand. Therefore a distal targeting device (Howmedica; Fig. 5) has been designed which facilitates

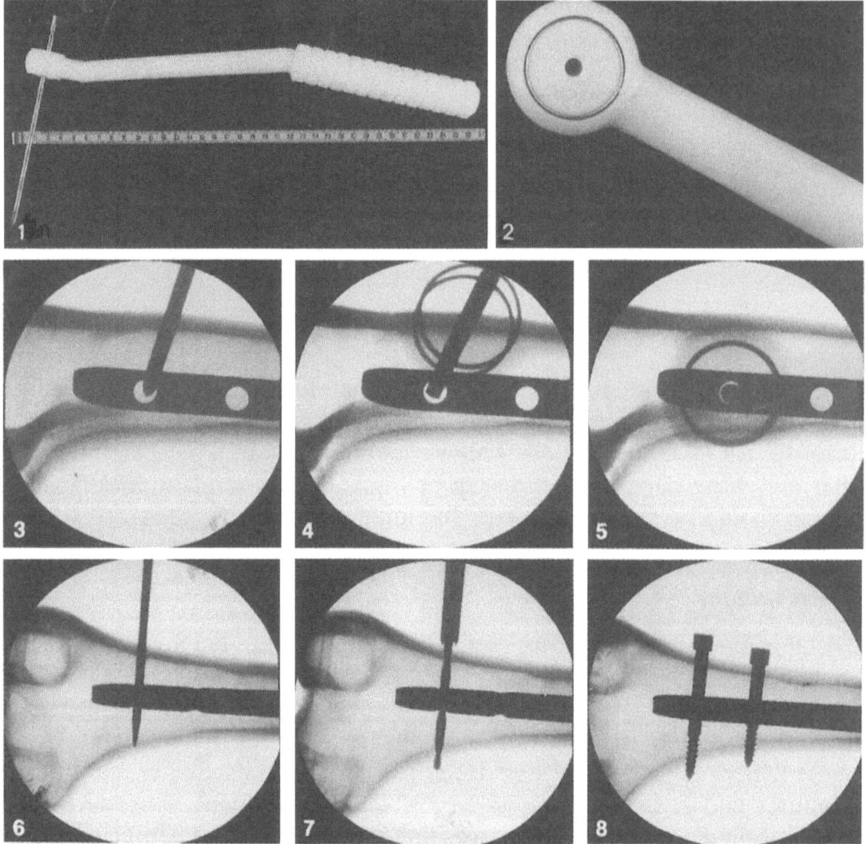

Fig. 5. Pennig-Brug free-hand target device (Howmedica, Germany). *1* With Steinmann pin in place. *2* Metal ring embedded on top and bottom of the cylinder. *3* After precise adjustment of the image intensifier, with the nail hole appearing as a circle, the guide wire pin is inserted and placed in the centre of this circle. *4* The target device with the two metal rings is manipulated. *5* Manipulation continues until only one ring is seen on the screen. *6* The anteroposterior view demonstrates only the correct positioning of the Steinmann pin without penetration of the far cortex. *7* Drilling of the far cortex and near cortex with the appropriate drill bits. *8* Correct length and placement of the distal cross-screws. (From [63,65])

insertion of the distal screws [63,65]. A prerequisite of successful distal locking in femur and tibia is correct alignment of the image intensifier. The images of the nail holes on the screen must be round, and a left/right movement along the leg must appear in the same direction on the image intensifier screen; otherwise handling of a targetting device becomes ineffective. The targetting device is made of medical grade plastic and consists of a handle, a stem and a cylinder. The cylinder accomodates a 4-mm Steinmann pin with a sharp tip. Metal rings are embedded on the top and bottom of this cylinder.

At the start of distal locking the position of the nail hole with reference to the skin must be established. An incision 15 mm long is made, and the soft tissues are divided down to the bone with scissors. The targetting device with the Steinmann pin in place is inserted so that the tip appears within the nail hole on the image intensifier screen. The device is now manipulated until the two metal rings are superimposed, and the Steinmann pin is therefore in line with the nail hole axis. The Steinmann pin, controlled with the targetting device, is now driven through the near cortex into the nail, and once again the position is checked with the image intensifier. The opposite cortex must not be penetrated since this may lead to an enlarged hole. The targetting device is now withdrawn and a 6.5-mm drill sleeve with a handle is pushed over the Steinmann pin. The Steinmann pin is removed, and the appropriate drill for penetration of the opposite cortex is chosen. The near cortex is enlarged with the suitable drill. The length of the required locking screw may be measured with a depth gauge.

Especially in the femur, where soft-tissue interposition renders correct measuring an impractical technique, this can be quite frustrating, and imitially the selected locking screw should not be inserted fully in order to facilitate exchange of this screw after an anteroposterior check. To overcome the problem of correct screw selection, a radiotransparent measuring device has been developed (Lukosch and Pennig, Richards). The use of this device is illustrated in Fig. 6. During the nailing procedure the last image prior to distal targetting which is checked is the position of the nail tip. At this point the radiotransparent measuring device is inserted, and on the level of the nail hole the distance from one cortex to another is measured. The correct point within the nail hole is the distal rim of the hole. The procedure is repeated for the second locking screw, and thereafter the image intensifier is repositioned for distal targetting. At the end of the locking procedure a check in both planes is made to ensure correct placement of the locking screws.

In osteoporotic bone a dowel bolt [81] has been designed which not only relies on anchorage in the bone but due to an expanding mechanism is secured inside the nail. This has also been a useful device in accidentally enlarged screw holes.

Before the operation is terminated a check of the whole nail in both planes is advisable.

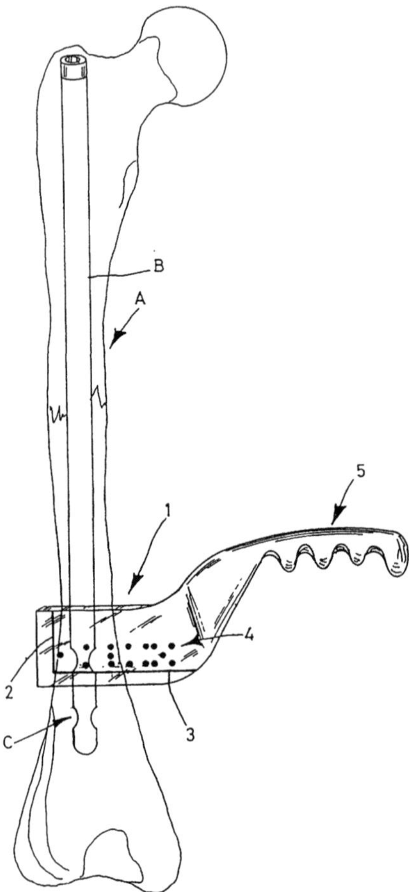

Fig. 6. Radiographic ruler for measuring the cross-screw length. After alignment of the device the required cross-screw length can be determined

Clinical Use of the Locking Nail

Femoral Shaft

Femoral fractures below the lesser trochanter and above the supracondylar region are suitable for closed nailing. Perhaps the easiest nailing is carried out in midshaft fractures where there is an intact portion of the tubular diaphysis above and below the fracture. This directs the nail down and makes valgus or varus displacement unlikely. With the diaphyseal tube widening towards the metaphysis proximally and distally, malalignment in valgus or varus presents a higher risk.

With a large area of comminution the correct length of the nail to be used can be assessed after taking a calibrated X-ray from the opposite femur. It is recommended to lock all midshaft fractures statically irrespective of the degree of comminution.

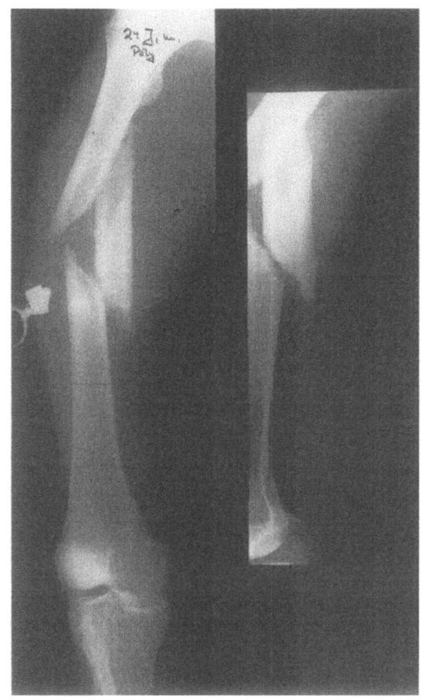

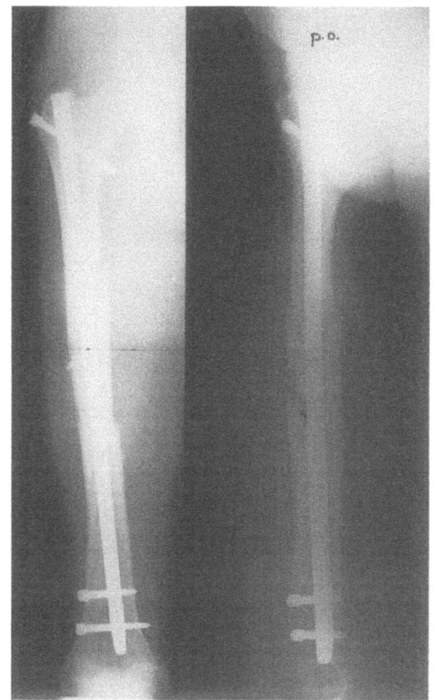

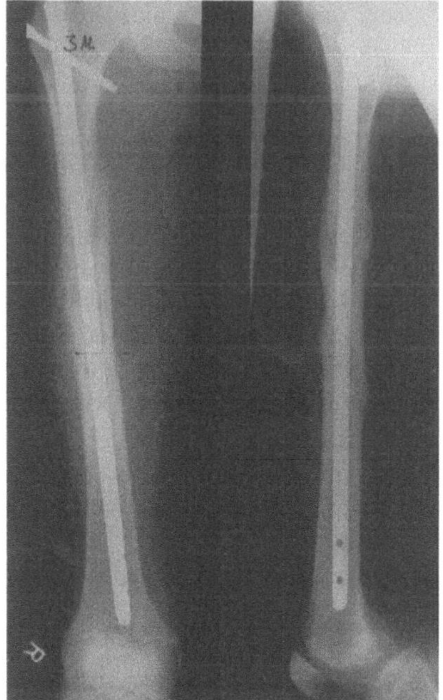

Fig. 7a–c. A 24-year-old patient. **a** Segmental fracture of the femur involving the femoral diaphysis. **b** Closed locked nailing, static mode. **c** After 3 months, callus healing, full weight bearing; distal locking screws were removed

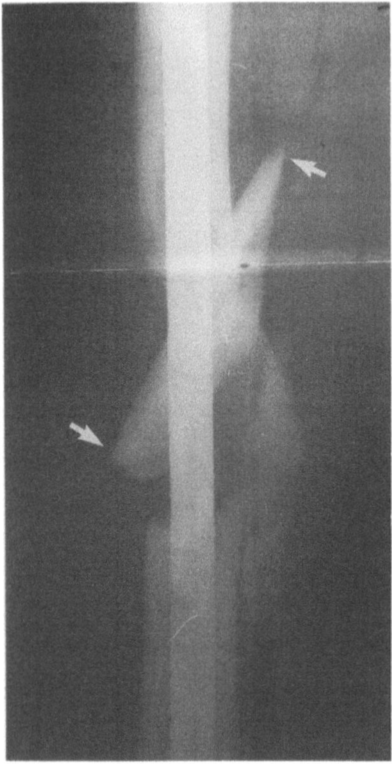

Fig. 8. Comminuted femoral shaft fracture with a severely rotated fragment (*arrows*). If left alone, the fragment becomes incorporated in the callus

In contrast to the meticulously restored fragments in plating techniques, locked nailing does not require the singular fragments to be in their anatomical position. The only aim of closed intramedullary nailing is the restoration of length and axis (Fig. 7). Due to the closed technique and the reaming products being distributed within the fracture area callus healing is almost guaranteed [39,42,62,75,85]. Even larger fragments rotated up to 180° should not be openly reduced [81] (Fig. 8), and cerclage wires certainly cannot be recommended to supplement a locked nailing procedure [13,14,30]. Reduction of a rotated fragment can be recommended only in cases in which a larger fragment penetrates, for example, the quadriceps muscle. If flexion and extension of the knee and hip joints are impaired, and this does not resolve after intensive physiotherapy, there is an indication either to remove this fragment or change its position so that the muscular function is no longer impaired. This, however, is extremely rare.

Femur: Proximal Fractures

As long as the lesser trochanter is completely intact, proximal fractures of the femur may be nailed (Fig. 9). Due to the short proximal fragment and the muscular pull, however, reduction of the fracture is more difficult. If

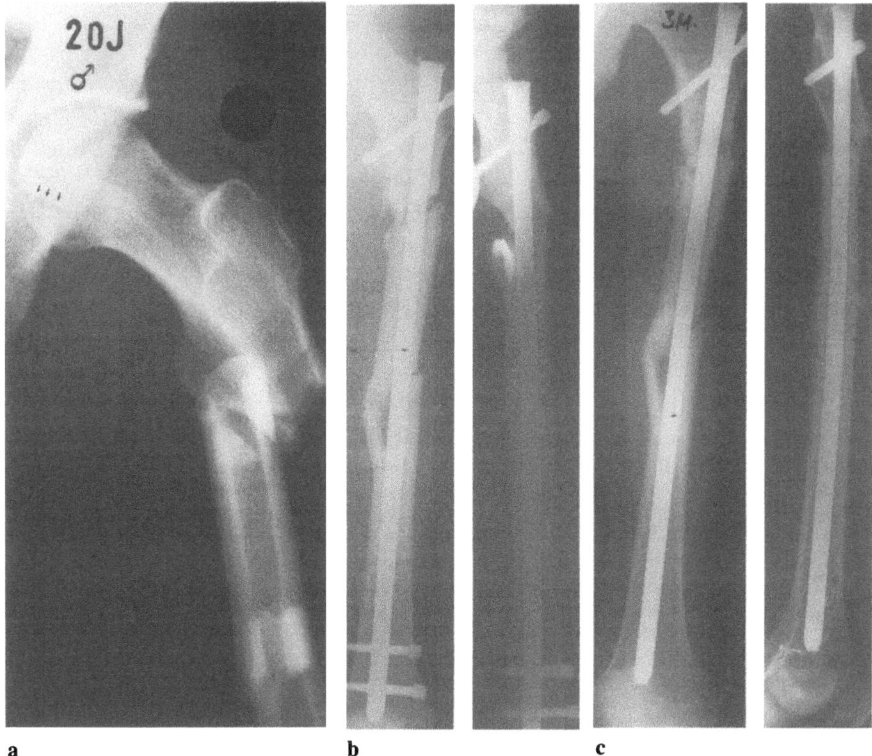

a   b   c

Fig. 9a–c. A young male. **a** Extremely proximal segmental fracture of the left femur. **b** Closed statically locked nailing. Note the slightly anterior point of entry. **c** After 3 months, callus formation, with full weight bearing

in the lateral view there is still a displacement of the proximal fragment anteriorly, this may be corrected intraoperatively after guide wire insertion into the proximal fragment and reaming to 10 mm with the assistance of a short 8- to 9-mm Küntscher nail. This is slit over the guide wire and the fragment manipulated until the guide wire can be inserted into the distal fragment. Nailing of proximal fractures requires considerably more expertise than nailing of shaft fractures and should not be attempted early in one's experience.

Pathological fractures are more common in the proximal part of the femur and may be stabilized with a statically locked nail provided the proximal locking screw sits in radiologically unaffected bone [36,61,71]. The technique has been described in detail elsewhere [61].

Femur: Distal Fractures

Most distal femoral fractures not extending into the condylar region can be nailed. In planning the procedure it is important to establish that the proximal of the two distal locking screws is below the fracture line. Steinmann pin insertion for traction should be performed under fluoroscopic control, and if there is any doubt whether the Steinmann pin may interfere with the distal locking procedure, it is safer to use traction through the proximal tibia. The ante- and retrocurvature of the distal fragment must be observed closely in the lateral view and is corrected by flexing or extending the tibia in the knee joint. The guide wire must be precisely above the condylar roof; otherwise valgus or varus deformities occur (Fig. 3). Since the whole diaphysis is intact in these fractures, the nail must pass this variably curved part of the femur. Therefore overreaming of 1.5–2 mm can be recommended. This avoids excessive hammering which may displace the distal fracture. The nail should be driven in under fluoroscopic control and should end at least 5 mm proximal to the cortex of the condylar roof. If it penetrates any further, cracks in the cartilage may occur. It is worth remembering that the nail ends anterior to the deepest point of the condyles. Locking should always be carried out using two screws since the use of only one screw might allow rotation of the distal fragment when the knee is flexed and extended [16].

Technically it is possible to nail fractures that extend even farther distally with fracture lines in the condylar region. This, however, requires considerable expertise and the use of supplementary techniques such as lag-screw fixation (Fig. 10) [3].

The operation usually begins with reconstruction of the condylar fracture, and the nail is used to bridge the supracondylar fracture portion. Meticulous operative technique is necessary for successful use of the locking nail in these situations.

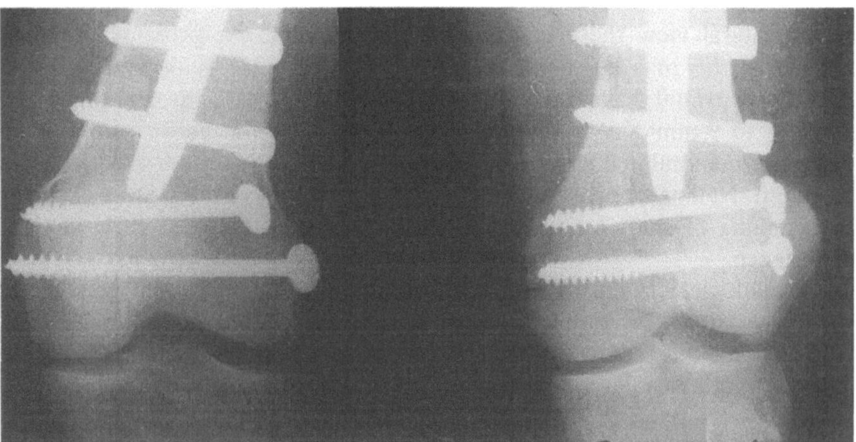

Fig. 10. Femoral shaft fracture associated with a pericondylar fracture of the femur. The lag screws were inserted prior to nail insertion

Femur: Combination Fractures [3]

A femoral shaft fracture in combination with a femoral neck fracture or a peritrochanteric fracture presents a challenging situation. Biomechanically the two fractures are very different and therefore require specific techniques [13,14]. Usually the femoral neck fracture is reduced in abduction and the femoral shaft fracture in adduction.

If the femoral neck fracture is not displaced, the medullary canal after cautious opening with the pointed awl is reamed at least 2 mm over the selected nail size. For the average patient the smallest possible nail size should be chosen, and the nail should be pushed into the medullary canal rather than being hammered, as hammering may displace the neck fracture. The point of entry should be in the centre of the greater trochanter at the

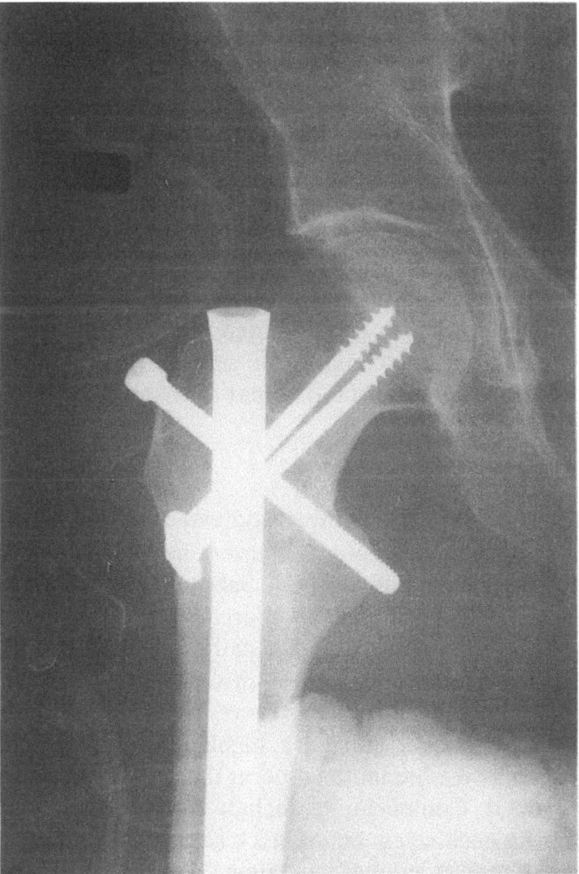

Fig. 11. Comminuted fracture of the femoral shaft associated with a femoral neck fracture. One screw in front and one screw behind the locking nail

piriform fossa. This leaves space for one screw inserted anterior to the nail and one inserted posterior to the nail (Fig. 11). It is recommended to first use a 2.5-mm Kirschner wire to establish the correct path for the drill. After checking in both planes the Kirschner wire can be removed, and after drilling with an appropriate drill bit a cancellous bone screw such as a lag screw should be inserted. Washers should be used in any case. In heavy patients three or even four screws may be inserted [22].

In a displaced fracture of the femoral neck, this fracture must be reduced beforehand. Reduction can be maintained with 2.5-mm Kirschner wires inserted so that they are unlikely to obstruct or interfere with the reamer. Again, a small-diameter nail should be used. The Kirschner wires are subsequently withdrawn one by one and replaced by two or more lag screws. The femoral shaft fracture in these combination fractures is treated according to the principles outlined above. Weight bearing should be delayed in these patients for at least 6 weeks, or until union has been established in the neck fracture.

The Richards reconstruction nail system [22] allows the placement of two screws through the nail at a fixed angle. This nail has reportedly been used successfully by some authors [22].

The centre line of the neck and the centre line of the diaphysis, however, do not match, and the neck is offset with regard to the diaphysis. Therefore screws inserted through the nail must compromise the normal anatomical relationships.

The incidence of combination fractures is less than 2%, and their importance may have been exaggerated in the past. It is certainly possible with the presently available nailing systems to treat isolated femoral fractures as well as combination fractures, but a technique for safe and reproducible placement of femoral neck screws around the nail may be helpful.

Peritrochanteric Femoral Fractures

The treatment of peritrochanteric fractures was addressed by Küntscher, who developed the Y nail. With some regret, however, he stated that the use of this device seems to be rather difficult [45]. Subsequently, based on the same principle, Zickel [6,87] developed another device with a single large-diameter screw for the femoral neck and a nail (unlocked) for the shaft. With this device peritrochanteric as well as inverse peritrochanteric and subtrochanteric fractures have been treated. There are few statistics on the Y nail, but reports on the Zickel nail have highlighted some of the problems that occur when a massive implant is used in the proximal femoral metaphysis and diaphysis [6,73]. Complications include fractures below the implant and cutting out of the neck screw or the neck screw/nail unit.

Based on the principle of locked nailing, the gamma nail was introduced in 1990 (Howmedica) [10,48]. Subsequently a similar device (Classic Nail) was presented by Richards. The principle of the gamma nail is that of a short intermedullary nail which permits distal locking and introduction of a single neck screw through the nail. This neck screw together with the instrumentation allows compression as well as a sliding movement. The basic instrumentation is similar to that of the femoral nail. Reduction is carried out on a traction table with the foot in a traction shoe. Most peritrochanteric fractures reduce in abduction and internal rotation. This necessitates the trunk of the patient to be moved away to the opposite site to permit unhindered instrumentation of the femoral canal. Since the gamma nail has a curvature of 10° (Howmedica) the point of insertion is the tip of the greater trochanter and not the piriform fossa.

After reaming down to the isthmus the proximal portion must be enlarged to 17 mm to allow the insertion of the gamma nail. In our experience the smallest gamma nail (11 mm) is adequate for most patients. Preoperatively on the opposite site the necessary angle for the neck screw must be measured. The standard angles to be used are 130° and 135°. After insertion of the gamma nail the neck screw is placed with the assistance of a jig. Prior to insertion of the neck screw the correct positioning of the guide wire is be

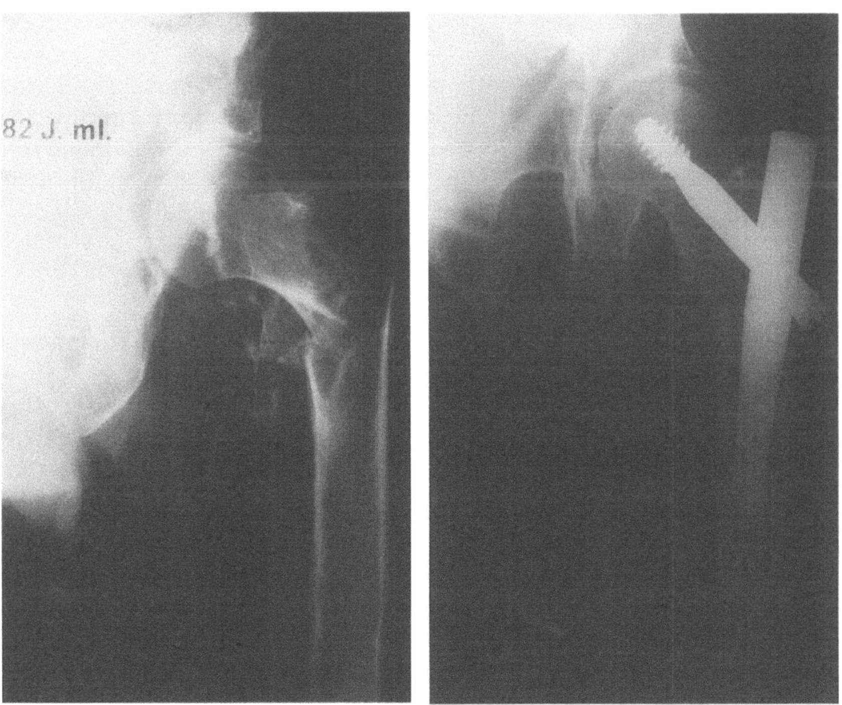

Fig. 12a,b. An 82-year old man with severe osteoporosis. **a** Unstable peritrochanteric fracture. **b** Closed nailing using a gamma nail with correct placement of the neck screw. One distal locking screw in the proximal position seems sufficient to control rotation and length

verified on both planes. In the Lauenstein view the guide wire should be placed centrally in the femoral head and in the anteroposterior view in the lower half of the femoral neck. In any case the neck screw must be long enough and should be anchored in the subchondral bone of the femoral head. In our opinion, one distal screw should be inserted in all cases in which the gamma nail is used, and we prefer to use the proximal hole for this screw (Fig. 12).

The main advantage of the gamma nail compared to other techniques [11,25,86] is completely unconstrained weight bearing postoperatively on day 1, due to the biomechanical advantage of an intramedullary implant. For subtrochanteric fractures the device may be used, but the standard locking nail is also an acceptable implant for this indication [13,34]. In cases of a combination between a peritrochanteric fracture and a femoral shaft fracture as well as for peritrochanteric fractures extending down into the diaphysis a long gamma nail is under investigation (Grosse and Taglang, personal communication). For Asian patients a modification with a medio-lateral curvature of 7° instead of 10° and a smaller distal portion has been developed [46].

Tibial Fractures

Whereas most surgeons agree on the benefits of intramedullary locked nailing for the femur, that in the tibia is somewhat more controversial [2,60]. The obvious difference between femur and tibia is evident in the soft-tissue situation. A large part of the tibia is covered by a thin soft-tissue envelope [57] which may be compromised by the fracture [20].

Tibial Shaft

In tibial shaft fractures assessment of the soft-tissue envelope is important for the timing and successful application of the nailing technique. Soft-tissue recovery is influenced positively by stabilization of the tibia. However, it is important to avoid additional damage due to overdistraction and excessive reaming [22]. The soft-tissue injury in closed fractures is best classified according to Oestern and Tscherne [57–61]. Closed fractures of types C-O and C-I with unstable fractures are probably ideal to gain early experience with the lock nailing technique. Type C-II (extensive bruising) and C-III (compartment syndrome) require considerable expertise in handling both the soft tissue and the nailing procedure and can perhaps be treated more safely with a unilateral external fixator [60]. Preoperative antibiotic prophylaxis can be recommended [8].

Soft-tissue injury in compound fractures is classified according to Gustilo [31,32]. Type I fractures have a similar prognosis as closed fractures and after soft-tissue débridement are nailed (static mode) without delay under antibiotic cover [23]. Type II fractures with more extensive soft-tissue damage require careful assessment, competent débridement [27,60] and a decision as to whether to use a nail or an external fixator [4,60,70]. If there is any doubt with regard to the viability of soft-tissues and bone, an external fixator appears safer. The same applies to fractures of type IIIa or IIIb. However, recent studies have shown that in skilled hands even type III fractures can be successfully nailed [24]. In any case, delayed closure of the soft-tissue envelope in all compound fractures is mandatory [20,31,32].

In nailing of tibial shaft fractures our current practice is to use small-diameter nails (11 or 12 mm). This avoids extensive reaming, shortens the procedure and enhances safety. All compound and unstable fractures should be nailed statically. In deciding whether to use a static or dynamic procedure, the potential for the fracture to shorten must be assessed. At least 50% of the cortex must be in contact in the midshaft area, and this cortical contact area should be perfectly reduced after nail insertion. If this is not the case, static locking is safer. In more distal fractures that are stable (transverse and short oblique) only distal locking may be carried out. Two locking screws should be inserted, but recent studies have shown that one locking screw distally may control the stability sufficiently [22]. In more proximal stable fractures (transverse and short oblique) proximal locking is carried out in both planes. We recommend the use of two screws to account for the longer lever arm and in recognition of the wider metaphysis proximally (Fig. 13). If the situation requires only one proximal locking screw, we prefer the mediolateral screw, which at least theoretically seems safer than the anteroposterior screw.

Proximal Fractures

Proximal fractures of the tibia are difficult to nail correctly since even a slight misplacement of the point of entry causes a malunion to occur. Unilateral external fixation should therefore be considered in extra-articular proximal fractures [60]. When a nailing procedure has been selected, anatomical reduction in both planes prior to insertion of the guide wire is compulsory. The point of entry is then of critical importance and must be checked using an image intensifier. Due to the bending forces in proximal fractures, a 12-mm nail may be selected as the implant, but in larger patients one of even larger diameter may be necessary. Correct insertion of both proximal locking screws with penetration of the opposite cortex is necessary to avoid loosening of those screws (Fig. 13). The increased mobility with inadequate proximal locking can lead to the development of a nonunion. If the fracture is unstable, distal locking is carried out using only one screw since the whole length of the diaphysis supports the nail. With proximal fractures the risk of compartment syndrome must be considered [76], and continuous monitoring is advisable [22].

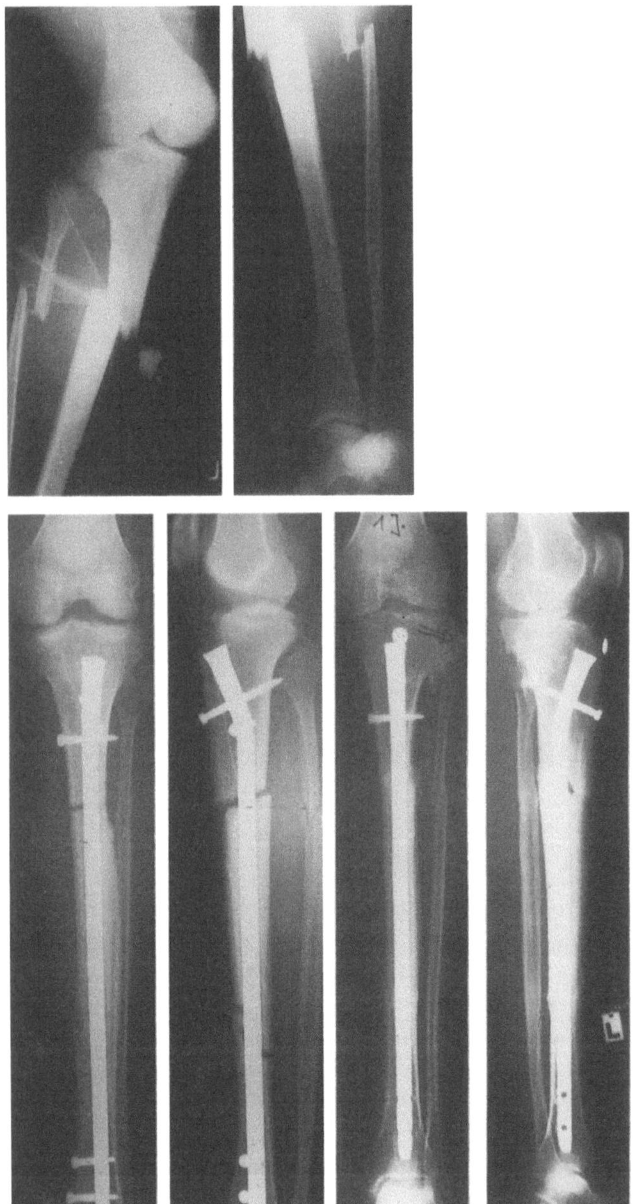

Fig. 13a–c. YOUNG man. **a** Segmental fracture of the tibia. Note displacement of the fibular head. Closed statically locked nailing with correct length of the proximal cross-screws. **b** The distal cross-screws are slightly short. **c** Follow-up after 1 year showing callus consolidation of the fracture; distal cross-screws were removed

Distal Fractures

As in distal fractures of the femur, care is taken to ensure free access to the distal locking holes, and draping should appreciate this. To apply the traction a foot plate or an os calcis pin may be employed. For the successful treatment of distal tibial fractures the correct placement of the guide wire in the centre of the distal articular surface is of utmost importance. Any placement to the medial or lateral side invariably causes malunion and may require a corrective procedure later. As with shaft and proximal fractures, the rotation must be carefully controlled, and the best way to achieve this is to have the distal femur strictly horizontal and the foot rotated externally by about 10°.

We recommend overreaming of 1–1.5 mm to facilitate nail insertion through the entire (intact) diaphysis. While hammering the nail through the medullary canal, the guide wire tends to move up as the nail moves down. This is avoided by maintaining constant pressure on the guide wire. In osteoporotic bone the progress of the nail, especially in the distal third, must be observed since involuntary penetration of the articular surface by a jammed guide wire may be possible. With static locking a single proximal screw inserted mediolaterally may be sufficient.

Ideally the more proximal of the two distal screws should not compromise the main fracture line. This requires careful preoperative planning to assess whether a nailing procedure is suitable for the fracture. After having gained considerable experience one can take the nail tip off with a hack saw to nail extremely distal fractures (Fig. 14). This, however, is an extension of the indication and bears additional risks. Preoperatively the correct nail length must be selected unless there are sterile facilities for taking the nail tip off and breaking the edges. It should be overreamed by 1.5 mm, and usually a 11- or 12-mm nail is selected. After preparation of the medullary canal a nail with a standard tip of the same diameter is used as a template and inserted into the medullary canal. This nail must progress easily through the canal; otherwise further reaming is necessary. The nail is inserted fully and is subsequently withdrawn. The cut nail is now inserted without applying undue force. If excessive resistance is felt, the nail is removed and further reaming performed. Use of the dowel bolt can be recommended to gain better purchase for distal locking [80].

Measurement of the correct locking screw length follows the principles outlined for the femur.

Fractures of the Humerus

Intramedullary nailing of the humerus was also pioneered by Küntscher [45], using a single hollow nail, and by Hackethal [33], using multiple nested nails of 3 mm diameter. Both used antegrade and retrograde nailing procedures depending on the fracture locations. Küntscher used a reamed

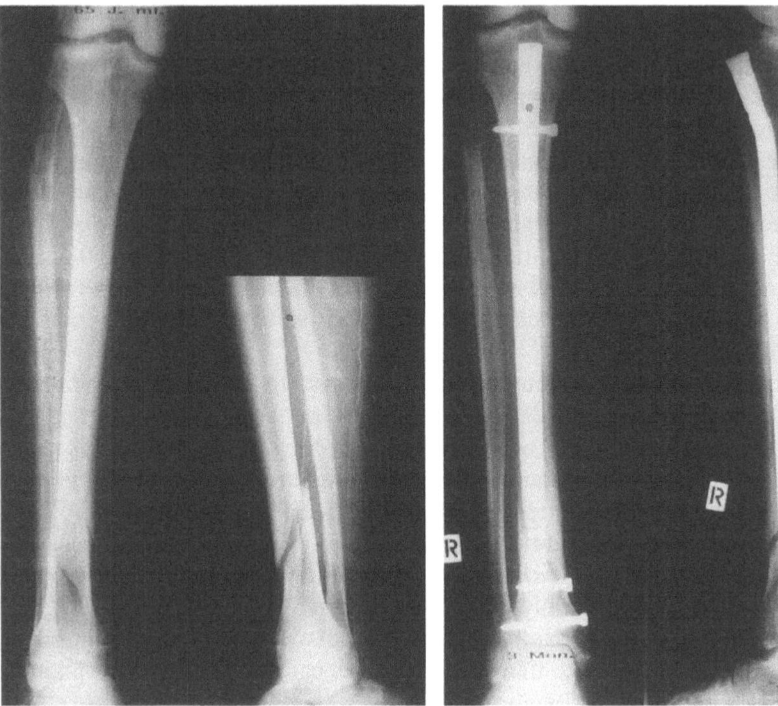

Fig. 14a,b. Locked nailing of an extremely distal tibial fracture with the tip of the nail being cut off preoperatively

procedure entering through the rotator cuff insertion at the greater tubercle, while Hackethal entered through the lesser tubercle and used an unreamed technique. Especially Hackethal's experience was later repeated using Rush pins and Ender's nails.

Following the development of locking nails for femur and tibia, a locking nail was also developed for the humerus by Seidel [72]. This nail has an anteroposterior and a lateromedial screw for proximal locking, and distal locking is achieved through an expansion mechanism by which nail flanges expand into the medullary canal.

Humerus: Shaft Fractures

The humeral locking nail as described by Seidel [72] has a diameter of 9 mm and requires reaming of up to 10 mm. Especially in comminuted fractures the reamer head must be pushed over the area of comminution with the motor switched off. There is an inherent risk of radial nerve damage when reaming is carried out under these circumstances. In general, the longest possible humeral nail should be used, and the entire medullary canal is reamed just above the fossa olecrani. The medullary canal of the humerus has a carrot shape and therefore differs considerably from the shape of the medullary canal encountered in femur and tibia. The nail is inserted more by pushing than by hammering and is buried below the cortex of the humeral head. The distal expansion screw is turned counter-clockwise to spread the flanges of the nail about 1 mm. This process must be checked with an image intensifier.

Proximal locking is then carried out with a nail-mounted jig. If there is an intact part of the diaphysis proximal to the fracture, and bone stock is within normal limits, one locking screw seems sufficient. For safety reasons we prefer the lateromedial screw. After a stab incision the soft tissues are divided down to the bone, and the guide sleeve is engaged firmly on the lateral cortex. The screws are predrilled, and care is taken not to injure the medial neurovascular bundle. The screws are self-tapping, and the correct length must be selected. If a second screw is necessary, this is performed through an extension of the nail-mounted jig. Care must be taken to avoid injury to the axillary nerve on the posterior aspect of the humerus when drilling for this screw. Anteriorly the biceps tendon can be damaged during

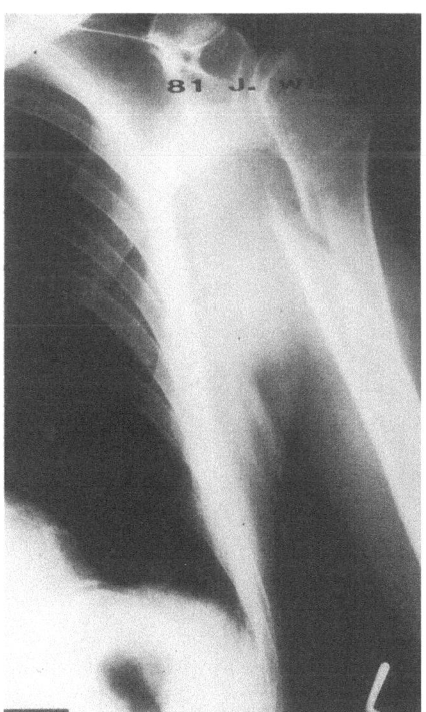
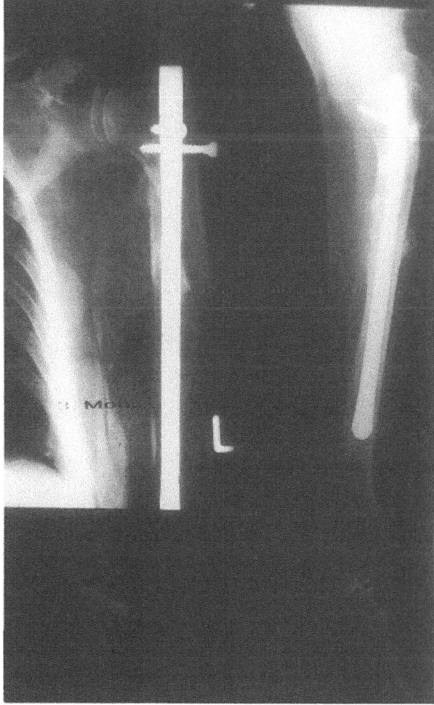

Fig. 15a,b. Fracture of the proximal humerus. Closed nailing using the Seidel nail (Howmedica)

drilling. Correctly measuring the length of the anteroposterior screw can present technical difficulties, but this should not be too long to avoid any irritation to the neural structure posteriorly.

Humerus: Proximal Fractures

Fractures of the proximal diaphysis and the metaphysis of the humerus can be nailed provided the nail end is buried below the cortical level of the insertion point. In proximal fractures it is particularly important to insert the two proximal locking screws to avoid any movement of the nail inside the wide metaphysis. The distal expansion is carried out prior to proximal locking as in shaft fractures (Fig. 15).

Postoperatively flexion, extension and elevation of the arm can be exercised. Rotational movements, however, should be restricted for at least

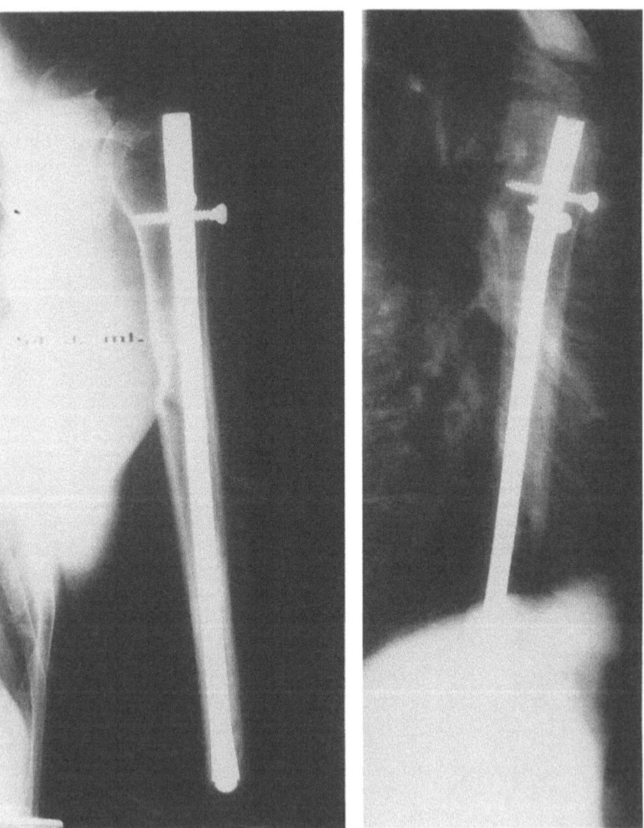

Fig. 16. Seidel locking nail in a shaft fracture of the humerus

3 weeks. With signs of early callus formation an assisted rotational movement may be employed (Fig. 16).

After both the point of insertion and the proximal locking mode have given rise to concern regarding later shoulder stiffness and weakness of the deltoid muscle injury to the axillary nerve or its branches. In osteopenic bone cutting out of the hole nail has been observed. Further investigations are needed to assess the long-term outcome with special reference to shoulder function.

Fractures of the Ulna

Management of forearm fractures continues to be a controversial topic. Plating has been most popular, but early and late failures and severe complications including infection have been reported [68]. Again, nailing of the ulna was performed by both Küntscher [45] and Hackethal [33]. Küntscher used a single nail, as for the humerus, whereas Hackethal used flexible nested solid nails of 2.5 mm diameter (Fig. 17). The point of entry for nailing of the ulna in Küntscher's approach was the olecranon, and he used cannulated reamers to widen the canal. Hackethal introduced two or more flexible bent solid nails through a window in the olecranon.

Lefèvre in Brest introduced the concept of locked nailing to the ulna. The point of entry, as in Küntscher's technique, is the olecranon, and a seating instrument is provided to enter the medullary canal correctly. Reaming of the medullary canal is followed by insertion of the locking nail with a single slot for distal locking. Due to a proximal sleeve that slides over the nail end the total nail length can be varied, and both compression and distraction are possible. The nail is locked proximally with a clamp and a screw.

Indications for this technique include fractures of the shaft of the humerus whereas proximal and distal metaphyscal fractures are not ideal. No statistics exist for the technique, but the general benefits of locked nailing seem applicable to the ulna (Fig. 18) as well as to other long bones. We see particular advantages in using this technique, especially the reaming prior to nail insertion, for refractures after plating (Fig. 19).

Locked Nailing in Nonunions

The salvage of nonunions using an intramedullary concept seems very attractive. Early concern that after plating with periosteal damage the stripping of the intramedullary blood supply might lead to large necrotic areas has not proven justified [13,14]. Nonunions occurring after conservative management have very little inherent risk of becoming infected [22]. After plating and especially after external fixation, one must be aware of possible chronic and subclinical infection [7,50,51,58,60].

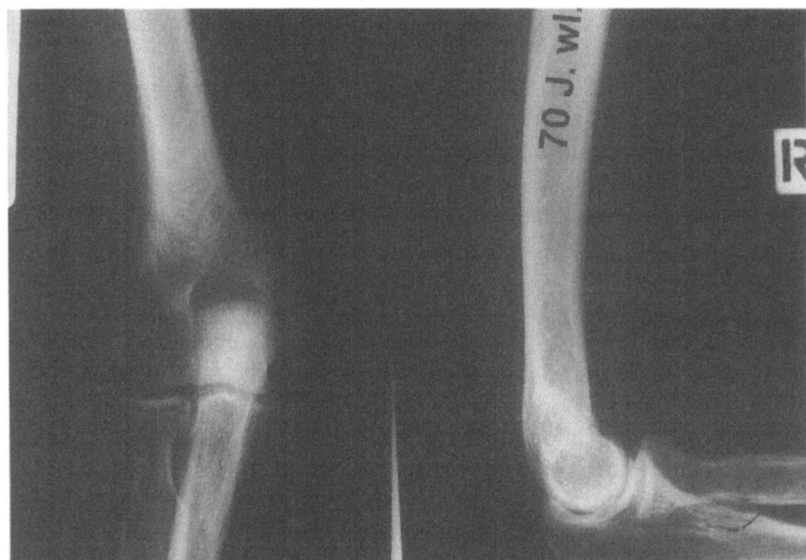

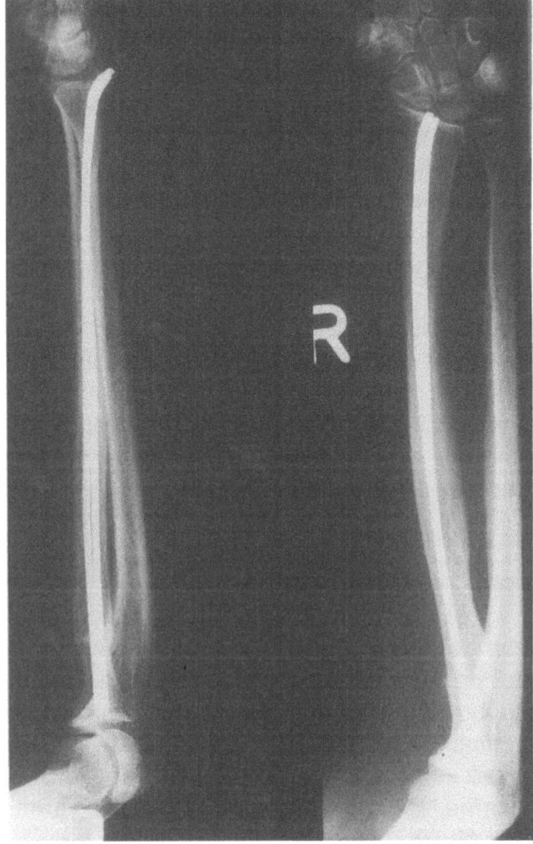

Fig. 17a,b. Hackethal nested nailing in a pathological fracture of the proximal radius. Immediate restoration of function

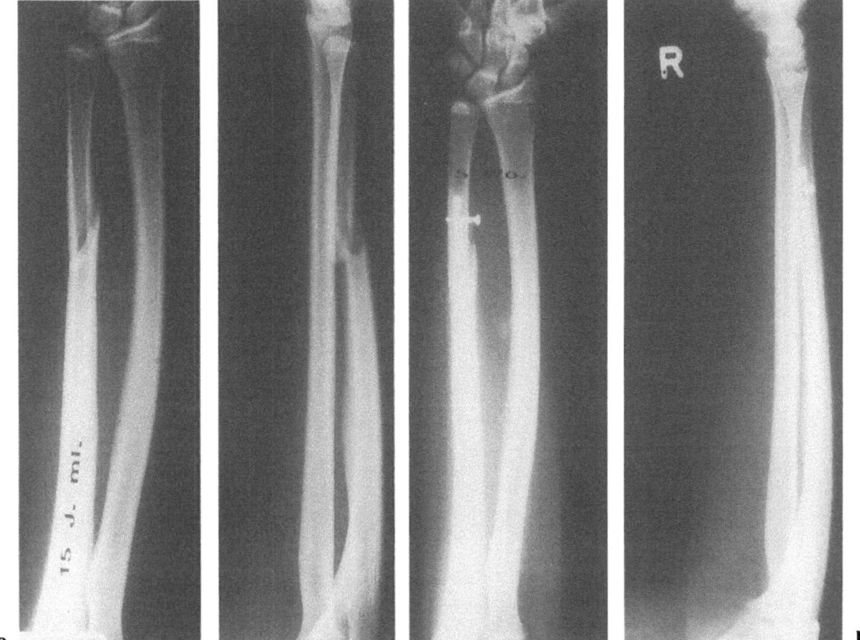

Fig. 18a,b. A 15-year-old boy. **a** Long oblique shaft fracture of the ulna with shortening. **b** Closed locked nailing with a Lefèvre locking nail showing consolidation 6 weeks after surgery and correct length of the ulna

Nonunion after conservative management usually accompanies malunion. Cortical overlap is common, and a closed procedure is rarely possible. In the femur it is usually necessary therefore to mobilize the nonunion with correction and open insertion of the guide wire to the distal fragment. Whenever possible, nonunions should be nailed dynamically to allow early loading of the nonunion site. Perhaps the most important intervention for the healing of nonunion is reaming of the medullary canal, with the bone chips from the reamer being pushed into the nonunion site [59].

The treatment of nonunion following plating is usually straightforward since major malalignment cannot be expected. It is important, however, to establish the aseptic nature of the nonunion, if necessary by aspiration biopsy. The operation begins with the patient being put on a traction table and the plate removed through the existing incision. No remaining hardware should obstruct the medullary canal, and the plating site should be irrigated thoroughly after a swab has been taken for bacteriology. The medullary canal is then opened from the greater trochanter, as for a standard nailing, and the guide wire inserted. After the guide wire has been successfully

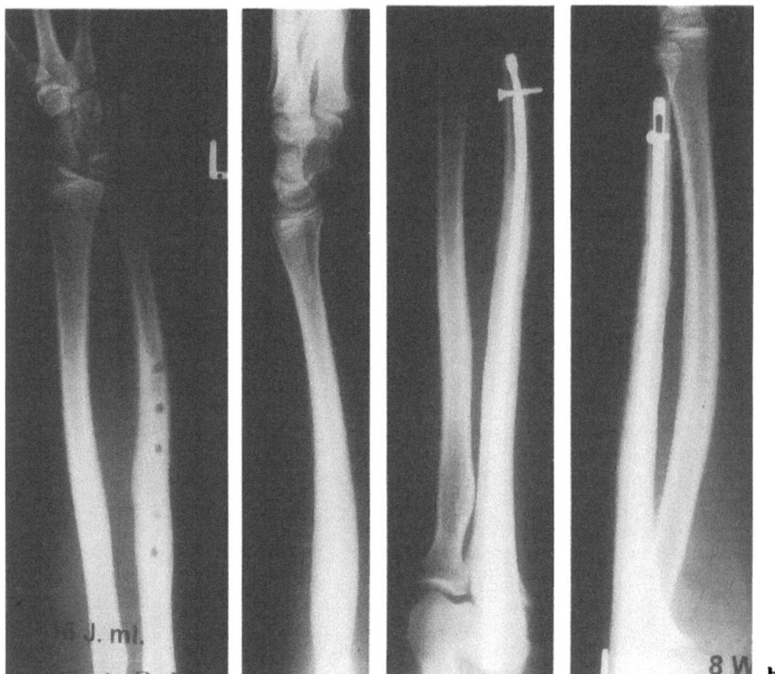

Fig. 19a,b. A 16-year-old boy. **a** Refracture after plate removal occurring after minimal trauma. The fracture did not occur through the original fracture site but through a screw hole. Closed locked nailing after reaming. **b** Consolidation 6 weeks postoperatively with Lefèvre locking nail

passed down to the distal fragment and correctly aligned distally, the wound through which the plate has been removed is closed over a drain. The rest of the technique follows the guide lines for closed nailing (Fig. 20).

The most common technical problem in nailing of nonunions is penetration of the nonunion site. The first step consists of insertion of the guide wire and reaming down to the nonunion. Sharp hand-held reamers which can also be hammered are used to overcome the nonunion site. If this is not possible, a 5-mm wire with a sharp cutting tip is used which can be driven down manually or by a motor. It is important to avoid misplacement of either of the devices since this via falsa is subsequently difficult to avoid. After the fibrous nonunion has been passed, the guide wire is inserted and standard reaming is carried out.

In the tibia an angular malalignment can often be corrected only when the fibula is cut at the level of the nonunion as the first step. If subsequent closed reduction is not successful, the nonunion site is entered through a small incision with a chisel and mobilized. Generally, correction of the

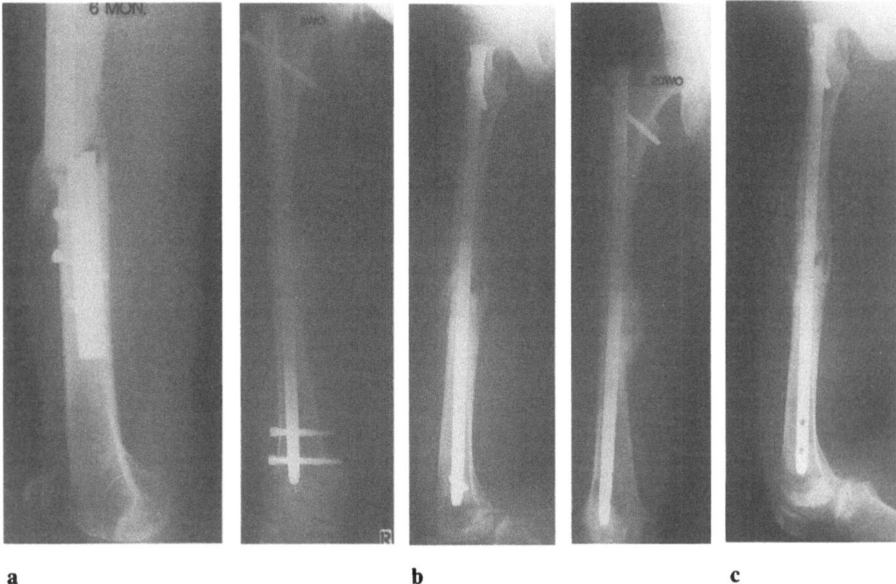

Fig. 20a–c. Fatigue fracture in a femoral plate. **a** Six months after surgery. **b,c** Plate removal, wound closure and closed nailing resulted in rapid consolidation without grafting

malalignment may now be carried out, and the wound is closed after the guide wire has been passed into the distal fragment. Nailing is then performed following standard procedures. In nonunion the medullary canal is often rather wide and accomodates a large implant. Due to the bending forces created by the frequently contracted soft tissues one should not hesitate to use a nail of larger diameter for better stability. Also, healing of a nonunion usually takes longer than that of a fresh fracture.

In atrophic nonunion of the tibia the procedure is carried out as described above. After the reaming is completed all bone chips harvested from the reamer heads should be collected and inserted into the atrophic nonunion site with the help of a nasogastric tube. Nailing is then carried out. If after 6–8 weeks there is no callus formation, laterodorsal bone grafting should be performed using corticocancellous bone chips. However, it is not uncommon even for atrophic nonunions to heal with nailing alone. Harvesting of bone from the iliac crest is not without problems [29].

Due to the poor bone quality in nonunions, especially of the tibia, the use of the dowel bolt [80] may be recommended.

Nonunion in the humerus presents a challenging situation. Especially in proximal nonunion sites, in addition to the nailing procedure a massive bone graft is usually necessary (Fig. 21). Secure locking proximally and distally is important for a successful outcome.

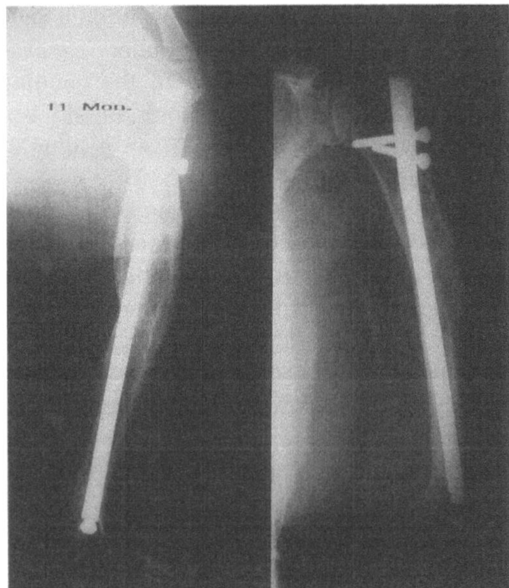

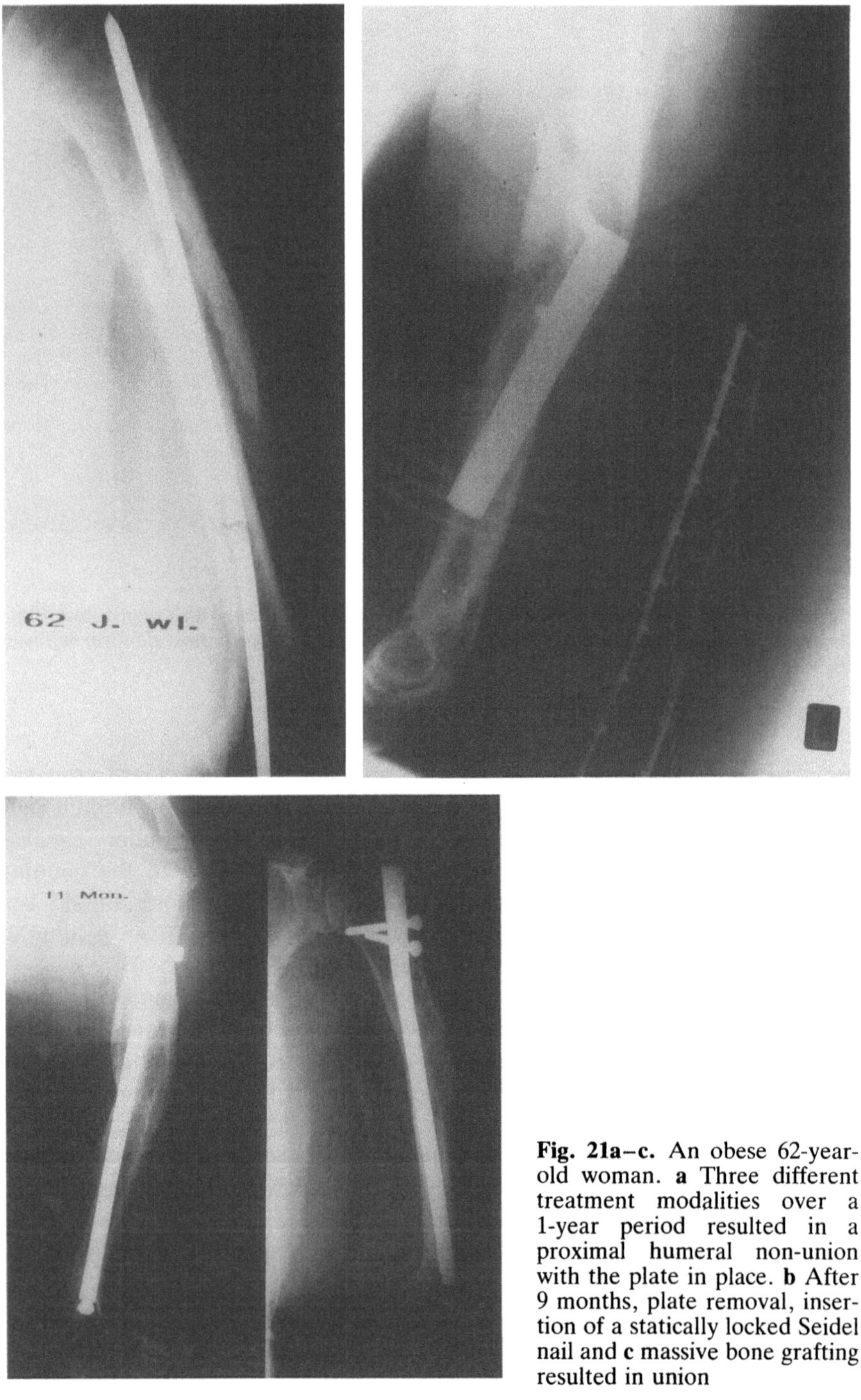

Fig. 21a–c. An obese 62-year-old woman. **a** Three different treatment modalities over a 1-year period resulted in a proximal humeral non-union with the plate in place. **b** After 9 months, plate removal, insertion of a statically locked Seidel nail and **c** massive bone grafting resulted in union

Exchange Nailing

Nonunion following previous nailing requires the procedure exchange nailing [22,45]. Exchange nailing may be necessary due to implant failure or nonunion – without the implant failing but with signs of loosening. In either instance it is obviously best to intervene early. After removal of the nail the guide wire is reinserted through the canal, and this is reamed for a larger nail. Again, dynamic nailing may be chosen. Infected nonunions in general should not be treated with locked nailing techniques, although one of the originators [44] has developed the tibial locking nail for treatment of infected nonunions. However, with the advent of suitable unilateral fixators this may be an unnecessary risk [4,60]. In infected and unstable nonunions of the femur this rule may be broken [22]. The sinus is excised, and all necrotic bone visible from the outside is removed. Gentamycin beads may be necessary, and a drain should be inserted. No closure of this wound is attempted. The rationale here is that a sinus may persist after locked nailing; however, the patient who otherwise had to use a splint may now ambulate freely. In these cases, after reaming of the medullary canal this is irrigated thoroughly using a nasogastric tube inserted down to the end of the medullary canal. The nail is always locked statically.

When using this technique, the patient must be warned of a potential superinfection and the possibility of early nail removal. As with all infected nonunions, informed consent of the patient must be upon the basis of advice concerning the possibility of subsequent amputation.

Locked Nailing of Malunions

Femur

Malunions are dealt with in the preceding section; however, one technique requires further explanation. Again, it was Küntscher – in his desire to have closed procedures exclusively for nailing techniques – who designed an intramedullary saw [45]. This device makes possible a closed osteotomy after reaming of the medullary canal. The osteotomy may be performed at any level of the femoral diaphysis, and theoretically in the tibia, but this is less suited. If an angular deformity exists, this should be corrected at its centre provided that there is an almost normal diameter of the medullary canal. The intramedullary saw cuts from the inside, and both correction of an angular deformity, with lengthening up to 2.5 cm, and a rotational correction are possible. After withdrawal of the intramedullary saw the correction is carried out with the traction table; a condylar Steinmann pin is mandatory with this technique. The nail is inserted when the correct position has been obtained. Locked static nailing is mandatory, and no dynamization is attempted [53–55].

An open corrective osteotomy has been described, but the technique is burdened with a higher complication rate [40]. Shortening is also possible with a closed osteotomy at two levels [54]. The femur is osteotomized at two levels, and the length of the segment to be cut out corresponds to the required shortening. A sharp hook is inserted and the segment cut on both the lateral and medial sides. The femur is now shortened, and, again, closed nailing with static locking is performed.

Knee Arthrodesis

The technique of closed and open knee arthrodesis using an intramedullary nail was described by Küntscher [45]. He used a closed procedure but also described partial resection of the knee joint. We now prefer to perform resection of the articular surfaces to allow the knee to be fused in the preferred position of 5°–8° of valgus and an antecurvature provided by standard antecurvature of the nail.

The femoral and tibial lengths are measured preoperatively with calibrated X-rays; the diameter of the medullary canal of femur and tibia is also measured. A custom-made nail is necessary; the most common combination is 14 mm for the femur and 12 for the tibia or 13 mm for the femur and 11 for the tibia. It is important that the gradation of the nail be in the distal part of the proximal tibial metaphysis and not at the level of knee joint. The technique can be used in primary destruction of the articular surfaces, in complex and totally unstable knee joints or after failure of a total joint replacement (Fig. 22).

Using standard-sized reamers the femur is reamed first, followed by reaming of the tibia. We overream 1.5–2 mm in both femur and tibia, and them nail is inserted in an open fashion. The resection surfaces of the knee joint are approximated under direct vision, and the nail is locked statically. Mobilization and weight bearing is allowed after healing of the soft tissues. Bone grafting may be necessary in large defects.

Postoperative Management

After surgery the traction pins are removed and the whole leg is wrapped using elastic bandages. There is no strict weight bearing regime, and we allow the patient to bear weight as much as is tolerable in fresh fractures. The pain threshold determines the amount of load which the patient can accept. The earlier that full function is restored the better it is for the patient, and the more uneventful the postoperative management will be. It can be expected that patients with stable fracture will be capable of full weight bearing 4–6 weeks after surgery, whereas in comminuted fractures this may take 8–10 weeks. If there is any soft-tissue compromise either in closed or in open fractures this must resolve before loading is permitted.

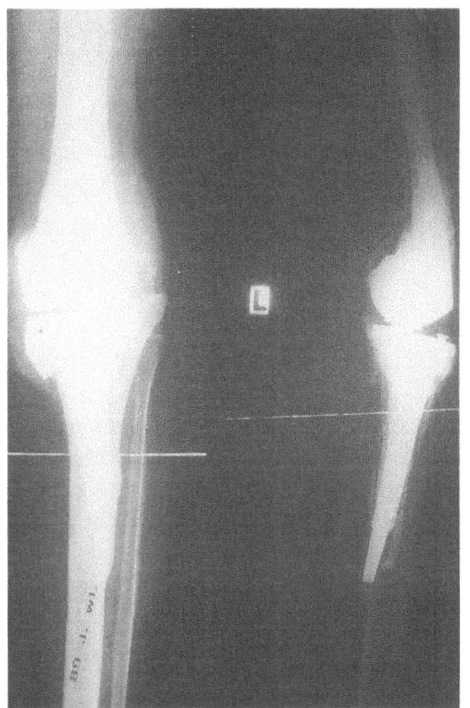

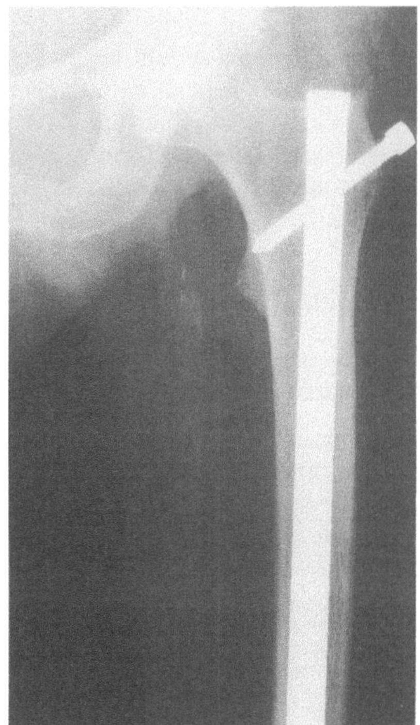

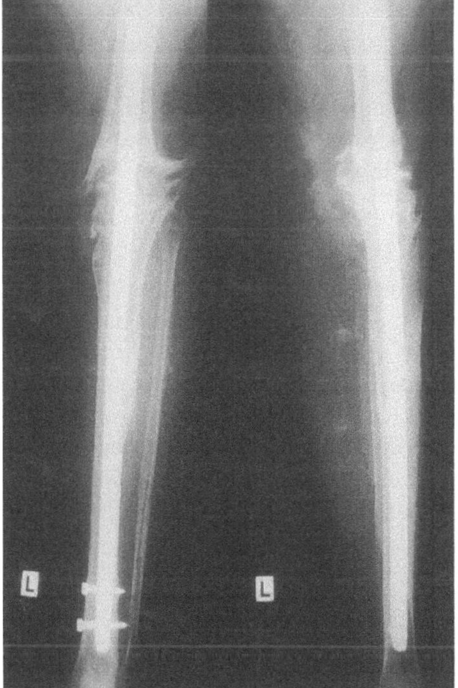

Fig. 22a–c. Loosening of both femoral and tibial components of a total knee joint with threatening penetration of the tibial component in two planes. Inability to walk. Insertion of a custom-made arthrodesis nail (Howmedica) after reaming of femur and tibia with standard instrumentation. Static locking. The procedure resulted in pain-free walking after anteromedial bone grafting secondarily

All adjacent joints should be mobilized immediately after surgery, and in general there should be no restriction. Dynamization is not carried out routinely; this is dealt with in previous sections.

Nail removal is performed in femoral fractures 18–24 months, in tibial fractures 12–15 months, and in humeral fractures 3–6 months after surgery. Follow-up with radiographic control is carried out after 6 weeks, 4 months, 12 months and prior to nail removal.

Complications

Intraoperative Femoral Neck Fracture

Neck fracture during insertion of an intramedullary nail is a serious complication, and an incidence of 1.5% has been reported [21]. In retrospect it may be somewhat difficult to decide whether the neck fracture was present prior to surgery or occurred during nail insertion and hammering. It is therefore of utmost importance to have a good X-ray in both planes of the entire femur including the femoral neck and head as well as the condylar region.

An incorrect starting point contributes to the development of an iatrogenic neck fracture [22]. Especially an insertion that is too medial presents dangers, as well as an extremely lateral starting point with a narrow femoral canal. The complication, however, can be treated with two or three cancellous lag screws inserted anteriorly and/or posteriorly to the nail (see Fig. 11). An extremely lateral starting point with a severe complication is illustrated in Fig. 23a. This resulted in the complete displacement of a proximal portion. It was salvaged by retrieval of the original nail, closed reduction and correct insertion of a locking nail (Fig. 23b).

Femoral Comminution

Of a similar nature but less serious is proximal femoral comminution due to an incorrect entry point. This usually occurs medially but occasionally anteriorly or posteriorly. In general this is without serious consequences if correct static locking is performed to prevent shortening, and healing is not affected.

Failure correctly to lock in a proximal fracture or a proximal comminution may result in a complex malunion, as illustrated in Fig. 24. In addition to the wrong implant, the wrong point of entry was also chosen here.

Nail Failure

Küntscher in his early account of intramedullary nailing reported that the use of small-diameter nails may lead to bending of the material [45]. Bending

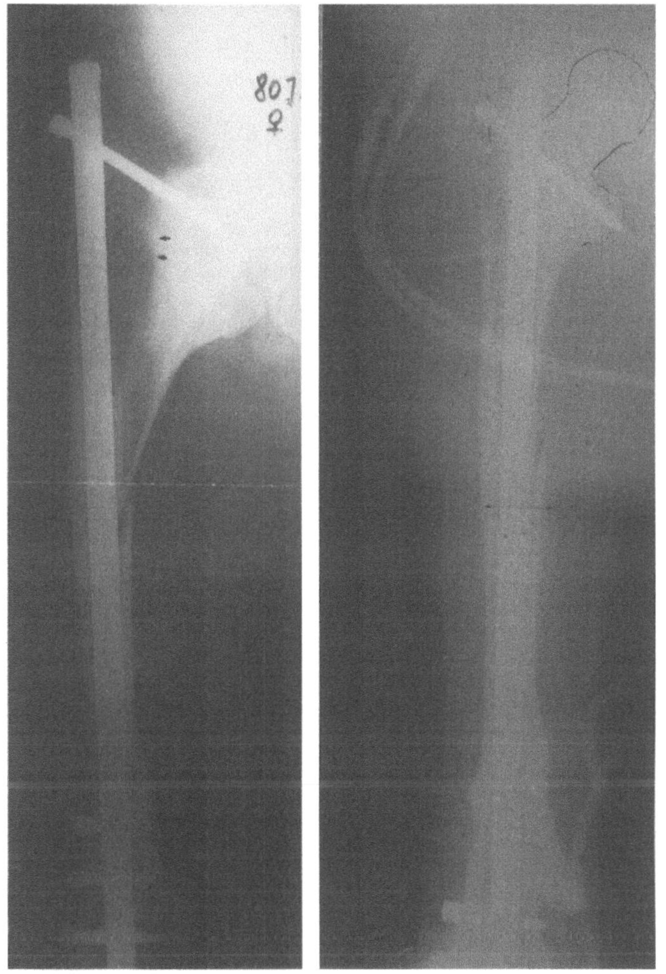

Fig. 23a,b. Incorrect point of entry at the innominate tubercle in an 80-year old woman with a femoral fracture. **a** Failure of the procedure. **b** Removal of the original nail, closed reduction and closed nailing to salvage the situation

of the nail may also occur after another injury. Either the fracture at this stage is not healed, or a new or additional fracture is present. This complication is treated by removal of the nail, and unless the bending is more than 45° this can usually be accomplished with the standard extraction tools. Renailing with a nail of larger diameter can overcome this problem.

Fatigue fractures of the nail have been reported, but these are extremely rare and are usually associated with improper techniques. A broken distal end of the nail may be difficult to retrieve [18].

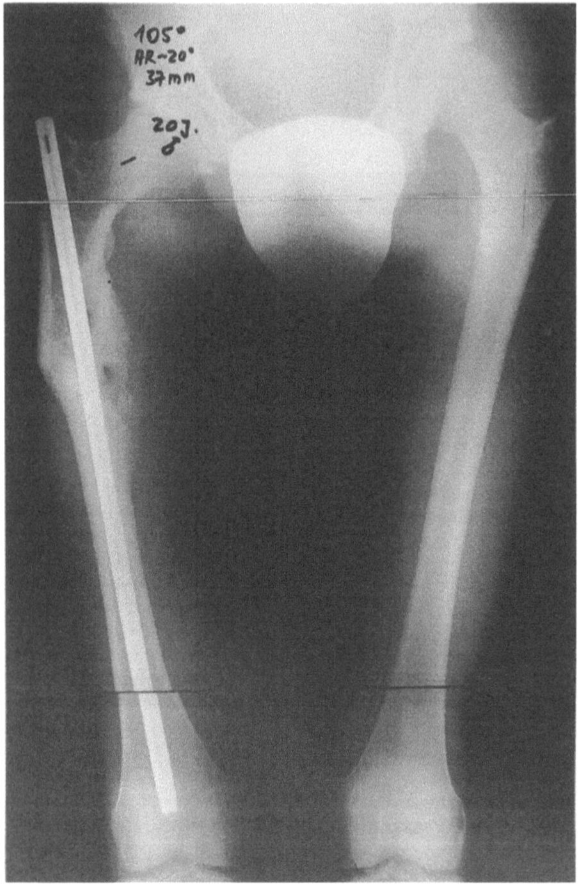

Fig. 24. A 20-year-old man. Incorrect use of a standard Küntscher nail without locking. Varus deformity, shortening and outward rotation occurred

Secondary Fractures

The most serious complication with the gamma nail is a fracture below the nail tip [19]. This may occur during surgery or, more likely, after surgery. The incidence of this complication has been reported to be as high as to 9%, but no biomechanical explanation of this phenomenon has yet been offered [19]. This problem may be salvaged with a longer gamma nail (Grosse and Taglang, personal communication), or, if the proximal femoral fracture is united, exchange nailing with a sufficiently large conventional locking nail is carried out (Fig. 25). The reconstruction nail may also be used in selected cases.

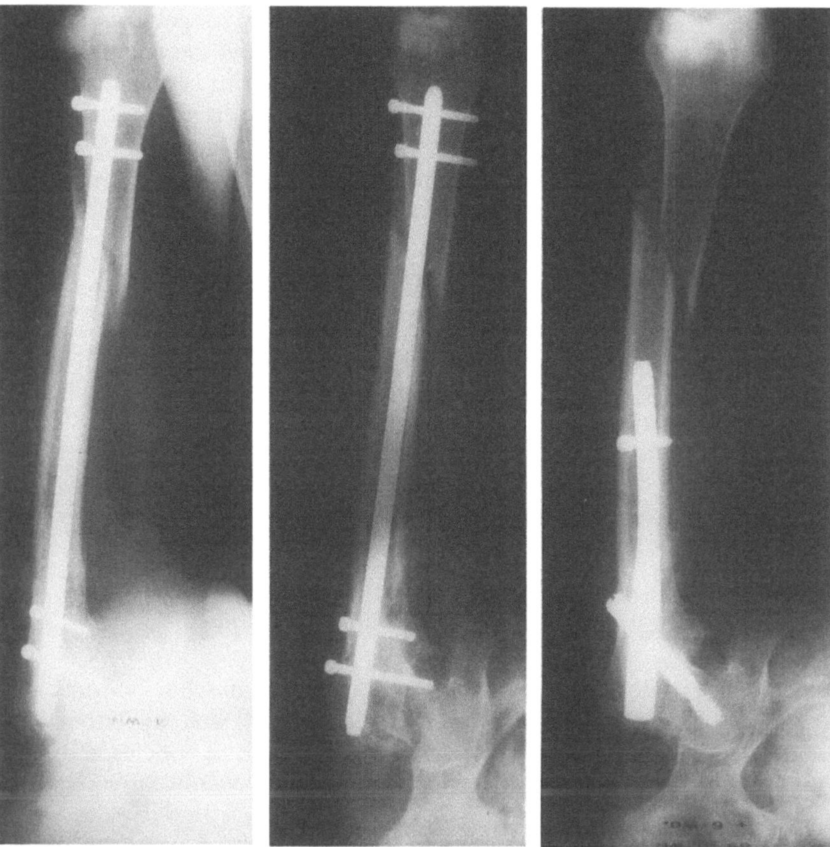

Fig. 25a,b. Femoral fracture below a gamma nail. **a** Six weeks postoperatively. **b** Removal of the gamma nail and insertion of a Colchero-type locking nail (independently of image intensifier) locking proximally and distally

Pudendal Nerve Lesion

Pudendal nerve neuropraxia has been a rare encounter in conventional locked nailing but seems to be more of a problem in reconstruction nailing [22]. The cause appears to be excessive traction on the leg, which creates high pressure on the skin imposed by the post of the orthopaedic table. According to Court-Brown [22], the incidence is 1.5%, and all the cases reported have resolved spontaneously.

Neurovascular Complications

Neurovascular damage in femoral nailing is highly unlikely [22]. In proximal locking of tibial fractures, however, the anteroposterior screw may damage the posterior neurovascular bundle, especially if the leg support is positioned wrongly in the popliteal fossa or the proximal tibia and thereby pushes the neurovascular bundle against the posterior tibial cortex. In any case, the anteroposterior screw must be drilled with extreme caution, and, if uncertain, a lateral view can verify correct penetration of the cortex. However, the incidence of this potential problem as reported in larger series has not been serious. Some nails employ oblique or mediolateral locking to account for the potential danger [22].

Locking Screws

Intraoperatively the locking screws must be inserted fully to avoid further irritation of the soft tissues. During the healing period some of the patients complain of cross-screw discomfort [22]. This now presents the most common reason for the removal of locking screws in our practice. Cross-screw failure may occur; however, the incidence is less than 1% [22]. No instances of cross-screw breakages reported in larger series have negatively effected the outcome of nailing [23].

Evaluation of the Current Locking Nail Concept

The technique of locked nailing as introduced by Küntscher [45] and subsequently perfected by Klemm and Schellmann [44] and by Grosse and Kempf [30,41] has become a highly successful surgical tool especially in femoral fractures. Most intra- and postoperative complications can be avoided by adhering to the technique. The most widely used locking nail is the Grosse-Kempf nail (Howmedica). In recent years other locking nail systems have been introduced, but none of those has shown a significant improvement with regard to nail performance or cross-screw insertion [37].

Despite the existence of reliable hand-held devices for insertion of locking screws this continues to be a conceptional problem. There is little doubt that without adequate technical assistance in handling the image intensifier this last part of the procedure can become tedious. Good training of operating room personnel in handling the image intensifier not only reduces the radiation but also shortens the operating time [42]. Ideally, locked nailing should be independent of the image intensifier after the guide wire has been inserted. One must also recognize that the majority of orthopaedic operating rooms around the world do not have ready access to a state-of-the-art image intensifier.

Several attempts have been made to produce nail-mounted jigs, which are designed to introduce the locking screws without the aid of an image intensifier [22]. Electromagnetic devices have also been developed but are not yet commercially available. Two problems have been observed with nail mounted jigs. Firstly, the jig itself is not sufficiently stable for instrumentation at its distal end. The second and more important problem lies in the nailing procedure and the nail itself. Hammering of the nail down the medullary canal may cause rotation of the nail when it engages in the medullary canal. In addition, deformation of the nail in its long axis may occur during insertion.

Based on the above observations a recent study was undertaken to evaluate and improve the nailing system originally developed by Colchero et al. [21]. This is based on Küntscher's conception of a straight nail. Since the curvature of the femur varies considerably [69], it is unlikely that a curved nail will facilitate introduction unless it perfectly matches this curvature in its entire length. Also, the curvature of the various commercially available and more commonly used nailing systems varies considerably [37]. The use of a straight nail design has the advantage of permitting a straight jig design. Since this nail, with a wall thickness of 3 mm, is highly stable, with a wider proximal portion it does not deform during nail insertion. The nail is not hammered down the medullary canal but is pushed down manually. This helps to avoid some of the complications encountered during nail insertion, including femoral neck fractures and proximal femoral comminution [22].

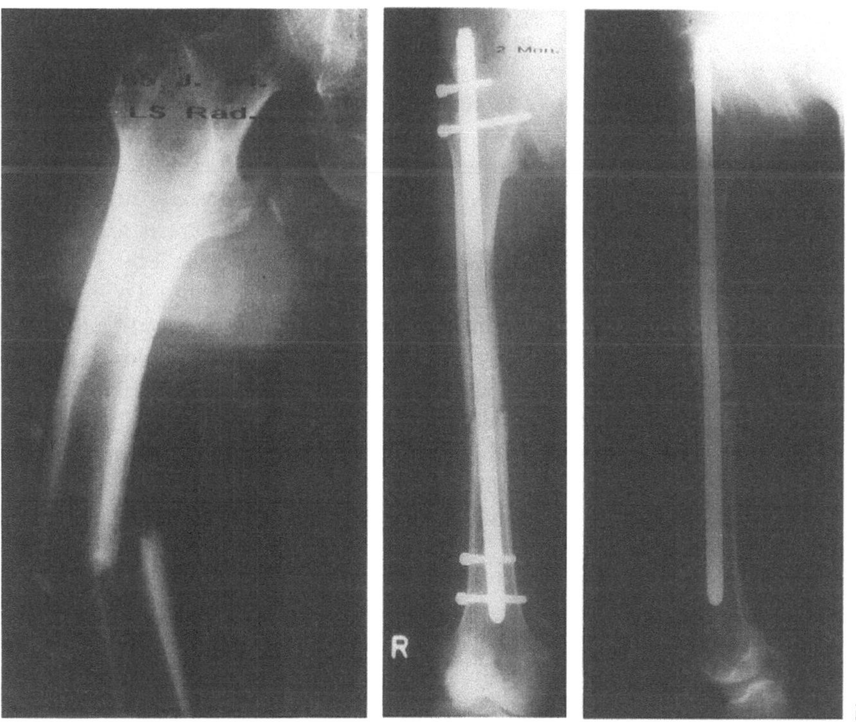

Fig. 26a,b. Proximal femur. a Impending pathological fracture. b Stabilized with a Colchero-type locking nail. Insertion of the distal locking screws, independent of image intensifier

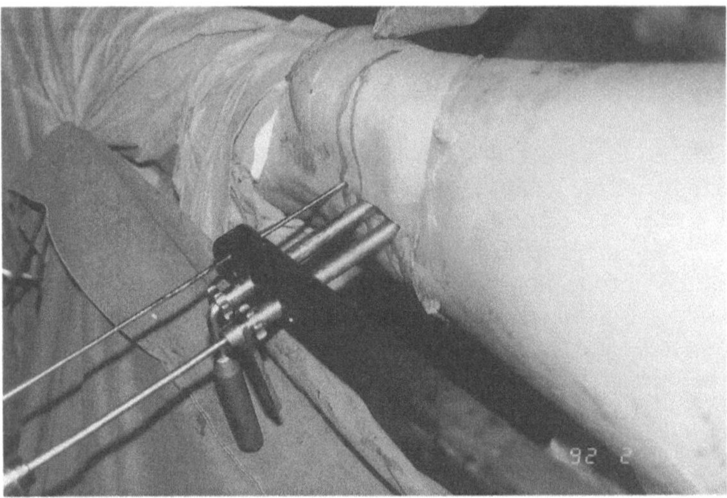

Fig. 27. Nail-mounted jig showing alignment of the straight nail and the straight jig to facilitate distal cross-screw insertion

The fit of the medullary canal can be tested prior to nail insertion using a template, which also helps to determine the nail length by direct measurement. After nail insertion the jig is mounted on the nail insertion handle, and proximal locking is carried out first. There are two locking screws in this nail system: the proximal one enters through the innominate tubercle and the lower one at the level of the lesser trochanter. Both screws are inserted transversely, as in the original Küntscher locking nail (see Fig. 1). Distal locking is carried out after the jig has been aligned distally. To avoid any involuntary movements two 3-mm Kirschner wires are used for additional fixation: the first is inserted through the jig in the coronal plane and the second after mounting an L-shaped extension from the anterior (sagittal plane). This produces the stability of a frame. After predrilling of the locking hole, with a smaller drill bit acting as a path finder, the appropriate drill bit is used to enlarge the hole in the near and far cortex.

This nailing system is intended to be independent of the image intensifier after the guide wire passes the fracture line. If an image intensifier is not available, the guide wire may be inserted in an open procedure, although most surgeons agree that nailing should be done in a closed fashion. With a stable and precise jig the distal locking procedure does not depend on the skill of the assisting radiographer. This also helps to reduce radiation and shorten the overall operating time.

Tests in larger series are required to evaluate the user-friendliness of this system. Early experience with it at the author's institution, however, is encouraging (Figs. 25–27).

Acknowledgements. I wish to thank Dr. T. Gausepohl for his assistance in preparing the clinical material and Mrs. C. Grümer for dilligently typing the manuscript.

References

1. Alho A, Ekeland A, Stomsoe K et al. (1990) Locked intramedullary nailing for displaced tibial shaft fractures. J Bone Joint Surg [Br] 72:805
2. Bach AW, Hansen ST Jr (1989) Plates versus external fixation in severe open tibial shaft fractures. Clin Orothop 241:89–94
3. Baranowski D, Pennig D (1988) Grenzindikationen der Verriegelungsnagelung. In: Nonnemann HC, Vécsci V, Lindholm R (eds) Osteosynthese International. Schnetztor, Konstanz, p 402
4. Bastiani G de, Aldegeheri R, Renzi-Brivio L (1984) Treatment of fractures with a dynamic axial fixator. J Bone Joint Surg [Br] 66:538
5. Behrmann SW, Fabian TC, Kudsk KA et al. (1990) Improved outcome with femur fractures: early versus delayed fixation. J Trauma 30(7):792–797
6. Bergman CD, Winquist RA, Mayo KA et al. (1987) Subtrochanteric fracture of the femur: fixation using the Zickel nail. J Bone Joint Surg [Am] 63:1032–1040
7. Blachut PA, Meek RN, O'Brien PJ (1990) External fixation and delayed intramedullary nailing of open fractures of the tibial shaft. J Bone Joint Surg [Am] 72:729
8. Bodoky A, Neff U, Heberer M et al. (1993) Antibiotic prophylaxis with two doses of cephalosporin in patients managed with internal fixation for a fracture of the hip. J Bone Joint Surg [Am] 75:61
9. Bone LB, Johnson KD, Weigelt J et al. (1989) Early versus delayed stabilization of femoral fractures. A prospective randomized study. J Bone Joint Surg [Am] 71:336–340
10. Boriani S, Bettelli G (1990) The gamma-nail. Chir Organi Mov 75:67
11. Bridle SH, Patel AD, Bircher M et al. (1991) Fixation of intertrochanteric fractures of the femur: a randomised prospective comparison of the gamma nail and the dynamic hip screw. J Bone Joint Surg [Br] 73:330–334
12. Brookes M (1990) Blood flow in the diaphysis of long bones and its biomechanics. Howmedica Publication, Schönkirchen/Kicl, pp 1–5
13. Brug E, Pennig D (1988) Standortbestimmung der Verriegelungsnagelung. In: Bünte H, Junginger T (eds) Jahrbuch der Chirurgie. Biermann, Münster, p 145
14. Brug E, Pennig D (1990) Indikation zur Verriegelungsnagelung. Unfallchirurg 93:492–498
15. Brug E, Pennig D, Gähler R et al. (1988) Polytrauma und Femurfraktur. Aktuel Traumatol 18:125
16. Brumback RJ, Reilly JP, Lakatos R et al. (1988) Intramedullary nailing of femoral shaft fractures. I. Decision-making errors with interlocking fixation. J Bone Joint Surg [Am] 70:1441–1452
17. Brumback RJ, Uwagei-Ero S, Lakatos R et al. (1988) Intramedullary nailing of femoral shaft fractures. II. Fracture-healing with static interlocking femoral fixation. J Bone Joint Surg [Am] 70:1453–1462
18. Bucholz RW, Ross SE, Lawrence KL (1987) Fatigue fracture of the interlocking nail in the treatment of fractures of the distal part of the femoral shaft. J Bone Joint Surg [Am] 69:1391–1399
19. Calvert PT (1992) The gamma nail – a significant advance or a passing fashion? J Bone Joint Surg [Br] 74:329–331
20. Caudle RJ, Stern PJ (1987) Severe open fractures of the tibia. J Bone Joint Surg [Am] 69:801–807

21. Colchero F, Orst G, Reboul C et al. (1983) Enclouage centro-médullaire claveté. Rev Chir Orthop 49:547–555
22. Court-Brown CM (1991) An atlas of closed nailing of the tibia and femur. Dunitz, London
23. Court-Brown CM, Christie J, McQueen MM (1990) Closed intramedullary tibial nailing: its use in closed and type I open fractures. J Bone Joint Surg [Br] 72:605
24. Court-Brown CM, McQueen MM, Quaba et al. (1991) Locked intramedullary nailing of open tibial fractures. J Bone Joint Surg [Br] 73:959–964
25. Davies TRC, Sher JL, Horsman A et al. (1990) Intertrochanteric femoral fractures: mechanical failure after internal fixation. J Bone Joint Surg [Br] 72:26–31
26. Eyre-Brook AL (1984) The periosteum: its function reassessed. Clin Orthop 189:300–307
27. Godina M (1986) Early microsurgical reconstruction of complex trauma of the extremities. Plast Reconstr Surg 78:285
28. Goodship AE, Kenwright J (1985) The influence of induced micromovements upon the healing of experimental tibial fractures. J Bone Joint Surg [Br] 67: 650–655
29. Grob D (1986) Probleme an der Entnahmestelle bei autologer Knochentransplantation. Unfallchirurg 89:339–345
30. Grosse A, Kempf I (1985) Handbuch der Verriegelungsnagelung bei Schaftbrüchen von Femur und Tibia. In: Grosse A (ed) Howmedica Publication, Schönkirchen/Kiel
31. Gustilo RB, Gruniger RP, Davis T (1987) Classification of type III (severe) open fractures relative to treatment and results. Orthopaedics 10:1781
32. Gustilo RB, Mendoza RM, Williams DN (1984) Problems in the management of type III (severe) open fractures: a new classification of type III open fractures. J Trauma 24:742
33. Hackethal KH (1961) Die Bündelnagelung. Springer, Berlin Göttingen Heidelberg
34. Halder SC (1992) The gamma nail for peritrochanteric fractures. J Bone Joint Surg [Br] 74:341
35. Heinz TH, Stoik W, Vecsei V (1989) Behandlung und Ergebnisse von pathologischen Frakturen. Unfallchirurg 92:477–485
36. Heitemeyer U, Kemper F, Hierholzer G et al. (1987) Severely comminuted femoral shaft fractures: treatment by bridging-plate osteosynthesis. Arch Orthop Trauma Surg 106:327–355
37. Johnson KD, Tencer A (1990) The mechanics of intramedullary nails for femoral fractures. Unfallchirurg 93:499
38. Johnson KD, Johnston DWC, Parker B (1984) Comminuted femoral shaft fractures: treatment by roller traction, cerclage wires and intramedullary nail, or an interlocking intremedullary nail. J Bone Joint Surg [Am] 66:1222–1235
39. Johnson KD, Cadambi A, Seibert GB (1985) Incidence of adult respiratory distress syndrome in patients with multiple musculoskeletal injuries: effect of early operative stabilisation of fractures. J Trauma 25:375
40. Kempf I, Grosse A (1985) "One Stage"-Verlängerungsosteotomie am Femur unter Verwendung der verriegelten Nagelungstechnik. Hefte Unfallheilkd 161:86
41. Kempf I, Grosse A, Lafforgue (1978) L'apport du verouillage dans l'enclouage centromédullaire des os longs. Rev Chir Orthop 64:635–651
42. Kempf I, Grosse A, Beck G (1985) Closed locked intramedullary nailing. Its application to comminuted fractures of the femur. J Bone Joint Surg [Am] 67:709–720
43. Klein MPM, Rahn BA, Frigg R et al. (1990) Reaming versus non-reaming in medullary nailing interference with cortical circulation of the canine tibia. Arch Orthop Trauma Surg 109:314
44. Klemm A (1983) Die Entwicklung der Verriegelungstechnik. Hefte Unfallheilkd 161:1–7

45. Küntscher G (1962) Praxis der Marknagelung. Schattauer, Stuttgart
46. Leung KS, So WS, Shen WY et al. (1992) Gamma nails and dynamic hip screws for peritrochanteric fractures. J Bone Joint Surg [Br] 74:345–351
47. Lhowe DW, Hansen ST (1988) Immediate nailing of open fractures of the femoral shaft. J Bone Joint Surg [Am] 70:812–820
48. Lindsey RW, Teal P, Probe RA et al. (1991) Early experience with the gamma interlocking nail for peritrochanteric fractures of the proximal femur. J Trauma 31:1649–1658
49. MacNab I, De Haas WG (1974) The role of the periostel blood supply in the healing of the tibia. Clin Orthop 105:27–34
50. Maurer DJ, Merkow RL, Gustilo RB (1989) Infection after intramedullary nailing of severe open tibial fractures initially treated with external fixation. J Bone Joint Surg [Am] 71:835
51. McGraw JM, Lim EVA (1988) Treatment of open tibial shaft fractures. External fixation and secondary intramedullary nailing. J Bone Joint Surg [Am] 70: 900
52. McKibbin B (1978) The biology of fracture repair in long bones. J Bone Joint Surg [Br] 60:150
53. Mockwitz J (1983) Probleme zur Verlängerungsosteotomie. Hefte Unfallheilkd 161:96–97
54. Mockwitz J, Küper R (1983) Posttraumatische Korrekturen: Korrektur von Längendifferenzen, Achsen- und Rotationsfehlstellungen mit dem Verriegelungsnagel. Hefte Unfallheilkd 161:79
55. Mockwitz J, Schellmann W-D (1978) Die gedeckte Osteotomie mit der Innensäge. In: Vecsei V (ed) Die Verriegelungsnagelung. Maudrich, Vienna
56. Moran CG, Gibson MJ, Cross AT (1990) Intramedullary locking nails for femoral shaft fractures in elderly patients. J Bone Joint Surg [Br] 72:19
57. Oestern H-J, Tscherne H (1984) Pathophysiology and classification of soft tissue injuries associated with fractures. In: Tscherne H, Gotzen L (eds) Fractures with soft tissue injuries. Springer, Berlin Heidelberg New York, p 1
58. Olerud S, Karlstrom G (1972) Secondary intramedullary nailing of tibial fractures. J Bone Joint Surg [Am] 54:1419
59. Pennig D (1990) Zur Biologie des Knochens und der Knochenbruchheilung. Unfallchirurg 93:488–491
60. Pennig D (1991) The place of unilateral external fixation in the treatment of tibial fractures. Int J Orthop Trauma 1(3):161
61. Pennig D (1992) Management of bony metastases. In: Newman RJ (ed) Orthogeriatrics. Butterworth-Heinemann, London, p 175
62. Pennig D (1992) Principles of fracture management in elderly patients. In: Newman RJ (ed) Orthogeriatrics. Butterworth-Heinemann, London, p 120
63. Pennig D, Brug E (1989) Das Einbringen der distalen Bolzen bei der Verriegelungsnagelung mit einem neuen Freihand-Zielgerät. Unfallchirurg 92:331
64. Pennig D, Brug E (1989) Femoral fractures in multiply injured patients. In: Pipino F (ed) La fissazione esterna. OIC Medical, Florence, p 213
65. Pennig D, Brug E, Kronholz HL (1988) A new distal aiming device for locking nail fixation. Orthopedics 11:1725
66. Reikeras O, Reigstad A (1985) Healing of stable and unstable osteotomies in rats. Arch Orthop Trauma Surg 104:161–163
67. Rhinelander FW (1974) Tibial blood supply in relation to fracture healing. Clin Orthop 105:34–81
68. Rosson J, Egan J, Monro P et al. (1990) Bone weakness after removal of internal fixation plates. J Bone Joint Surg [Br] 72:160
69. Rubin PJ, Leyvraz PF, Heegaard JH (1989) Radiological variations in the anatomical parameters of the proximal femur in relation to rotation. Fr J Orthop Surg 3(2):121–127
70. Russell GG, Henderson R, Arnett G (1990) Primary or delayed closure for open tibial fractures. J Bone Joint Surg [Br] 72:125

71. Schmidt-Neuerburg KP, Klaes W (1990) Chirurgische Therapie bei pathologischen Frakturen. In: Bünte H, Junginger T (eds) Jahrbuch der Chirurgie. Biermann, Münster, p 151
72. Seidel H (1989) Humeral locking nail: a preliminary report. Orthopaedics 12:219
73. Strachan RK, McCarthy I, Fleming R et al. (1990) The role of the tibial nutrient artery. J Bone Joint Surg [Br] 72:391
74. Thomas WG, Villar RN (1986) Subtrochanteric fractures: Zickel nail or nail plate. J Bone Joint Surg [Br] 68:255–259
75. Thoresen BO, Alho A, Ekeland A et al. (1985) Interlocking intramedullary nailing in femoral shaft fractures. J Bone Joint Surg [Am] 67:1313–1320
76. Tischenko GL, Goodman SB (1990) Compartment syndrome after intramedullary nailing of the tibia. J Bone Joint Surg [Am] 72:41
77. Trueta J (1974) Blood supply and the rate of healing of tibial fractures. Clin Orthop 105:11–26
78. Tscherne H, Trentz O (1977) Operationstechnik und Ergebnisse bei Mehrfragment- und Trümmerbrüchen des Femurschaftes. Unfallheilkunde 80:221
79. Van Linge B (1985) Fracturen statistiek van het Gemeenschappelijk Administratiekantoor. Ned Tijdschr Geneeskd 130:2019
80. Vecsei V (1978) Verriegelungsnagelung. Maudrich, Vienna
81. Vecsei V, Mockwitz J, Börner N et al. (1983) Fehlerhafte Technik und Komplikationen. Hefte Unfallheilkd 161:143–152
82. Whittle AP, Russell TA, Taylor JC et al. (1992) Treatment of open fractures of the tibial shaft with the use of interlocking nailing without reaming. J Bone Joint Surg [Am] 74:1162
83. Winquist RA, Hansen ST (1980) Comminuted fractures of the femoral shaft treated by intramedullary nailing. Orthop Clin North Am 11:633–648
84. Winquist RA, Hansen ST Jr, Clawson DK (1984) Closed intramedullary nailing of femoral fractures. J Bone Joint Surg [Am] 66:529–539
85. Wiss DA, Fleming CH, Matta JM et al. (1986) Comminuted and rotationally unstable fractures of the femur treated with interlocking nail. Clin Orthop 212:35–47
86. Wolfgang GL, Bryant MH, O'Neill JP (1982) Treatment of intertrochanteric fracture of the femur using sliding screw plate fixation. Clin Orthop 163:148–158
87. Zickel RE, Mouradian WH (1976) Intramedullary fixation of pathological fractures and lesions of the subtrochanteric region of the femur. J Bone Joint Surg [Am] 58:1061

5 Problems in Compound Fractures

N.P. Suedkamp and H. Tscherne

Introduction

Due to the soft-tissue injury involved, compound fractures represent surgical emergencies and require a sophisticated management protocol and appropriate grading to achieve uncomplicated healing and complete functional restitution. Compound fractures are very often associated with additional injuries, and the primary care and priorities of multiply traumatized patients must be considered. The difficulty lies in determining what steps and procedures should be instituted and in what sequence. Therefore the surgeon must be familiar with the relative timing, risks, and benefits of the available treatment options, not only for a single injury but for the patient's overall profile of injuries and areas at risk.

Immediately after resuscitation and establishment of the patient's cardio-pulmonary stability, with special concern to possible massive haemorrhage, an assessment of musculo-skeletal injury is necessary. This includes the aetiology of the injury and a complete diagnosis of the bone and soft-tissue injury. This furnishes the data which the surgeon needs for a correct classification of the limb injury and is thus the basis for the resulting treatment philosophy which seeks to guarantee an optimal outcome.

Classification of Fractures with Soft-Tissue Injury

Tscherne [44] and Yaremchuk et al. [46] have emphasized the importance of establishing a complete aetiology. To determine the appropriate choice and timing of treatment the surgeon needs to know when, where and how the injury occurred. For instance, prolonged entrapment in a car suggests a possible compartment syndrome, and barnyard accidents a high risk of infection. Most important of all is knowledge of the amount and direction of the force or energy that caused the injury. The greater the force was, the more serious the damage and sequelae. The causative force determines both the extent of the injury and the necessary steps in treatment.

The fracture pattern can be identified by plain antero-posterior and lateral radiographs, and it adds additional information. A comminuted fracture results from a severe force which – prior to damaging the bone –

destroyed the covering soft tissues. The radiographs also provide data about the soft-tissue injury if foreign bodies, dirt, denser soft-tissue or entrapped air at a distance from the actual fracture site is found. Assessment of vascular integrity is determined with inspection (color), palpation (temperature, peripheral pulses) and in doubtful cases Doppler sonography or angiography (incomplete/complete ischaemia). The examination of neurological status covers distal sensations and motor functions and can be completed by checking the patient's ability to respond to pain stimuli, follow commands and accurately report sensations. The degree of wound contamination is an important factor affecting the course and prognosis of the injury. Foreign bodies and dirt particles provide useful information and assist in the grading of contamination. High-velocity shotgun wounds and farming accidents must be considered as severely contaminated. Definite determination of the extent of soft-tissue injury must be made by the surgeon at the time of operation because the amount of soft-tissue destruction – with respect to avital muscle tissue, avital subcutaneous tissue, degloving, periosteal stripping, and vascular or nerve injuries – is often evident only at this time. Assessment of soft-tissue damage influences the treatment protocol as well as the type of fracture fixation.

In Tscherne's classification (Table 1), soft-tissue injuries are grouped according to severity into four categories, with the fracture labelled, in addition, as open or closed by an "O" or "C". Open fractures of *grade I* (O-I) represent skin lacerations through a bone fragment from the inside. There is no or only little contusion of the skin, and fractures are thus the result of indirect trauma to A fractures of the AO classification. Even in cases of minor skin wound size or no visible soft-tissue damage a fracture resulting from direct trauma, such as B and C type fractures in the AO classification, must be classified as second-degree open. *Grade II* open fractures (O-II) are characterized by any type of skin laceration with a circumscribed skin or soft-tissue contusion and moderate contamination. This injury can be accompanied by any type of fracture. Any severe soft-tissue damage without

Table 1. Classification of fractures with concomitant soft-tissue injury

Grade	Skin: open (+) or closed (−)	Soft-tissue damage	Fracture type	Contamination
O-I	+	+	+ to + +	+
O-II	+	+ +	+ to + + +	+ +
O-III	+	+ + +	+ to + + +	+ + +
O-IV	+	+ + +	+ to + + +	+ to + + +
C-O	−	−	+	−
C-I	−	+	+ to + +	−
C-II	−	+ +	+ to + + +	−
C-III	−	+ + +	+ to + + +	(+)

+, Little; + +, medium; + + +, severe.

injury to a major vessel or peripheral nerve is categorized in this group. To classify a fracture as *grade III* (O-III) the open fracture must have extensive soft-tissue damage, often with an additional major vessel injury and/or nerve injury. Every open fracture accompanied by ischaemia and severe bone comminution belongs in this group. Farming accidents, high-velocity gunshot wounds and manifest compartment syndromes are also graded as third-degree open because of their extremely high risk of infection. *Grade IV* open fractures (O-IV) include subtotal and total amputations. Subtotal amputations are defined by the Replantation Committee of the International Society for Reconstructive Surgery [3] as separation of all important anatomical structures, especially of the major vessels, with total ischaemia. The remaining soft-tissue bridge may not exceed one-fourth of the circumference. Any case of revascularization must be classified as grade III open.

Hanover Fracture Scale

The type of compound fractures treated have tended over time to the high-velocity injury patterns. The currently most frequently used classifications [15,44] have shown limitations in these types of injuries. Therefore Gustilo et al. [16] have subclassified type III injuries as III-A, III-B and III-C to improve management control.

Tscherne has developed the Hanover Fracture Scale, based on an analysis of approximately 1000 open fractures from 1972 to 1982 (Table 2). This considers every injury of the concerned extremity and consists of a checklist. The total score on this scale adds assessments of fracture type according to the AO classification [30], skin laceration, underlying soft tissues, vascularity, neurological status, contamination, compartment syndrome, elapsed time between injury and treatment and total injury severity of the patient. The category of *bone loss* represents bone fragments that were lost with the injury. The longest axis of the missing piece of bone is measured and graded as shorter or longer than 2 cm; for example, in a missing butterfly fragment the length on the outside and not the thickness is graded. For the evaluation of *soft tissues* the score provides three different criteria: size of the skin wound, extent of the skin loss, and damage to deep soft tissues such as muscles and tendons. Due to the varying diameter and thickness at different levels in the involved extremities the extent of soft-tissue damage is related to the circumference at the level of injury. This enables a comparison of different compound fractures. The three criteria allow evaluation of both superficial and of deep injury. The category *amputation* serves for a primary judgement of the amputation mechanism in respect to a possible replantation.

An exact evaluation of the neurological status at the time of admission is often difficult, but control of reflexes allowes a gross estimation of possible neurological damage. This can be important in the decision-making process

Table 2. Hanover Fracture Scale

Fracture type		Ischemia / compartment syndrome	
Type A	1	No	0
Type B	2	Incomplete	10
Type C	4	Complete	
Bone loss		<4 h	15
<2 cm	1	4–8 h	20
>2 cm	2	>8 h	25
Soft tissues		Nerves	
Skin (wound, contusion)		Palmar/plantar sensations	
No	0	Yes	0
<1/4 Circumference	1	No	8
1/4–1/2	2	Finger/toe motion	
1/2–3/4	3	Yes	0
>3/4	4	No	8
Skin defect		Contamination foreign bodies	
No	0	None	0
<1/4 Circumference	1	Single	1
1/4–1/2 Circumference	2	Multiple	2
1/2–3/4 Circumference	3	Massive	10
>3/4 Circumference	4	Bacteriological smear	
Deep soft tissues (muscle, tendon,		Aerobe, 1 germ	2
ligaments, joint capsule)		Aerobe, >1 germ	3
No	0	Anaerobe	2
<1/4 Circumference	1	Aerobe/anaerobe	4
1/4–1/2 Circumference	2	Start of treatment	
1/2–3/4 Circumference	3	(Only if soft tissue score >2)	
>3/4 Circumference	6	6–12 h	1
Amputation		>12 h	3
No	0		
Sub-/total guillotine	20		
Sub-/total crush	30		

2, 3 points, O-I; 4–19 points, O-II; 20–69 points, O-IV; >70 points, O-IV.

of salvage versus amputation. At the time of admission a bacteriological evaluation of smears is not available, but bacteriological contamination is still a component of the score to remind the treating surgeons to consider this.

The score assists in injury management and therapy supervision. In particular, partial scores based on the bone or soft-tissue criterion are valuable for treatment decisions and prediction of possible complications.

Treatment Protocol

Compound fractures require a treatment protocol to achieve good results and minimize complications. Tscherne [44] published a protocol for open fractures in 1983.

Scene of Accident

After gross reduction of the fracture a sterile dressing is applied and splinting performed by paramedics. Since open fractures often result from severe trauma, many patients with open fractures are polytraumatized. Resuscitation is therefore initiated at the scene of the accident and completed upon admission to hospital.

Admission to Hospital

The patient is evaluated, as required, both overall and as regards resuscitation. At no time is the sterile dressing over the open fracture opened; however, splints, etc. are removed for careful and full evaluation of the involved extremity, with special consideration to the circulation and nerve function. In doubtful cases emergency angiography must be carried out. As expeditiously as possible, the patient is transferred to the operating room for definitive care of the open fracture.

Operating Room Management of the Open Fracture

Only when the patient is in the operating room and under anaesthesia is the sterile wound dressing removed and a thorough wound evaluation conducted by the surgical team. Sterile preparation of the injured extremity consists of depilation and aggressive mechanical cleansing with a sterile brush and soap followed by an alcohol disinfectant of the open wound. Standard iodine and alcohol preparation of the limb and sterile draping follows. Radical débridement of all contaminated and non-viable soft tissues and jet lavage irrigation with at least 9 l irrigation solution is routinely performed. Débridement often requires enlargement of the primary wound, and the extent is determined according to the degree of contamination, the extremity involved, the required approach and the implants used (Fig. 1). Following aggressive débridement and jet lavage irrigation the extremity is again prepared with iodine and alcohol and then re-draped. The surgical team re-gowns and re-gloves, and new sterile instruments are used.

Most open fractures – as a result of the energy absorbed, the comminution of the bone and the soft-tissue injury – are inherently unstable. In addition, many of these patients have suffered multiple trauma and have other complicating injuries. Therefore the treatment protocol recommends immediate bone stabilization to avoid further damage to already compromised soft tissues and bone and to allow subsequent and adequate bone débridement and access to the soft-tissue envelope. The choice of bone and limb stabilization type is obviously that of the senior treating surgeon, but follows the protocol outlined in Table 3.

Following bone stabilization all the primary open wounds are left open, and temporary coverage is achieved with artificial skin (Epigard), which

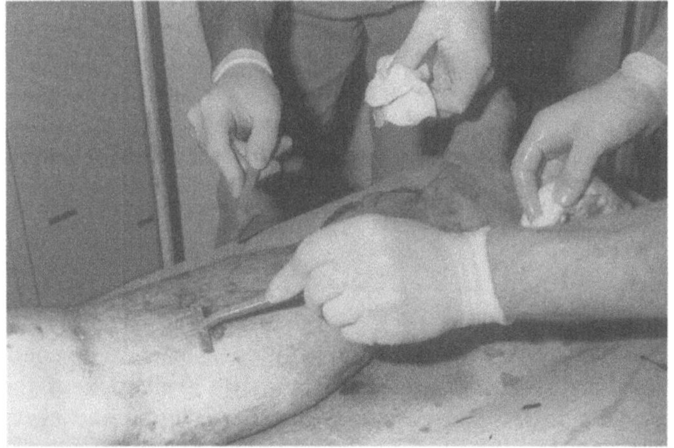

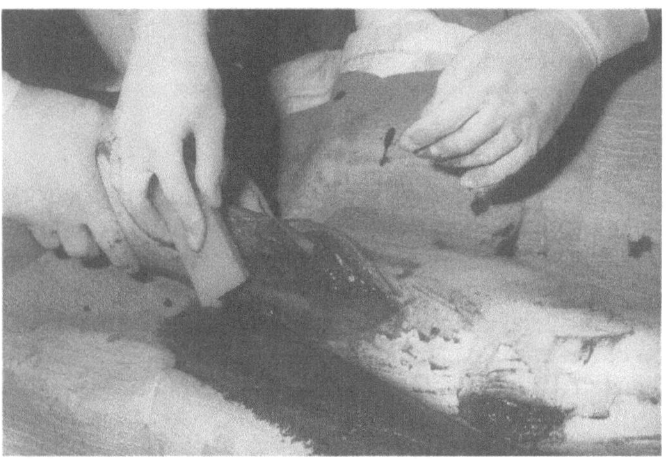

Fig. 1a–d. Operating room management of open fractures. **a** Depilation. **b** Mechanical cleansing with a sterile brush and soap. **c** Radical débridement and irrigation. **d** Wounds after débridement prior to stabilization of the fracture

prevents soft-tissue desiccation at the same time as providing a barrier to secondary contamination from the outside. Once soft-tissue control is achieved by serial débridement, delayed, primary or secondary closure or split-thickness skin graft is used to restore the soft-tissue envelope (Fig. 2). In cases with skin defects or exposed bone, classical procedures including soft-tissue transfers and/or free tissue flaps must be performed, usually 2–5 days after the injury (Fig. 3).

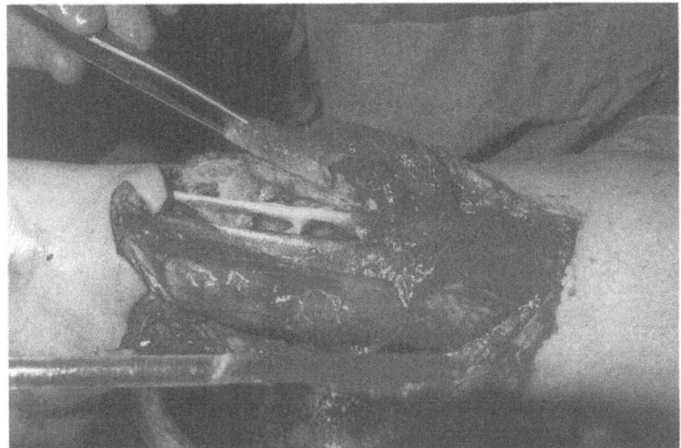

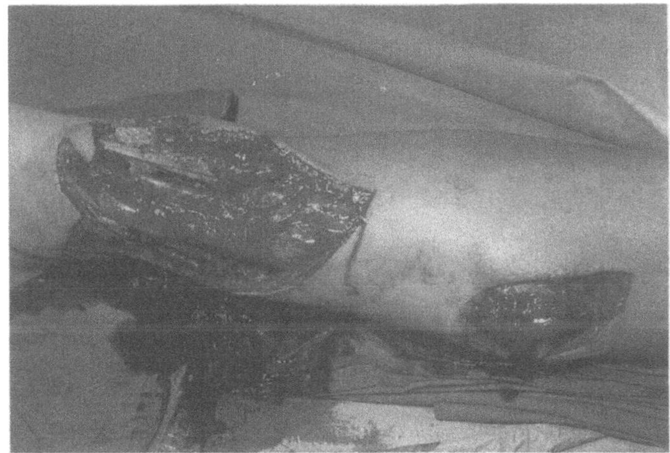

Fig. 1c,d.

Table 3. Type of fixation by soft-tissue damage and fracture location

Grade	Femur	Tibia	Humerus	Forearm
O-I C-O C-I	Interlocking nail, (plate)	Nail, interlocking nail, plate, external fixator		
O-II C-II			Plate	Plate
O-III C-III	Unreamed nail, plate	Unreamed nail, external fixator		
O-III (gross contamination)	External fixator		External fixator	External fixator

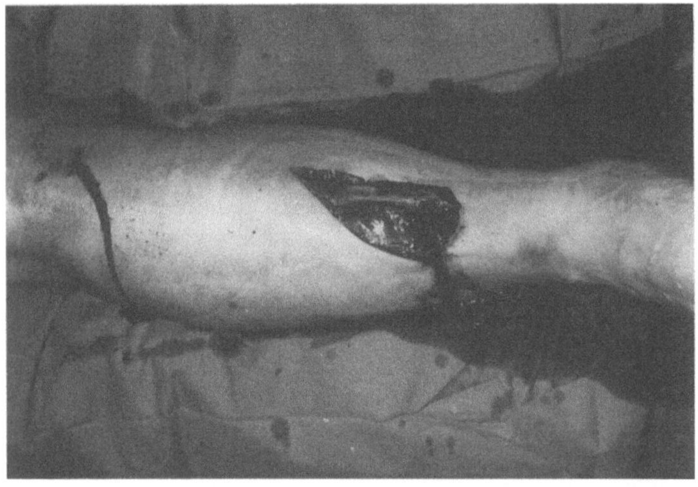

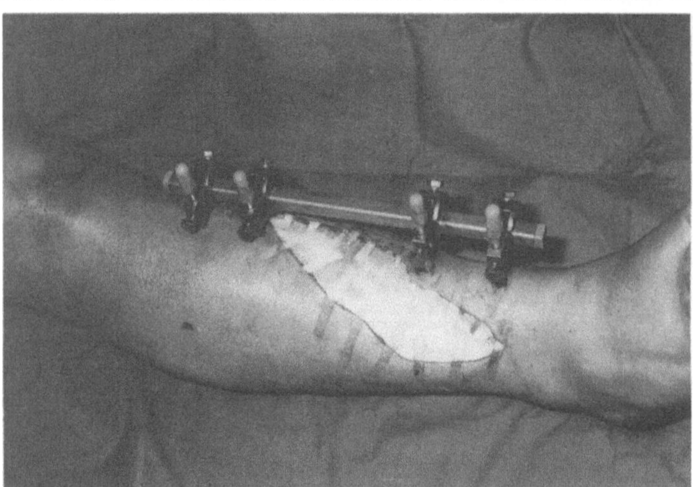

Fig. 2a–d. Soft-tissue treatment of open fractures. **a** Grade II open tibial fracture. **b** Primary soft-tissue coverage with artifical skin and fracture stabilization with external fixator. **c** Secondary closure with split skin graft. **d** Healed fracture and soft-tissue

Emergency Evaluation

Vascular Status

In the assessment of an injured limb the vascular status is a mandatory examination. The clinician must check peripheral pulses and, comparatively, extremity temperature and capillary refill. Although the absence of a palpable pulse is important information for a possible vascular impair, the presence of a pulse or capillary refill does not necessarily guarantee an intact

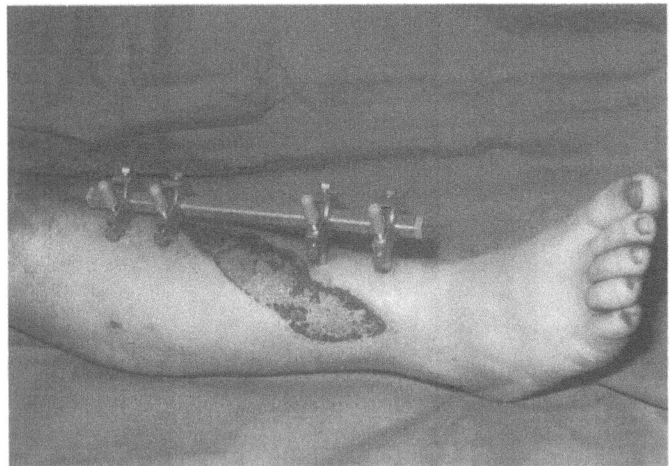

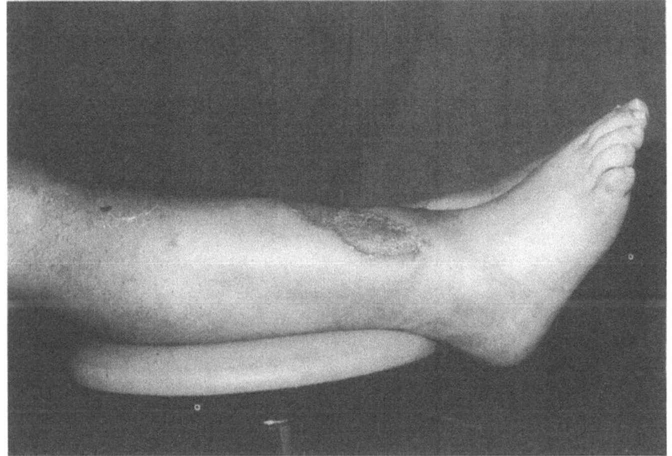

Fig. 2c,d

vascular tree. Therefore comparative Doppler examination of the injured
and unharmed extremities should be carried out. In all cases in which the
history of trauma, physical examination or radiographic fracture pattern indicates a vascular impairment an additional angiography should be performed.

Neurological Status

Gross neurological assessment can be difficult in the multiply injured patient
because of unconsciousness, lack of response for motor function and sensations. However, the reflex status and the responses to strong pain stimuli
give at least an orientation in respect to possible major deficits. This check-
up must be performed routinely because information on an existing neuro-

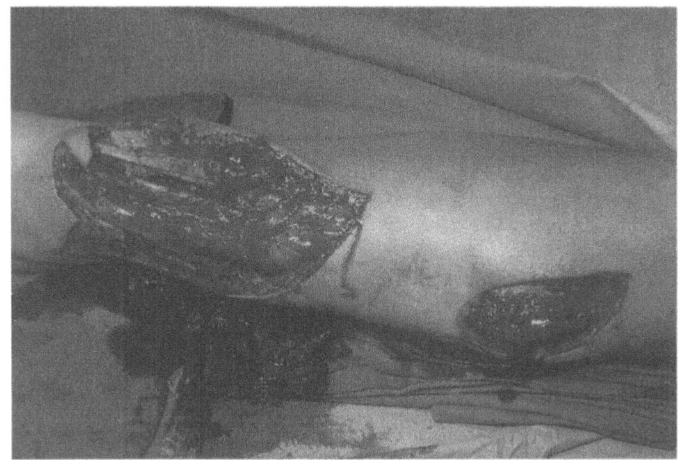

a

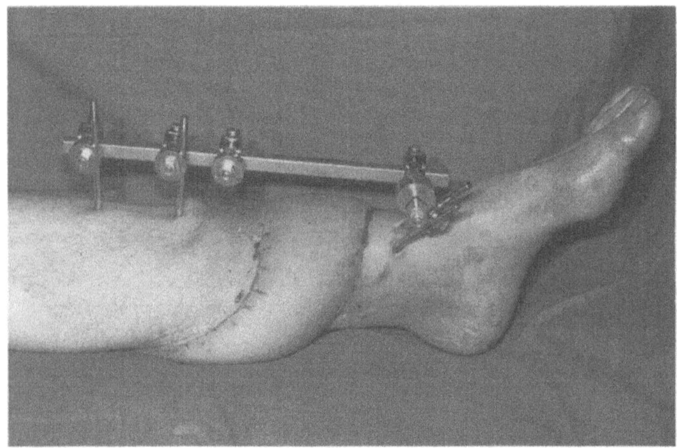

b

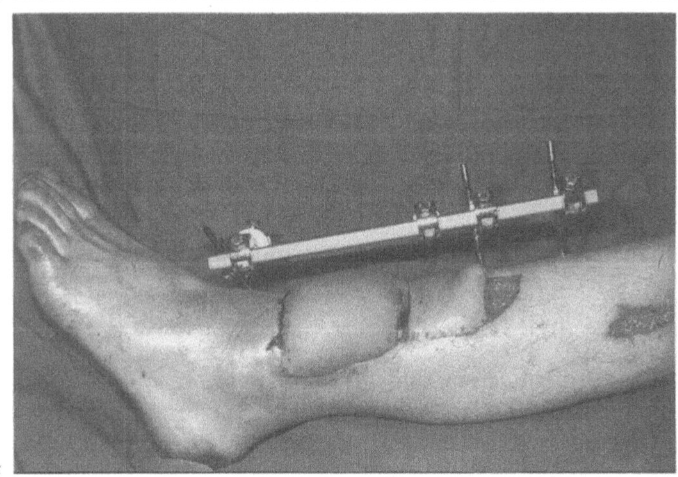

c

logical deficit can be influential in the decision of salvage attempt versus amputation in severely injured extremities.

Soft-Tissue Status

Since the skin wound is draped sterilely at the site of the accident, and the draping is not removed prior to arrival of the patient to the operating room, exact evaluation of the complete soft-tissue damage is carried out at that time. After formal surgical preparation and necessary extension of traumatic wounds a gentle manipulation under sterile operating conditions gives the best information concerning bone conditions as well as skin wound and deep soft-tissue damage – in addition to the surgical débridement, which becomes a diagnostic modality as skin edges, muscle borders and fascial elements are checked for viability and bleeding.

Bone Status

At the time of débridement the careful inspection of bone fragments, their relationship to the soft-tissue envelope and the information obtained from radiographs optimize the assessment of the bone damage.

Compartment Syndrome

Definition

Compartment syndrome is defined as an increase in interstitial fluid pressure of sufficient magnitude to compromise the micro-circulation and neuro-muscular function [23,24,28]. If the magnitude and duration of the increase in this interstitial pressure are great enough, it will lead to irreversible tissue necrosis. Patients who have suffered an untreated or over-looked compartment syndrome develop a Volkmann's ischaemic contracture that manifests clinically as a contracted non-functional limb. For preservation of function in severe extremity trauma the treating surgeon must have thorough knowledge and appreciation of the compartment syndrome to pevent its inevitable devastating functional loss.

Aetiology

Envelopes surrounding a given space in which a pressure increase can occur include the epimysium, an osseofibrous sheath, a fascia, the skin or a

---

Fig. 3a–c. Open fracture with exposed skin and bone. **a** Fracture at the end of débridement. **b,c** Healed free tissue transfer (latissimus dorsi flap)

constrictive dressing which creates a limiting boundary. The increased pressure may result from an increase in volume within a given compartment by haemorrhage, perivascular infusions, or fluid loss due to abnormal capillary permeability such as in prolonged ischaemia.

There is general agreement that the blood flow to the muscles is determined by the relationship of the intracompartmental to the blood pressure and not by the absolute pressure within a fascial compartment. Hypotension can also result in compartment syndrome [47]. Therefore multiply injured patients are predisposed to the development of compartment syndrome due to their decreased peripheral blood flow. Certain injuries entail a high risk of developing compartment syndrome, and patients can be divided into low-risk and high-risk groups. The low-risk group includes trauma patients with no shock-induced peripheral hypoxia and a simple fracture pattern without concomitant injuries. The high-risk group includes the following conditions or injuries – where the treating surgeon must consider the possibility of developing compartment syndrome: vascular injuries with peripheral ischaemia, high-energy trauma, severe soft-tissue injury, comminuted fractures of the tibia [4] and polytraumatized patients.

Treatment

The treatment of choice is dermato-fasciotomy since the intact skin acts as a limiting membrane, prolonging the compartment syndrome [13]. There are several techniques, but the most commonly used are the double-incision technique of Mubarak and Owen [29] and the parafibular dermato-fasciotomy of Matsen et al. [24]. Both techniques provide a release of all four compartments in the lower leg. Even if the pressure is increased in only one or two compartments, it is mandatory to release all. This is true for every possible location of compartment syndrome in the upper or lower extremity. Fibulectomy fasciotomy as described in the vascular surgical literature [12,22] is obsolete and contra-indicated for trauma patients; this must be considered a severe treatment error.

Soft-Tissue Treatment

Analysis of open fracture studies shows that about 10 years ago surgeons were reluctant to perform radical débridement, fearing soft-tissue defects and healing failures. However, the results were bone infections and multiple operations. Therefore it is necessary to perform radical débridement with removal of all non-viable soft-tissues and dead bone. The use of jet lavage, scheduled redébridements, and a low threshold for early plastic procedures are also part of the treatment protocol as outlined.

Primarily, skin defects are covered with artificial skin. Once soft-tissue control is achieved, wound closure is attempted by delayed, primary or secondary closure or split-thickness skin graft. In all cases with a remaining skin defect or exposed bone, classical procedures including soft-tissue transfers and/or free tissue flaps must be performed, usually 2–5 days after the injury. In open fractures of grade I primary wound closure is usually possible. In a number of cases of grade II open fractures primary closure can also be performed, usually in fractures of the humerus, forearm or femur. In all other cases secondary wound treatment is necessary.

The maximum soft-tissue score on the Hanover Fracture Scale (Table 2) is 14 points for any soft-tissue injury. The soft-tissue score is helpful in considering possibly necessary plastic procedures in those cases in which it is less obvious. Scores of 1–4 points usually allow secondary suture of the wound. Scores of 5 or 6 points require split skin grafts, and a score of 7 points or higher requires a local or free flap.

Fracture Treatment

After aggressive débridement of all non-viable tissue attention is turned to the fracture. Since most compound fractures are inherently unstable and have a tendency to secondary redislocation even after a good reduction, further damage to the already compromised soft tissues is inevitable, leading to pressure on damaged tissues, necrosis and secondary infection. Optimal conditions for an undisturbed recovery and healing of injured soft tissues are provided only with a totally stable fixation of the fractured bone.

Exceptions to operative fracture treatment are very rare: cases in which only a minimum of muscular and periosteal damage is found, the fracture

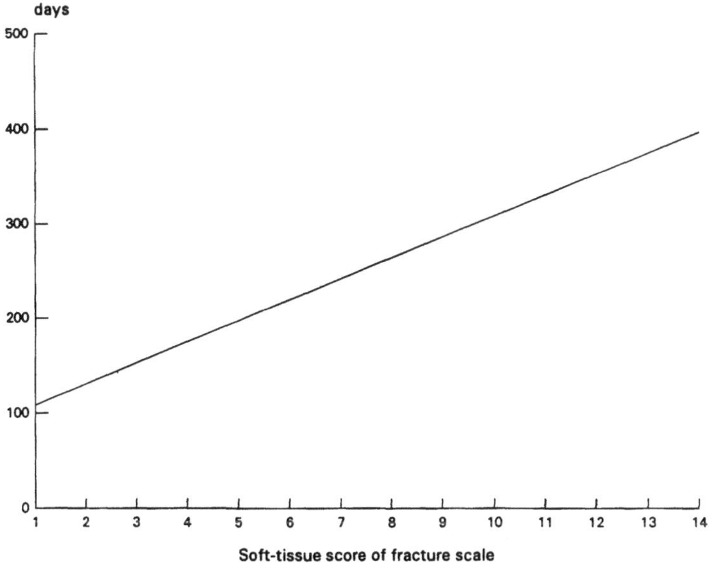

Fig. 4. Relationship between time to union in tibia fractures and soft-tissue damage

itself is reasonably stable, and retention is possible through adequate immobilization by conservative means (e.g. humeral and tibial shaft fractures, periarticular fractures).

Selection of the type of fixation depends on numerous factors, discussed in Chaps. 2–4 and 7–15 in this volume. The primary goal in all cases of open fractures is rigid fixation with a minimum amount of hardware to prevent further compromise of the damaged soft tissues and to preserve the vascularity of the bone. Table 3 gives an overview of preferred implants for different fracture locations and the concomitant soft-tissue injury.

In considering the type of fixation it is helpful to recall that the time to union is a function of the concomitant soft-tissue injury. Figure 4 illustrates the linear function between healing time and soft-tissue score on the Hanover fracture scale in open tibial shaft fractures.

Complications

Osteitis

The incidence of post-traumatic osteitis is multifactorial and related both to the injury and the treatment [1,2,8–10,15–20,25–27,32–34,36–38,40,42,45]. A discriminant analysis of 948 open fractures treated by the authors from 1981 to 1989, revealed the following factors to be the most influential and of statistical significance: bone loss, deep soft-tissue damage, primary contamination in terms of bacteriological smear, occurrence of soft-tissue infection, skin loss, compartment syndrome and ischaemia. Figure 5 illustrates that incomplete or complete ischaemia is followed five times as often by post-traumatic osteitis than is a normally perfused extremity. Undisturbed vascularity had an osteitis rate of 0.8%, while in cases of an incomplete/ complete ischaemia the bone infection rate was 4.1%.

The much more radical débridements in recent years with improved soft-tissue reconstructive procedures have still not been able to eliminate osteitis, but primary damage to the soft tissue must exceed one-half the circumference of the involved extremity to entail a significant rise in the frequency of post-traumatic osteitis (Fig. 6). In cases of extensive soft-tissue damage the bone infection rate was 3.9%.

The type of bacteriological contamination in terms of the results of bacteriological smear prior to antibiosis and soft-tissue débridement has a significant influence on the development of post-traumatic osteitis, as illustrated in Fig. 7. Cultures with more than one aerobe germ or mixed aerobe/anaerobe cultures had a increased rate of bone infections of 3.8% and 4.0% in comparison to 1.5% in those cases in which only a single germ was cultured.

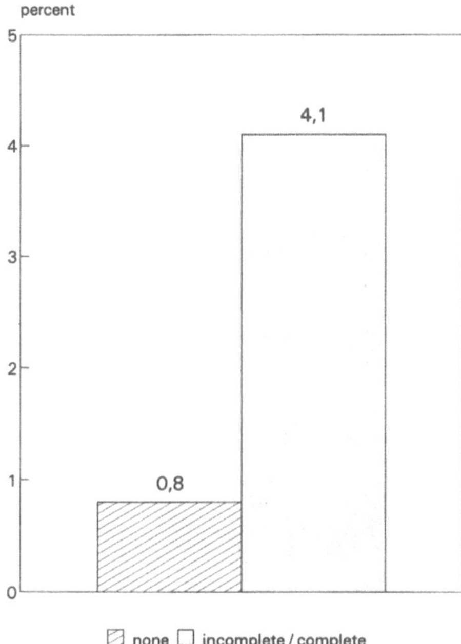

Fig. 5. Relationship between osteitis and ischaemia

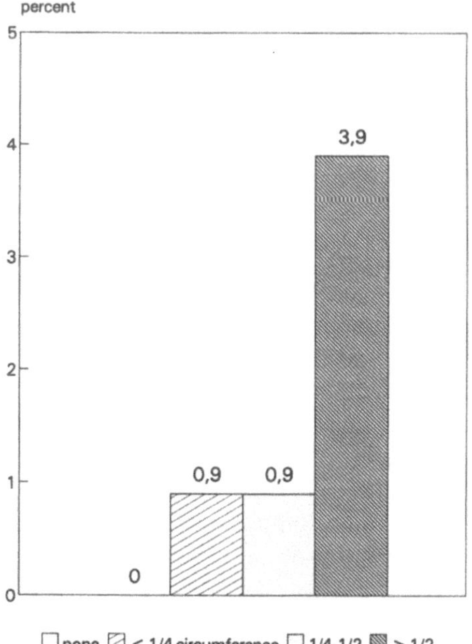

Fig. 6. Relationship between osteitis and soft-issue injury

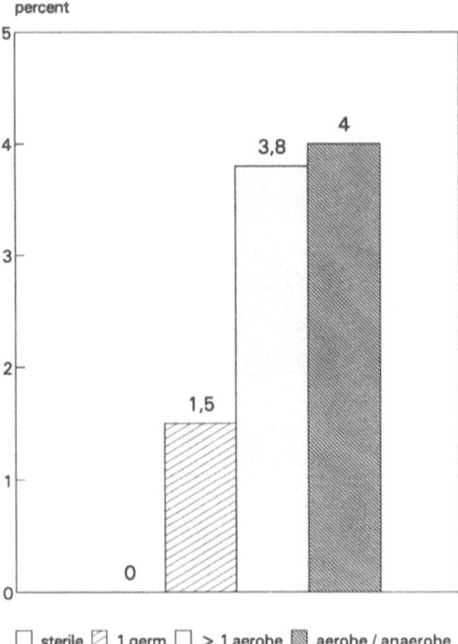

Fig. 7. Relationship between osteitis and contamination

The above figures illustrate the dependence of post-traumatic osteitis on various aspects of the injured extremity. Exact estimation of the damage to the different structures of a concerned extremity is necessary to optimize treatment and prospective outcome.

Non-Union

According to the literature [5–7,11,14,21,31,35,39,41,43], high-velocity trauma with severely comminuted and unstable fractures are the most important factors in non-union. Type of fixation and fracture location are also thought to have an effect. A discriminant analysis of 948 open fractures showed the following factors to be statistically significant: amount of bone loss (Fracture Scale variable), fracture type (according to AO classification) and severity of fracture (torsion, oblique, butterfly, comminuted, defect). The fracture scale variable of bone loss was the most influential variable (Fig. 8). Non-union rates in cases of no or minor bone loss of less than 2 cm were 3.8% and 3.0%, respectively, while in cases of more than 2 cm the rate was 10.6%.

According to the AO classification of fractures, non-union rates in A, B and C fractures were, respectively, 2.4%, 2.7%, and 7.5% ($p < 0.03$; Fig. 9). In contrast to opinions expressed in the literature, we did not find a

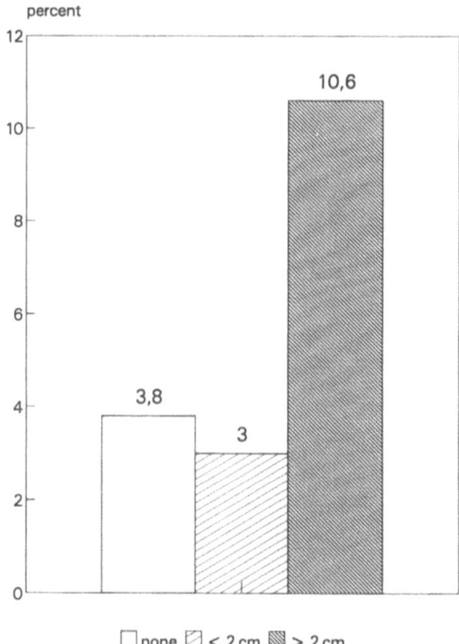

Fig. 8. Relationship between osteitis and bone loss

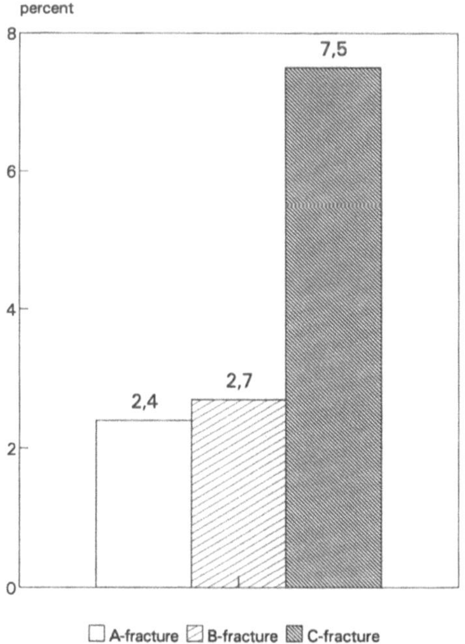

Fig. 9. Relationship between osteitis and fracture type

significant correlation between soft-tissue damage and the incidence of non-union. Soft-tissue damage does, however, influence the time necessary for fracture consolidation (Fig. 4).

Knowledge of the factors affecting non-union in open fractures assists the surgeon in taking appropriate measures for their prevention.

References

1. Bach AW, Hansen ST Jr (1989) Plates versus external fixation in severe open tibial shaft fractures. A randomized trial. Clin Orthop 241:89–94
2. Benson DR, Riggins RS, Lawrence RM, Hoeprich PD, Huston AC, Harrison JA (1983) Treatment of open fractures: a prospective study. J Trauma 23(1): 25–30
3. Biemer E (1982) Internationale Definitionen im Gebiet der Replantationschirurgie und Möglichkeiten eines Bewertungsschemas der funktionellen Ergebnisse. Handchirurgre 14:161
4. Blick SS, Brumback RJ, Poka A et al. (1986) Compartment syndrome in open tibial fractures. J Bone Joint Surg [Am] 68:1348
5. Boyd HB, Lipinski SW, Wiley JH (1961) Observations on non-union of the shafts of the long bones with a statistical analysis of 842 patients. J Bone Joint Surg [Am] 43:159–168
6. Chan KM, Leung YK, Cheng JC, Leung PC (1984) The management of type III open tibial fractures. Injury 16(3):157–165
7. Clancey GJ, Hansen ST Jr (1978) Open fractures of the tibia: a review of one hundred and two cases. J Bone Joint Surg [Am] 60(1):118–122
8. Clifford RP, Beauchamp CG, Kellam JF, Webb JK, Tile M (1988) Plate fixation of open fractures of the tibia. J Bone Joint Surg [Br] 70(4):644–648
9. Dellinger EP, Caplan ES, Weaver LD, Wertz MJ, Droppert BM, Hoyt N, Brumback R, Burgess A, Poka A, Benirschke SK, Lennard ES, Lou MA (1988) Duration of preventive antibiotic administration for open extremity fractures. Arch Surg 123(3):333–339
10. Dellinger EP, Miller SD, Wertz MJ, Grypma M, Droppert B, Anderson PA (1988) Risk of infection after open fracture of the arm or leg. Arch Surg 123(11):1320–1327
11. Edwards CC, Simmons SC, Browner BD, Weigel MC (1988) Severe open tibial fractures. Results treating 202 injuries with external fixation. Clin Orthop 230:98–115
12. Ernst CB, Kaufer H (1971) Fibulectomy – faciotomy. J Trauma 11:365
13. Gaspard DJ, Kohl RD (1975) Compartmental syndromes in which skin is limiting boundary. Clin Orthop 113:65
14. Gershuni DH, Pinsker R (1982) Bone grafting for nonunion of fractures of the tibia: a critical review. J Trauma 22(1):43–49
15. Gustilo RB, Anderson JT (1976) Prevention of infection in the treatment of one thousand and twenty-five open fractures of long bones: retrospective and prospective analyses. J Bone Joint Surg [Am] 58(4):453–458
16. Gustilo RB, Mendoza RM, Williams DN (1984) Problems in the management of type III (severe) open fractures: a new classification of type III open fractures. T Trauma 24(8):742–746
17. Gustilo RB, Gruninger RP, Davis T (1987) Classification of type III (severe) open fractures relative to treatment and results. Orthopedics 10(12):1781–1788

18. Gustilo RB, Merkow RL, Templeman D (1990) The management of open fractures. J Bone Joint Surg [Am] 72(2):299–304
19. Haas NP, Suedkamp NP, Tscherne H (1990) Infektionshäufigkeit: Ursachen und Vermeidung in der Unfallchirurgie. Aktuel Probl Chir Orthop 34:8–26
20. Jahna H (1982) Die konservative Behandlung des Oberschenkelschaftbruches. Hefte Unfallheilkd 158:106–111
21. Karlstroem G, Olerud S (1974) Fractures of the tibial shaft; a critical evaluation of treatment alternatives. Clin Orthop 105:82–115
22. Keays AC (1981) Fibulectomy – fasciotomy. J Bone Joint Surg [Br] 63:478
23. Matsen FA III (1980) Compartmental syndromes. Grune and Stratton, New York
24. Matsen FA III, Winquist RA, Krugmire RB Jr (1980) Diagnosis and management of compartmental syndromes. J Bone Joint Surg [Am] 62:286
25. McGraw JM, Lim EV (1988) Treatment of open tibial-shaft fractures. External fixation and secondary intramedullary nailing. J Bone Joint Surg [Am] 70(6): 900–911
26. Merritt K (1988) Factors increasing the risk of infection in patients with open fractures. J Trauma 28(6):823–827
27. Moore TJ, Mauney C, Barron J (1989) The use of quantitative bacterial counts in open fractures. Clin Orthop 248:227–230
28. Mubarak SJ, Hargens AR (1981) Compartment-syndromes and Volkmann's contracture. Saunders, Philadelphia
29. Mubarak SJ, Owen CA (1977) Double-incision fasciootomy of the leg for decompression in compartment-syndromes. J Bone Joint Surg [Am] 59:184
30. Mueller ME, Nazarian S, Koch P (1988) The AO classification of fractures. Springer, Berlin Heidelberg New York
31. Nicoll EA (1964) Fractures of the tibial shaft: a survey of 705 cases. J Bone Joint Surg [Br] 46:373–387
32. Patzakis MJ, Wilkins J (1989) Factors influencing infection rate in open fracture wounds. Clin Orthop 243:36–40
33. Patzakis MJ, Wilkins J, Moore TM (1983) Considerations in reducing the infection rate in open tibial fractures. Clin Orthop 178:36–41
34. Patzakis MJ, Wilkins J, Moore TM (1983) Use of antibiotics in open tibial fractures. Clin Orthop 178:31–35
35. Reckling FW, Waters CH (1980) Treatment of non-unions of fractures of the tibial diaphysis by posterolateral cortical cancellous bone-grafting. J Bone Joint Surg [Am] 62(6):936–941
36. Rittmann WW, Schibli M, Matter P, Allgöwer M (1979) Open fractures. Long-term results in 200 consecutive cases. Clin Orthop 138:132–140
37. Rojczyk M (1981) Keimbesiedlung und Keimverhalten bei offenen Frakturen. Unfallheilkunde 84(11):458–462
38. Rommens P, Broos P, Theunis P, Willemen P, Gruwez JA (1985) The operative treatment of tibial shaft fractures: a review of 277 cases. Acta Chir Belg 85(4):268–273
39. Rosenthal RE, MacPhail JA, Oritz JE (1977) Non-union in open tibial fractures. J Bone Joint Surg [Am] 59(2):244–248
40. Russell GG, Henderson R, Arnett G (1990) Primary or delayed closure for open tibial fractures. J Bone Joint Surg [Br] 72(1):125–128
41. Schmelzeisen H (1979) Infektpseudarthrosen des Tibiaschaftes – klinische Studie an 252 Fällen. Hefte Unfallheilkd 138:167–168
42. Schreinlechner P (1982) Infekthäufigkeit nach Plattenosteosynthesen offener Unterschenkelfrakturen. Hefte Unfallheilkd 157:86–89
43. Simpson JM, Ebraheim NA, An HS, Jackson WT (1990) Posterolateral bone graft of the tibia. Clin Orthop 251:200–206
44. Tscherne H (1983) Management offener Frakturen. Hefte Unfallheilkd 162:10–32

45. Weise K, Holz U, Sauer N (1983) Zweit- bis drittgradig offene Frakturen langer
    Röhrenknochen – therapeutisches Management und Behandlungsergebnisse.
    Aktuel Traumatol 13(1):24–29
46. Yaremchuk MJ, Burgess AR, Brumback RJ (1989) Lower extremity salvage and
    reconstruction. Elsevier, New York
47. Zeifach SS, Hargens AR, Evans KI, Gonsalves MR, Smith RK, Mubarek SJ,
    Akeson WM (1980) Skeletal muscle necrosis in pressurized compartments as-
    sociated with hemorrhagic hypotension. J Trauma 20:941

6 Microvascular Reconstruction in Limb Trauma

L.K. HUNG

Microsurgical techniques enable the reimplantation of amputated limbs, the precise repair of severed vessels and nerves, and to a certain extent a more refined repair of tendons. Microsurgery also adds to the armamentarium of the trauma surgeon a flexibility in the transplantation of composite tissues for the reconstruction of multilated limbs: vascularised bone graft or vascularised skin coverage. On a more selective basis, especially for the mutilated hand, vascularised tendon grafts, vascularised muscles, vascularised joint or a whole digit and vascularised nerves can also be transplanted. A vascularised growth plate transplantation in a growing limb is also a not too theoretical possibility.

Replantation and Revascularisation

Replantation or revascularisation of the amputated limb is a well-established technique. There are replantation centres in almost every major city of the world. Success rates for replantations are reported in the range of 80%–90% depending on the nature of the injury and the level of amputation [1–4] (Fig. 1). Certain aspects of replantation and revascularisation need to be looked at in greater detail.

Replantations in the Hand

It is becoming increasingly clear that some digital amputations are not suitable for replantation and fare better with primary revision amputation and closure of the stump [5]. The decision requires experience and confidence on the part of the surgeon. When the amputation occurs in the region of the "no man's land", the result of replantation is usually unsatisfactory: tendon adhesion is almost inevitable, and nerve regeneration is imperfect. The end result may be a stiff and numb finger which the patient avoids using. Therefore a primary revision amputation may return him to work sooner. This is especially true for the index finger [4] (Fig. 2).

Similarly, the prognosis of ring avulsion amputation is so poor that the consensus of opinion is not to replant it [6]. However, the residual deformity

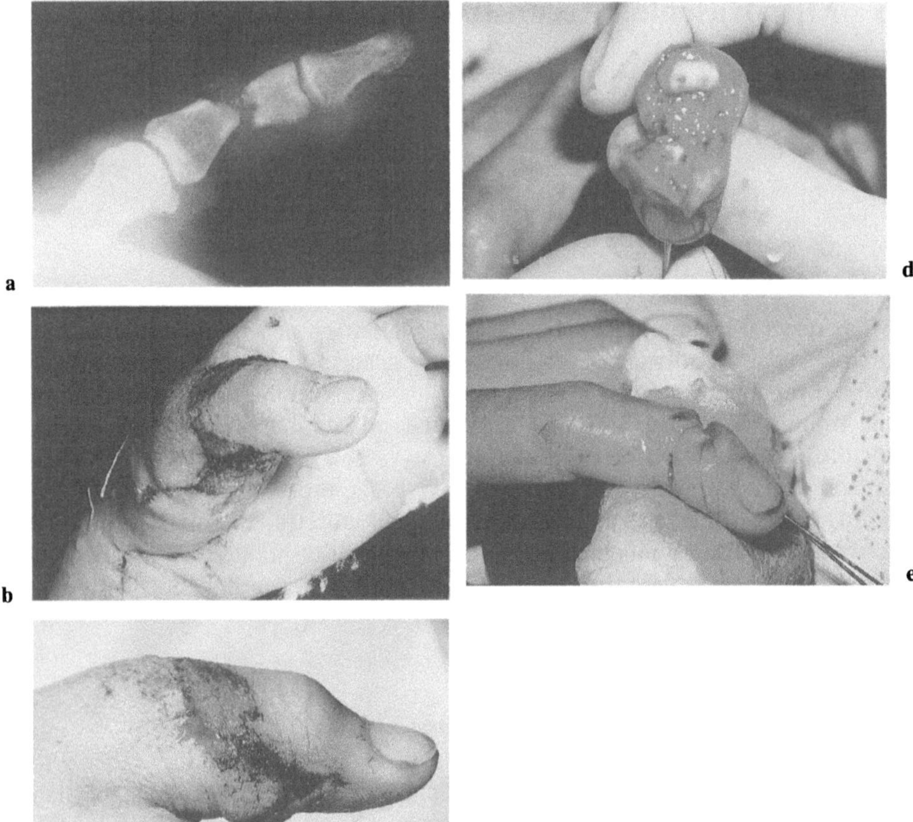

Fig. 1a–e. Two successful examples of replantation/revascularisation. **a,b,c** Amputation of the thumb through the proximal phalanx, with successful replantation. **d,e** Near amputation of the index finger through the distal interphalangeal joint, which was successfully revascularised

after amputation of the ring finger is unacceptable and is difficult to correct. One must therefore look for alternative surgical options.

We still favour replantation of ring avulsions especially for manual workers. The technique that we use [7] converts the amputated part into a skin tube by opening up on the ulnar side, enabling excision of the distal part of the phalangeal bone which has come off (Fig. 3). This allows good decompression of the vessels and very ample shortening. There is no need for any vessel grafts. The end result is a short finger (roughly the same as the little finger) with about a 50° range of movement of the remaining interphalangeal joint. There are obvious limitations to this technique, but it may be considered when the suitable situation arises. When this technique cannot be used, and when the amputated ring finger cannot be replanted,

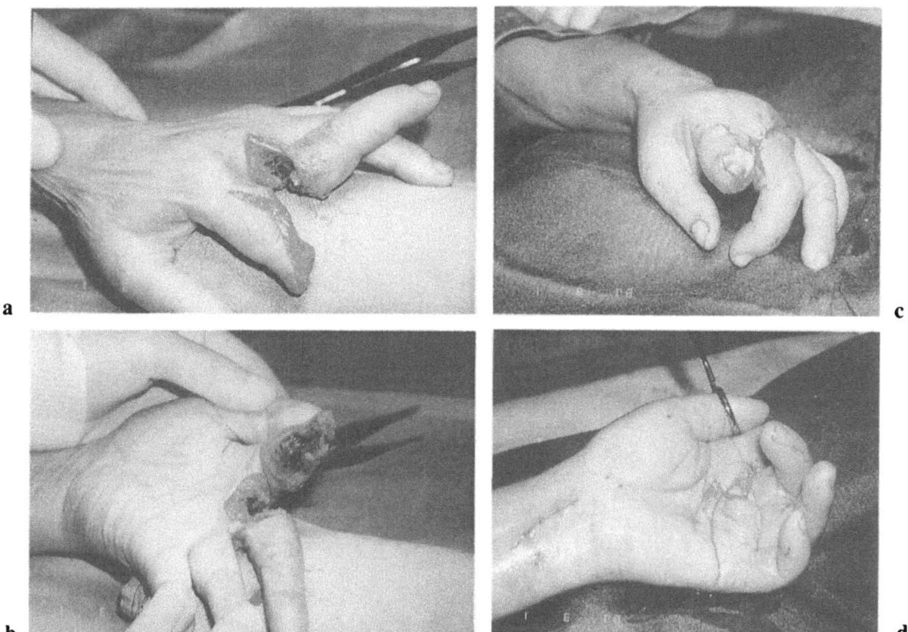

Fig. 2. a,b Two views of an oblique amputation of the index finger and a near amputation of the middle finger. **c,d** The index finger was not replanted, and the stump closed. The middle finger was successfully revascularised

one is faced with a difficult situation of reconstructing the gap left by the missing ring finger. The manual worker may find it inconvenient since small objects may drop and the grip is weakened. It may therefore be necessary to transpose the little finger by means of a carpal ostcotomy [8]. Amputation of the middle finger poses similar problems although the solution is simpler: transposition of the index finger, which is relatively straightforward.

In summary, the general indications for digital replantation are: amputations occurring in children, those involving the thumb, amputation through the metacarpal bones, amputation through the wrist and selectively in multiple digital amputations. The general contraindications include amputations through the "no man's land" (zone II), especially in the index finger, and avulsion amputations.

Replantations in the Arm and Forearm

Replantations of proximal upper limb amputations are full of dilemmas and controversies [2,9]. The nature of injuries around the arm is frequently that of avulsion or crush. Damage to muscles and soft tissues makes the prognosis very poor. Many of these patients also have other major injuries, such as to

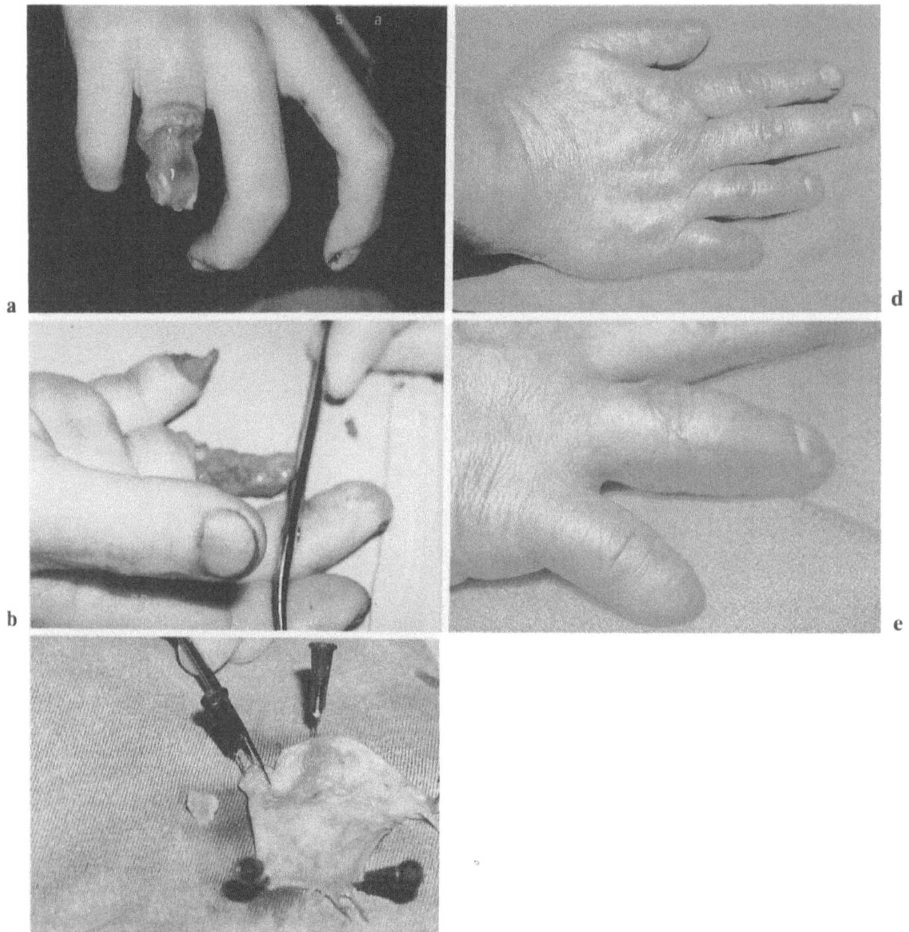

Fig. 3a–e. Ring avulsion injury. **a,b** Two views of a case of ring avulsion amputation of the ring finger. **c** The amputated part was opened up along the ulnar side, with removal of any bone remnant and adequate decompression of neurovascular bundles. This skin flap was replanted onto the proximal finger stump. **d,e** Postoperative views of the same patient. The little finger was shortened for a concomitant tip injury

the head and neck or to the abdomen. Ischaemic time is inevitably prolonged. With all these factors in mind, it is not easy to make a decision whether to replant an amputated arm. On the other hand, amputation above the elbow is not well accepted by patients. Prosthetic compliance is low, and in developing countries where prosthetic support is not adequate many patients eventually become non-users. Under such circumstances one can perhaps cautiously attempt a replantation with the limited aim of preserving the function of the elbow. When this is decided, perfusion and refrigeration of the arm may be necessary. Temporary shunting between the amputated part and the proximal vessels is essential to reduce the ischaemic time when the bone is being fixed (Fig. 4).

Amputation through the forearm also leaves many structures to repair and reconstruct. If the amputation passes through the muscle bellies, satisfactory repair is difficult, and healing of the muscle mass eventually results in fibrosis. Repair in the tendinous portion of the muscles is also challenged by the problem of fibrosis. The nerves after repair take over 1 year for good sensation to recover. A recent review [9] failed to show a relationship between the nature of injury and the eventual functional outcome, and this has added to the controversy of below-elbow amputations. Set against replantation, which requires lengthy rehabilitation with an unpredictable result, one has the alternative of a primary below-elbow amputation. When prosthetic support is good, a prosthesis can be fitted in 2 months, and the patient can quickly return to useful activities. Myoelectric prosthesis fitting takes about the same duration of time, and the results are even more gratifying (Fig. 5).

When the amputation occurs through the wrist or the palm, replantation is the only option since there is presently no viable alternative. Despite the high likelihood of tendon adhesions, nerve function can be expected to recover faster and better than more proximal amputations and usually takes 6 months (Fig. 6). Emergency flap coverage of the hand may also be performed at the same time (Fig. 7).

Lower Limb Replantations

The replantation of lower limbs is fraught with controversies. Despite sporadic reports of gratifying results [10] the general feeling at present is that for amputations below the knee the results of replantation are not comparable to well-fitted below-knee prostheses and are therefore generally not indicated for replantation. The reasons are usually apparent, as most of these injuries result from severe crushing, avulsion or degloving associated with significant degrees of contamination of the wounds. Nerve regeneration in such situations is obviously very poor, and frequently the limb remains hypo-aesthetic. Healing of muscles and tendons is also associated with substantial fibrosis. In addition, the skin coverage of the distal part of the leg is rather poor, and very often there are problems with bone union.

Similar considerations also apply to severe open fractures of the lower limbs. The type III-C open fracture with extensive soft-tissue injuries and compromise of the circulation poses the dilemma of salvage or amputation. Reports from a few renowned trauma centres in developed countries have shown the generally poor outcome of many of these cases and have thrown serious doubt on the merits of salvaging these limbs initially since many of these eventually result in amputation [11–14]. A major consideration in the justification for amputation is in fact socioeconomic and cultural [15]. Similar

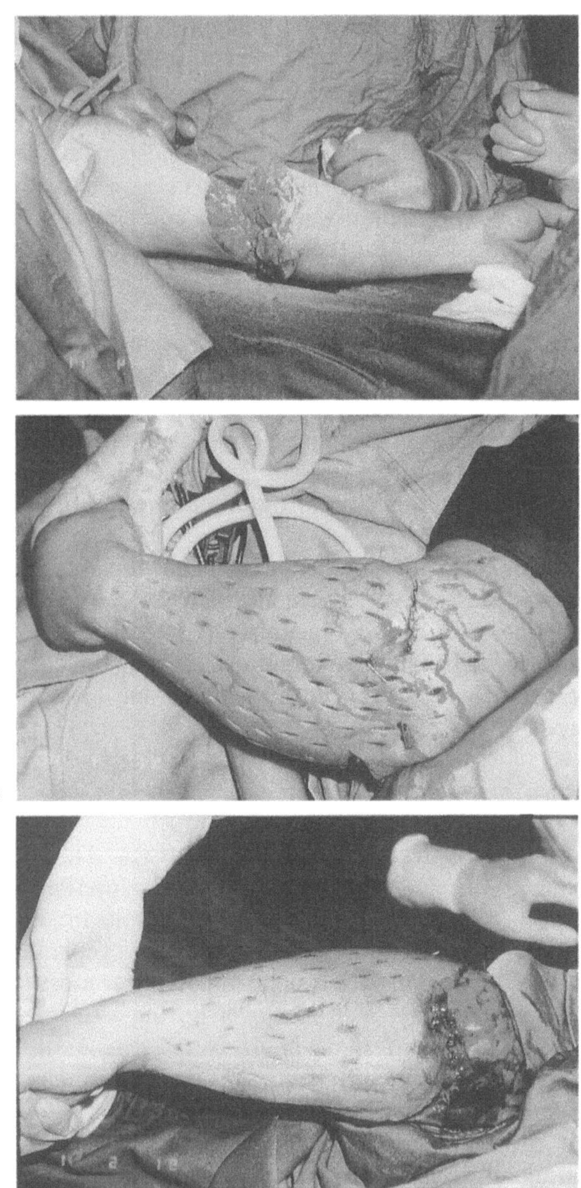

Fig. 4. a,b Nearly complete amputation of the arm through the elbow. It was successfully revascularised although multiple skin incisions were required for decompression and reduction of swelling. **c** Appearance at 10 days. With shrinkage of the swelling the incisions closed up spontaneously. The wound around the elbow required skin grafting

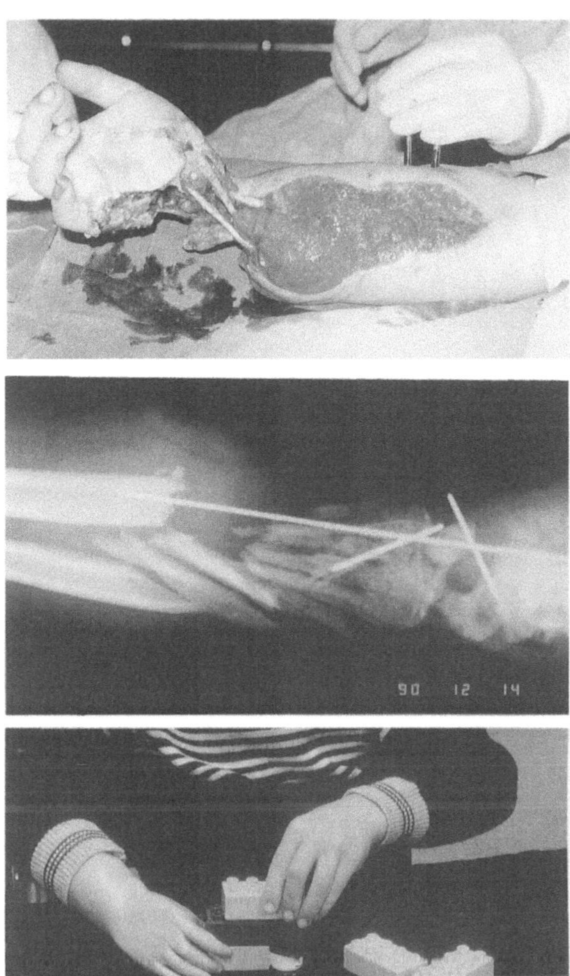

Fig. 5. a Severely crushed forearm showing extensive bone and soft-tissue defect. **b** Radiograph showing the badly comminuted fracture of the radius and the segment of bone lost from the ulnar. The wrist joint was also grossly disrupted. A below-elbow amputation was preformed. Myoelectric prosthesis was subsequently fitted successfully. **c** An example of a myoelectric prosthesis for forearm injury

long-term studies from the developing countries on open fracture are lacking. Of course, in situations in which resources are very limited or poorly organised the choice is obvious. However, when the situation is not so depressing, what is the better option?

The case of leprosy patients may provide insights regarding the choice between amputation and salvage of a defective leg. In leprosy one

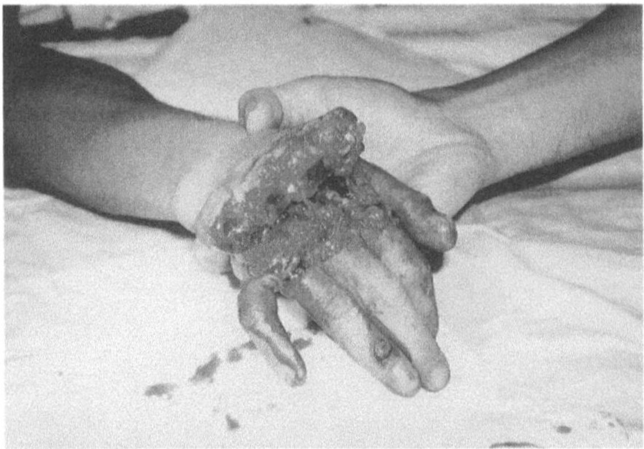

a

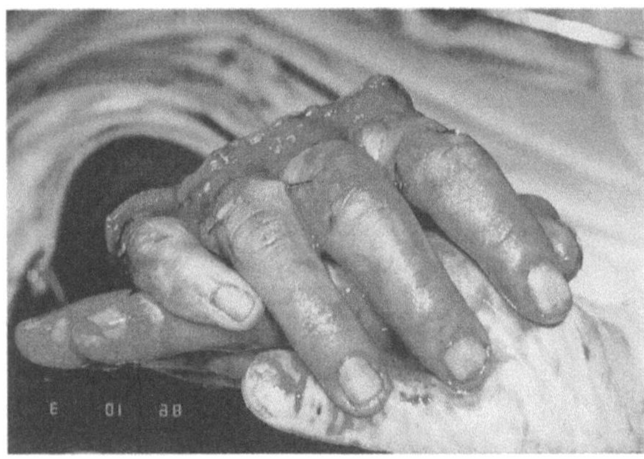

b

Fig. 6. a Near amputation of the hand through the metatarsal heads with division of all neurovascular bundles. **b** The hand was successfully revascularised

endeavours to conserve the limb, and is usually successful. It is well documented that many of these patients retain reasonable functional use of their limbs for a long time. In developing countries, where farming is still the principle economic activity, and transportation is poorly developed, the priority for retaining the limb is far higher, as few artificial limbs can withstand such rough handling. There is seldom ischaemia in leprosy, however, and therefore the analogy is valid only if one can ensure very good repair of the vessels and reperfusion of the replanted limb. A favourable factor in developing countries is the generally warm weather and therefore decreased risk of vasospastic complications.

Careful consideration of amputations at or above the knee level suggests replantation or some modified form of it may be a better option. Above-knee prostheses are not as yet entirely satisfactory, and few patients enjoy a very normal life with them. Conserving the knee joint by replantation is more beneficial to the patient. Of course, for the knee to be functional it requires the presence of sufficiently innervated muscles proximally.

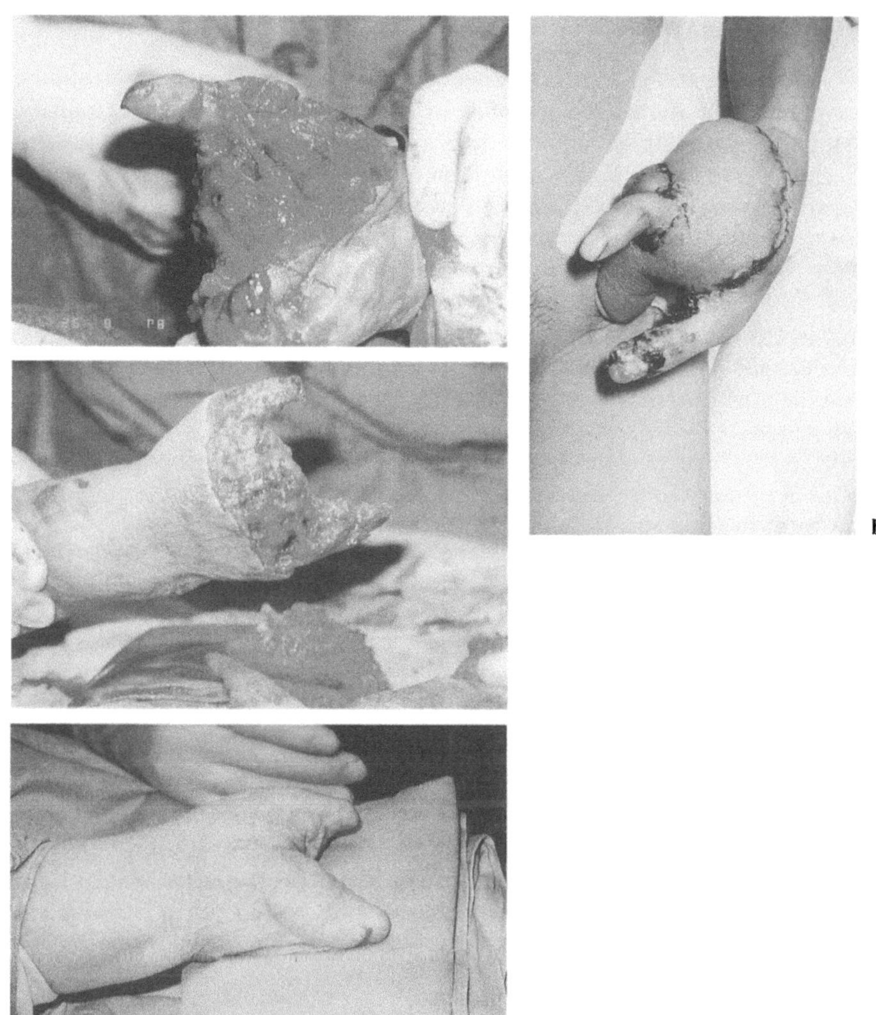

Fig. 7. a Severely crushed hand with multiple amputation of digits and degloving of the hand. **b** One digit was replanted back to the first metacarpal to become a new thumb and the large wound resurfaced by a pedicled groin flap. **c** Another case of severely crushed hand with loss of three digits which were not salvagable. **d** A free dorsalis pedis flap with the first toe web was transplanted to resurface the large wound. The toe web was wrapped around the remnant of the proximal phalanx of the thumb to build it up

Salvage Replantations

For injuries slightly distal to the knee joint in which a complete replantation is not justified, it may be possible to perform a salvage replantation by retaining parts of the amputated limb to fashion a good below-knee stump. An emergency free-flap transplantation may also be performed to cover and preserve or construct a sufficient below-knee segment, therefore retaining a functional knee joint and enabling the fitting of a below-knee prosthesis. There are a few successful reports on the transplantation of a segment of fibula to lengthen the stump or on the transplantation of musculocutaneous flaps to cover degloved below-knee segments (Fig. 8) [16]. This concept has been expanded to the "banking" concept whereby amputated parts, usually from the upper extremity, are temporarily revascularised to an untraumatised area of the body with readily accessible vessels. This keeps the amputated parts alive while awaiting stabilisation of the patient's general condition before a proper reimplantation can be carried out to reattach the amputated part to its original site [17] (Fig. 9).

The Open Fracture

Severe open fracture of the extremities poses multiple problems in managing the bone defect, sometimes involving the joint, skin coverage, reconstruction of nerve function, vascularity and tendon function – which is frequently overlooked in the lower extremities [18]. A recent classification divides these fractures into five grades (Table 1), but a more practical classification may still be the more established concept of Gustilo, with grades I–III and subgroups A, B and C for grade III open fractures, the latter of which are badly contused fractures with large open wounds and ischemia [19–21].

Soft-Tissue Coverage

It has long been recognised that the wound in open fractures can be closed primarily or early with vascularised tissue, such as the gastrocnemius muscle flap for proximal tibia; this entails no increased risk of infection [22–24]. For large wound defects in type III open fractures, microvascular transplantation of skin, muscle or a musculocutaneous flap is the best means to cover the wound, although some "simpler" local flaps may be used (Fig. 10). The best quality of skin is provided by the free-flap transplantation; this brings the least disturbance of the local wound and structures and immediately improves vascularity [25–27]. The best functional and aesthetic results can be achieved. In the presence of gross contamination or even low-grade infection, if the wound can be thoroughly débrided and cleaned, closing the wound with a vascularised tissue flap is not a problem [28]. In fact the vascularised tissue transplant promotes local vascularity, which is also beneficial to leucocyte function [29].

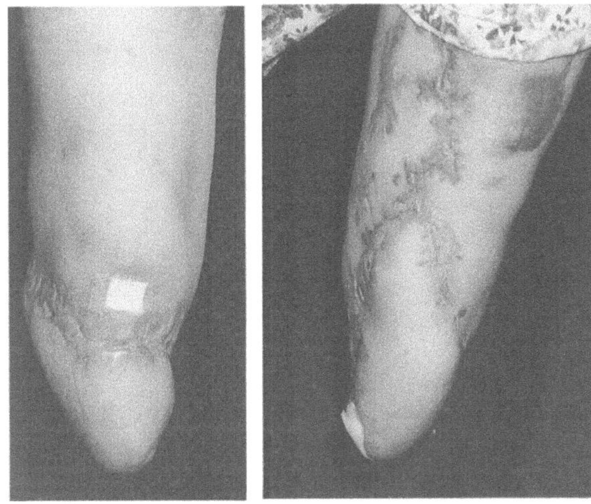

a,b

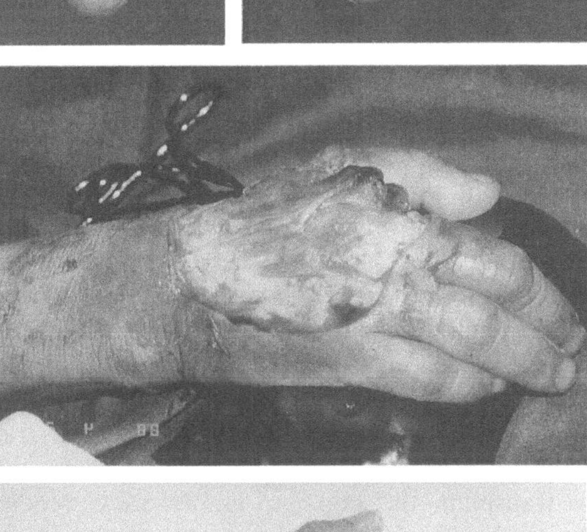

c

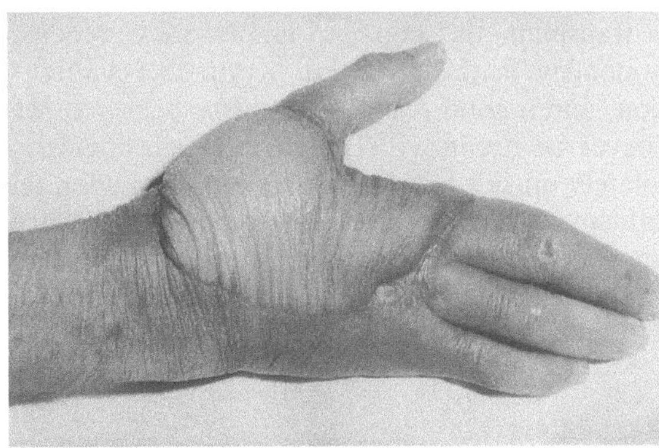

d

Fig. 8a–d. Severely crushed injury of the leg with extensive soft-tissue injury around the knee and proximal tibia. A below-knee amputation was mandatory, and the tibial stump was salvaged by coverage with the Tensor Fascia Lata flap. The knee joint was therefore preserved. The appearance at 5 years after the operation. **a** Anterior view. **b** Posterior view. The knee joint range of movement was 0°–90°. A below-knee prosthesis was fitted with a suprapatella harness to improve stability. The patient, a young woman in her 20s, enjoyed a wide range of social life. A second case is also illustrated. Gangrene of the hand in a diabetic patient who also required an above knee amputation for an infected exposed knee joint (**c**) Posterior tibial skin flap harvested from the amputated leg was used to cover the defect in the hand after thorough debridement. The hand is salvaged. Appearance after operation (**d**)

Timing and Emergency Free Flaps

It is now generally agreed that the open wound should be covered as soon as possible once it is certain that the wound is adequately débrided [26,30]. Repeated débridements may be necessary [31]. Some authors even advocate immediate free-flap coverage. In the study by Godina [32] free-flap trans-

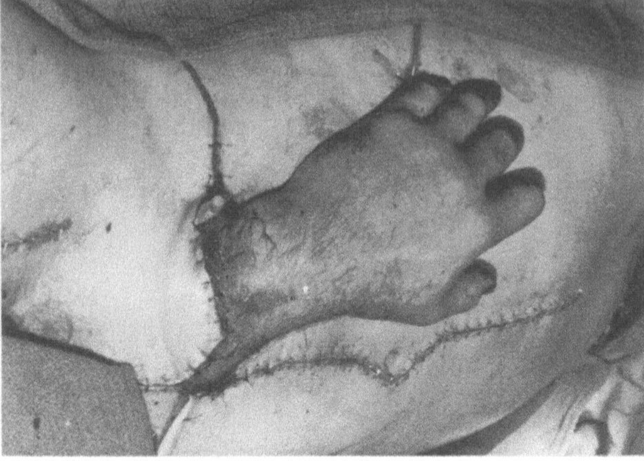

Fig. 9. "Banking" of an amputated hand on the inferior epigastric artery and vein. (From [17])

plantation to cover the open wound after 72 h was associated with a much higher failure rate. A good explanation for this observation is still lacking, but it is believed that débridement may not have been adequate so that there was local infection and vasculitis of the vessels with proximal extension. In many centres free-flap transplantation is carried out immediately upon stabilisation of the fracture [33]. When an external fixator is used for stabilisation, it is important that the microsurgeon be present so that the external fixator is not located at a site that may jeopardise the subsequent transplantation of the flap.

If it is not possible to transplant the skin flap immediately, repeated wound inspection and débridement in the operating theatre is essential to control any possible infection, and a good result may still be achieved [31]. Prolonged waiting should never be necessary. The vascular anastomosis is also planned at a site completely outside the field of trauma, including that of muscle contusion beneath intact skin. Venous anastomosis to the deep veins and venae commitantes is preferred to superficial veins since these may be involved in inflammatory processes and be easily compressed by external pressure.

Choice of the Type of Soft-Tissue Coverage

The optimal coverage for an open fracture should consist of muscle. This provides bulk and good soft-tissue cushioning around the fracture to fill up dead spaces and a good environment to support cancellous grafts; it also ensures excellent vascularity around the fracture and wound. Most of the known donor muscles have large and reliable vascular pedicles [34–36].

Table 1. Orthopaedic Trauma Hospital Association's coding for fracture type (after [56])

Type	Wound size	Contamination	Tissue crush	Tissue loss	Bone stripping	Fracture comminution	Vascular injury
O	Closed						
I	<1 cm	Minimal	None	None	None	Minimal	None
II	1 cm	Moderate	Minimal	Minimal	Minimal	Moderate	No repair required
III	Usually >5 cm	Severe	Moderate	Moderate	Moderate	Severe	No repair required
IV	Usually >5 cm	Severe	Severe	Severe	Severe	Severe	No repair required
V	Usually >5 cm	Severe	Severe	Severe	Severe	Severe	Repair required

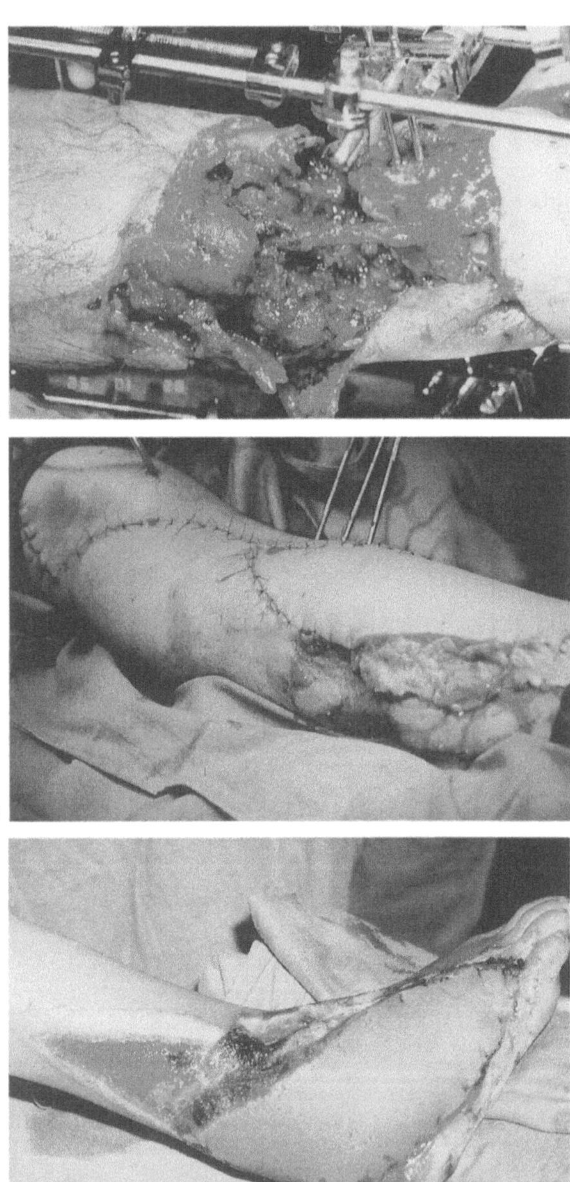

Fig. 10. a Type III-B (Gustilo) open fracture of the tibia with extensive soft-tissue damage. **b** A free latissimus dorsi flap was transplanted to cover the critical part of the wound. **c** Degloved injury of the ankle in a boy which was resurfaced by a free latissimus dorsi flap

The pure skin flap lacks many of the advantages of the muscle flap. An additional drawback is that most donors have small pedicles, making them more precarious. The few donors which have large vascular pedicles are located in the leg or foot, which are commonly involved in open fractures, and they are thus not always available for transplantation [37].

In the past it was customary to transplant a musculocutaneous composite flap since the skin overlying the donor muscle is usually well supplied by the same vascular pedicle. However, experience has indicated that this is not the best choice. The reason for this may be that taking the overlying skin with the muscle complicates the procedure of raising the muscle flap, increases donor morbidity, and sometimes provides insufficient skin to cover all the recipient wound. Once the skin is raised, there is a reduction in size of about 10%. The bulk of the muscle also adds to the area of the wound to be covered. Either a very large donor defect must be created, or additional skin grafts are needed. Partial necrosis of the skin is not unusual. Therefore transplantation of the muscle alone is becoming the preferred option [38]. Without the skin it becomes much easier to tailor the amount of muscle to be taken, thus involving the least donor morbidity. Further release of the muscle fascia or aponeurosis after transplantation allows the muscle to expand and better to adapt to the recipient wound. Direct observation of

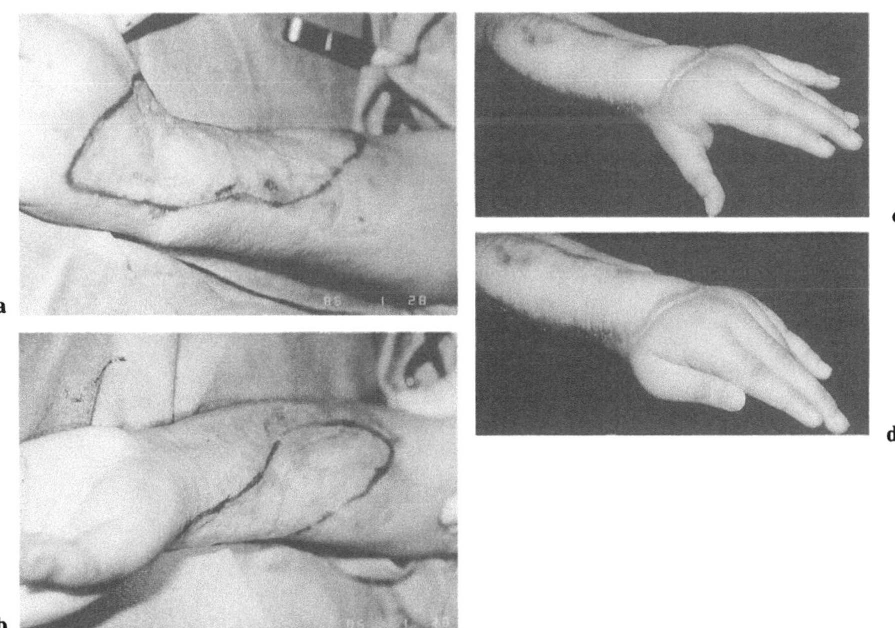

Fig. 11a–d. A free latissimus dorsi flap was used to replace the sensitive and contracted skin of the forearm of a young woman sustained after a road traffic accident. Tendon transfers were performed together with the flap transfer. **a,b** Preoperative views. **c,d** Postoperative views

the viability of the muscle is also easier. The muscle is covered with meshed split-skin grafts with a ratio of 1:1.5, applied in an unspread manner.

The latissimus dorsi muscle remains the best donor site for soft-tissue transplantation because a very large piece of skin can be taken, and with careful dissection of the vascular pedicle the whole or part of the muscle can be transplanted (Fig. 11). The pedicle is particularly large. As discussed above, the current trend is to transplant the muscle alone. When there is the need to provide skin coverage without much bulk, the muscle can also be tailored down to a small trunk bearing the vascular pedicle alone and perfusing the skin by perforators. The rectus abdominis is also a convenient muscle to take, with the patient supine, as is the gracilis muscle, when the thigh is not involved. However, many patients with severe extremity injuries also have abdominal injuries, and laparotomy may – albeit not usually – jeopardise the blood supply to the rectus abdominis flap. Similarly, an

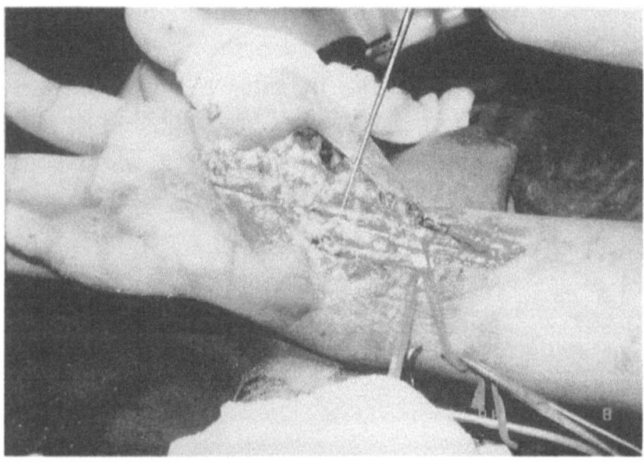

a

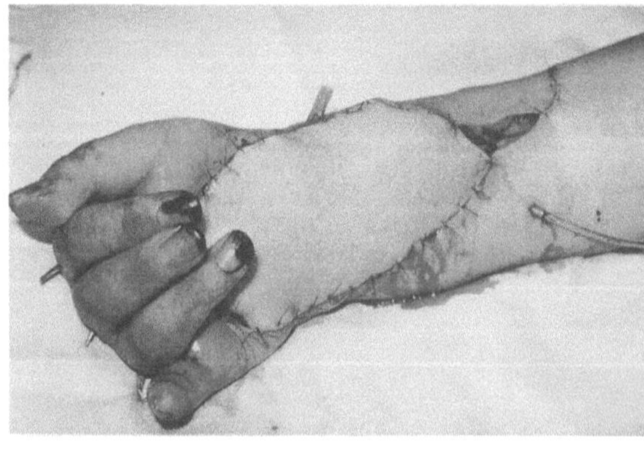

b

Fig. 12. a Exposed wound on the front of the wrist due to a chopped wound injury, after necrosis and breakdown of the skin. There were multiple tendon injuries, and the median nerve was also divided. **b** A free posterior tibial skin flap was transplanted to resurface the wound together with tendon and nerve graftings abdominal wound should not be exacerbated in a patient who already has a breathing problem, such as in chest contusion.

When only skin is desired, the free groin flap is another alternative, although the vascular pedicle is less constant and is usually small [39,40]. In addition, a large bulk of fat may be transplanted. The inferior epigastric flap offers another possibility [41].

In multiply injuried patients with chest and or abdominal injuries one may not be able to obtain a donor flap from the trunk. Peroneal or posterior tibial flaps [42] or very occasionally free gastrocnemius flaps from one intact leg may be used (Fig. 12). The Tensor Fascia Lata flap also presents a useful alternative (Fig. 13).

Occasionally the condition of the patient precludes a lengthy microvascular procedure, and one must consider stabilising the skeleton first and leave the soft-tissue damage to a later stage. A large number of artificial skin substitutes are now available which allow one to "close" the wound for up to 3 weeks while the patient overcomes the initial severe trauma before an elective procedure of free composite tissue transplantation is carried out.

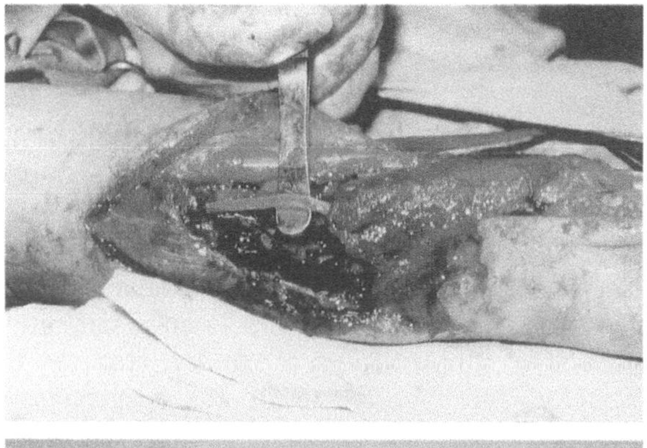

a

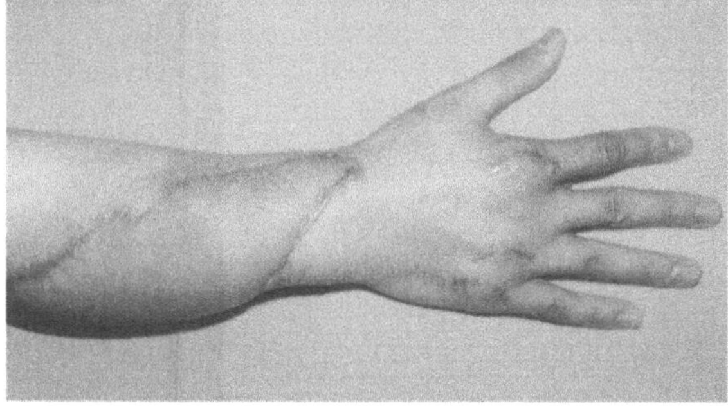

b

Fig. 13. a Open fracture of the forearm (Gustilo type III-B) and multiple tendon avulsions. **b** The wound was resurfaced by a Tensor Fascia Lata flap after plate fixation of the bone and tendon transfers

Bone Grafting

Although there have been reports in the past on the successful use of nonvascularised bulk autografts [43], onlay grafts [44] and cancellous grafts [45,46], these procedures are inferior to microvascular free bone grafts [47–51]. There are some cases of stress shielding in vascularised bone grafts or excessive movements resulting in failure to achieve hypertrophy [52] and stress fracture or delayed union at the repair site; however when these factors are controlled or eliminated, vascularised bone grafts lead to much faster union and incorporation than other techniques. A vascularised graft also survives better in infected situations.

Microvascular techniques enable the transplantation of vascularised bone graft for large bone defects. This can be transplanted either at the time of composite soft-tissue transplantation during the acute stage, at a later stage when the soft tissue has healed, or when there is established nonunion with or without segmental bone loss (Fig. 14). The current opinion is that when the trauma was one of low energy, one-stage osteocutaneous transplantation is indicated. When the trauma was a high-energy one with extensive tissue damage, it is preferable to heal the soft tissue by soft-tissue transplantation followed by bone grafting [53–56].

The osteocutaneous "groin flap" – consisting of the iliac crest bone and overlying skin and supplied by the deep circumflex iliac artery – is the best donor when one needs both skin and bone [40,57]. This easily damages the blood supply to the skin and therefore results in a high incidence of skin necrosis; however, this can be improved if one takes the superficial circumflex iliac pedicle as well. The iliac crest is ideal for bone grafting and in the adult has much more red marrow than the fibula. Its only limitations are the difficulty in harvesting a piece of graft longer than 15 cm and overcoming the curvature of the iliac crest. A large graft usually results later in significant morbidity of the donor site, whereas the curvature of the iliac crest can be corrected by an osteotomy before the bone is fixed to the recipient site. Alternatively, the iliac crest may be taken with a flap of the internal oblique muscle for dead space obliteration or wound coverage, which can be skin grafted.

The fibula offers another alternative for vascularised bone transplant [48]. The bone is straight, and a very long segment can be raised measuring well over 20 cm depending on the height of the individual. The bone can therefore be used for bridging very long defects. The overlying skin on the peroneal aspect of the leg can also be raised together for transplantation, or the soleal muscle may be transplanted with the bone. The only criticisms are the cortical nature of the bone and the relatively narrow diameter. Bone regeneration is slow, and prolonged protection of the bone is required after transplantation. Because of stress shielding the fibula occasionally shows inadequate hypertrophy, and stress fracture then becomes likely and problematic.

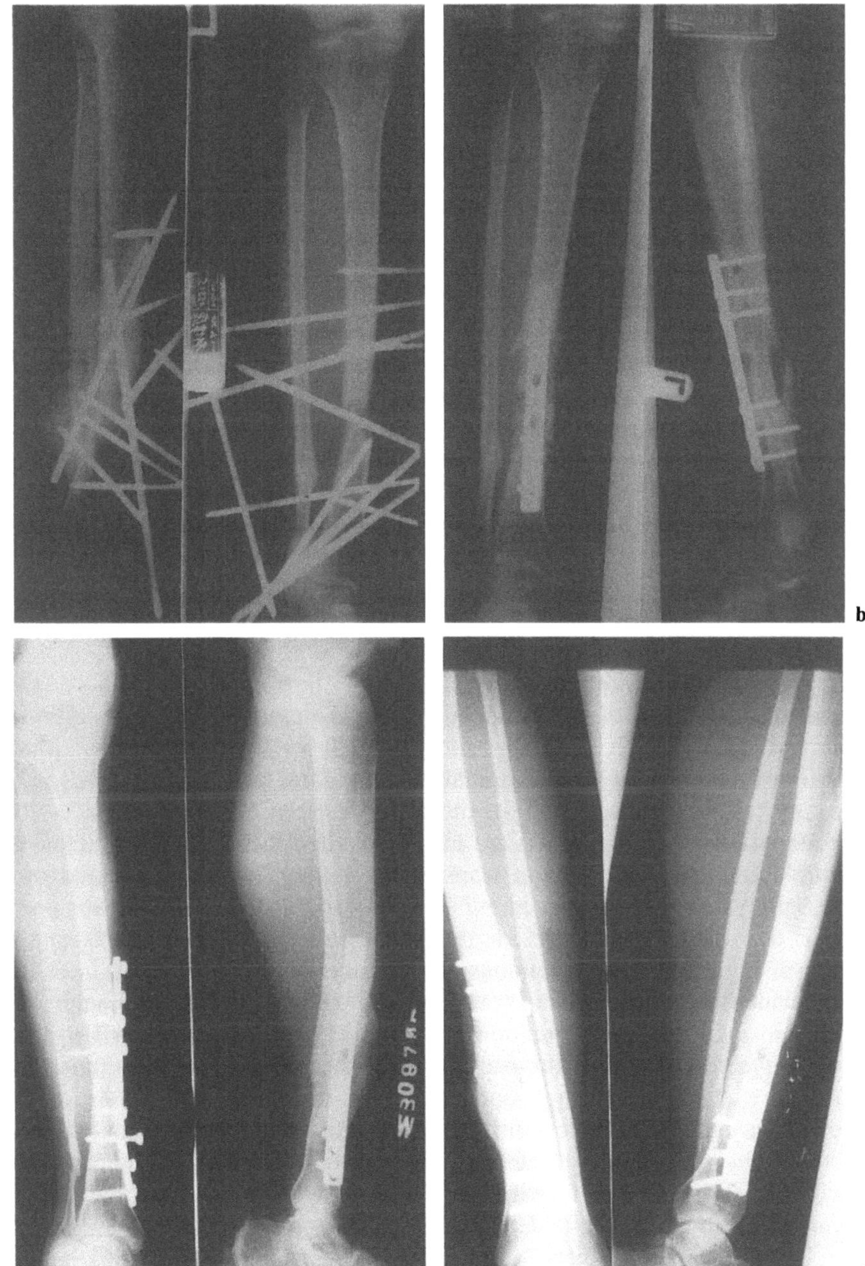

Fig. 14. **a** Open fracture of the tibia which was inappropriately fixed and resulted in nonunion. **b** The nonunion was resected. The gap was bridged by a free vascularised iliac crest graft and fixed in place by a plate. **c,d** Two other examples of successful union of open tibial fractures with bone loss by free vascularised iliac crest grafts

In the lower limb when the bone loss is not extensive, the bone may be stabilised with the interlocking nail or an external fixator, which gives sufficient stability even for weight bearing before the bone graft is transplanted.

Alternative Bone Grafting Techniques

Worth mentioning here is the fibular pro-tibia technique, where the intact fibula is shifted sideways to replace a missing tibial segment [58]. Provided the extent of soft-tissue damage is not great, this is a useful technique in situations in which microvascular bone transplant cannot be performed.

Recently the technique of "bone transport" has been introduced [59–61]. Theoretically this technique enables the closure of large bone defects. At its present state of art, taking everything into consideration, it appears that the results of bone transport cannot rival those of microvascular bone transplantation. The greatest drawback with this technique is the long duration of distraction required. Its potential is great, and with time the technique of bone transport may be further refined. This is discussed further below (see "Microsurgical Procedures for Complications in Musculoskeletal Trauma").

The Mutilated Hand

The mutilated hand presents a special category in trauma management. The sophisticated nature of the hand puts great demand on the techniques of reconstruction [62]. It is in this situation that vascularised tendon, joint, nerve or functional muscle transplantation are sometimes required. A toe or toes may also be transplanted for the reconstruction of missing digits.

Vascularised tendon grafts are indicated when there is segmental loss of multiple tendons, and tendon transfer or sharing cannot be carried out, especially when there is associated skin loss or fracture. The dorsalis pedis flap is the ideal flap tailored for this situation [63]. Long segments of the extensor digitorum longus tendons can be taken with the dorsal skin of the foot, which therefore provides a very nice gliding surface (although one must still take care of the tendon bed; Fig. 15). In fact, one can also take short segments of the metatarsals, usually the second and sometimes the third as well, for replacing bone defects in the hand. The whole of the second toe can also be taken with the tendocutaneous flap for reconstruction of the digits. This flap is therefore very versatile. The flap fits the extensor surface of the hand and forearm very well, as well as the volar part of the forearm, although it is less ideal for the palm.

The metatarsophalangeal joint, usually the second or the third, or the proximal interphalangeal from the second or the third toe, can be transplanted to replace those badly damaged in the hand [64,65]. The surgery itself is not very complicated. This is justifiable in the young manual worker with a badly damaged metacarpophalangeal joint and more selectively when the proximal phalangeal joint is involved (Fig. 16).

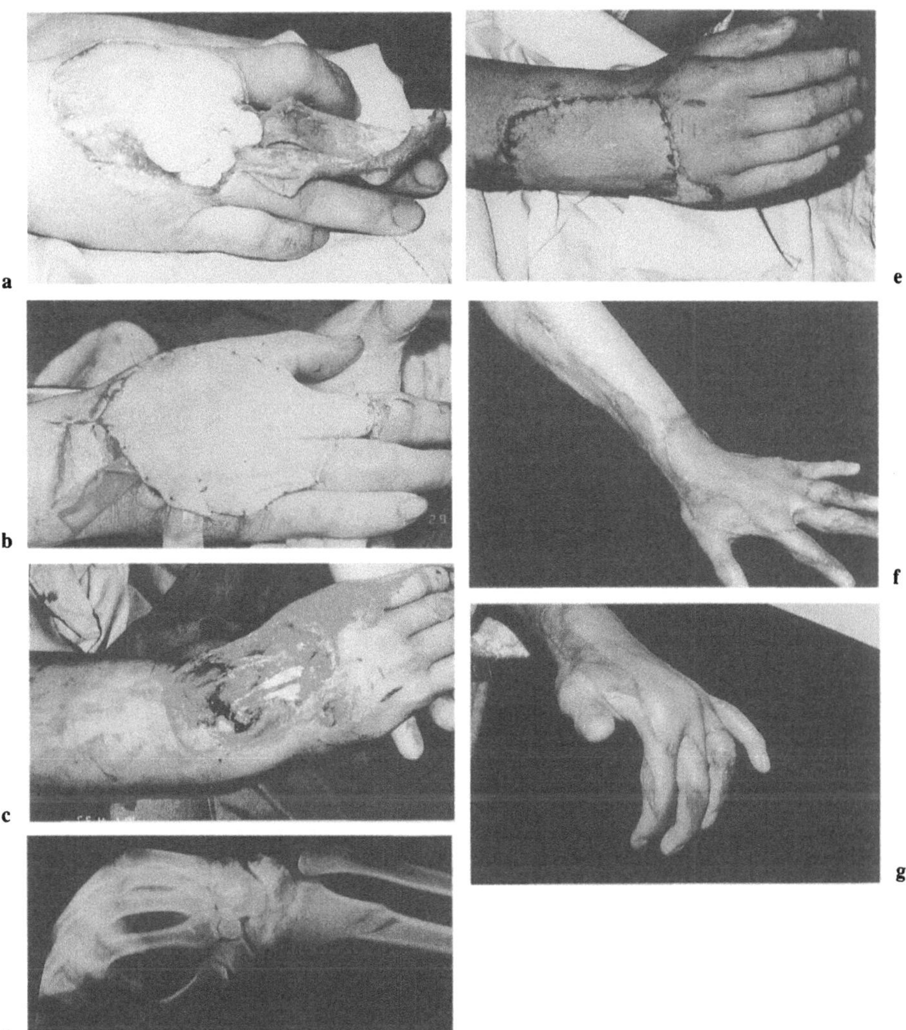

Fig. 15. a Thermal crush of the hand. The white object was a block of consolidated plastic which was injected into the dorsum of the hand. **b** The wound was thoroughly débrided and resurfaced by a free dorsalis pedis flap with toe extensor tendon segments to bridge the severed finger extensor tendons. **c** Degloved injury of the hand with multiple tendon avulsions, and fracture of both forearm bones. **d,e** The wound was resurfaced by a free dorsalis pedis tendocutaneous flap with toe extensor tendon segments transplanted to bridge the avulsed extensor tendons. The forearm bones were plated. **f,g** Extensive card injury of the back of the hand which was repaired by a large dorsalis pedis tendocutaneous flap with repair of all long finger extensor tendons. Extension of the proximal interphalangeal joints was recon-structed by transposition of a tendocutaneous flap from the ulnar side of the finger to the dorsal aspect of the proximal interphalangeal joint

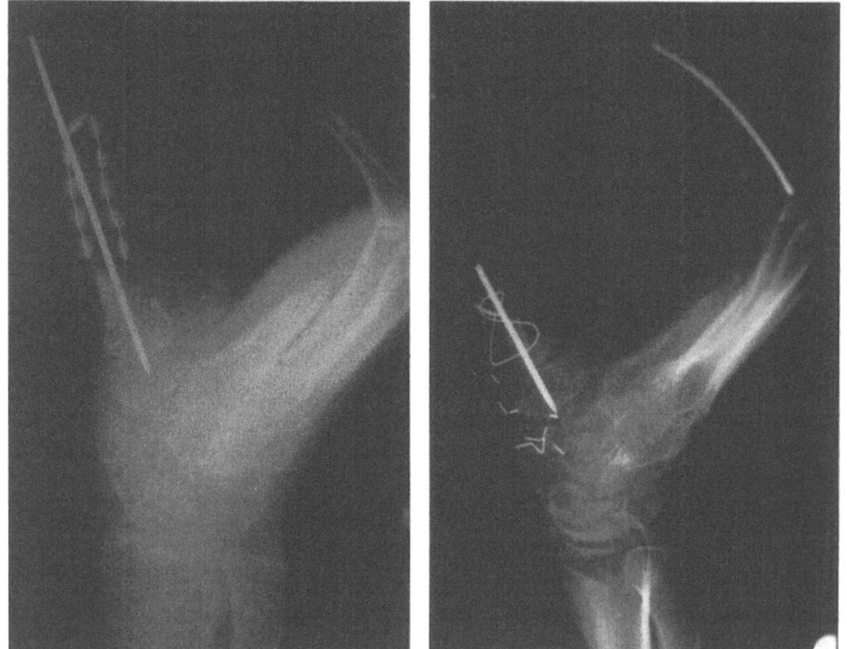

Fig. 16. a A groin skin tube was used to resurface the crushed thumb in this severely injured hand. Unfortunately, chronic osteomyelitis developed and most of the bone was excised. The skin tube was preserved. b A free second metatarsophalangeal joint was transplanted into the skin tube to construct a thumb with some movement at the joint

The sural nerve can be raised with the peroneal artery as a vascularised nerve graft. It may also be raised in continuity with the short saphenous vein and while the nerve is reversed for the nerve grafting the vein is reversed at the same time, giving rise to a good vessel graft for anastomosis. Due to mechanisms not fully understood, the nerve is also vascularised in this manner [66].

When the forearm is badly crushed, with loss of muscles, free functional muscle transplantation may offer the only option for restoration of motor function. The gracilis muscle is the first choice, although its strength is less than that of the latissimus dorsi [67].

A single toe or multiple toes may be transplanted for the reconstruction of pincer function. This form of surgery remains one of the most gratifying operations both for the patient and for the surgeon (Fig. 17). Special considerations, however, are required for the thumb when there is loss of the thenar muscles. In such case pollicisation may yield a better functioning digit.

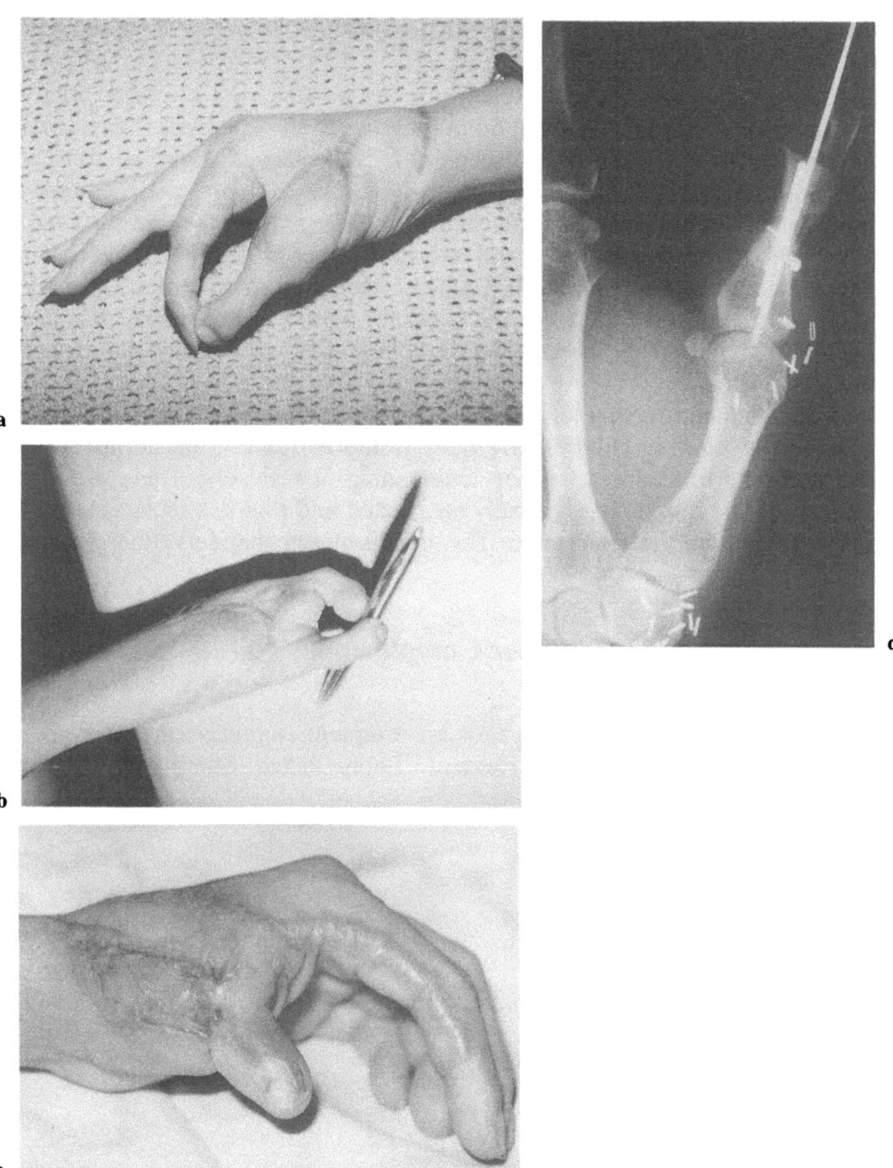

Fig. 17. a A very successful example of second toe transplantation for thumb reconstruction in a young woman. Both functional and cosmetic results were good. **b** A case of double second toe transplantation for pincer reconstruction in a transcarpal amputation. The functional result was very good. **c,d** Free toe wrap transplantation for avulsion injury of the thumb

Microvascular Procedures for Children

Children with serious musculoskeletal trauma benefit from the same micro-vascular procedures as do adults. Sometimes when the epiphysis is damaged, there is limited potential for replacement by vascularised transplantation of autogenous epiphysis and growth plates [68]. For example, the metatarsal heads can be transplanted for replacement of damaged epiphyses in the hand, and the fibula head may be transplanted for larger bones [69]. Experience with replantations in children also indicate that the growth potential of the epiphyses may suffer little from the transient period of ischaemia, although the real outcome of the vascularised epiphysis has yet to stand the test of time (Fig. 18).

Ischaemic contracture of muscles (Volkmann's contracture) still occurs from time to time in children. In many instances this can be improved by muscle-sliding procedures, tendon lengthening or transfers. There are also times when the muscle is very badly contracted and requires replacement by functional muscle transplantation. The gracilis muscle may serve this purpose well [70].

Microsurgical Procedures for Complications in Musculoskeletal Trauma

Nonunions and chronic osteomyelitis are frequent complications after open fractures. There is also a varying extent of bone deficit. Microvascular bone

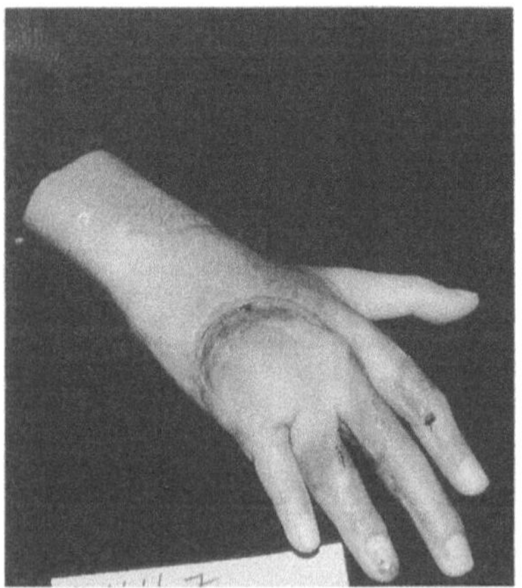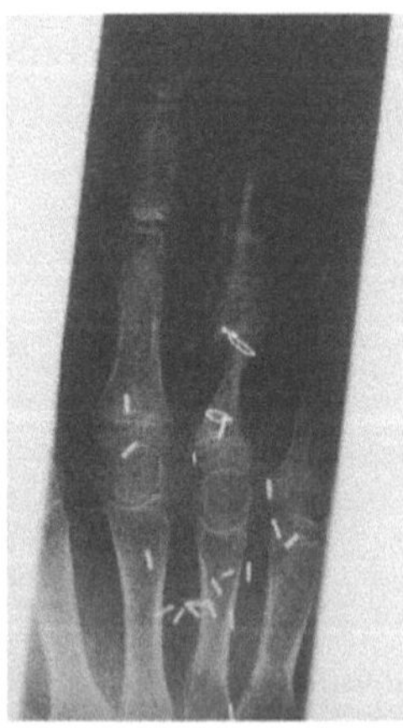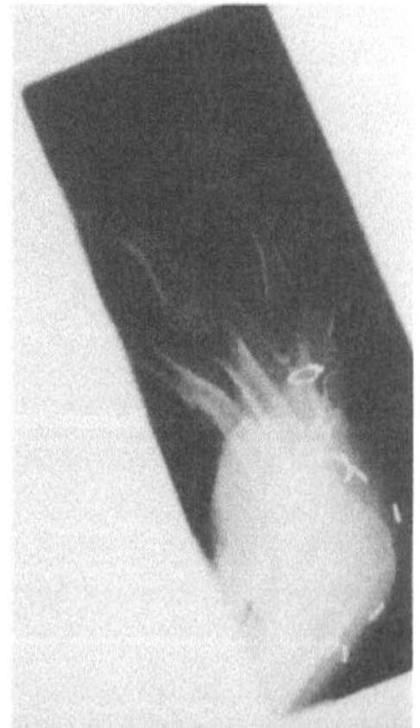

Fig. 18a,b. The right hand of this 8-year-old boy suffered a severe degloving injury in a road traffic accident. The metacarpophalangeal joints of the middle, ring and little fingers were exposed, and a segment of the proximal phalanx of the ring finger was lost, although the proximal growth plate was preserved. A free osteo-tendocutaneous flap of dorsalis pedis was transplanted to reconstruct the defect. A segment of the proximal phalanx of the second toe was used to replace the missing phalanx of the hand. Segments of toe extensors were transplanted to replace missing extensors in the hand. Although there was residual stiffness, the result was graftifying and soft-tissue transplantation has a definite place in the management of such problems. Nonunions can be classified according to whether there is a large bone gap, and whether there is shortening and deformity. Treatment should be tailored to each category [54]. In chronic osteomyelitis there is frequently associated bone defects or dead spaces and poor vascularity. These may be classified according to the extent of involvement of the medullary cavity and the circumference of the bone [71].

In the past there have been numerous attempts to handle such problems. The most noteworthy are Phemister's technique of autogenous onlay grafts [44], cancellous grafting through the posterior approach [72] and Papineau's technique of radical débridement and cancellous bone grafting, which are left exposed and may be repeated [45,46]. When there is significant deformity, bone loss and shortening, such techniques are not able to deal with all the problems.

It has been demonstrated in animal experiments and clinical studies that a well-vascularised soft-tissue transplantation helps to control the infection and close the wound and enables a primary or a secondary bone grafting for repair of the bone defect [28,73,74]. With microsurgical techniques distant and more dispensible tissues can be transplanted to the wound, thus avoiding further morbidity to the limb, increasing the flexibility and expanding the indications to the whole of the leg and also the upper limb.

In established chronic osteomyelitis after saucerisation a free vascularised muscle provides good soft-tissue coverage and good vascularity to the region, which help to eradicate infection. When there is a large bone defect which requires bone grafting, vascularised bone grafting produces a more guaranteed result [71,75,76]. It is proposed that if the bone defect is longer than 8 cm, the following procedure should be performed [54]: a vascularised soft-tissue transplantation, usually a muscle flap because of its good space filling property, followed after 6 weeks by a second vascularised bone or cancellous bone grafting procedure.

Reconstructions of the lower extremities can be classified as follows [60]:

Soft tissue
    Clean
    Infected
Soft tissue and bone (<8 cm)
    Clean
    Infected
Massive soft tissue and bone (>8 cm)
    Clean
    Infected
Bone only
    Clean
    Infected

It is unclear as yet whether the new technique of bone transportation will solve the problem of infected nonunions with large defects [59,60]. It certainly appears to be a very useful alternative to microvascular bone transplantation. Early experiences show that the procedure takes a long time, and that complications are frequent. Most of these complications may be minor, but repeated procedures are commonly required. Although experiments suggest that the newly formed bone requires an average of 1 month to consolidate [60], this usually takes longer, and the site of nonunion or bone defect may also have difficulties uniting despite being brought together and compressed. The advantage of microvascular bone transplantation is that it is a one-stage procedure. Bone union is usually rapid in 6 weeks time. When stress shielding is not serious, the bone graft shows rapid hypertrophy, and weight bearing of the limb can usually be started in 3 months. This is much shorter than the time required in bone transportation. In bone transportation there is more than one procedure, and this takes at least 1 day for each millimeter of transportation, plus 10 days of waiting for the callus to form and 3 months after the last transport for the bone to consolidate and the distal union to heal. One must therefore await more data on bone transportation before this can be strongly recommended. The technique certainly warrants attention but requires further refinement and a better definition of indications. One thing is certain: the technique offers greater versatility in correcting bone deformities, length deficiencies and large bone defects in a scarred bed, which may not be effectively tackled with microvascular procedures alone. In principle, bone transportation techniques may be combined with microvascular tissue transplantation: a muscle flap may be transplanted first to cover any skin defect, followed by the bone transportation.

The same principles also apply in noninfected nonunions. For small defects routine bone grafting after rigid fixation usually leads to healing of the fracture. When the defect is large and a large segment of bone is required, one can consider either microvascular bone transplantation or bone transportation.

Microvascular Procedures in Pathological Fractures

It is seldom necessary to employ microvascular bone transplantation in pathological fractures. There are two exceptions to this: congenital pseudoarthrosis of the tibia and bone cyst occurring in the proximal femur.

Experience in the use of vascularised grafts for congenital pseudarthrosis of the tibia is accumulating, and it seems to be proving itself as the procedure of choice for this particular condition [77]. Both free vascularised fibula and iliac crest block have been used. Defects larger than 7–8 cm require the free fibular rather than iliac crest block because the latter is not straight. A word of caution is necessary regarding the timing. For very young children the vessels in the involved limb may be very hypoplastic, and the procedure can be very difficult. Bone transportation has also been reported for this condition, but further clinical data are awaited.

Bone cysts around the proximal femur, especially those occurring in the calcar region, require a strong piece of bone graft to maintain the integrity of the bone architecture after their removal; otherwise fracture easily follows. The iliac crest, based on the deep circumflex iliac vessel, is ideal for this purpose. We have found in most occasions that a pedicled bone block from the ipsilateral iliac crest yields the best bone graft material, and this procedure eliminates the need for microvascular repair. The bone graft with its intact vascular pedicle is tunnelled beneath all the hip flexors to reach the proximal femur [78,79]. Healing is very rapid because the vascularised bone flap and adjacent bone unite as healing fractures.

Conclusion

Limb trauma is frequently threatened by ischaemia resulting from vascular damage sustained during the injury. If the ischaemia is transient, as in the case of compartment syndrome, no serious consequence results as long as the ischaemic factors are removed. If, on the other hand, the ischaemia is permanent, as in case of multiple vascular damages, not only is bone healing affected, but soft-tissue coverage may also become defective. Under such circumstances, procedures either to reconstruct the feeding arteries or to introduce new blood supply to the widely damaged soft tissues must be successful; otherwise the traumatised ischaemic limb undergoes gangrene or a natural process of atrophy. Although survival may still be maintained, the functional results are disappointing.

Microsurgical procedures offer means of revascularisation in the acute phase and later allow the effective introduction of new blood supply into the ischaemic area by free vascularised tissue transfers. The success with free vascularised skin flap, composite tissues and bone transfer illustrates the versatility of the technique. In the present era of orthopaedics, when new techniques are offering so many treatment options to difficult problems, microsurgical manoeuvres should not be forgotten as a useful option in the treatment of difficult limb trauma. Indeed orthopaedic surgeons tend to be either conventional or gadget dependent, and there appears to be an under-utilisation of microsurgical techniques in limb trauma. It is the author's wish that more awareness and exploration be given by colleagues to the application of microsurgical techniques in the treatment of fractures and dislocations.

References

1. Morrison WA, O'Brien BMcC, MacLeod AM (1978) Digital replantation and revascularisation. A long term review of one hundred cases. Hand 10:125
2. Wong SH, Young KF, Wei JN (1981) Replantation of severed limbs – clinical analysis of 91 cases. J Hand Surg 6:311
3. Tamai S (1982) Twenty years' experience of limb replantation – review of 293 upper extremity replants. J Hand Surg 7:549
4. Urbaniak JR, Roth JH, Nunley JA, Goldner RD, Koman LA (1985) The results of replantation after amputation of single finger. J Bone Joint Surg [Am] 67:611
5. Jones JM, Schenck RR, Chesney RB (1982) Digital replantation and amputation – comparison of function. J Hang Surg 7:183
6. Urbaniak JR, Evans JP, Bright DS (1981) Microvascular management of ring avulsion injuries. J Hand Surg 6:25
7. Hung LK, Leung PC (1989) Salvage of the ring-avulsed finger in heavy manual worker. Br J Plast Surg 42:43
8. DeBoer A, Robinson PH (1989) Ray transposition by intercarpal osteotomy after loss of the fourth digit. J Hand Surg [Am] 14(2):379
9. Axelrod TS, Buchler U (1991) Severe complex injuries to the upper extremity: revascularisation and replantation. J Hand Surg [Am] 16(4):574
10. Chen ZW, Zeng BF (1983) Replantation of lower extremity. Clin Plast Surg 10:103
11. Keblish PA (1986) Amputation alternatives in the lower limb, stressing combined management of the traumatized extremity. Clin Plast Surg 13(4):595
12. Hansen ST (1987) The type IIIC tibial fracture. Salvage or amputation (Editorial). J Bone Joint Surg [Am] 69:799
13. Hansen ST Jr (1987) Overview of the severely traumatized lower limb: reconstruction versus amputation. Clin Orthop 243:17
14. Lange RH (1989) Limb reconstruction versus amputation decision making in massive lower extremity trauma. Clin Orthop 243:92
15. Bondurant FJ, Cotler HB, Buckle R, Miller-Critchett P, Browner BD (1988) The medical and economic impact of severely injured lower extremities. J Trauma 28:1270
16. Colen SR, Romita MC, Godfrey NV, Shaw WW (1983) Salvage replantation. Clin Plast Surg 10:125
17. Chernofsky MA, Sauer PF (1990) Temporary ectopic implantation. J Hand Surg [Am] 15:910
18. Chapman MW (1991) Open fractures. In: Rockwood CA, Green DP, Bucholz RW (eds) Fractures in adults. Lippincott, Philadelphia, pp 223–264
19. Gustillo RB, Anderson JT (1976) Prevention of infection in the treatment of one thousand and twenty-five open fractures of long bones. J Bone Joint Surg [Am] 58:453
20. Gustilo RB (1983) Management of infected fractures. In: Evarts CM (ed) Surgery of the musculoskeletal system, vol 4. Churchill Livingstone, New York, pp 105–134
21. Gustilo RB, Mendoza RM, Williams DN (1984) Problems in the management of type III (severe) open fractures: a new classification of type III open fractures. J Trauma 24:742
22. Ger R, Efron G (1970) New operative approach in the treatment of chronic osteomyelitis of the tibia diaphysis: a preliminary report. Clin Orthop 70:165
23. Barford B, Pers M (1970) Gastrocnemius-plasty for primary closure of compound injuries of the knee. J Bone Joint Surg [Br] 52:124
24. Ger R (1977) Muscle transposition for treatment and prevention of chronic post-traumatic osteomyelitis of the tibia. J Bone Joint Surg [Am] 59:784
25. Cannon B, Constable JD, Furlaw LT, Hayhurst JW, McCarthy JG, McGraw JB (1977) Reconstructive surgery of the lower extremity. In: Converse JM (ed) Reconstructive plastic surgery, 2nd edn. Saunders, Philadelphia, p 3521

26. Shaw WW (1986) Acute management of severe soft tissue damage accompanying open fractures of the lower extremity: editor's discussion. Clin Plast Surg 13(4):631
27. Throne CHM, Siebert JW, Grotting JC, Vasconez LO, Shaw WW, Sauer PF (1990) Reconstructive surgery of the lower extremity. In: McCarthy JG (ed) Plastic surgery. Saunders, Philadelphia, pp 4029–4092
28. Feng LJ, Eaton C (1986) Soft tissue infection in lower extremity trauma. Clin Plast Surg 13(4):735
29. Feng L, Price D, Hohn D et al. (1983) Blood flow changes and leukocyte mobilisation in infections: a comparison between ischemic and well perfused skin. Surg Forum 34:603
30. Byrd HS, Cierny G, Tebbetts, JB (1981) The management of open tibial fractures with associated soft tissue loss: external pin fixation with early flap coverage. Plast Reconstr Surg 68:73
31. Yaremchuk MJ (1986) Acute management of severe soft tissue damage accompanying open fractures of the lower extremity. Clin Plast Surg 13(4):621
32. Godina M (1986) Early microsurgical reconstruction of complex trauma of the extremities. Plast Reconstr Surg 78:285
33. Quaba A (1990) Management of soft tissue defects. Edinburgh International Trauma Symposium, Aug 22–24, Edinburgh
34. Cormack GC, Lamberty BGH (eds) (1986) The arterial anatomy of skin flaps. Churchill Livingstone, Edinburgh
35. Strauch R, Vasconez LO, Hall-Findlay EJ (eds) (1990) Grabb's encyclopedia of flaps. Little Brown, Boston
36. Buncke HJ (ed) (1991) Microsurgery: transplantation – replantation. Lea and Febiger, Philadelphia
37. Taylor GI, Daniel RK (1975) The anatomy of several free flap donor sites. Plast Reconstr Surg 56:243
38. Gorman PW, Barnes CL, Fischer TJ, McAndrew MP, Moore MM (1989) Soft tissue reconstruction in severe lower extremity trauma. Clin Orthop 243: 57
39. Ohmori K, Harii K (1975) Free groin flaps: their vascular basis. Br J Plast Surg 28:238
40. Taylor GI, Townsend P, Corlett R (1979) Superiority of the deep circumflex iliac vessels as the supply for free groin flaps: experimental work. Plast Reconstr Surg 64:595
41. Taylor GI, Corlett RJ, Boyd JB (1984) The versatile deep inferior epigastric (inferior rectus abdominis) flap. Br J Plast Surg 37:330
42. Hung LK, Chen SZ, Leung PC (1990) Resurfacing difficult wounds – selective use of the posterior tibial flap. J Reconstr Microsurg 6(1):13
43. Enneking WF, Eady JL, Burchardt H (1980) Autogenous cortical bone grafts in the reconstruction of segmental skeletal defects. J Bone Joint Surg [Am] 62: 1039
44. Phemister DB (1947) Treatment of ununited fractures by onlay bone grafts without screw fixation and without breaking down of the fibrous union. J Bone Joint Surg 29:946
45. Papineau LJ (1973) L'excision greffe avec fermeture cutanée retardée deliberée dans l'ostermyélite chronique. Nouv Presse Med 2:2753
46. Green SA, Dlabal TA (1983) The open bone graft for septic nonunion. Clin Orthop 180:117
47. Cutting CB, McCarthy JG (1983) Comparison of the residual osseous mass between vascularized and nonvascularized onlay bone transfers. Plast Reconstr Surg 72:672
48. Weiland AJ, Moore JR, Daniel RK (1983) Vascularised bone autografts. Experience with 41 cases. Clin Orthop 174:87
49. Shaffer JW, Field GA, Goldberg VM, Davy DT (1985) Fate of vascularized and nonvascularized autografts. Clin Orthop 197:32

50. Tessier J, Bonnel F, Allieu Y (1985) Vascularization, cellular behaviour and union of vascularized bone grafts: experimental study in the rabbit. Ann Plast Surg 14:494
51. Wood WB, Cooney WP III, Irons GB Jr (1985) Skeletal reconstruction by vascularised bone transfer: indications and results. Mayo Clin Proc 60:729
52. Fujimaki A, Suda H, Yasuma T, Yamauchi Y (1988) Experimental study and clinical observation on the hypertrophy of the vascularised bone graft. 9th Symposium of the Interational Society of Reconstructive Microsurgery, Lake Kawaguchi, Japan
53. Cierny G, Byrd HS, Jones RE (1983) Primary versus delayed soft tissue coverage for severe open tibial fractures. A comparison of results. Clin Orthop 178:54
54. Swartz WM, Mears DC (1985) The role of free tissue transfers in lower extremity reconstruction. Plast Reconstr Surg 76:364
55. Bieber EJ, Wood MB (1986) Bone reconstruction. Clin Plast Surg 13:645
56. Swartz WM, Mears DC (1986) Management of difficult lower extremity fractures and nonunions. Clin Plast Surg 13:633
57. Taylor GI, Watson N (1978) One stage repair of compound leg defects with free vascularised flaps of groin skin and iliac bone. Plast Reconstr Surg 61:494
58. Chacha PB (1984) Vascularised pedicular bone grafts. Int Orthop 8:117
59. Aronson J, Johnson E, Harp JH (1989) Local bone transportation for treatment of intercalary defects by the Ilizarov technique. Clin Orthop 243:71
60. Paley D, Catagni MA, Argnani F, Villa A, Benedetti GB, Cattaneo R (1989) Ilizarov treatment of tibial nonunious with bone loss. Clin Orthop 241:146
61. Mast JW, Teitge RA (1990) Nonunion and malunion of fractures. Orthop Clin North Am 21:4
62. Breidenbach WC (1989) Emergency free tissue transfer for reconstruction of acute upper extremity wounds. Clin Plast Surg 16(3):505
63. Ohmori K (1976) Free dorsalis pedis sensory flap to the hand with microneurovascular anastomoses. Plast Reconstr Surg 58:546
64. Foucher G (1988) Vascularised joint transfers. In: Green DP (ed) Operative hand surgery, 2nd edn. Churchill Livingstone, New York, pp 1271–1294
65. Ellis PR, Tsai TM (1989) Management of the traumatized joint of the finger. Clin Plast Surg 16(3):457
66. Towsend PLG, Taylor GI (1984) Vascularised nerve grafts using composite arterialised neuro-venous systems. Br J Plast Surg 37:1
67. Manktelow RT (1986) Functioning muscle transplantation. In: Manktelow RT (ed) Microvascular reconstruction. Springer, Berlin Heidelberg New York, p 151
68. Mathes SJ, Buchannan R, Weeks PM (1980) Microvascular joint transplantation with epiphyseal growth. J Hand Surg 5:586
69. Pho RWH, Lee YS, Kour AK, Kumar VP (1988) Free vascularised epiphyseal transplantation in upper extremity reconstruction. J Hand Surg [Br] 13:440
70. Zuker RM (1989) Volkmann's ischemic contracture. Clin Plast Surg 16(3):537
71. Weiland AJ, Moore JR Daniel RK (1984) The efficacy of free tissue transfer for osteomyelitis. J Bone Joint Surg [Am] 66:181
72. Harmon PH (1945) A simplified surgical approach to the posterior tibia for bone grafting and fibular transference. J Bone Joint Surg 27:496
73. Chang N, Mathes SJ (1982) Comparison of the effect of bacterial inoculation in musculocutaneous and random patterned flaps. Plast Reconstr Surg 70:1
74. Luk KDK, Zhou LR, Chow SP (1987) The effect of established infection on microvascular surgery. Plast Reconstr Surg 80(3):423
75. May JW Jr, Gallico GG III, Lukash FN (1982) Microvascular transfer of free tissue for closure of bone wounds of the distal lower extremity. N Engl J Med 306:253
76. Moore JR, Weiland AJ (1986) Vascularised tissue transfer in the treatment of osteomyelitis. Clin Plast Surg 13:657

77. Leung PC (1983) Congenital psendarthrosis of the tibia – 3 cases treated by free vascularised iliac crest graft. Clin Orthop 175:45
78. Leung PC (1983) Reconstruction of a large femoral defect using a vascular pedicle iliac graft – case report. J Bone Joint Surg [Am] 65:1179
79. Leung PC, Chow YYN (1984) Reconstruction of proximal femoral defects with a vascular – pedicled graft. J Bone Joint Surg [Br] 66:32

Further Reading

Chang TS, Zhu SX, Wang ZC (1986) Principles, techniques and applications in microsurgery. World Scientific, Singapore
Hung LK, Cheng J, Leung PC (1988) "Let there be flesh" – application of microsurgery to upper limb degloving injuries. Proceedings of the Centennial Conference, Faculty of Medicine, University of Hong Kong. Hong Kong University Press, Hong Kong, pp 301–304
Lau RSF, Leung PC (1982) Bone graft viability in vascularized bone graft transfer. Br J Radiology 55:325
Leung PC, Ma GFY (1982) Digital reconstruction using the toe flap – report of 10 cases. J Hand Surg 7(2):366
Leung PC (1985) Thumb reconstruction using second-toe transfer. Hand Clin 1(2):285
Leung PC (1986) Malignant giant cell tumour of the distal end of the radius treated by resection and free vascularised iliac crest graft. Clin Orthop 202:232
Leung PC (1987) Double toe transplants. J Hand Surg [Br] 12(2):162
Leung PC (1987) Pincer reconstruction using second toe transplantation. J Hand Surg [Br] 12:159
Leung PC (1988) Vascularised bone graft from the iliac crest. In: Pho RWH (ed) Microsurgical technique in orthopaedics. Butterworth, London, pp 135–145
Leung PC (1989) Restoration of the thumb. In: Lamb D, Hooper G, Kuczynski K (ed) The practice of hand surgery. Blackwell, Oxford, pp 374–390
Leung PC (1989) Thumb reconstruction using the second toe. In: Landi A (ed) Reconstruction of the thumb. Chapman and Hall, London, pp 205–212
Leung PC (1989) Current trends in bone grafting. Springer, Berlin Heidelberg New York
Leung PC (1989) Bone reconstruction using vascularised bone grafts: a 7-year review. In: Yamamuro T (ed) New developments for limb salvage in musculoskeletal tumors. Springer, Berlin Heidelberg New York, pp 431–436
Leung PC, Hung LK (1989) Bone reconstruction after giant cell tumour resection at the proximal end of the humerus using vascularised iliac crest graft – a report of 3 cases. Clin Orthop 247:101
Leung PC, Gu YD, Ikuta Y, Narakas A, Landi A, Weiland AJ (1991) Microsurgery in orthopaedic practice. World Scientific, Singapore

7 Problems in Children's Fractures

J.C.Y. CHENG

Introduction

Fractures in children differ significantly from those in adults; there are basic differences anatomically, physiologically, biomechanically and clinically [1–5]. Failure to realize such differences often leads to mistakes in diagnosis and treatment strategy, which can result in unnecessary morbidity and long-term consequences.

Anatomically, the most unique feature in children is the presence of the growth plate and ossification centres. This accounts for specific patterns of injury and the resulting growth disturbances. The blood supply to certain epiphysis such as the femoral head is precarious, and damage to it can lead to serious complications of avascular necrosis and growth arrest. The periosteum is much thicker and stronger and produces abundant callus at a more rapid rate compared with adults.

Physiologically, the rate of healing of fractures is more rapid the younger the child is. Reduction should be achieved early, before the fracture becomes too "sticky" to manipulate. Bone overgrowth is a commonly observed phenomenon associated with diaphyseal fractures of the long bone. Remodelling can potentially correct an angular deformity of up to 30° in the plane of motion of an adjacent hinge joint in young children. However, one must realize that such potential is not without its limitations; rotational deformities, displaced intra-articular fractures and angular deformities not in the plane of joint movement do not remodel easily, if at all [6].

Biomechanically, the porosity of bone can result in unique compression fracture (torus or buckling fracture). Plastic deformation and greenstick fracture in children can be accounted for by the thick periosteum and underlying elastic bone. The presence of different ossification centres and growth zones also alters the mechanical strength of the bone, leading to unique patterns of fractures [7,8].

Clinically, the mechanism of injury and the pattern and type of fracture are quite different from those in adults. The clinical presentation can be misleading and non-specific, especially in younger children. The clinical approach, physical examination of the child and the handling of anxious parents demand special skills and patience. Subsequent diagnosis and management of children's fractures also necessitate additional caution, technique and a well-organized system of follow-up care.

Relative Incidence of Fractures

Results from our own series in 1986–1990 on the relative incidence among 2500 fractures in children under 12 years of age are presented in Table 1. Comparable results from the study by Landin [9] are given in Table 2 and those from the study by Worlock and Stower [10] in Table 3. It is obvious from the figures in these tables that the fracture pattern can vary among different places as a result of such differences as physical activities, environment and socioeconomic factors. However, when one groups these in categories, the commonest fractures in children are still those of the distal radius, forearm, and supracondylar fracture of the humerus and tibia [11,12].

Common Pitfalls in Management of Fractures in Children

Certain fractures in children are well known as giving rise to problems and difficulties in treatment, for example, growth plate injuries, spinal fractures, fractures of the femoral neck and fractures in neuromuscular disease. However, the majority of problems and complications in clinical practice come from pitfalls in the management of common fractures that one encounters from day to day, such as forearm fractures and fractures around the elbow and lower limb. The situation is further complicated by the fact that such fractures are often managed by inexperienced junior physicians who tend to underestimate the problems or to overlook them [3].

Pitfalls in Diagnosis

Missed diagnosis can result from:

- Poorly taken history and inadequate physical examination. This is particularly true in the case of a crying child and anxious parents. Most fractures produce clear physical signs of soft-tissue swelling, tenderness, deformity and loss of function of the affected limb, which are revealed on careful direct or indirect observation and palpation.
- Associated injuries in the same limb and other regions. These should be looked for carefully to avoid complications resulting from them.

Misinterpreted radiographs commonly occur in the following situations:

- Poor radiograph quality and inadequately covered field.
- Poor positioning and inadequately splinted fracture.
- Fractures not shown on standard views (Fig. 1).

Table 1. Relative incidence of children's fractures: Hong Kong series

Fracture	Percentage
Distal radius ulna	19.88
Supracondylar humerus	19.33
Radius ulna shaft	13.45
Tibial shaft	13.45
Finger hand	5.37
Lateral condyle humerus	4.55
Femoral shaft	3.69
Olecranon	2.12
Distal radius epiphysis	1.73
Ulna	1.57
Monteggia	1.41
Foot toe	1.25
Medial condyle/epicondyle humerus	1.25
Patella/dislocation	1.18
Humerus shaft	1.02
Clavicle	0.98
Ankle/malleolus	0.86
Elbow dislocation	0.78
Proximal humerus	0.71
Radius head/neck dislocation	0.67
Distal tibia epiphysis	0.63
Femur condyle/supracondylar	0.55
Pelvis	0.31
Galleazzi's	0.31
Proximal femur	0.24
Miscellaneous	2.71

Table 2. Relative incidence of children's fractures: Malmö series (from [9])

Fracture	Percentage
Distal forearm	22.7
Hand, phalanges	18.9
Carpal-metacarpal (scaphoid excluded)	8.3
Clavicle	8.1
Ankle	5.5
Tibia, diaphysis	5.0
Tarsal-metatarsal (talus, os calcis excluded)	4.5
Foot, phalanges	3.4
Radius-ulna, diaphysis	3.4
Supracondylar region of the humerus	3.3
Proximal end of the humerus	2.2
Facial skeleton	2.1
Skull	1.8
Femur shaft	1.6
Radial neck fracture	1.2
Vertebral fracture	1.2

Table 3. Relative incidence of children's fractures: Nottingham series (from [10])

Fracture	Percentage
Distal radius/ulna	35.8
Hand (including carpus)	14.7
Distal humerus	7.7
Foot	7.7
Radius/ulna (shaft)	6.5
Clavicle	6.3
Tibia/fibula (shaft)	4.3
Ankle	4.0
Skull	3.6
Radial neck	2.7
Proximal humerus	1.7
Femur (shaft)	1.2
Olecranon	1.0
Supracondylar femur	0.8
Proximal tibia	0.8
Ribs	0.7
Patella	0.4
Humerus (shaft)	0.2

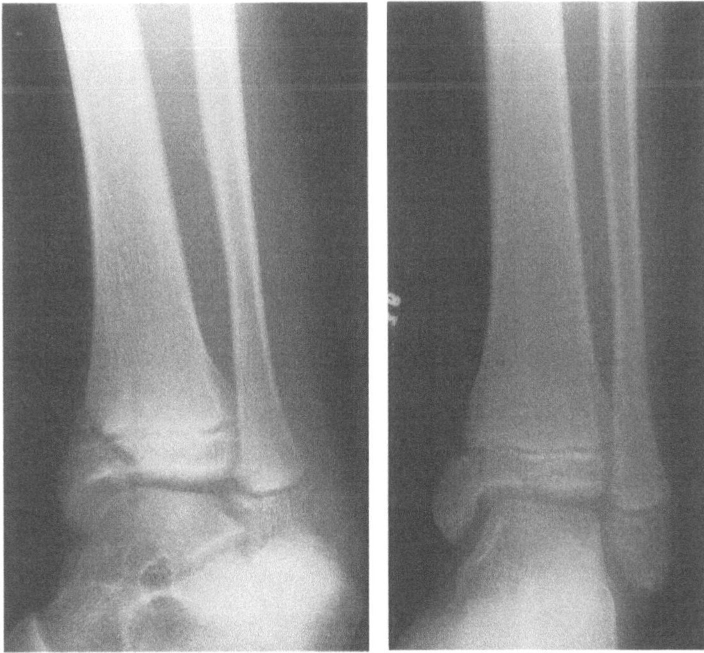

a   b

Fig. 1a,b. Epiphyseal fracture Salter-Harris of type IV. **a** Fracture clearly shown on oblique view. **b** Fracture easily missed on standard view of the ankle

- Fractures that are obvious but not recognized (Figs. 2, 3).
- Failure to look for soft-tissue signs, which always occur adjacent to the fracture site.
- Fat-pad sign is particularly important for diagnosing fracture around the elbow joint (Fig. 4).
- Failure to understand and locate unossified epiphysis.
- Failure to obtain a comparison view of the contralateral limb. This should not be a routine practice, but for certain fractures such as the supracondylar fracture of humerus it helps greatly in measuring the actual angulation (Fig. 5).
- Overdiagnosis of fractures can result from failure to recognize the nutrient vessels, accessory bones, Harris' lines, and unusual ossification centres (Fig. 6).
- Failure to correlate radiological signs with clinical findings is the most important pitfall in the diagnosis of fractures in children.

Pitfalls in Treatment

The pitfalls in manipulation and reduction are:

- Insufficient relaxation of the child and the fractured limb. Most displaced fractures require proper general anaesthesia to allow careful manipulation and reduction.

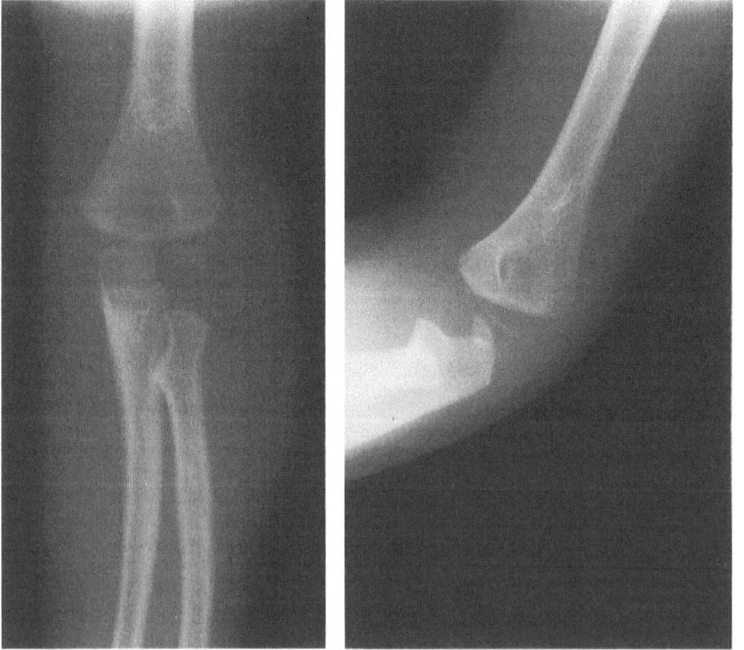

a   b

Fig. 2a,b. Lateral condyle fracute of humerus. A frequently missed fracture

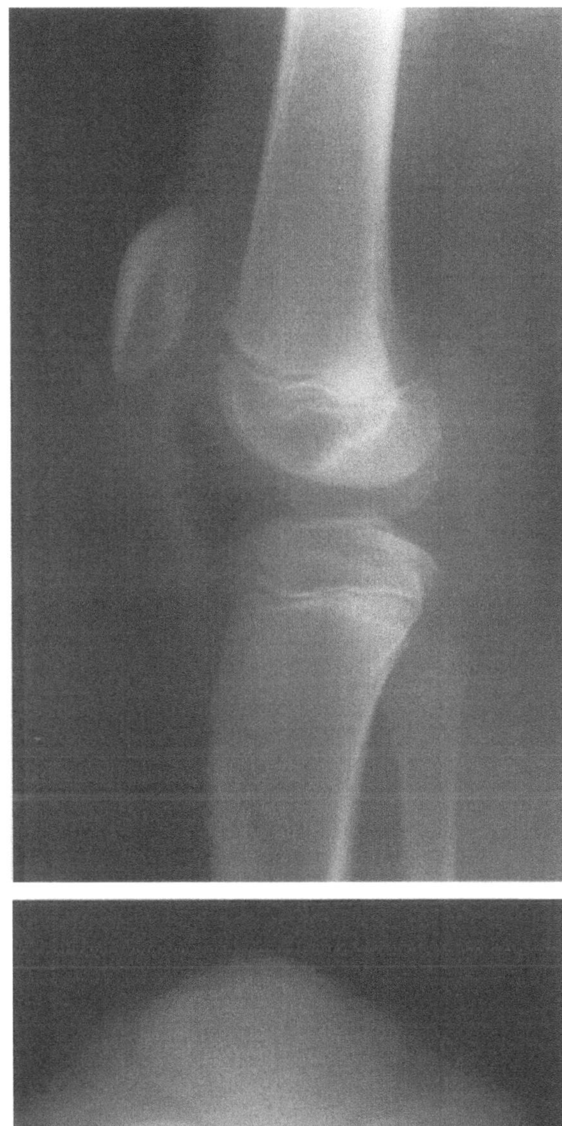

Fig. 3a,b. Osteochondral fracture of patella with haemarthrosis. **a** Lateral view. **b** Skyline view

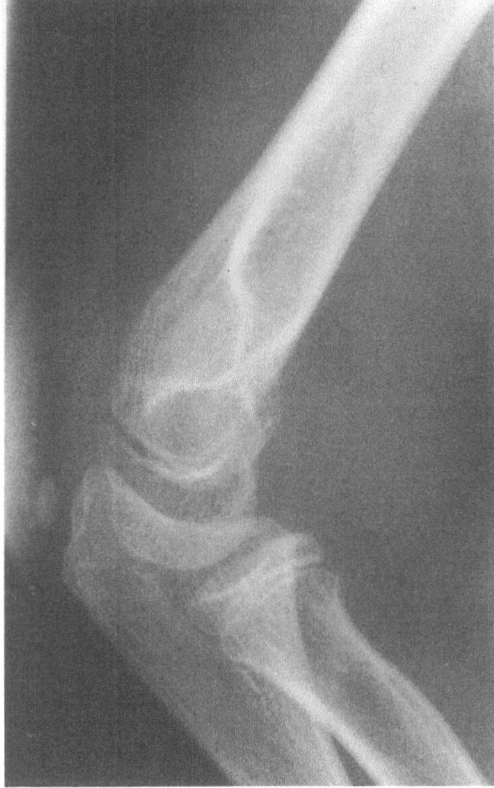

Fig. 4. Positive anterior and posterior "fat-pad" sign showing haemarthrosis in elbow joint

- Failure to achieve adequate reduction. Not every fracture can be reduced perfectly, but an acceptable reduction and alignment should be achieved by proper technique and checked with an image intensifier. For greenstick fractures one needs to break the remaining intact opposite cortex to achieve a proper reduction [13].
- Inadequate countertraction by assistant or special frame. This can lead to great difficulty in reducing some fractures, for example, displaced supracondylar fracture of the humerus.
- Poor understanding of fracture mechanics. This can lead to inadequate reduction, for example, not increasing the fracture angulation in distal radial fracture and radial shaft fracture can result in failure of reduction, and not locking the supracondylar fracture humerus in pronation or supination can easily result in loss of reduction.
- Poor timing of reduction. When the treatment is unduly delayed, the onset of oedema and swelling can cause great difficulties in manipulation and reduction.

The pitfalls in immobilization after closed reduction are:

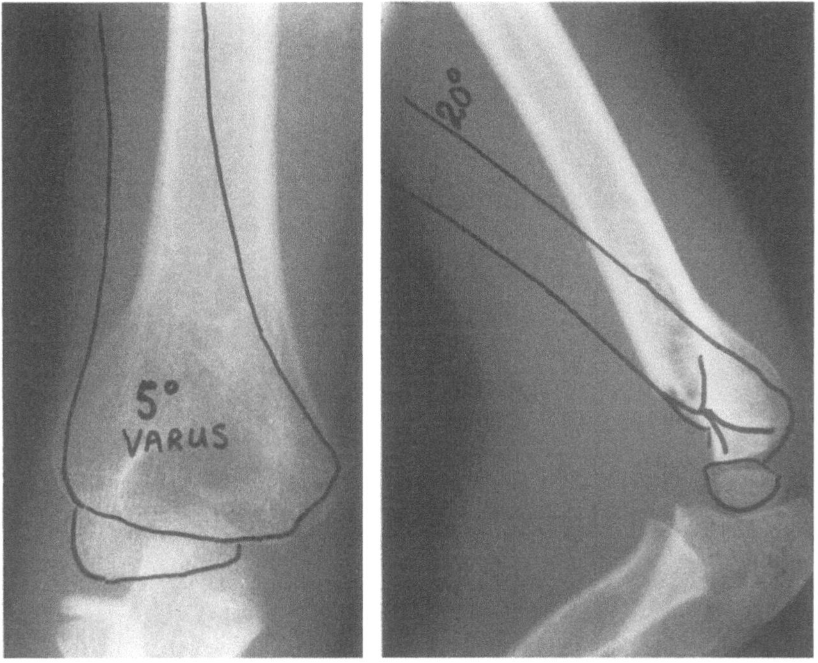

Fig. 5a,b. Overlapping the comparison view from the contralateral humerus gives a more accurate measurement of the degree of angulation in supracondylar fractures of the humerus

- Failure to lock the fracture with the three-point locking principle. This can result in loss of reduction [13].
- Poor plastering technique. Various faults in the use of plaster of paris can lead to poor immobilization and complications: for example, too thin or too thick paddings, poor moulding technique with poor contouring and lamination, poor positioning, tightness or looseness, indentation of plaster at the joint level (Fig. 7) [13].
- Inadequate length of plaster. The short arm type of plaster cannot be relied upon in young children; it is much better to immobilize joints adjacent to the fracture.
- Use of plaster slab. This never works in children except for fractures not requiring immobilization such as the torus fracture.
- Fibreglass cast. When using the newer synthetic fibreglass materials in place of traditional plaster of paris, one must observe that in general the moulding property is not as good, contouring is more difficult, and they are more liable to form sharp compressing edges especially at the elbow cubital fossa and dorsum of ankle joint. The radiological appearance, however, is superior.

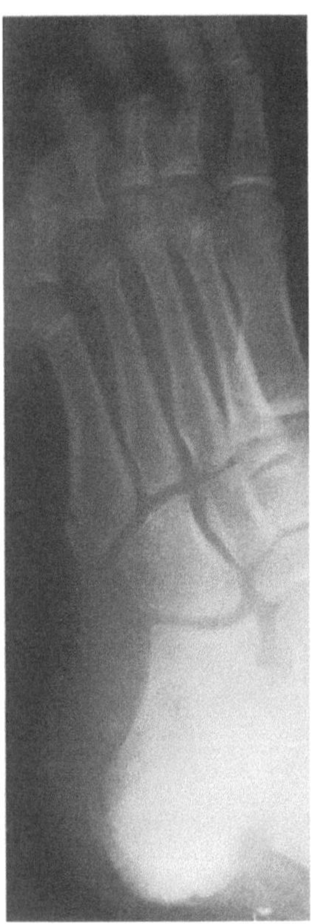

Fig. 6. Apophysis at base of 5th metatarsus, misdiagnosed as avulsion fracture. (Note the absent soft-tissue signs)

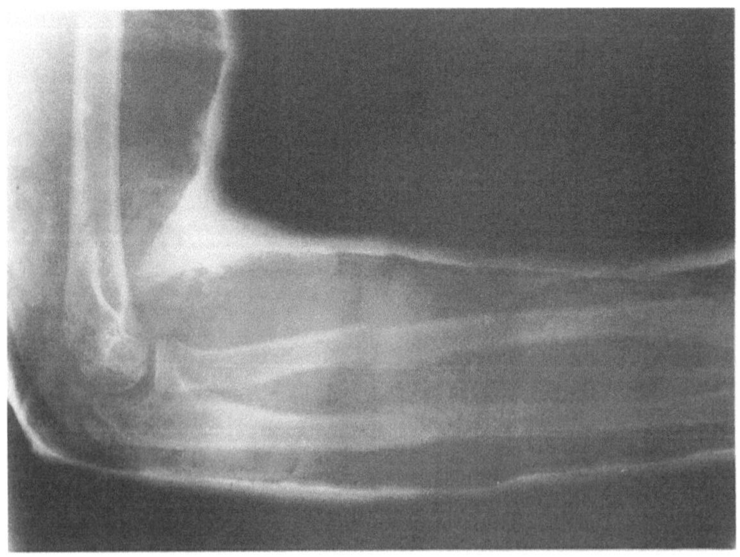

Fig. 7. Marked indentation of plaster at cubital fossa causing pressure sore and other pressure phenomena

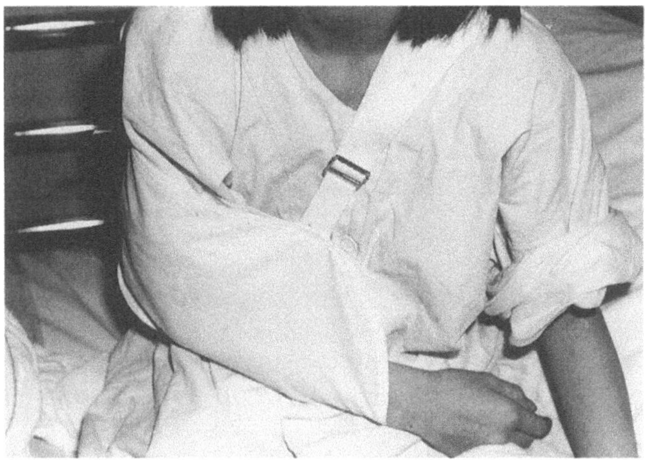

Fig. 8. Shoulder immobilizer with cross-shoulder, posterior and around waist strappings. These are better than simple slings

- Holding the plaster cast. The usual practice is to give a sling to the plaster cast in upper limb fractures, which in children is often unsatisfactory. A shoulder immobilizer certainly gives better support and prevents the child from excessively moving the injured limb with resulting re-displacement of the fracture inside the cast (Fig. 8).

The pitfalls in open reduction are:

- Bias in indications. For the majority of children with fractures open reduction is not necessary; a careful closed reduction under good relaxation can usually achieve the goal.
- Percutaneous pinning. In fractures that are difficult to hold after reduction, such as supracondylar fractures of the humerus and distal radius fractures, percutaneous pinning under imaging can often replace open reduction and internal fixation [14]. Closed flexible intramedullary nails have been used as an alternative treatment of forearm shaft fractures and femoral shaft fractures [15].
- Technique of open reduction. Open reduction is not fool-proof in fracture treatment. There are many cases of poor reduction even after open technique. Typical examples are observed in supracondylar fracture of the humerus, epiphyseal fractures around the ankle, etc.
- Pin tract care. Failure properly to release the pin tract and bend the pin outside the skin with good padding can result in pin tract infections, granulation and migration. An alternative is to cut the pin short and bury it beneath the skin, but the obvious disadvantage is that one must remove it under anaesthesia later.
- Poor immobilization after open reduction. In children's fractures the fixation is usually not rigid, and children never follow the rules. To

avoid re-displacement it is appropriate to have proper immobilization with cast and support post-operatively.

Pitfalls in Follow-Up Care

The pitfalls during follow-up care include:

- Timing and frequency of follow-up. Children with fractures should be followed-up more frequently than adults. Most re-displacements of fractures occur in the first 2 weeks. Swelling and complications of plastering should be monitored carefully in the first few days.
- Organization and channelling of records. This is important because without the initial records and radiographs the follow-up physician is not able properly to manage the child, especially in a busy clinic.
- Failure to check status of plaster. The plaster come get loose by the first to second weeks after oedema after the fracture site has subsided. Children can easily break or deform their plasters. One may have to carefully adjust or change to new set of plaster.
- Failure to detect re-displacement of fracture. Proper radiography is important in detecting change of position and state of union of the fracture. A common mistake is failure to observe the fact that greenstick fracture can deform progressively if the initial reduction is inadequate.
- Timing for removal of plaster. Premature removal of plaster cast can lead to malunion or nonunion of fracture. This is particularly common in lateral condylar fractures of the humerus and in femoral shaft fractures.
- Failure to talk to the parents. One cannot over-emphasize the fact that an inadequate explanation to the parents is usually the cause of poor follow-up attendance and of complications and accusations.
- Failure to follow and detect late complications. For fractures near the growth plate, ossification centres and joint surfaces, and special fractures such as proximal tibial fracture a much longer period of follow-up is necessary to detect any late growth disturbances, deformities, length discrepancies or joint complications.

Common Children's Fractures Presenting with Treatment Problems

The most frequently committed mistakes in the management and treatment of common fractures in children are discussed below.

Fractures of the Distal Radius

Fractures of the distal radius constitute the commonest group of fractures in children, ranging from 18% to 36% in various series and representing 20%

in our series of 2500 fractures in children under 12 years of age. These can be divided into epiphyseal fractures, the commonest of which is the Salter-Harris type II fracture, followed by type I, and metaphyseal fractures consisting of buckling fractures, greenstick fractures and complete fractures [16–18].

Greenstick Fractures. The most frequently encountered problem in treating greenstick fracture is the misconception that greenstick fractures are stable, and even if they are not perfectly reduced, remodelling can do the job. This is certainly not true. In most angulated greenstick fractures one must reduce the fracture by breaking the intact opposite cortex (Fig. 9). This is possible only with an efficient three-point correcting force over a short lever arm with the child under adequate anaesthesia and relaxation. The surgeon's knee or a well-padded wooden block may serve as the volar correcting force against the two hands of the surgeon, to the dorsal distally and the dorsal

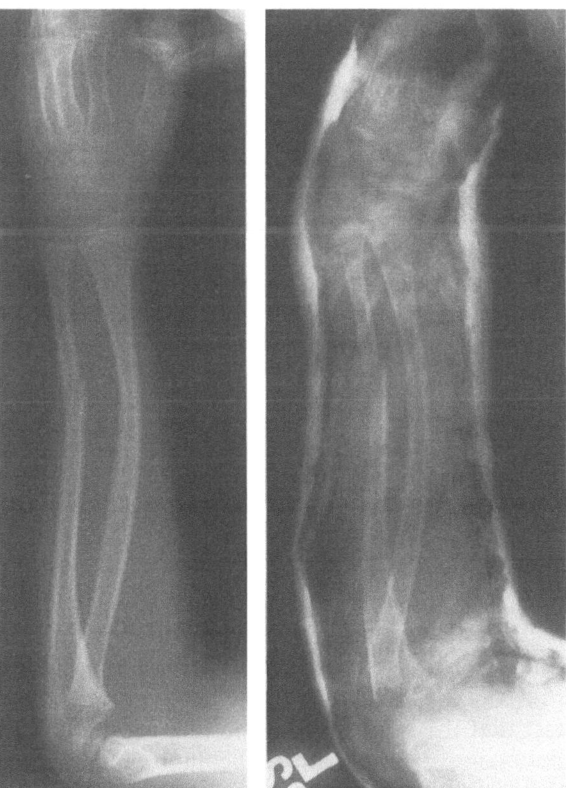

Fig. 9. Greenstick fracture of radius not properly reduced. The intact cortex was not broken during the reduction

proximally. The fracture after reduction should be locked in some degree of volar flexion of the wrist with pronated forearm inside a well-contoured three-point moulded cast. For younger children the long-arm cast gives more reliable holding than the short-arm cast. Post-manipulation swelling is common 12–36 h after and may require controlled splitting of the plaster. Very close follow-up in the first 2–3 weeks is necessary to detect plaster loosening or re-displacement of the fracture.

Complete Fractures. The distal fragment is displaced dorsally and radially with varying degree of overriding. The fracture can be accompanied by greenstick or displaced fracture of the distal ulna. Reduction can be difficult and usually requires adequate relaxation and hyperextension to disimpact the fracture. The plastering technique for a short, chubby forearm can be difficult (Fig. 10). Because of the short, fractured distal segment maintaining the reduced fracture in place in a cast is difficult. Moreover, subsidence of the marked swelling around the fracture site in the first 2 weeks following the reduction can easily lead to re-displacement. Of the 195 cases of fractured distal radius in our series, 35 had completely displaced fracture. Follow-up at an average of 3 years showed that one-third of all such fractures treated by closed reduction had re-displacement significant enough to require secondary procedures, all within the first 3 weeks. Among the whole group of completely displaced fractures, 40% ended up with either open reduction or percutaneous Kirschner's wire fixation. On the basis of our own and others' experiences, closed reduction followed by percutaneous pinning under image intensifier should have a definite place in the treatment of unstable, completely displaced fracture of the distal radius (Fig. 11). The pins can be removed with the cast after 4–5 weeks. Open reduction may still be required for delayed cases but can be avoided in most early cases and should be replaced by closed percutaneous pinning whenever possible to avoid unnecessary scarring and complications.

Shaft Fractures of the Forearm

Diaphyseal fractures of the forearm are the third commonest fracture in our series of children's fractures, and together with distal radius fractures they account for 33.33% of all fractures.

The most important principle in the treatment of forearm shaft fractures is to aim at restoring normal rotation, i.e. supination-pronation of 180° in children. The concept of rotational deformity is often not well appreciated since the plain radiographs reveal only angulation in the anteroposterior and lateral planes alone. The fact that the normal radius bowing is essential for the smooth pronation-supination movement points to the important principle that shaft fractures should be reduced three-dimensionally to restore the normal rotation of the forearm. In addition, compared with fractures in the metaphyseal region, remodelling power is much poorer: "rounding off" of

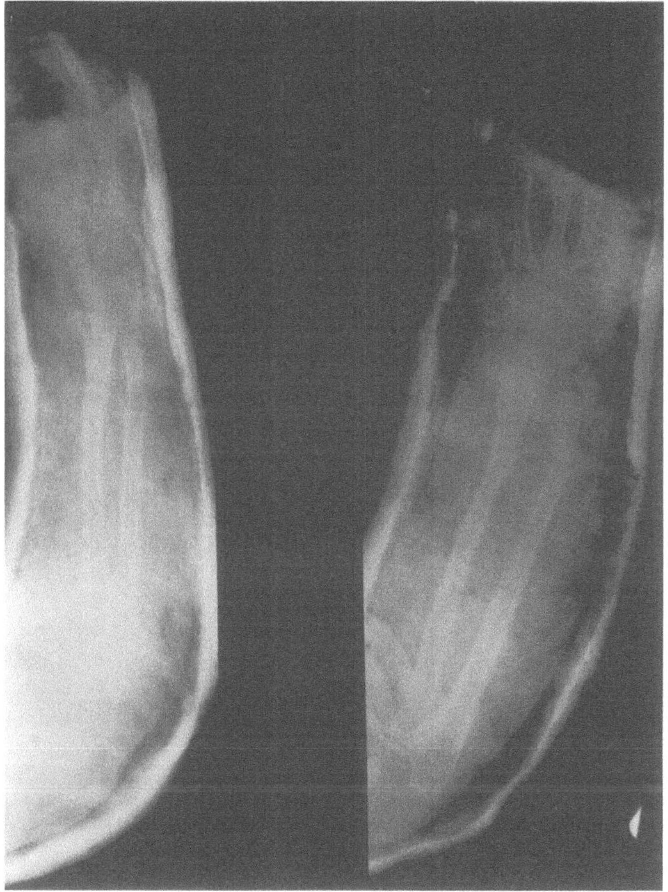

Fig. 10. Poor plastering technique. Too loose, laminated and poorly moulded plaster

malunion occurs, but not true rotational realignment. Studies have shown that 10° of residual angulation can limit rotation by 20° [6,19–22].

Greenstick Fractures. A very common complaint by young surgeons dealing with greenstick fractures is "Why has the fracture displaced again? I definitely manipulated and reduced the fracture!" The problem is that they did not break the intact cortex on the side opposite to the angulation by overcorrecting and completing the fracture. An audible "click" is commonly felt and heard on completing the fracture, especially at the mid-shaft region. Re-angulation can be prevented by holding the forearm in a complete long-arm cast in the correct degree of rotation and moulded with due respect to the three-point principle (Fig. 12). One must remember to apply the "squeeze grip" during moulding of the cast to create an oval cross-section which acts

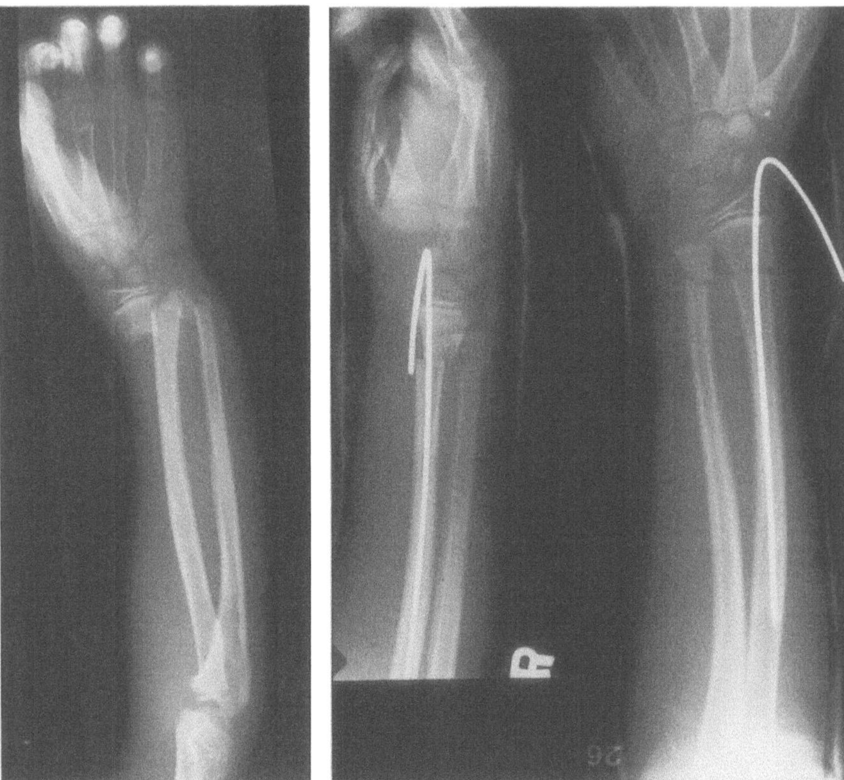

Fig. 11. Fracture of distal radius and ulna. Percutaneous Kirchner's wire through metaphyseal region can prevent the high incidence of redisplacement afterwards

to restore the anatomy of the radius and ulna more accurately (Fig. 13). Minimally displaced greenstick fractures are not uncommon and can usually be corrected by applying the proper pressure while the cast is setting.

Plastic Deformation in Shaft of Radius and Ulna. This can occur in young children without any radiological evidence of fracture. Such microstructural failure if not reduced may lead to significant deformity since no remodelling can occur (Fig. 14). Reduction can be very difficult and must be carried out under general anaesthesia with great sustained corrective force acting on a three-point fulcrum principles sequentially in different planes of the deformity [23,24].

Complete Fractures of the Radius and Ulna. This type of fracture is very unstable since the periosteal cuffs are ruptured and partial tear of the interosseous membrane has occurred. Malunion with rotational limitation can easily result from inadequate treatment.

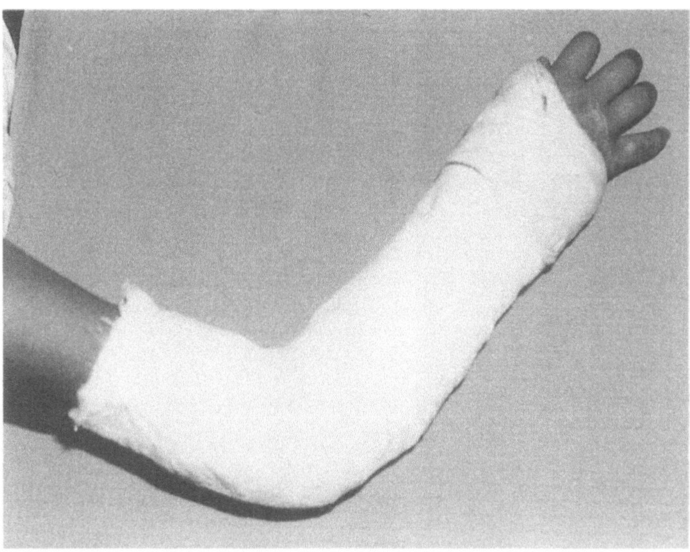

Fig. 12. A long-arm plaster ending only at mid-arm level giving poor holding for fracture at lower end of humerus

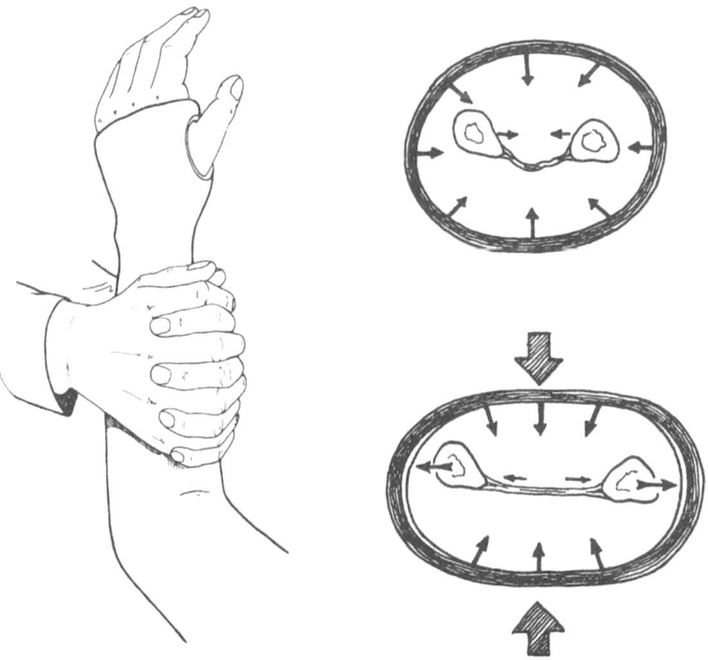

Fig. 13. "Squeeze grip" on the plaster is essential for restoring the anatomical cross-section to the forearm

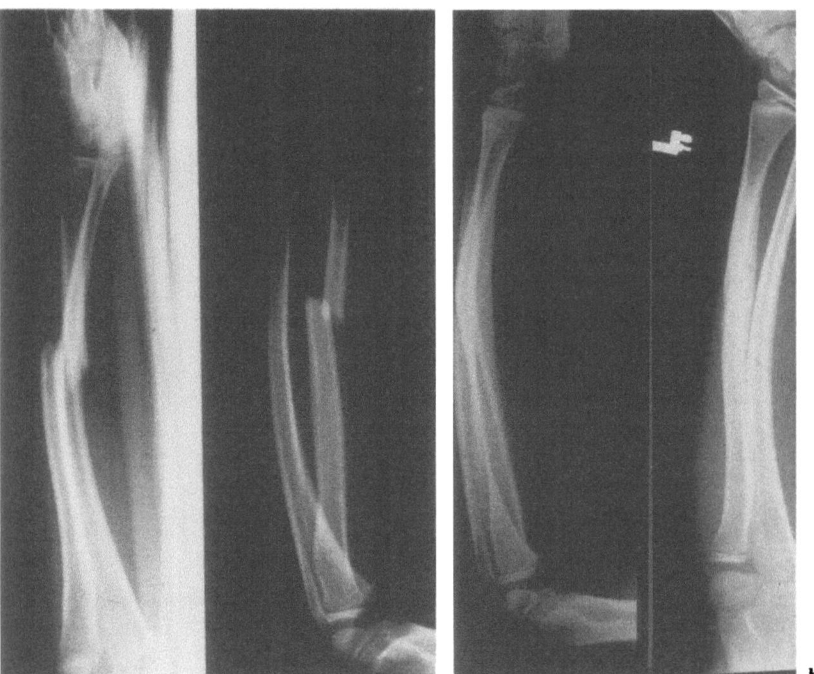

Fig. 14a–d. Fracture of radius shaft with plastic deformation of ulna. Not diagnosed and initially reduced, resulting in marked limitation of supination pronation and ugly bowing of forearm

For the reduction, preliminary traction to correct the shortening under general anaesthesia with Chinese finger-trap suspension system is highly recommended as it allows the surgeon's hands to be freed for manipulating the fracture under distraction longitudinally (Fig. 15). The criteria for satisfactory closed reduction are that the fracture ends are in end-to-end contact, angular deformity is corrected, interosseous space is preserved, and rotational deformity is eliminated. With regard to the rotational alignment, the classically recommended position to immobilize these fractures is that of full supination for the upper third fracture, neutral for the middle third and pronation in the lower third; however, these should only act as guidelines rather than be followed rigidly. The proper position is the one which yields the best alignment and stable reduction. Moulding of the cast after reduction is of utmost importance, and the oval cross-section must be maintained, and a proper long-arm cast from the axilla down to the palm should be applied. The palm region should also be properly moulded to prevent undue rotation of the forearm. One useful way is to apply the arm and elbow section of the cast first to obtain a well-moulded proximal segment before going down to the forearm and hand. The newer fibreglass cast material should not be used in this type of fracture because of the significantly poorer moulding property.

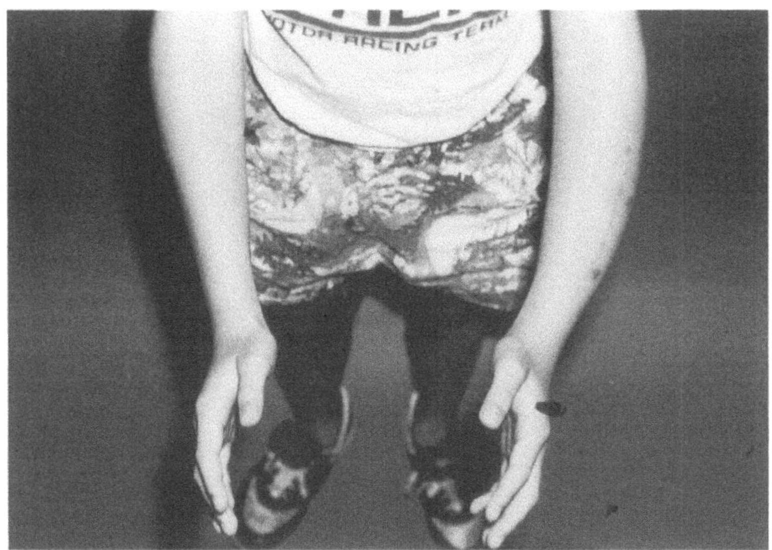

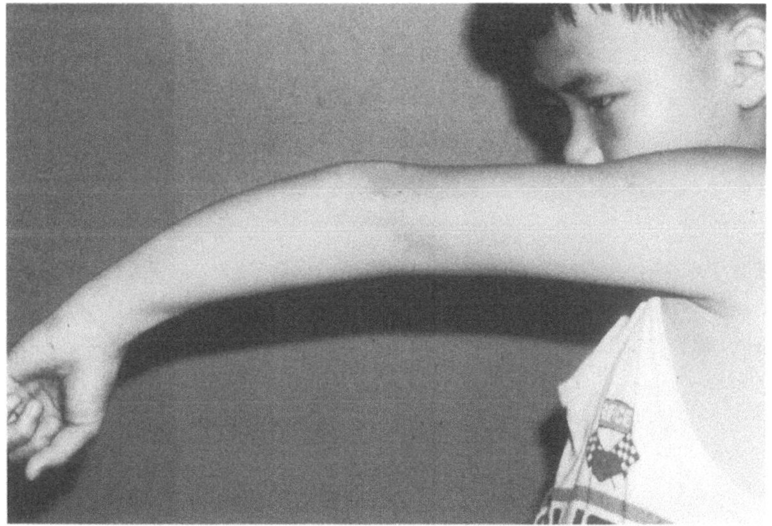

Fig. 14a,d.

One cannot over-emphasize the fact that all these fractures need very careful and frequent follow-up checks of the cast and radiographs (Fig. 16). Minor displacement can usually be corrected in up to 4 weeks after injury by manipulating the sticky callus under image intensifier, and parents should be warned right at the beginning of the possibility of secondary procedures.

When facing the difficult situation of not being able to reduce or hold the reduction under closed means, one should be prepared to carry out open

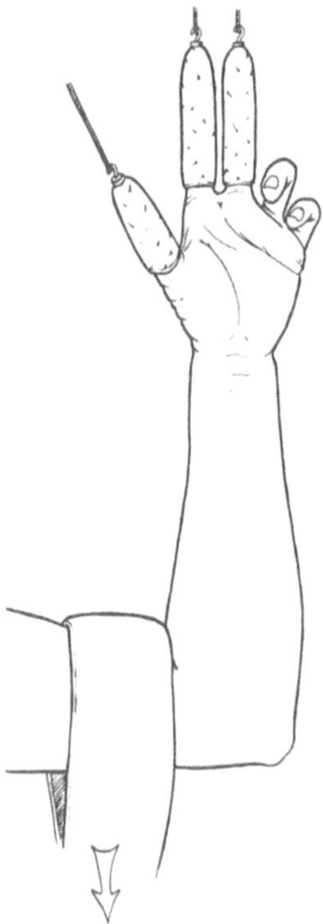

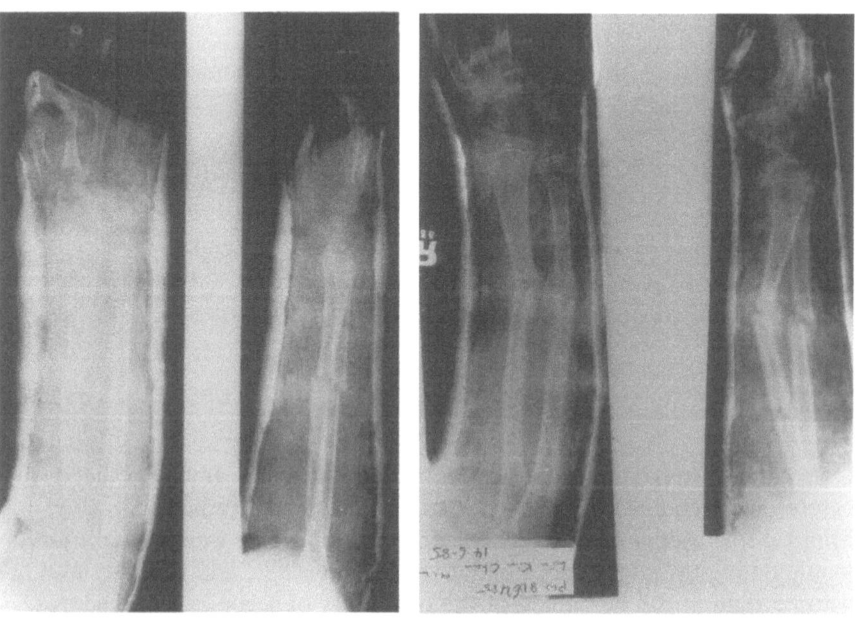

Fig. 15. Using Chinese finger-trap traction on the radial three fingers with weight counter traction at arm level allows the surgeon to have both hands free for manipulation and reduction of forearm shaft fracture

Fig. 16a,b. Fracture of radius and ulna. **a** Well reduced in plaster at 1 week. **b** At 2 weeks redisplacement and angulation can be seen reduction and internal fixation or percutaneous pinning techniques. Flexible intramedullary nails introduced through the metaphyseal region under image intensifier across the fracture site can act as an effective aligning internal splint without going through the more drastic open reduction and plating. Open reduction with cross Kirschner's wire fixation is difficult and gives poor fixation expecially in transverse fractures. One need only align the fractures by intramedullary splinting and putting the forearm in the proper rotation and cast. For older children and adolescents there may be a place for open reduction and plating in difficult cases as a primary procedure [15,25].

Monteggia's Fractures

By definition Monteggia's fracture is a fracture of the ulna with simultaneous dislocation of the head of the radius. Although Monteggia's fracture is not very common (1.64% of our series), it is included here for discussion since it is one of the commonly mismanaged fractures. The associated dislocation of the radial head occurs anteriorly in 85%, posteriorly in 10% and laterally in 5%. The type of the fracture of the ulna ranges from greenstick type to completely displaced type and occurs proximally in 0.67% of cases and in mid-shaft or distally in the rest. It is the proximal greenstick ulna fracture with a mild anterior radial head type of dislocation that frequently escapes the detection of inexperienced surgeons. For practical purposes, all isolated fractures of the ulna should be treated as Monteggia's fracture "until proven otherwise", and all such cases should have proper anteroposterior and lateral views, including those of the elbow and wrist.

In the reduction of Monteggia's fractures one should accept only a perfect alignment of the radial head, i.e. a line drawn along the longitudinal axis of the radius should always pass through the centre of the ossification centre of the capitellum in all radiographic projections. Anything less than this always means an improper reduction (Fig. 17). Reduction of the ulna fracture can be difficult. With a greenstick type of fracture the short lever arm of the proximal segment may cause difficulty in reduction. For complete fracture of the ulna, shortening at the fracture site may be difficult to restore. One should not hesitate to openly reduce and internally fix the ulna fracture to achieve a proper reduction of the dislocated radial head (Fig. 18). The ulna fracture can be fixed by intramedullary splinting with Kirschner's wire or flexible nail or in older children and adolescents with plating. In fresh fractures the radial head dislocation can usually be reduced adequately by properly reducing the ulna fracture. In delayed cases open reduction with or without reconstruction of the annular ligament is required. The proper long-arm cast must be used with forearm in supination, and close follow-up checks for cast loosening and proper position of the radial head are important to detect early re-displacement [26–29].

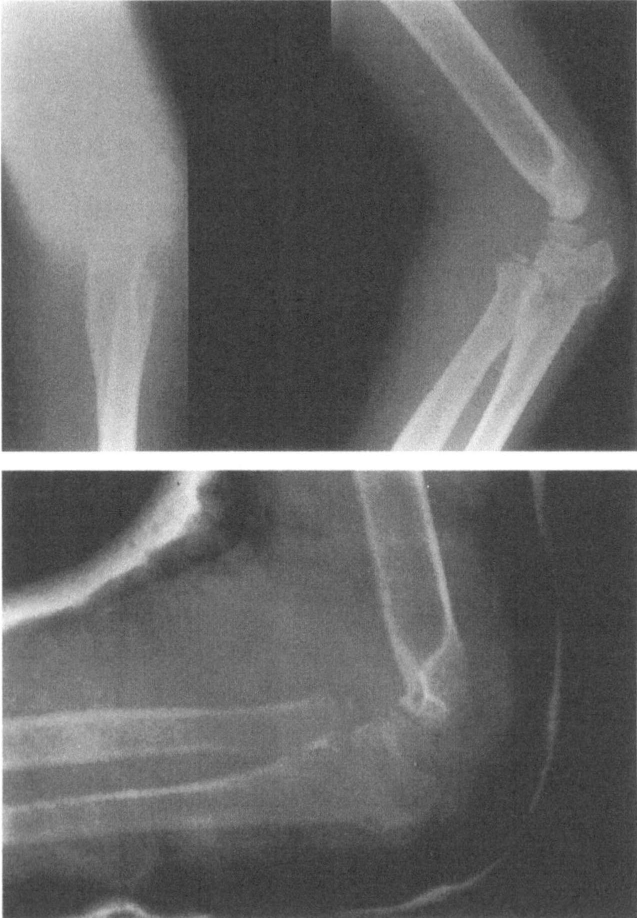

Fig. 17. Monteggia's fracture inadequately reduced in plaster. The radial head epiphysis should point perfectly to the capitulum rather than superiorly as in this case

Pulled Elbow

Probably one of the commonest musculoskeletal injuries in children under the age of 4 is the pulled elbow, or subluxation of the radial head. The actual incidence is difficult to document since many cases of them are reduced spontaneously either by the child, their parents or radiographers during the positioning for radiograph of the elbow in an accident and emergency department. It is classically produced by sudden traction of the hand with the elbow extended and forearm pronated. The sudden traction is thought to tear part of the annular ligament, which then slips over the radial head and becomes jammed between the radial head and the capitellum, thus

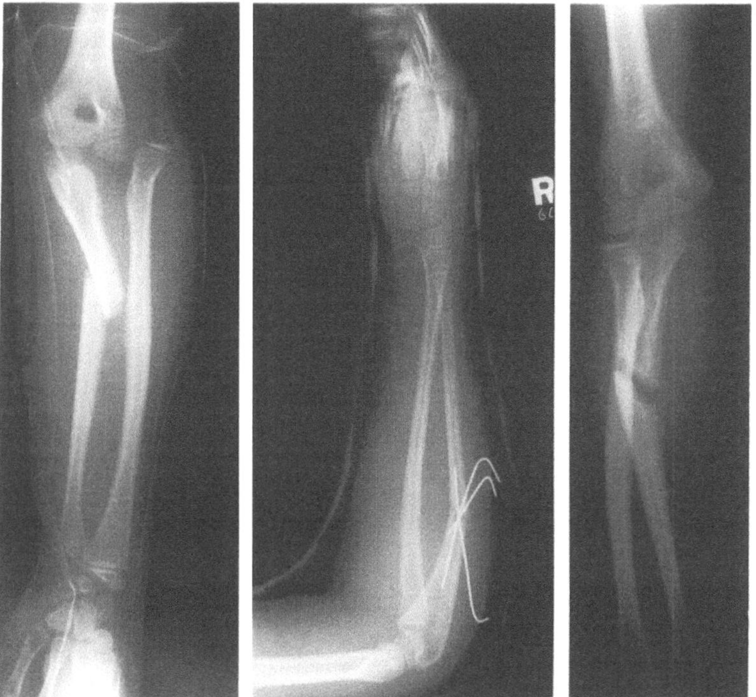

Fig. 18a–c. Monteggia fracture. **a** Open reduction and cross Kircher's wire. **b** Open reduction failed to stabilize the ulna fracture. **c** The result was non-union at 5 months

preventing the relocation of the radial head (Fig. 19). Following the injury the child typically cries and refuses to move his entire upper limb which is held with the forearm in pronated position and elbow slightly flexed. The inexperienced physician who does not take a proper history may diagnose this injury as contusion of the elbow, sprain of the elbow, pseudoparalysis of the limb after traction, injury to the arm, etc. Radiographs are then ordered which show no abnormality, and the crying child is then sent home without a proper diagnosis. Most of these cases are reduced spontaneously. However, if one knows of this condition, it can be one of the most dramatic "cures" that a surgeon can offer, simply by flexing the elbow to over 90° and supinating the forearm with a thumb pressing over the subluxed radial head. In nearly all cases, reduction is accompanied by a palpable or audible click. A few minutes later the child can move his elbow normally. Failure of reduction is usually a result of inadequate supination of forearm or flexion of elbow. Post-reduction immobilization is not necessary except for multiple recurrent cases [30–32].

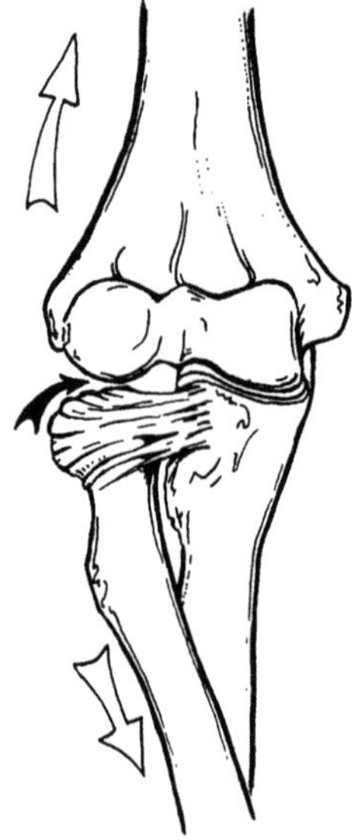

Fig. 19. Hyperpronation of forearm with forceful longitudinal pull can result in partial tear and slipping of the annular ligament over the radial head into the joint

Supracondylar Fracture of the Humerus, Lateral Condyle Fracture of the Humerus

Both supracondylar and lateral condyle fractures of the humerus are very common fractures in children, forming 19.33% and 4.55% in our series, respectively. These fractures are also two of the most commonly mismanaged fractures in children. They are discussed in detail in Chap. 10 of this volume.

Femoral Shaft Fractures

Femoral shaft fracture is the second commonest fracture of the lower limb in our series (94 cases, 3.69%). This fracture usually results from a major deforming force such as in traffic accidents and falls from a height, although in children under the age of 5 years the possibility of child abuse must also be considered. Association with other major injuries and fractures is common and should be carefully ruled out in clinical examination. The fractured middle third of the shaft forms the commonest subgroup – 65% in our series, similar to the figure in most other series – followed by fracture of the proximal third (18%) and the distal third (17%). It is important to understand the deforming muscle force in different sites of fracture as this helps in the reduction of such fractures. Upper third fractures usually result in a flexed, abducted and externally rotated proximal fragment and an abducted distal fragment. Middle third fractures lack a constant pattern of displacement. Distal third fractures commonly give rise to an anteriorly displaced proximal fragment and posteriorly displaced distal segment. Many studies have shown that remodelling potential following femoral shaft fracture is greatest for anterior posterior angulation, less for varus valgus angulation and practically nil for rotational deformities. Longitudinal overgrowth can be a problem especially in those aged 3–9 years. Thus, the aim of treating femoral shaft fractures in children is to align the fracture to less than 15° angulation in varus valgus or anteroposterior plane, with no rotation and with shortening of 1–1.5 cm. These aims are readily achieved by non-operative means in the majority of cases. Operative treatment is indicated only in multiply injured patients, those with neurovascular injury and in older children or adolescents over 12 years of age.

For children under 2 years of age, Gallow's skin traction for 2–3 weeks followed by spica gives satisfactory results. However, one should be very careful when using this method, the vascular status should be checked frequently, skin sores at the mallolar region should be prevented, and a fixed traction system should never be used. It is safer to use balanced traction with pulleys and weights. For children aged over 2 years, we recommend skeletal traction in the 90°–90° position (Fig. 20). A few common pitfalls with the skeletal pin are poor positioning of the pin, pins placed too near the growth plates, oblique insertion of the pin and wrong choice of size of pin. The pin should preferably be inserted in the distal femoral shaft away from but parallel to the growth plate under image intensifier control with the knee bent to 90° to facilitate the proper positioning of the pin in the coronal plane. Movement of the pin and the resulting pin tract infection can be eliminated by the addition of a tailor-made segmental femoral brace with a pin-guard extension (Fig. 21). In a 90°–90° traction, alignment of the fracture is easily achieved by first over-distracting the fracture and gradually reducing the weight in the first few days with X-ray checks. Rotational alignment is achieved automatically by this method of traction. Additional corrections of angulation can be made by adjusting the tension in the lateral or medial traction cord attached to the pin or positional paddings in the segmental brace. When early callus is formed in 2–3 weeks, an ambulatory functional ischial weight-bearing brace with pelvic extension and lockable hip and knee hinges can be applied, and the child can be started on weight-bearing walking with aids (Fig. 22). This method is, in our opinion, much better than spica cast or cast brace since for the spica cast ambulation would be very difficult, and in hot and humid countries it is usually poorly tolerated by the children and the parents. For children aged over 12 years, closed flexible or rigid intramedullary nailing can be a good alternative in the treatment of femoral shaft fractures in allowing a more anatomical reduction and quicker rehabilitation process [33–38].

Fracture Shaft of Tibia

Tibial shaft fracture is the commonest fracture in the lower limb in children, forming 13.45% (343 cases) of all fractures in our series. In younger children

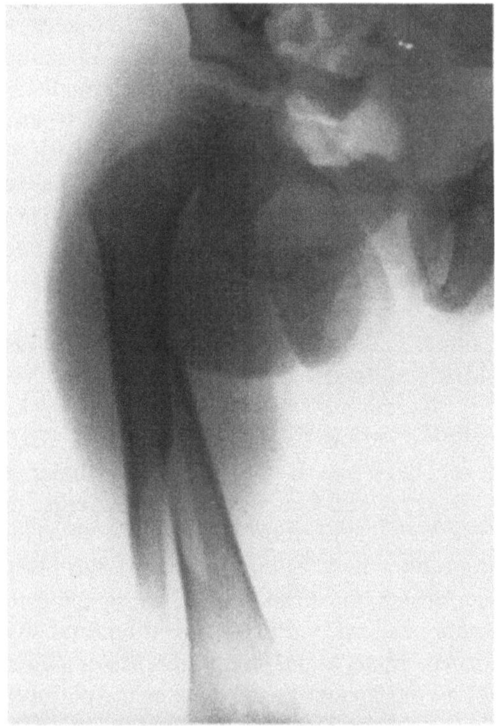

a

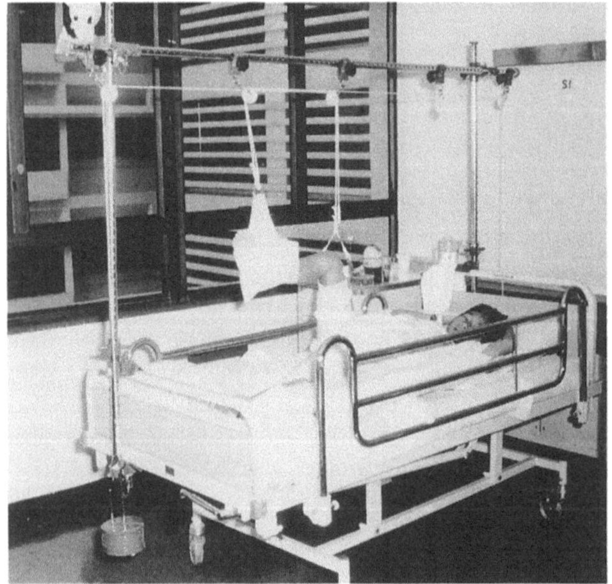

b

Fig. 20a,b. A 90°–90° skeletal traction in bed for femoral shaft fractures

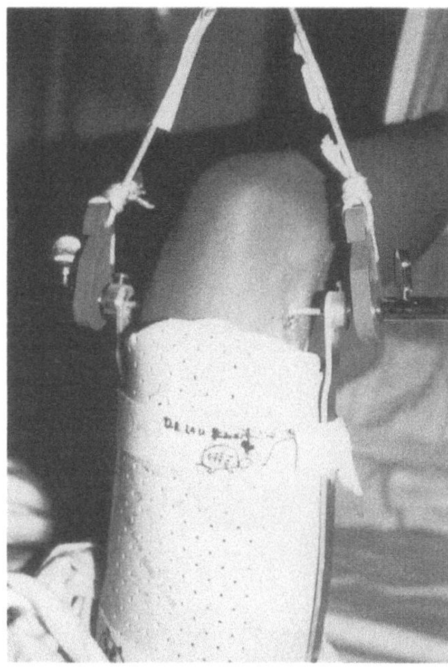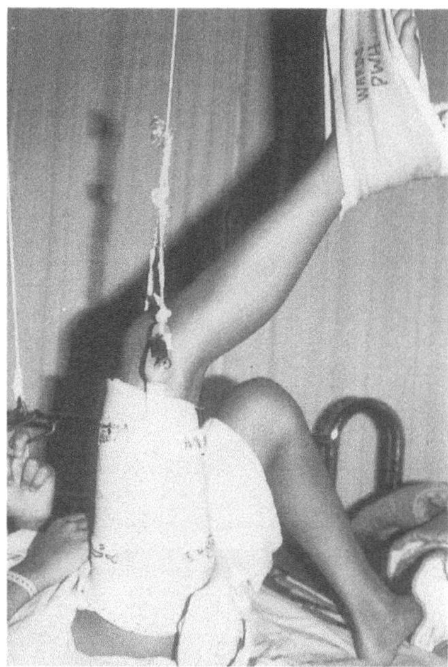

Fig. 21. Segmental brace with pin guard to allow adjustment and stabilization of femoral shaft fracture and prevent pin migration

70%–80% are stable undisplaced spiral fractures. Because of the absence of any significant swelling or deformity it is not uncommon to see small children with such fractures presenting with limp and pain a few days after the injury where the diagnosis was not made or even suspected at the time of initial injury. The treatment of this group is usually simple with a long leg cast immobilization for 3 weeks, mainly for the pain. The remaining 20%–30% of our cases had displaced fractures requiring reduction and casting. When the fibula is intact, which is usually the case in younger children, reduction is usually easily achieved and maintained. For those with both the tibia and fibula fractured, it is not uncommon to find difficulties in reducing and holding the fractures. If the legs are swollen with a displaced fracture, they may be supported with a three-quarter plaster slab and elevated for a few days before the definitive reduction and cast is given. Reduction is much easier when one hangs the leg over the side of the table and lets gravity help in the traction realignment (Fig. 23). Then the tibia, ankle and foot portion are first casted with proper rotational, anteroposterior and varus valgus alignment. The above-knee segment is then completed with the knee joint in slight flexion, or in difficult small children the knee can be kept in 90° flexion. Minor corrections can be made afterwards by wedging of the cast.

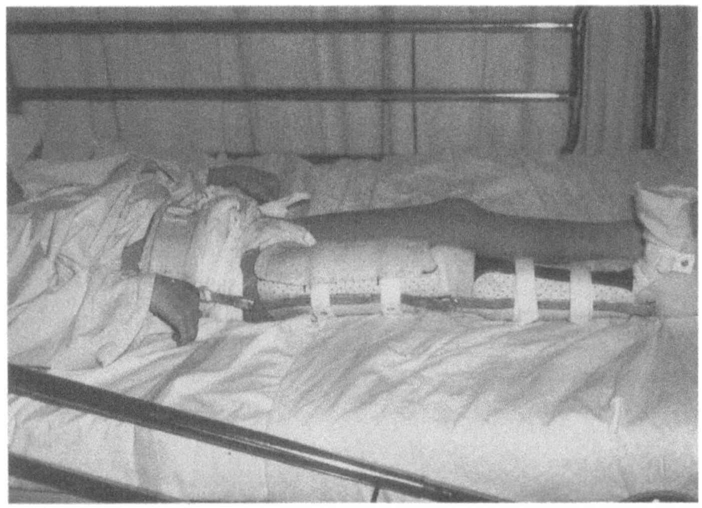

a

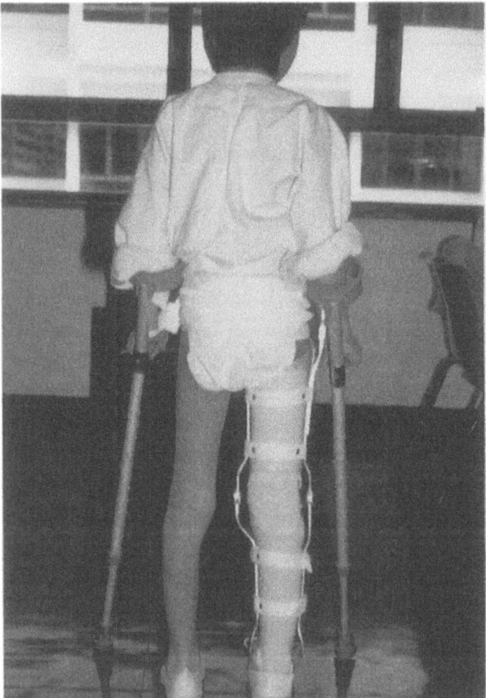

b

Fig. 22a,b. Ischial weight-bearing functional femoral brace with hip hinge and pelvic band for ambulatory treatment of femoral shaft fractures

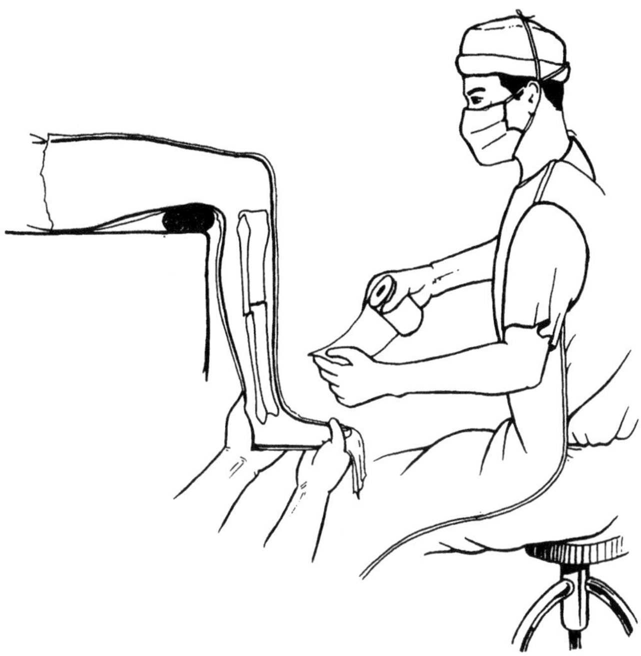

Fig. 23. Surgeon seated and facing the fracture with the assistance of gravity and the knocked knee. The tibial shaft fracture can be reduced and held in place for plaster application first below knee and then above knee. The ankle and foot can be stabilized in plantigrade position by an assistant holding a long stockinette tube

A very frustrating experience in treating such fractures is that during follow-up the children return with broken, deformed and worn plaster since they begin walking with the cast once the pain is gone. We have found that the newer fibreglass cast material is much stronger and can tolerate the abuse by children better. In most cases, we can shorten the fibreglass cast in 3 weeks to a short leg patella tendon bearing cast without changing the cast and allow weight-bearing walking with aids. Excessive angulation inside the cast when detected in the first 2 weeks can be manipulated back into position with or without anaesthesia depending on the age of the child. We can usually accept an angulation of no more than 10° in either anteroposterior or varus valgus plane and a shortening of no more than 1 cm. Fracture of the upper tibial shaft near the metaphyseal region can classically give rise to progressive valgus deformity afterwards and should be carefully reduced and followed-up for a few years to avoid missing such deformities. Open reduction and internal fixation is almost never required except in complicated situations such as multiple trauma, neurovascular damage or compound fractures.

Conclusion

The proper care of children with fractures demands a sound knowledge of the basic science of the growing skeleton and fracture and of mechanics, an observant clinician with great attention to detail and a caring attitude towards the patients and parents, in addition to a well-organized system of delivery of such care. This chapter highlights briefly the common mistakes made by physicians attending children's fractures and provides a check-list for them to use in the day-to-day care of such problems. Children are not "small adults". The proper attention to their fractures requires special considerations and modifications in the basic philosophy and techniques of general fracture management.

References

1. Ogden JA (1990) Skeletal injury in child. Saunders, Philadelphia
2. Tachjian M (1990) Pediatric orthopaedics. Saunders, Philadelphia
3. Rang M (1983) Children's fractures. Lippincott, Philadelphia
4. Rockwood CA Jr, Wilkins KE, King RE (1984) Fractures in children. Lippincott, Philadelphia
5. Weber EG, Brunner CL, Frenler F (1980) Treatment of fractures in children and adolescents. Springer, Berlin Heidelberg New York
6. Friberg S (1983) Remodelling after fractures healed with residual angulation in problematic musculoskeletal injuries in children. Butterworth, London, pp 77–100
7. Currey JD, Butler G (1975) Mechanical properties of bone tissues in children. J Bone Joint Surg [Am] 57:810–814
8. Bright RW, Burstein AH, Elmore SM (1974) Epiphyseal plate cartilage. A biomechanical and histological analysis of failure modes. J Bione Joint Surg [Am] 56:688–703
9. Landin LA (1983) Fracture patterns in children: analysis of 8682 fractures with special reference to incidence, etiology, and secular changes in Swedish urban populations. Acta Orthop Scand Suppl 202
10. Worlock P, Stower M (1986) Fracture patterns in Nottingham children. Pediatr Orthop 6:656–661
11. Gallagher SS, Finison K, Guyer B, Goodenough S (1984) The incidence of injuries among 87000 Massachusetts children and adolescents. Am J Public Health 74:1340–1347
12. Garraway WM, Stauffer RM, Karland LT (1979) Limb fractures in a defined population. I Frequency and distribution. Mayo Clin Proc 54:701–707
13. Charnley J (1980) The closed treatment of common fractures. Churchill Livingstone, Edinburgh
14. Flynn JC, Matthew JG, Benoit RL (1974) Blind pinning of displaced supracondylar fractures of the humerus in children. Sixteen year's experience with long term follow up. J Bone Joint Surg [Am] 56:263–272
15. Lascombes P, Prevol J, Ligier JN, Metaizean JP, Poncelet T (1990) Elastic stable intramedullary nailing in forearm shaft fractures in children: 85 cases. J Pediatr Orthop 10:167–171
16. Roberts JA (1968) Angulation of the radius in children's fractures. J Bone Joint Surg [Br] 68:751–754
17. Carr CR, Tracy HW (1964) Management of fractures of the distal forearm in children. South Med J 57:540

18. Ansorg P, Graner G (1985) Effectiveness of conservative treatment following distal radius epiphyses injuries. Zentralbl Chir 110:360–365
19. Knight RA, Purvis GD (1949) Fractures of both bones of the forearm in adults. J Bone Joint Surg [Br] 31:755
20. Evans EM (1951) Fractures of the radius and ulna. J Bone Joint Surg [Br] 33:548–561
21. Gandhi RK, Wilson P, Mason Brown JJ, MacLeod W (1962) Spontaneous correction of deformity following fractures of the forearm in children. Br J Surg 50:5–10
22. Undeland K (1962) Rotational movements and bony union in shaft fractures of the forearm. J Bone Joint Surg [Br] 44:340
23. Blankstein A, Liberty E, Itay S et al. (1985) Biomechanical aspect of traumatic bowing of the forearm in children. Orthop Rev 14:61
24. Sanders WE, Heckman JD (1984) Traumatic plastic deformation of the radius and ulna. Clin Orthop 188:58–67
25. Vainionpaa S, Bostman O, Patiala H, Rokkanen P (1987) Internal fixation of forearm fractures in children. Acta Orthop Scand 58:121–123
26. Bado JL (1967) The Monteggia lesion. Clin Orthop 50:71–86
27. Boyd HB, Boals JC (1969) The Monteggia lesion. A review of 159 cases. Clin Orthop 66:94–100
28. Tompkins DG (1971) The anterior Monteggia fracture. J Bone Joint Surg [Am] 53:1109–1114
29. Kalamchi A (1986) Monteggia fracture-dislocation in children. J Bone Joint Surg [Am] 68:615–619
30. Quan L, Marcuse EK (1985) The epidemiology and treatment of radial head subluxation. Am J Dis Child 139:1194–1197
31. Ryan JR (1969) The relationship of the radial head to radial neck diameters in fetuses and adults with reference to radial-head subluxation in children. J Bone Joint Surg [Am] 51:781–783
32. Salter RB, Zaltz C (1971) Anatomic investigations of the mechanism of injury and pathologic anatomy of "pulled elbow" in children. Clin Orthop 77:134–143
33. Hedlund R, Lindgren V (1986) The incidence of femoral shaft fractures in children and adolescents. J Pediatr Orthop 6:47–50
34. King J, Diefendorf D, Apthorp J, Negrete VF, Carlson M (1988) Analysis of 429 fractures in 189 battered children. J Pediatr Orthop 8:585–589
35. Viljanto J, Kiviluoto H (1975) Remodeling after femoral shaft fracture in children. Acta Chir Scand 141:360–365
36. Shapiro F (1981) Fractures of the femoral shaft in children – the overgrowth phenomenon. Acta Orthop Scand 52:649–655
37. McCollough NC, Vinsant JE, Sarmiento A (1978) Functional fracture bracing of long-one fractures of the lower extremity in children. J Bone Joint Surg [Am] 60:314–319
38. Cheng JCY, Cheung SSC (1989) Modified functional bracing in the ambulatory treatment of femoral shaft fractures in children. J Pediatr Orthop 9:547–462

8 Hand Fractures: Controversies and Dilemmas

L.K. HUNG and P.C. LEUNG

Basic Concepts

Introduction

Since basic hand function forms the major support to all activities of daily living and bread-winning occupations, injuries to the hand are naturally common occurrences. Despite the increasingly developed automation and computerised programmes that have substantially simplified not only occupational procedures but also household routines, until some future time when the human hand may be totally discarded in these activities, it will remain the most vulnerable organ to external hazards. A discussion of the management of hand fractures is therefore a priority in any systematic consideration of human fractures.

The hand is a complicated organ. It consists of the most complicated collection of musculoskeletal components, namely bones and joints, tendons and muscles, arteries and nerves – all contained within thin bags of skin and soft tissues. Not only is the space available limited, but the arrangements tend to be more complicated than in other anatomical structures. The bones and joints are arranged in complicated systems which easily turn stiff when mobilisation becomes limited. The tendons are so tightly packed that injuries readily lead to adhesions and loss of gliding ability. The vessels consist of end-arteries and multiple small veins, and injuries easily obstruct the arterial flow (which leads to ischaemia) and slow down the venous return (which leads to venous congestion and tissue oedema). The surgeon responsible for the management of hand fractures must be aware of this basic background, which makes the job difficult and perfect functional results not readily achievable. Otherwise, swollen and stiff hands are the immediate result.

Because of the complex nature of the structures of the hands and fingers, some procedures which are considered basic in the routine management of long-bone fractures, for example, external splintage and cast making, become impossible. Instead of searching for alternative methods to achieve the same outcome of fracture management, compromising procedures are adopted. Results of such treatment, expectedly, are also compromised and far from satisfactory.

Modern fracture management endorses the classical demands of reduction, immobilisation and rehabilitation. At the same time it emphases the importance of immediate mobilisation to preserve the function of muscles, tendons and joints. Fracture treatment in general has been turning increasingly towards operative procedures for the simple reason of functional preservation. Under most circumstances operative procedures yield a perfect reduction of fracture fragments, supply accurate implant fixation and allow immediate joint mobilisation. Nevertheless, operative treatment is always traumatic and produces more damage to the already injured tissues. It is therefore accepted that unless an operation satisfies all requirements of reduction, internal fixation and immediate joint motion, it should not be performed at all.

Management of hand fractures has often been criticised as being either overly conservative or overly aggressive. The former criticism is related to a failure to endorse the basic requirement for fracture treatment while the latter could be due to an over-estimation of surgical promises and under-estimation of the surgical limitations. Surgeons should accept that the choice of management technique in hand fractures need to be governed by the same principles in fracture treatment – without exceptions. But more flexibility, more demanding technique and more careful observations are mandatory for a satisfactory restoration of hand function [1,2].

General Principles of Management

As is pointed above, the general principles of management should be identical with those of fracture treatment for long bones; nevertheless, difficulties in their application are real. Rather than weighing conservative versus operative treatment, as is discussed in most books on hand surgery, it may be more revealing to young surgeons to analyse some of the dilemmas that exist.

Can Perfect Reduction Be Achieved with Closed Means for Displaced Hand Fractures? With healthy soft tissues perfect reduction can be achieved for unstable fractures that are not comminuted and occur linearly across the bone. However, when there is comminution and soft-tissue damage, notably of skin and extensor tendon expansions, reduction may become very difficult or impossible.

Can Reduced Fractures Stay Reduced with External Splintage? After perfect reduction for the transverse and spiral types of fracture, sufficient friction across the fracture lines do keep the fragments together. This, however, does not apply for oblique or comminuted fractures. Apparently stable reduced fractures still displace within an external splint or cast as oedema of the injured part subsides, and when the patient moves the other fingers, which causes a chain-reaction movement of the flexor/extensor tendons, thus producing displacing strain on the fracture sites. When soft-tissue damage or reaction is extensive, losing stability and re-displacement become more likely.

Can External Splintage Maintain Reduction and Yet Allow Controlled Joint Motion so as To Prevent Joint Stiffness? For the undisplaced and the most stable jammed-back fractures, Sarmiento's principle of holding fracture ends with a tight tissue cylinder can be applied by means of a thin plaster or thermoplastic cylinder and joint motion continued. However, this cannot be applied with multiple finger involvement and soft-tissue damage. Two good examples of exceptions are (a) simple strapping of one finger to its adjacent partner to enforce movement (in spite of pain) in a solitary undisplaced, cracked fracture of a phalanx, and (b) volar basal fracture of the middle phalanx by applying a dorsal splint which allows flexion but limits extension of the joint to 30°–45° (Fig. 1). Most hand fractures may well fall beyond these examples.

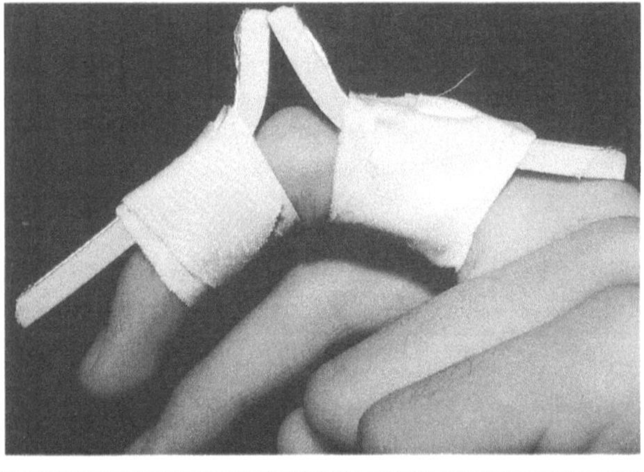

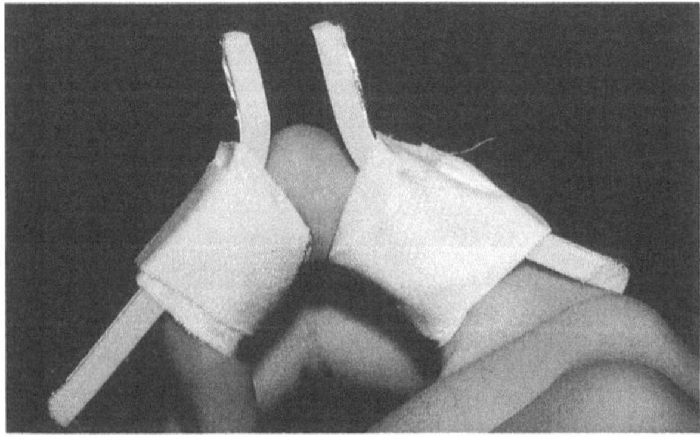

Fig. 1a–b. Dorsal splint made of aluminium, which prevents extension but allows unrestricted flexion for dorsal dislocation of the proximal interphalangeal joint. **a** Extension of the joint. **b** Flexion of the joint

Can Comminuted Fractures Be Reduced? This depends on the degree of comminution, extent of separation and soft-tissue situation. Very often these factors are not promising. When the soft tissues are injured and oedematous, even apparently favourable comminuted fractures do not join. Moreover, reduction may appear reasonable and yet collapse and displacement follow immediately after removal of the distraction force because of empty spaces within the site of the fracture. As long as these gaps exist, reduction is impractical.

Can Comminuted Fractures Be Fixed Externally or Internally? Feasibility of fixation depends on the success of reduction. External means of fixation are therefore extremely difficult. Internal means of fixation, given the best technique, is also difficult. Filling the bone gaps with different types of spacers, for example, bone grafts and bone substitutes, makes the procedures more practical. The presence of soft-tissue damage is an adverse factor.

Should Juxta-artcular Fractures Be Considered Separate Categories? The general principles of fracture management advocate operative treatment for all juxta-articular fractures so that the joint architecture is preserved and motion started immediately. An exception to this rule is noted above [under point (b): "Can External Splintage Maintain Reduction and Yet Allow Controlled Joint Motion so as To Prevent Joint Stiffness"]. Under other circumstances the immediate fixation and mobilisation principle can still be applied. If reduction and fixation are technically impossible, the choice is a stiff, painful joint or early compromise. The compromise consists of early fusion of the joint, which produces a slightly short finger with the injured joint in a functionally flexed position. All juxta-articular fractures of the hand should therefore enjoy special considerations, and surgical intervention generally deserves the priority.

How Much Do the Available Implants Achieve in Procedures of Internal Fixation? Kirschner wires (K-wires) are still the most commonly used implants in hand fracture fixation. Longitudinal introduction of K-wires produces good alignment but no rigid fracture fixation. If K-wires can be crossed over a fracture, the rigidity is reasonable. However, the tough cortical diaphysis of small dimensions usually do not allow the effective introduction of K-wire. If the K-wire crosses a joint, it does provide a little more stability through the control of joint motion. However, one pays the price of infection, adhesions and motion loss. When the K-wire passes percutaneously, as most surgeons prefer because of easy removal, the pin tract is not only the site of infection, but the pain related to finger motion at the pin site hinders functional training.

Mini- and micro-screws and plates offer more versatile alternative means of interval fixation. These are good for linear fractures and large fragments but still work badly with comminuted ones without bone grafting. Wire loops are useful as supportive or additional means of fixation to limit rotation and give tension band effects. Solitary loops hold small, indispensable fragments well, but their application is technically difficult. It is therefore apparent that no single entity of implant is capable of satisfying all the need and flexibility in the choice of management. All implants carry the common disadvantage of inducing more soft-tissue trauma, more tendon adhesions, joint stiffness and secondary procedures of implant removal. When applied to open fractures with significant tissue damages, these become dangerous.

Against this background of the general dilemmas facing surgeons in treating hand fractures, it may now be easier to decide about conservative versus operative treatment.

Closed Treatment

Closed treatment is confined to those fracture types that do not require reduction or can be reduced perfectly, and those for which the external splint or cast can be applied. The fingers must be able to move immediately after the reduction, and the finger movements should not re-displace the fracture ends. Any situation not fulfilling these requirements deserves consideration for operative treatment. Evidently only a small group of hand fracture patients fall into this category in most trauma hospitals.

Open Operative Treatment

All patients excluded from the closed treatment group should be considered. It should be emphasized that consideration for operative treatment may not mean for immediate surgery. Hand fractures are very often associated with open wounds and extensive soft-tissue damage. The principle of delayed primary operation not only lowers the incidence of infection but also gives more time to the damaged tissues to settle down so that surgeons may be more confident in their attempts at dédridement. It must also be pointed out that the purpose of surgical intervention is not only fixing the fracture, but that the fixation should achieve a sufficient degree of rigidity to allow immediate joint motion. If this aim is not fulfilled, the operation is a failure. If this aim cannot be fulfilled, a better alternative may have been closed reduction and conservative treatment. If this aim is only partially achieved, rehabilitation will be delayed, and the results may be as bad as those of closed, conservative treatment. Once operative treatment is selected as the method of choice, all efforts must be made for rigid fixation and immediate mobilisation. This often involves the sacrifice of a joint in juxta-articular comminutions (arthrodesis) and the immediate coverage of skin and soft-tissue defects (flap surgery).

It must be stressed again that the choice between a closed and an open method is a functional consideration with technical challenges, not a sheer technical decision. The following sections discuss the details of different categories of hand fracture. Readers are advised to bear in mind, however, this important concept.

Controversy and Dilemmas of Hand Fracture Management

Controversy 1: Stability

The classification of large-bone fractures can broadly be applied to fractures in the hand (Fig. 2). The configuration of the fracture and its displacement reflects the mechanism producing the fracture and therefore the extent of bone and soft-tissue damage. They also help the managing surgeon to assess the inherent stability of the fracture before or after a closed reduction.

Except in the case of a few classical fractures such as the Bennette, Mallet and those involving the carpal bones, there has been no detailed study on the stability of different configurations of fractures in the hand.

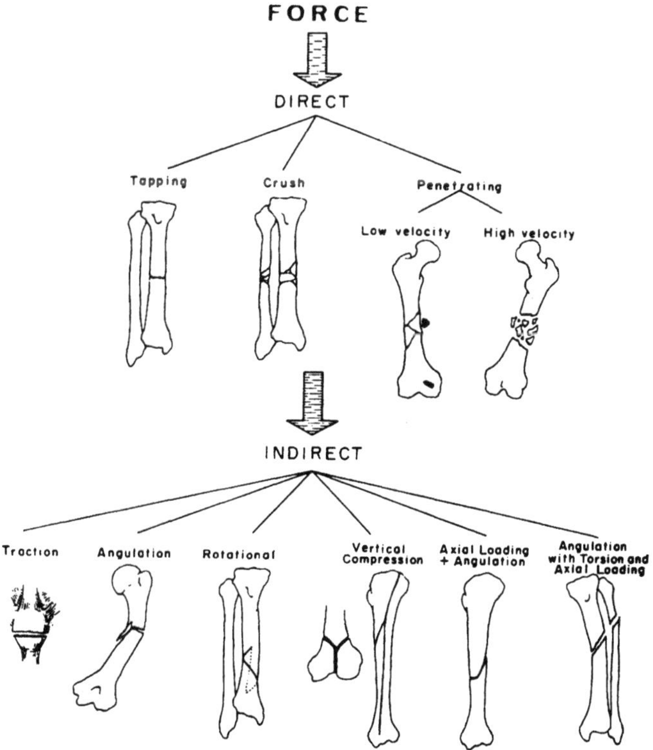

Fig. 2. Schematic drawing of the relationship between force and different configurations of long-bone fractures. (From [114])

The implication is obvious: if the fracture is inherently stable or can be converted into a stable fracture with closed manipulation, it can be managed with early mobilisation and can expect good functional recovery. The true definition of a stable fracture is therefore one that with or even without a closed manipulation requires only the simplest means of support, and which permits almost immediate mobilisation. This is a functional definition and requires a functional test: the fracture is manipulated under local anaesthesia, and the patient is instructed to move the digit or hand immediately. This may be screened by fluoroscopy or followed by a radiograph. A stable fracture does not become displaced, and the digit or hand can thus be safely allowed to move at an early stage. Those that are displaced are unstable and must be treated accordingly. Subsequent displacement of the fracture means that the fracture then requires treatment. This normally occurs within the first week, and such a delay should not affect the subsequent course of the fracture.

In a carefully designed prospective study by Pun et al. [3] on digital fractures, a closed reduction was attempted on all fractures. During the early stage of the study some of the fractures liable to displace after reduction were splinted by external splintage. However, it was soon recognised that this group had the highest failure rate and the worst functional outcome. This arm of the protocol was quickly dropped. All subsequent fractures which were liable to displace were fixed with implants. The functional outcome was greatly improved. It therefore appears that functional stability must be present immediately after closed reduction or be achieved with open reduction and fixation so that mobilisation can be started immediately.

Some feel that most closed finger fractures can be reduced adequately by closed means and the reduction maintained by splintage. Frequently in order to overcome the deforming force the finger must be kept flexed acutely. Although the finger is not in a functional position, and mobilisation is not started early, this is still being practised by some physicians. That such an approach can still produce acceptable clinical results indicates only that there is case selection in the reported series. Supple hands suffering fractures produced by relatively minor, indirect, low-energy forces may escape permanent stiffness from immobilisation in flexion. However, manual labourers' hands are more susceptible to stiffness from any period of immobilisation, even in the optimal position. Besides, fractures sustained by them are usually the result of more vigorous forces and are usually associated with some form of soft-tissue injury.

The main aim of any treatment protocol is to achieve early mobilisation [4–8]. It is therefore necessary to review again the concept of fracture stability: that the fracture is stable or can be made stable by manipulative or operative means to allow immediate mobilisation. When this cannot be achieved by closed means, open reduction is required.

Controversy 2: The Ideal Fixation Device

Perhaps one of the first considerations in the choice of best fixation device for finger fractures is the degree of stability that the device can offer. Just as stability of finger fractures cannot always be determined adequately, there are no direct scientific data on how rigidly a finger fracture should be fixed. Most of the currently available fixation methods afford different degrees of stability, and it can only be inferred that, if applied carefully according to the right indications, all of them provide sufficient stability to the fracture that mobilisation can be started immediately [6,9–20]. However, there is obviously a very wide margin here, and not infrequently one sees a fracture fixed with an inappropriate means producing diastrous results. Therefore it is still a matter of controversy how one interprets the stability of a fracture, and how one should fix it.

Biomechanically a mini-plate and screw system offers the most rigid internal fixation for hand fractures (Fig. 3) [21–24]. Interfragmentary compression may also be achieved by this system. However, this technique is highly sophisticated, is technically demanding, requires experienced nurses and a full range of up-to-date instruments and implants, has a narrow margin of safety [25,26] and requires relatively more soft-tissue exposure, which may not always be feasible. The dissection required may reduce the vascularity of the fracture, resulting in an increased risk of nonunion. The advantages of the plate and screw system, on the other hand, are its versatility in suiting almost all kinds of fracture configuration while still providing good fracture reduction and stability, and its ability to span a bone gap – when there is bone loss or comminution, the defect can be bridged by the plate, and bone graft may be incorporated (Fig. 4) [27,28]. Primary fusion of joints can also be achieved. This kind of versatility is not matched by other implants or devices, with the possible exception of external fixators.

One major drawback with the mini-plate and screw system is its size. Currently the profiles and sizes for most mini-plates average 1 mm in thickness. These are actually too large for the fingers and impede the extensor tendon function. Newer plates have been developed which are 0.6 mm in thickness; the screw heads are much reduced in size and do not protrude much from the plate (Fig. 5). This would probably diminish most of the problems associated with size. At the same time, although interfragmentary compression can be provided with the screws, the margin of error is very narrow because of the small size of the implants. If one is not sufficiently careful, the screw threads can easily become fractured, and stability is lost. It is also very difficult to provide compression with the mini-plate. If the plate is not moulded to the contour of the bone, rotation or angulation of the fragments can easily occur when the screws are tightened. Prebending the plate to achieve additional compression as in large bones is impossible for the small finger bones, and hence when the plate is applied to a concave

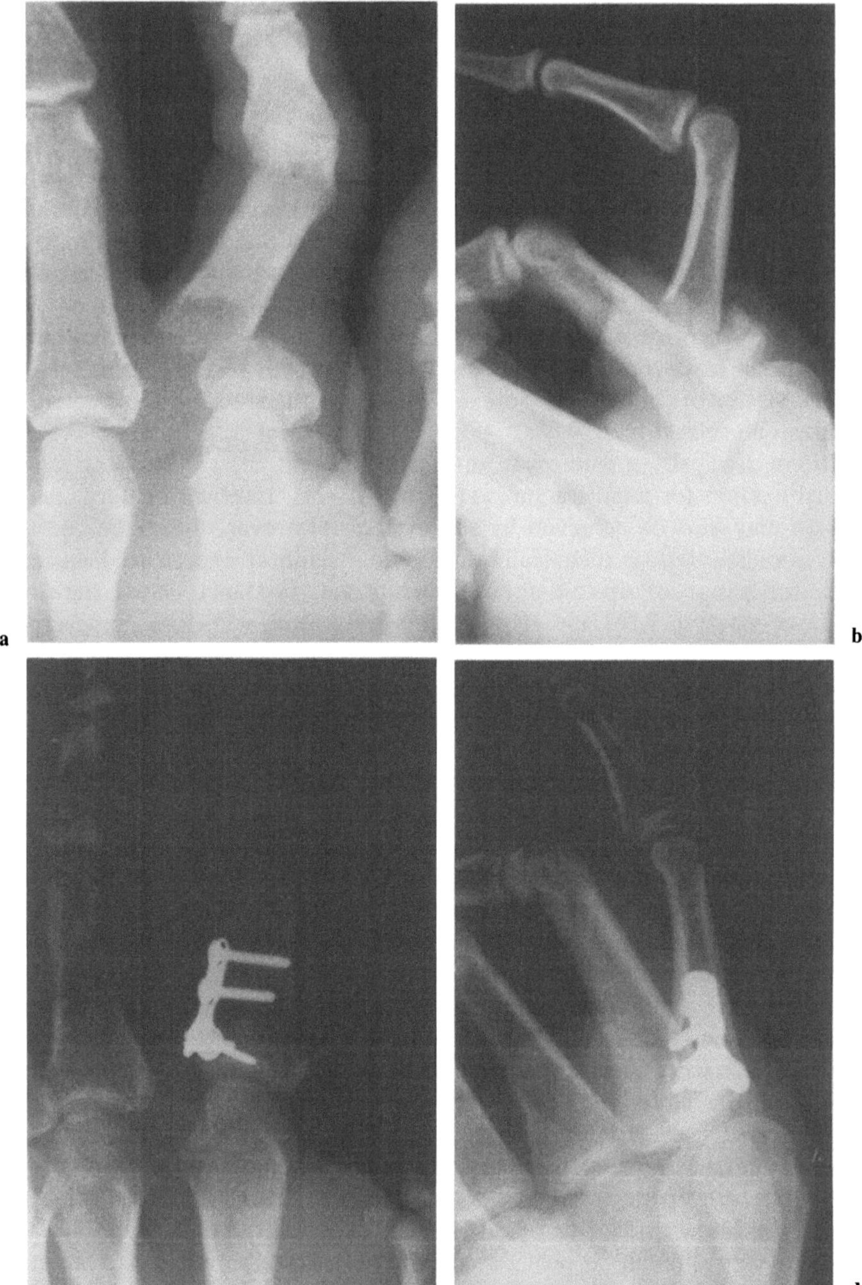

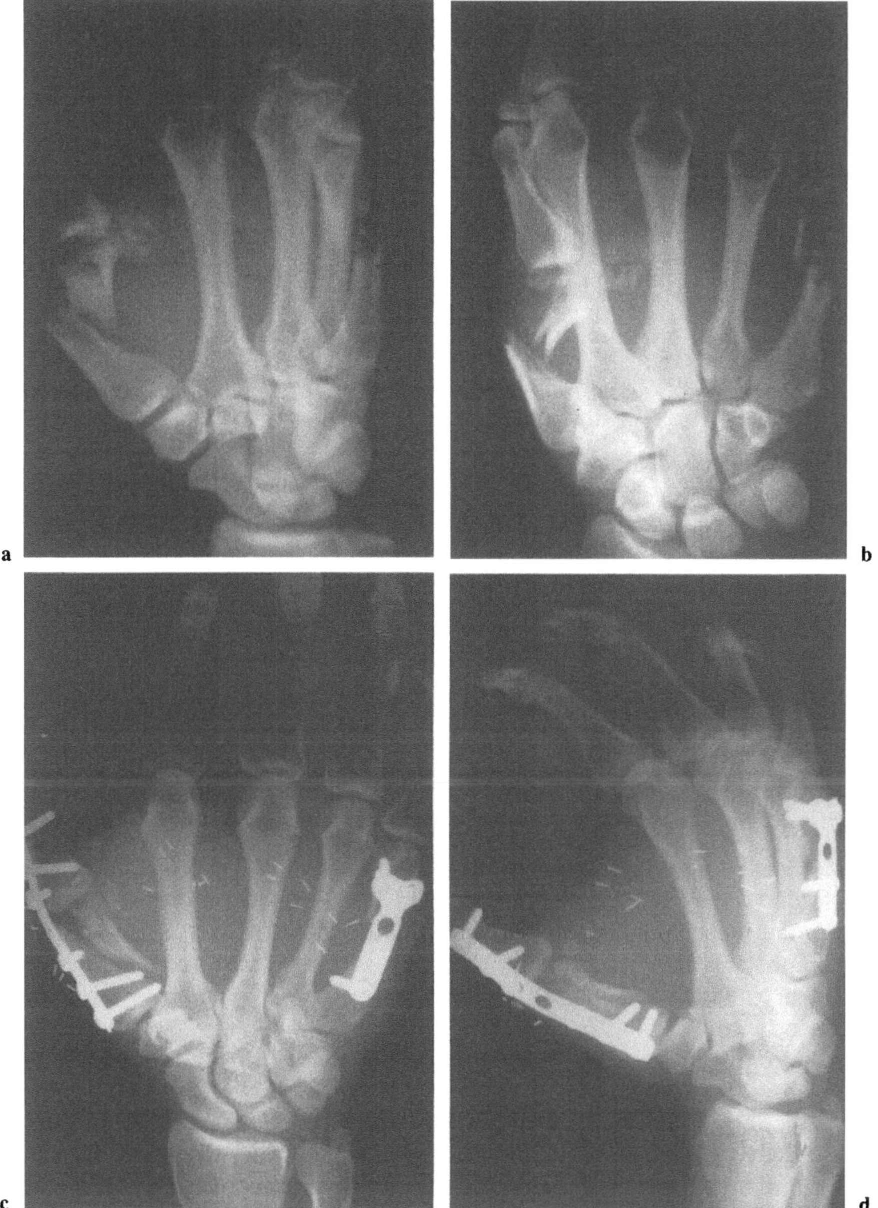

Fig. 4a–d. Severely crushed hand with comminuted fracture of the first and fifth metacarpals and concomitant soft-tissue injury requiring revascularisation. The metacarpophalangeal joint of the thumb was fused with a long plate spanning the comminuted segment, thus preserving length and ensuring correct aligmment. The comminution in the fifth metacarpal bone was also spanned by a plate. Preoperative (**a,b**) and Postoperativc radiographs (**c,d**)

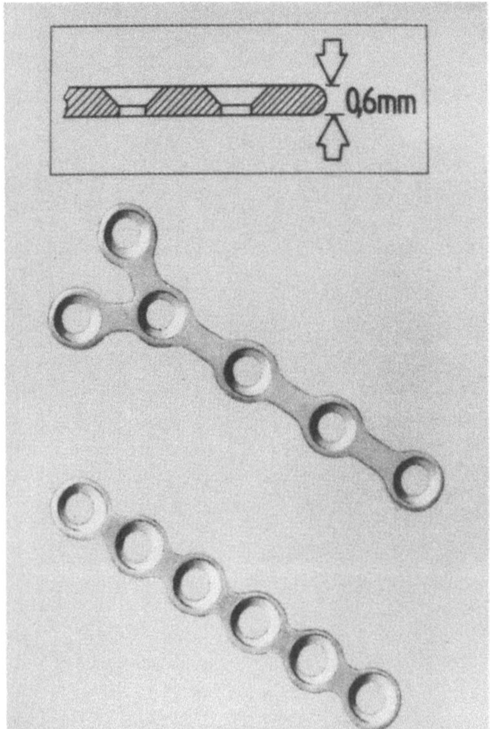

Fig. 5. A new plate of very low profile and only 0.6 mm thick, made of titanium. (Courtesy Oswald Leibinger, Germany)

surface such as on the lateral surface of the bone, there is a possibility that the fracture may not be compressed and may instead be distracted, with subsequent delayed union or nonunion. Mainteinance of instrumentations is also important. It is particularly important to have sharp and straight drill bits (especially the 1.1-mm bit for the 1.5-mm screws) in order to insert the screws accurately.

Alternative means of fixation include various forms of intraosseous wiring [29,30], intramedullary implants [31–34] and percutaneous pinning [35–37]. The combination of an intraosseous wire loop plus either an intramedullary K-wire (Fig. 6) [12] or one driven obliquely across the fracture seems the most convenient method to use in most situations. This method is undemanding and fast and does the least damage to soft tissues. The stability provided by this system is sufficient to allow immediate, unresisted mobilisation. This technique works best for transverse or slightly oblique fractures. On the other hand, it does not work well for long spiral fractures or when there is comminution.

Various versions of intramedullary devices with or without an additional transosseous element are also available (Fig. 7) [31,32]. Basically these can provide quite a rigid fixation. For individual techniques there are problems with the introduction of the device, the possibilities of distracting the fracture, and the removal when the need arises.

K-wires, either nonthreaded or threaded, still enjoy great popularity. By modifying the technique of insertion they can provide sufficient stability to allow early mobilisation. However, even strong supporters of their use realise the potential for complications [37]. These wires work best for oblique and spiral fractures of the diaphysis with little comminution. Although apparently very handy for condylar fractures, they often cause irritation or tethering of the collaterals and skin that make them less than ideal. A more subtle worry is the potential for distraction of the fracture. Interfragmentary compression can be achieved only by external means and must be maintained while the wires are being driven through the bone. This is not always easy, and either fragmentation of the fragment results, or the fracture is distracted.

There are various kinds of external fixators (Fig. 8). These are best used for open fractures or severely comminuted intra-articular fractures [27,28,38–45]. Theoretically they can be used to align any fractures [46]. Biomechanically, since the rigid components of the system are set at a distance from the bone, they are not very rigid systems and do not provide sufficient compression at the fracture site. At the same time, because the axis is so far from bone, angulation or rotation is also likely to occur. Some of the systems are also quite complicated to set up. In view of all these factors together, these systems do not appear the best means for routine fractures.

It therefore appears that there is no ideal fixation device. The choice relies on the fracture configuration, whether the fracture is open or closed, the age of the patient, the availability of instruments and the training and experience of the surgeon. If one has the competence and requires versatility, the mini-plate and screw system offers the best option.

Controversy 3: The Optimal Exposure

A dorsal midline longitudinal incision has long been the utility incision for most hand fractures. The extensor tendon may either be split in the midline longitudinally or incised at the junction with one retinaculum band. This is obviously an over-simplified approach and works only for closed, minimally displaced fractures at the midshaft of the proximal phalanx. It causes substantial extensor tendon problems for directly contussed hands.

What probably happens after a dorsal midline incision in the extensor tendon in the mid-diaphyseal portion of the proximal phalanx is: when the finger extends, the slit in the tendon closes up as a purse. The substance of the extensor tendon in this area is also thick enough for repair and suturing. However, when the fracture occurs at the distal diaphyseal-metaphyseal junction, the complex central band structure is violated, especially when one

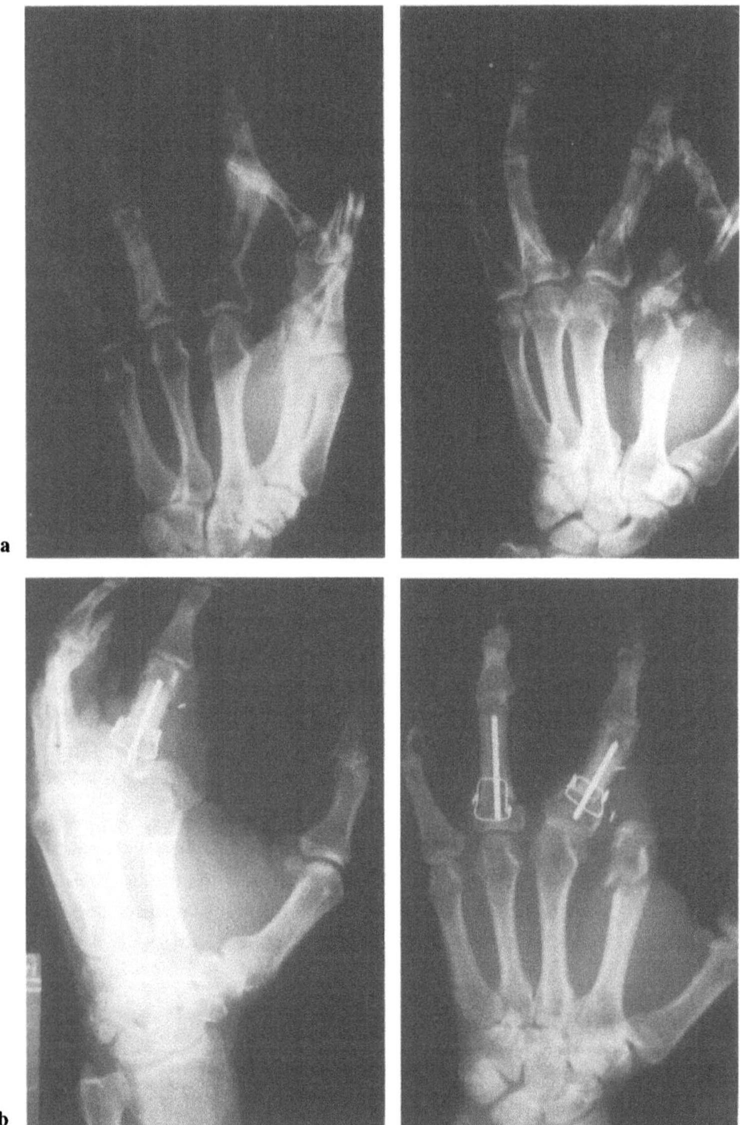

Fig. 6. a,b Severely crushed hand, which required amputation of one digit and revascularisation of the others. The bones were fixed with intramedullary Kirschner wire and intraosseous wire loop. **c,d** Multiple fracture of the proximal phalanges, fixed with intraosseous wireloop and oblique Kirschner wire. **e,f** Fracture base of proximal phalanx of the little finger, fixed with a simple intraosseous wireloop

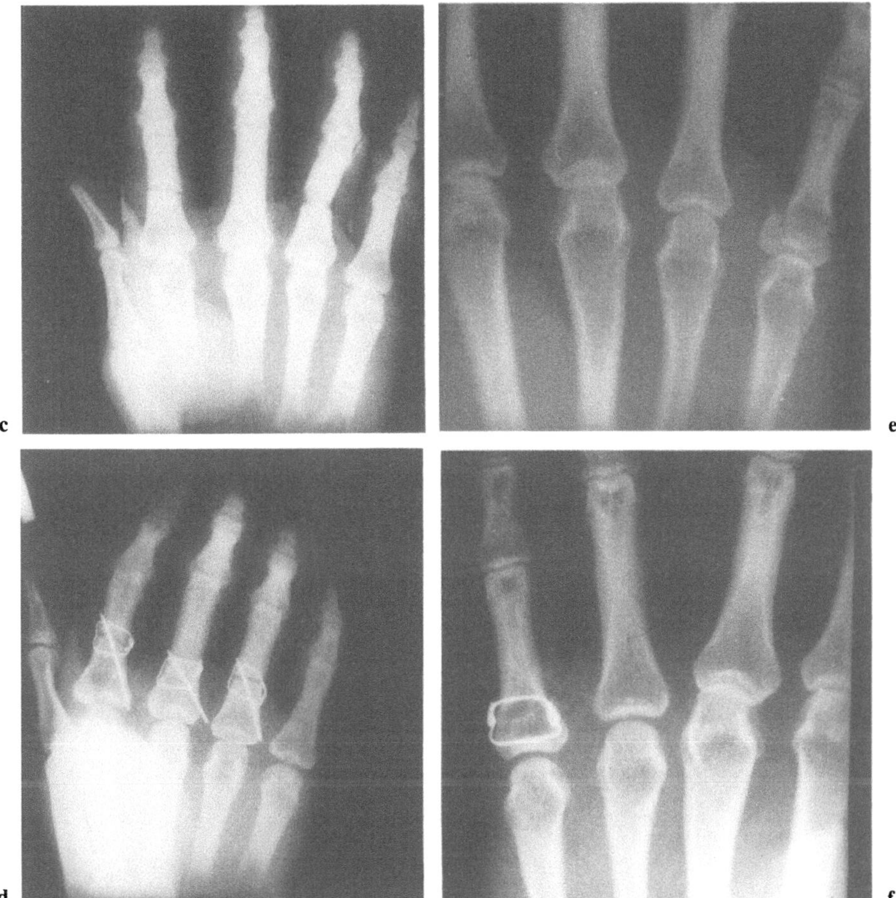

Fig. 6c–f.

applies a plate. The best approach for fractures in this region is a mid-lateral
incision (Fig. 9). The lateral margin of the extensor tendon and the retinaculum, i.e. tendon of the intrinsic muscle on one side, is identified and
retracted to permit exposure of the bone. For fractures extending into the
joint, the joint may also be opened by an incision dorsal to the collateral
ligament for direct inspection into the joint.

When the fracture occurs at the base of the proximal phalanx, a dorsal
longitudinal incision on the ulnar side of the central extensor with retraction
of the tendon radially provides good access to the bone. The mid-lateral
incision is a good alternative for exposure of proximal phalanx diaphyseal
fractures. The retinaculum fibre is retracted or incised obliquely along
the direction of its fibres and therefore preserves the integrity of most of
the intrinsic tendon. This avoids the subsequent difficulty of repairing the

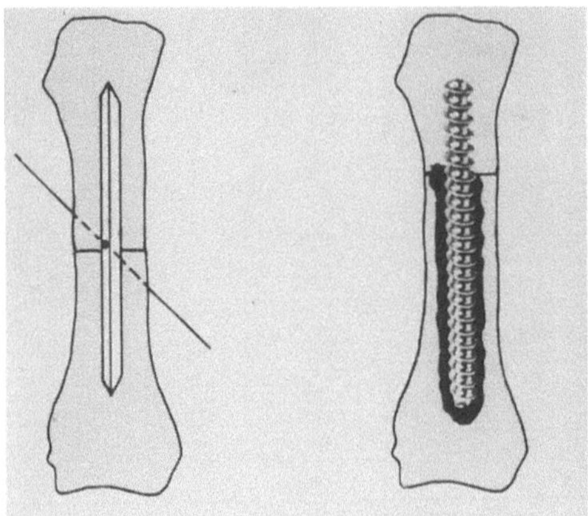

Fig. 7. Schematic representation of intramedullary fixation devices. Prismatic rod and an oblique Kirschner wire (*left*) and an intramedullary threaded pin (*right*). (Courtesy of Osteo, Switzerland)

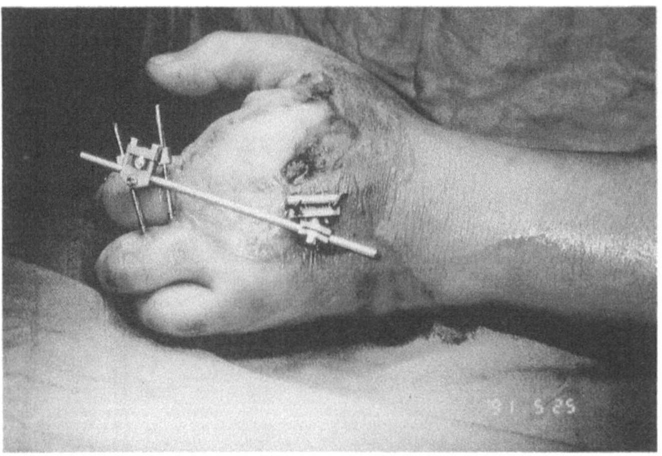

Fig. 8. Degloving injury of the hand with comminuted fracture base of the proximal phalanx, stabilised by a mini-Hoffmann external fixator

retinaculum. However, there is still a very high chance of the intrinsic tendon being damaged, and attrition over a plate is still very likely when one is used.

The mid-lateral incision is the best exposure for the middle phalanx. The thinness of the central extensor tendon makes the dorsal midline incision unfavourable, whereas the lack of a large lateral retinaculum makes the lateral approaches rather straightforward. Towards the base of the middle phalanx, however, the oblique retinaculum fibre passes from the flexor sheath to the dorsal extensor tendon, and care must be taken to limit damage and scarring to this structure; otherwise movement of the distal interphalangeal joint may be affected.

Controversy 4: Intra-Articular Fractures

Although it is generally agreed that intra-articular fractures require open and accurate reduction, there are times when traction and mobilisation may be the only feasible means, such as depressed tibial fractures in an elderly woman. For fractures of the hand, because of the small size of the bones, open reduction can be difficult to achieve, and there is a definite place for nonintervention and expectant treatment [47]. Some of the fractures are too minute to be fixed stably with metallic implants. Skeletal traction was practised in the past but had almost become obsolete until a recent improvement in technique revived the concept (Figs. 10, 11) [48,49]. When well-balanced traction can be maintained, the fracture remains in reduction, and early mobilisation can be started as well.

Miniaturised external fixators also present an alternative, although at the expense of motion of the involved joint. Some of these fixators are actually quite complicated to apply. A new design has built-in elasticity in the system so that some degree of movement can be achieved. However, whether this will reduce stability remains to be studied (Fig. 23) [50].

The use of tissue adhesive, in particular fibrin, has a definite potential in the fixation of minute intra-articular fragments [51]. Its use has been demonstrated successfully in capitellum fractures [52], and theoretically it should also be very useful in phalangeal fractures. Some form of unloading of the joint is required for phalangeal fractures after the fragments are stabilised by the tissue adhesive. This can be achieved with a dynamic form of external fixation.

Another recent trend for fixing osteochondral fractures in large joints such as the knee is the use of biodegradable pins which can be inserted through the articular cartilage and burried within it [53]. At the moment the smallest pins have a diameter of approximately 1.3 mm. Therefore any fracture in the hand which can be stabilised by a conventional K-wire can theoretically also be fixed with such a pin (Fig. 12). The advantage is obvious: there is no need to remove the pin, and the pin can be carefully inserted through the joint surface since it will be slowly dissolved. However, there are technical questions to be answered before such pins can be used widely. For example, at present such pins are either too elastic or too brittle. The elastic ones require multiple pin insertion in some form of triangulation to achieve stability, and this may not be feasible for small intra-articular fractures. The hard, brittle ones are not yet as sharp and strong as stainless steel K-wire, and their insertion can be difficult. Another more far-reaching question is the behaviour of such materials inside the joint. Whether the parts exposed to the synovial environment are met-

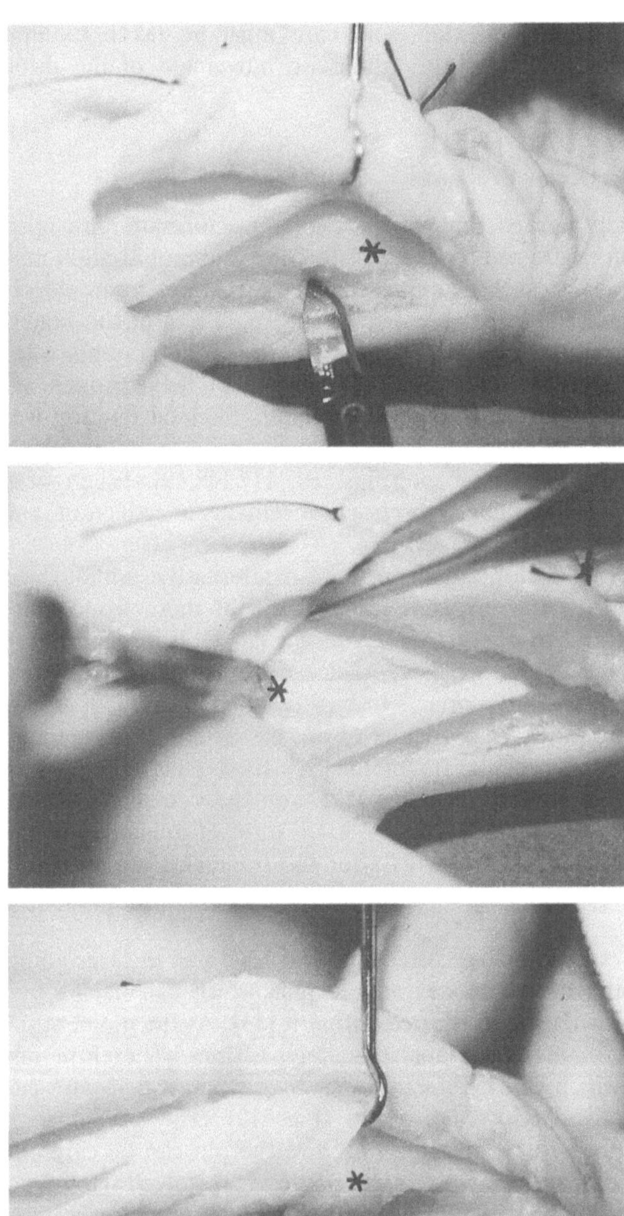

Fig. 9a–c. Cadaveric dissections to demonstrate surgical approaches for exposure of the proximal and middle phalanges. **a** A latero-dorsal incision was used and the extensor expansion, in particular the free margin of the intrinsic tendon, was dissected free and retracted dorsally for exposure of the head and neck of the proximal

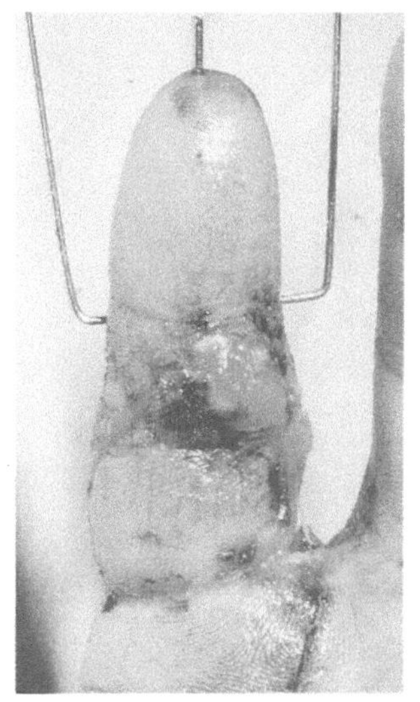

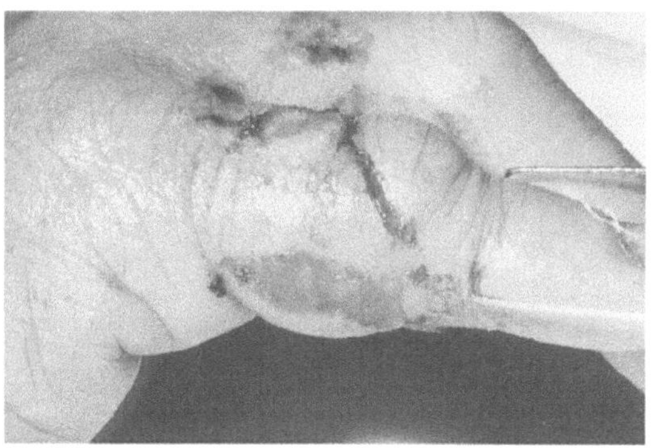

Fig. 10a–b. Multiple fractures of the little finger with comminution at the base of the proximal phalanx, stabilised by skeletal traction with a Kirschner wire driven through the neck of the middle phalanx. **a** Frontal view. **b** Side view

abolised as readily as those in contact with soft tissues or bone remains to be clarified. If not, such particles left in the joint cavity may be shed as a free body and may cause mechanical or chemical problems. Furthermore, the cyclical pressure changes in the joint cavity during movement may also pump synovial fluid into the tract surrounding the biodegradable pins and alter the degradation process. It therefore seems at present that the indications for the use of biodegradable implants for intra-articular fractures of the hand are limited. More careful and scientific studies should be carried out.

Continuous passive mobilisation has been used with success for intra-articular fractures in some of the large joints, especially in the knee and the hip, although it is less successful in the elbow. There have been a few reports on its use in the hand [54,55]. The difficulty remains with the design of an appropriate machine. It is also difficult to maintain external pressure on the fingers to control oedema and at the same time moving them, i.e. if there is oedema of the hand, the application of continuous passive

---

phalanx (*). **b** When approach to the base of the proximal phalanx is required, the extensor expansion is split along the direction of fibres of the intrinsic tendon, which is kept carefully intact, and the bone is exposed (*). **c** A mid-lateral incision was used for exposure of the middle phalanx. Care is taken to mobilise and retract forward the oblique retinacular tendon when exposure of the base (*) is required

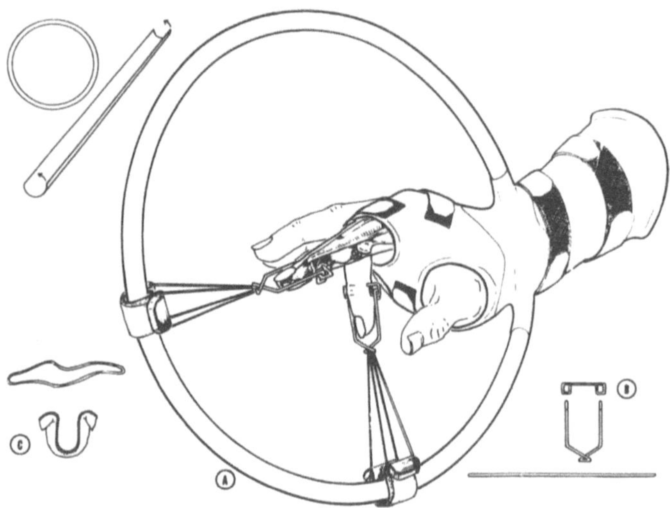

Fig. 11. Schematic drawing of a special splint configuration that maintains skeletal traction on a comminuted phalangeal fracture and at the same time permits passive mobilisation by moving the traction along the arc of the splint. (From [49])

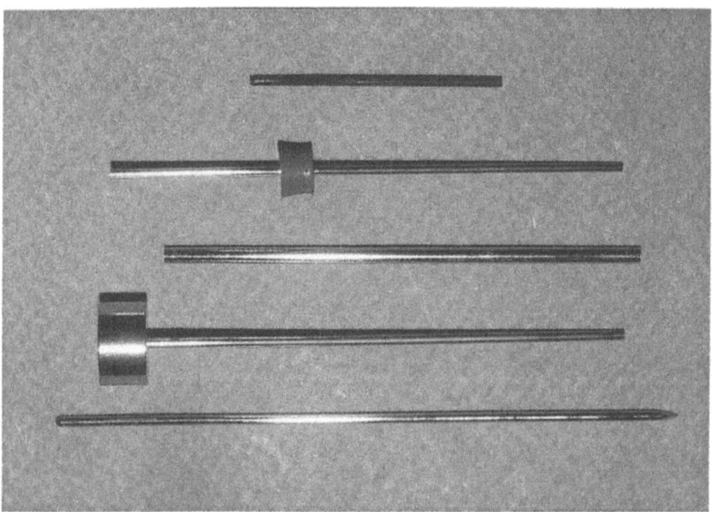

Fig. 12. The Orthosorb (Johnson and Johnson) biodegradable pin system. The fracture is pinned with Kirschner wire and the track prepared with pins 1.3 mm in diameter. The depth is measured by the depth gauge bearing the rubber stopper. The pins are housed in metal cylinders, and after the appropriate length is cut (measured by inserting the reversed end of the depth gauge into the metal cylinder) the pin can be inserted with the assistance of the punch. The pin is also 1.3 mm in diameter

mobilisation can be difficult. Actually, for the first 2 days after any surgery the hand should be kept bandaged in the functional position and elevated.

Primary Fusion

There are times when the fracture is so comminuted that reduction by whatever means is extremely difficult, and the final outcome may be a very stiff joint, and it may be better for the patient to have the joint fused primarily (Fig. 13). This would hasten the rehabilitation process and ensure a faster return to work. This approach works particularly well for the distal interphalangeal joint, the interphalangeal joint of the thumb, and sometimes for the proximal interphalangeal joint or the metacarpophalangeal joint of the thumb. However, it is not appropriate for the metacarpophalangeal joint of the fingers. It is also very important for the surgeon to have a full understanding of the vocation of the patient and his wishes about the position in which he would prefer his finger to be fused. This is an important point and may influence the patient's acceptance of the fusion and therefore

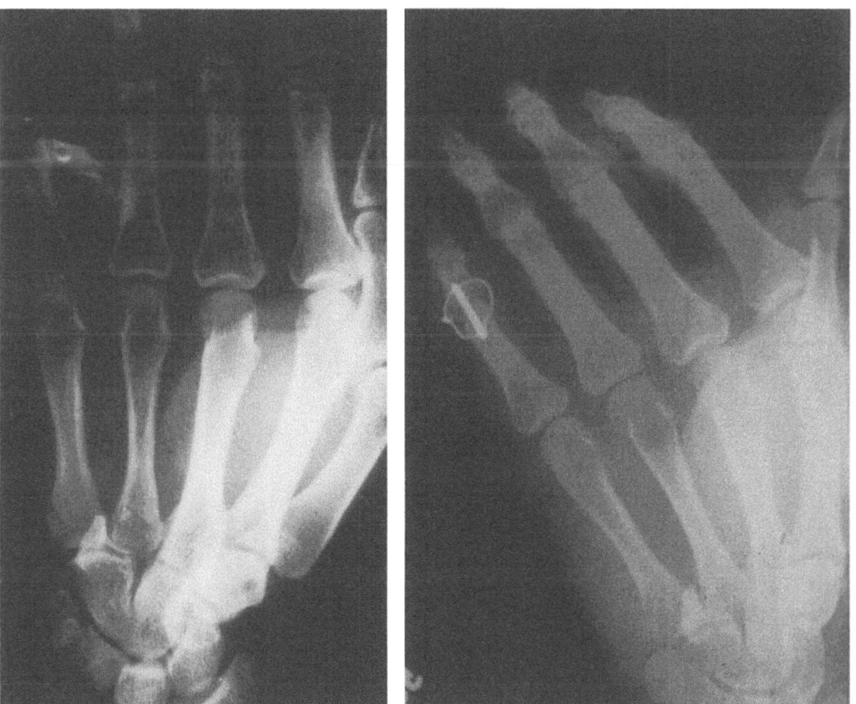

Fig. 13. a Comminuted fracture of the proximal interphalangeal joint of the little finger. b Primary arthrodesis with an intramedullary Kirschner wire and intraosseous wire loop

the eventual success of the operation. It may sometimes be better to defer the fusion 1–2 weeks to enable a more in-depth discussion with the patient. However, in developing countries, especially for patients with poor educational background, it may be wiser to carry out everything in one operation (the primary one) since it may be difficult to convince him of the necessity for a second operation and the reason for waiting.

Toe Joint Transplantation

There have been a few reports of successful microvascular toe-joint transplantation to salvage destroyed metacarpophalangeal and even the proximal interphalangeal joints [56–58]. It remains controversial whether this is applicable in most cases. At present our own indications are severe joint injuries in children and injuries associated with bone loss in young and active adults (Fig. 14). For the latter group fusion may result in a very short finger.

Dilemma 1: Open Fractures

Hand fractures are commonly open. Many of them are also part of a severe crushing injury that results in extensive soft-tissue damages. Some of these injuries also require revascularisation, and most of them therefore fall into

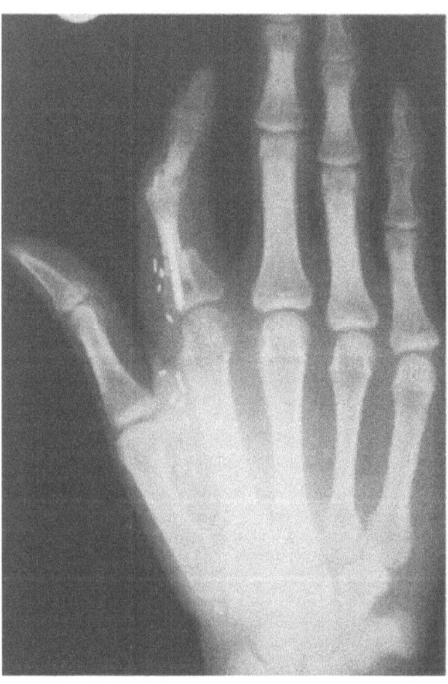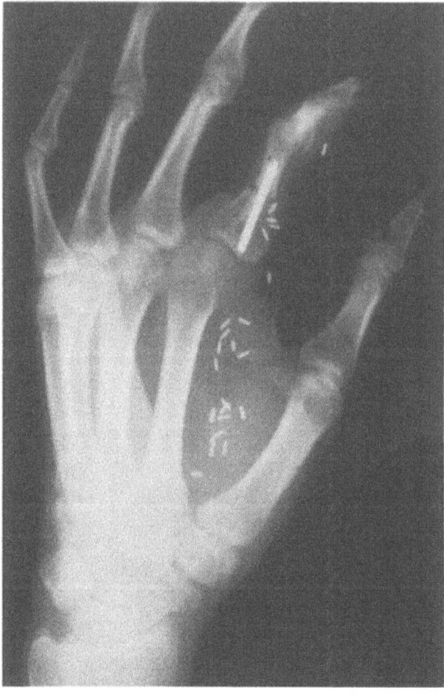

Fig. 14. Comminuted fracture of the proximal interphalangeal joint of the index finger, salvaged by free vascularised transplantation of the second toe proximal interphalangeal joint, giving a stable pain-free joint and 30° movement

the category of type III-B or -C open fractures. Currently there is a wealth of evidence for not retaining a type III-C limb in major limb fractures. What about the hand? For type III open hand fractures the considerations in the hand must be entirely different from those in the lower limb. They must also be very different when only a single digit or multiple digits are involved than when the whole limb is involved. Obviously the thumb warrants higher priority.

Strickland [59] has proposed a scoring system for grading digital injuries. He found that if the score is above 10 for any single digit, the prognosis is so bad that it is better for the patient to have the digit removed primarily. This system works well for a single digit and probably for two adjacent fingers but is very difficult to apply to more extensive injuries or to injuries occurring at a more proximal level.

Amputation for a severely injured "central" digit is also fraught with undesirable problems [60–62]. When either the middle or ring or both digits are removed, the patient is left with a space in the hand which is unsightly, and through which small objects will drop. One may transpose the index finger for a missing middle finger with little consequence. The same technique may also be applicable for an absent ring finger, although the result is less assured [63].

When the injury occurs at a more proximal level, the decision is difficult. At such level the functional losses are significant. On the other hand, the mechanisms of injury are frequently crushing or avulsion, and the prospect for good functional outcome is poor. When the injury occurs at the arm level, one can look upon it as the equivalent to a partial brachial plexus palsy. Recent data indicate that intercostal nerve neurotisation and phrenic nerve neurotisation, sometimes together with free muscle transplantation, give some useful function to the limb in brachial plexus palsy. These techniques can certainly be applied for other traumatic conditions to the arm. When the injury occurs at the forearm level, there is the dilemma of salvaging the limb or performing a below-elbow amputation and prosthesis fitting. Myoelectric hands have become a very reliable and easy-to-use device, and they offer very good cosmetic appearance and function. Of course, one must put things into perspective. To make the use of the myoelectric prosthesis successful one needs good technical support. The heat and humidity of most developing countries make the prosthesis a nuisance to wear and a burden to maintain. When the injury occurs around the wrist or at the palm, surgical reconstruction remains the only and the better solution.

When the decision for retaining the injuried digit or a mutilated hand is made, one faces the dilemma of the priority of management of the many different structures involved. It is generally accepted that a good stable bony fixation is the cornerstone to the success of salvaging the functions of the hand. It seems that the additional time required in stabilising the bony skeleton in the hand does not normally compromise survival even if revascularisation is required. The golden rule for ischaemic time of 6 h in major limb ischaemia is still true for proximal level hand injury involving muscles, but for injuries distal to the main muscle bulk of the forearm this time can be stretched. The length of time spent in fixing the bone is also well spent since it has become recognised that without a good stable fixation of the bony skeleton control of pain and oedema is difficult. The position of the hand is difficult to maintain, and mobilisation cannot be implemented early. The original goal of salvaging the function of the hand is thus never achieved.

Indications for internally fixing type III open long-bone fractures are being explored, but most physicians are generally very cautious about it.

One is naturally concerned about the risk of infection after internally fixing open hand fractures [40,64,65]. The same approach to open long-bone fractures should also be applied to hand fractures. In severely crushed and contaminated fractures the incidence of infection approaches 20% [65]. The aim of treatment is first to achieve skeletal stability by external fixation, followed by a policy of delayed closure in heavily contaminated wounds [66]. The wounds should be inspected frequently within the first 48 h and early closure with grafts or flaps carried out as soon as feasible. The conventional belief that the hand tolerates infection well because of its good vascularity and relative freedom of muscle bulk should not be held rigidly, and meticulous attention must be paid to débridement, stabilisation and revascularisation.

Fixation of the bone by the mini-plate and screw system provides rigid stability. In addition, alignment can be controlled precisely. The system can also provide compression osteosynthesis or can be used to maintain length or alignment in comminuted fractures even when significant bone is lost. Primary fusion of joints can also be achieved with relative ease. Thus the system is quite versatile. A major drawback of the system is the soft-tissue dissection required. This is undesirable when there is already significant soft-tissue contusion, or when there is already some degree of soft-tissue degloving. In replantation a modified square plate with two transverse holes on each side of the fracture can be used [67]. Stability is compromised slightly, but the system simplifies the fixation procedure.

One can perhaps put the plate and screws directly on exposed bone together with some form of skin flap coverage. For a single digit this usually means a cross-finger island flap. This can be a flag flap, but for a large defect one may take a digital artery island flap from a large area of the dorsal skin of an adjacent finger. The digital nerve is left behind (Fig. 15). When several digits are involved, or when the injury is on a proximal part of the hand, the groin flap or the reversed radial forearm flap must be considered. If the injury involves the dorsum of the hand, there is usually concomitant skin and extensor tendon damage, and a vascularised dorsalis pedis tendocutaneous flap provides ideal coverage. On the other hand, when the injury occurs on the palm, a vascularised medial plantar flap is best.

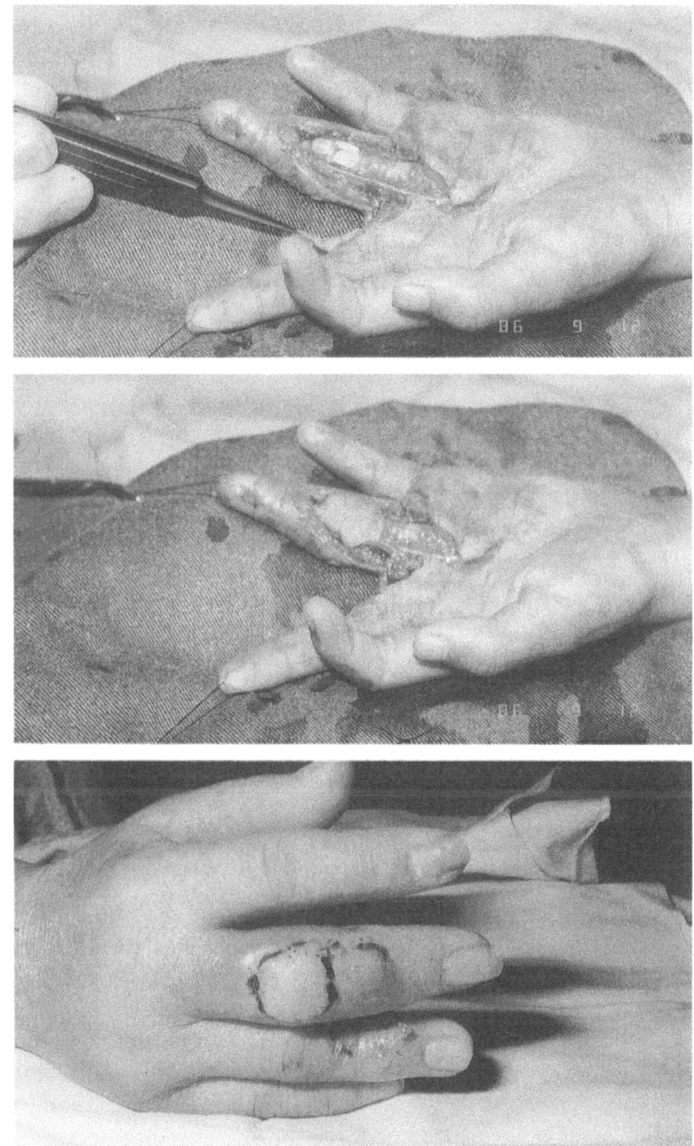

Fig. 15. a Open injury of the front of the ring finger with skin loss, resurfaced by an island flap from the ulnar aspect of the middle finger. **b** The flap was based on the ulnar digital artery of the middle finger with the nerve left undisturbed. **c** Another case of open wound of the back of the proximal interphalangeal joint, covered by an island flap from the radial side of the ring finger

Mini-external fixators such as that of Hoffmann is another option for managing open hand fractures [45] (Fig. 31e–g). The system is most suitable for multiple bone involvement in a single digit and for very comminuted fractures. It is less suitable when multiple fingers are involved and should be combined then with the plate and screws. Control of alignment is also less good, especially when there is large intervening comminution or a missing segment. The system does not produce good compression or good arthrodesis. Although an external fixator system such as the mini-Hoffmann can be quite complicated and confusing to use, once mastered, it allows fixation to be achieved with relative speed and ease.

Other fixation systems include intramedullary rods of various designs, different techniques of intraosseous wiring and the traditional K-wire. K-wire is unsuitable for open hand fractures. Although it is apparently simple to insert, in certain fracture configurations it may be very difficult to insert properly and stably. Many of the rehabilitation goals cannot be achieved. In such a situation requiring a quick procedure which least disturbs the soft tissues or joints an mini-external fixator should be used instead. Intraosseous wiring is unsuitable for comminuted fractures. They also require another adjunctive fixation such as an additional K-wire for stability. Intramedullary devices can be difficult to insert and are unsuitable for comminuted fractures. The lack of rotatory stability is often cited as a disadvantage, but in practice the fracture ends can interdigitate together, and rotatory deformity is usually a result of failure to achieve a good alignment from the very beginning. Intramedullary devices made of materials other than metal may have an increased risk of infection in open hand fractures.

Dilemma 2: Early Mobilisation in Associated Tendon Injuries

It is generally accepted that flexor tendon injuries should be mobilised early (either with the Klinert splint or actively) to reduce adhesions and to promote gliding and healing. When there is flexor tendon injury associated with finger fracture, it may be difficult to meet the rehabilitation requirements for both of the lesions. To enable early controlled mobilisation of the flexor tendons it has become routine to openly reduce and fix the fracture. If one can fix the fracture stably, early mobilisation can be initiated for both the fracture and the tendon to the benefit of both. This policy would influence the choice of fixation device, and in order to meet the force exerted on the bone by some of the splints mobilising the finger (for the tendon), the mini-plate and screw system is the most guaranteed device. If the force is not great, or if there is little oedema, and the joints are not stiff, the intraosseous wire loop plus an oblique K-wire offers a useful alternative.

Finger fractures are actually more commonly associated with extensor tendon lacerations since many of these injuries are from direct contussion by rugged or sharp objects onto the dorsum of the fingers resulting in damage to both. It had been routine to immobilise extensor tendon injuries in some degree of extension for up to 4 weeks. However, this defeats the goal of early mobilisation for finger fractures. Recently there has been an increasing trend towards instituting early mobilisation for extensor tendon injuries by following the same philosophy as for flexor tendon injuries. This has also become a routine for the authors' Department [68]. When the fracture is associated with extensor tendon injury, it is also routinely reduced openly and fixed with a device of sufficient stability so that early mobilisation of the finger can be started.

Management of Different Hand Fractures

Fractures of the Terminal Phalanx

There is a very close relationship between the nail plate and the terminal phalanx. When one is pinching, part of the force is actually borne by the nail plate and then through the terminal phalanx. These also provide stability to each other. Fracture of the terminal phalanx is also usually open through an associated laceration of the nail bed. Therefore one cannot separate the discussion of the management of one from that of the other [69,70].

Management of nail bed laceration requires suturing with 6'0' absorbable suture, with or without free nail bed graft taken from a big toe. The nail bed is then splinted by a silastic sheet. This is anchored by stitches to the nail folds and also through the depth of the eponychium. Once the nail injury is managed, most of the terminal phalanx fracture is readily reduced and heals. However when there has been a severe crushing injury to the finger tip, when there is comminution of the bone in a transverse shaft fracture, or when the bone ends are far apart, it is necessary to fix the bone primarily to ensure a higher chance of union [71]. An axial K-wire driven through the tip of the finger to splint the fracture is a commonly practised method. This often does not need to be driven through the distal interphalangeal joint, and early movement in that joint can be implemented. However, the fragments may not be adequately reduced by the K-wire, and nonunion is still likely [72].

A newly developed technique to fix a fracture of the shaft of the terminal phalanx is the use of a pull-out wire. This is first passed through the base of the phalanx, which comprises the proximal fragment, and then passed either through the medullary cavity of the shaft of the distal fragment or subcutaneously by the sides of the phalanx to emerge at the finger tip and be secured over a dental swab and a button. The wire loop provides compression of the fragments. This wire loop is retained for 3 weeks, after which the fracture is usually sufficiently stable (Fig. 16).

Avulsions of either the extensor or the flexor tendon from the base of the distal phalanx requires reattachment for preservation of tendon functions [73,74]. This is achieved by pull-out wiring through the distal phalanx which emerges through the distal part of the nail or the tip of the finger. We

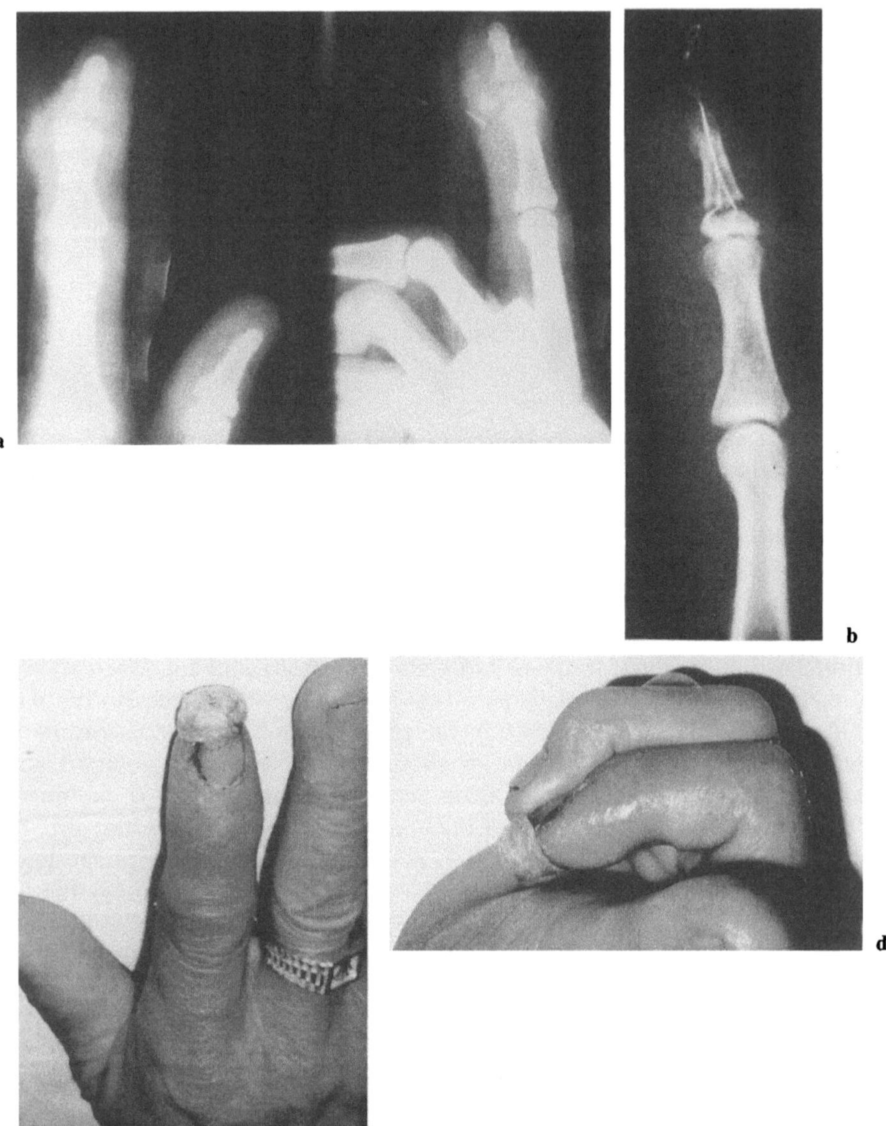

Fig. 16. a Comminuted fracture base of the terminal phalanx of the index finger. **b** Fixation achieved by a pull-out wire. **c** Post-operative appearance and flexion range. **d** After 1 week in a similar case. **e,f** Similar fixation for a fracture in the thumb

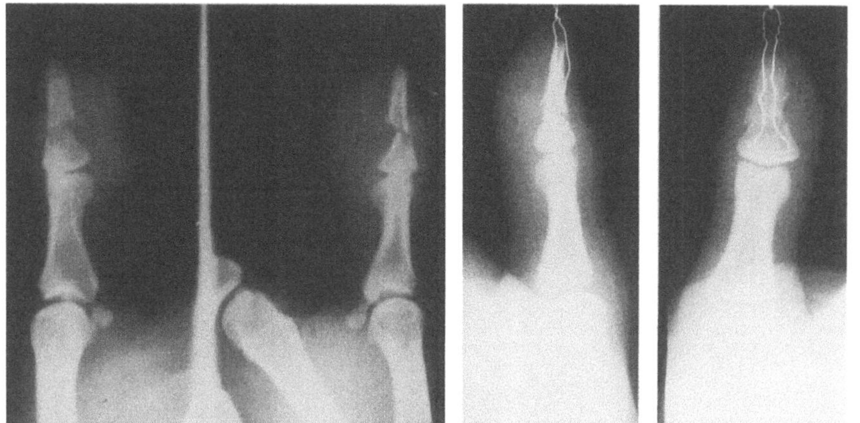

Fig. 16e,f.

cannot accept a pull-out wire passing through the pulp of the finger since the skin here does not withstand persistent pressure well, and scarring is likely. On the other hand, the pulp is also too soft and does not provide sufficient holding strength to the wire. We have not found it necessary to use the retrieval wire for pulling out the pull-out wire. We simply use a single pull-out wire, of 4'0' size, through the tendon in one single criss-cross (half figure-of-eight) and then through the bone and out from the nail or the tip of the finger. When there is no kink or knot in the wire, removal by gentle and persistent tension on one end of the wire after 3 weeks is without problem.

Fixation of the bone fragment in tendon avulsion is a difficult procedure, and the consideration is purely technical. For a small bone fragment of less than one-third of the joint surface it may be better to disregard the reduction of the fragment (but making sure that it does not protrude into the joint) or even trim it, and concentrate on the reattachment of the tendon. Retaining a small amount of bone facilitates reattachment of the tendon since it holds stitches better. Once the tendon can be reattached with stability, early mobilisation can be implemented. The end result of this is better than that with attempts to reduce and fix the bony fragment. In this manner part of the articulating surface is occupied by the tendon. This behaves as a form of arthroplasty.

When the fragment is larger, in addition to reattaching the tendons, the fragment needs to be reduced and fixed. Perhaps the simplest way is to stabilise the distal interphalangeal joint with a K-wire driven obliquely across the joint (since the medullary cavity is occupied by the pull-out wire for the tendon attachment) and then fix the fragment with either small biodegradable pins or adhesives. Adhesives appear at the moment preferable since they have a longer history, and fibrin is a proven nonirritant. A

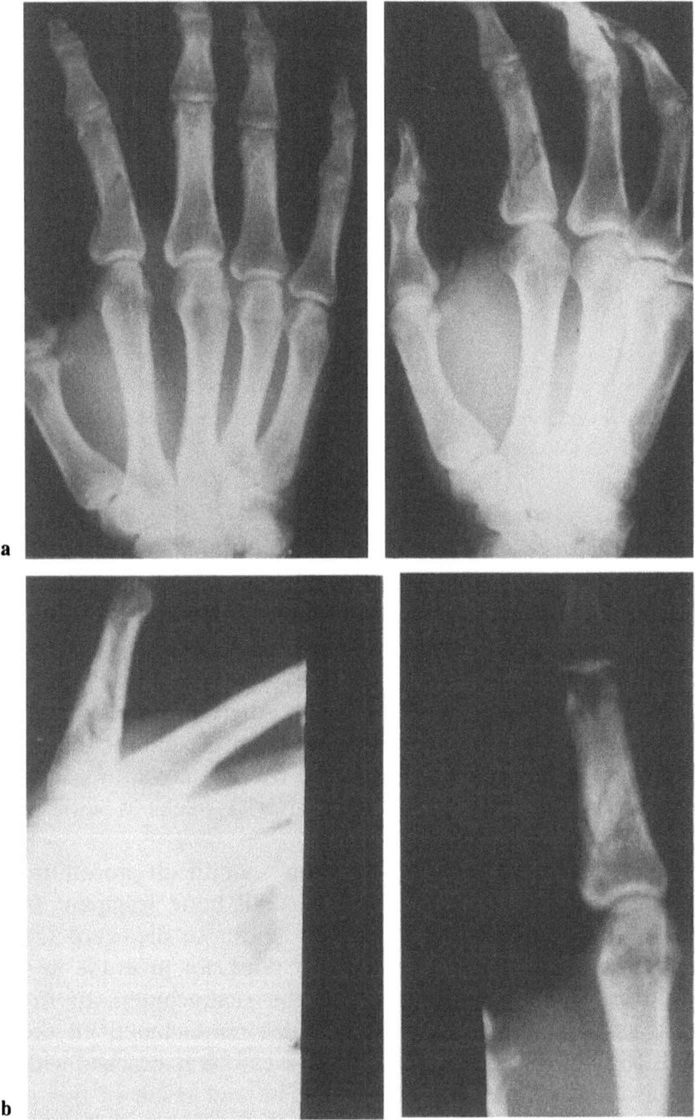

Fig. 17. a Apparently comminuted fracture of the base of the proximal phalanx, which remained stable to permit immediate mobilisation after a simple closed reduction. **b** No operation was required

hole is required for the biodegradable pins, which complicates the procedure and poses the risk of fracturing the fragment.

Fractures of the Middle and Proximal Phalanges

The differences between the middle and proximal phalanges are their sizes, their distances from the metacarpophalangeal joint and their tendon attachments, which influences the pattern of their fractures, the surgical approaches and the choice of implants when open reduction and internal fixation are required.

There are more indirect fractures in the proximal phalanx since they are longer, farther from the finger tip and more susceptible to torsional or angular forces applied to the finger tip. These injuries result in closed long oblique or spiral fractures in the proximal phalanx which are frequently stable, and conservative management after a closed reduction is usually sufficient. We prefer the functional definition of stability, i.e. that the fracture should be sufficiently stable to allow immediate mobilisation after the closed reduction, and we employ the least amount of splintage, which is cross-finger taping (Fig. 17). If this degree of stability is not achieved, open reduction and internal fixation is required [75–78].

Fractures of the middle phalanx usually occur after direct trauma and are frequently associated with extensor tendon injury. Such fractures are likely to be transverse and are unstable. We prefer open reduction and internal fixation. This also enables early mobilisation for the extensor tendon injury. An intraosseous wire loop (0.56 mm) plus either an intramedullary pin (1.6 or 2 mm) or an oblique K-wire (1.2 mm) is the simplest means to fix most middle and proximal phalangeal fractures (Fig. 18). In competent

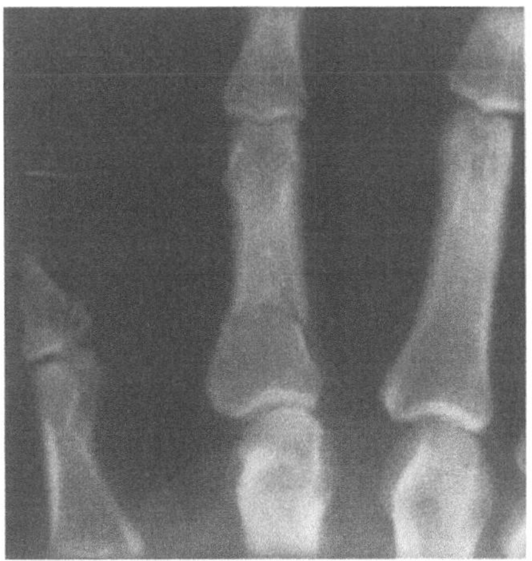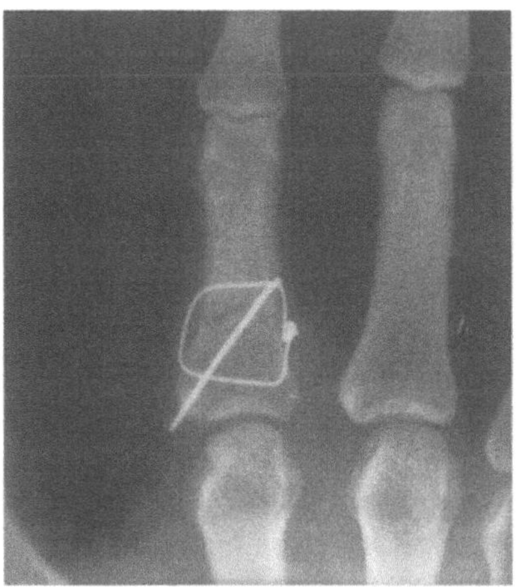

a   b

Fig. 18a,b. Fracture of the proximal phalanx, fixed with an oblique Kirschner wire and an intraosseous wire loop. Preoperative (**a**) and postoperative (**b**) radiographs

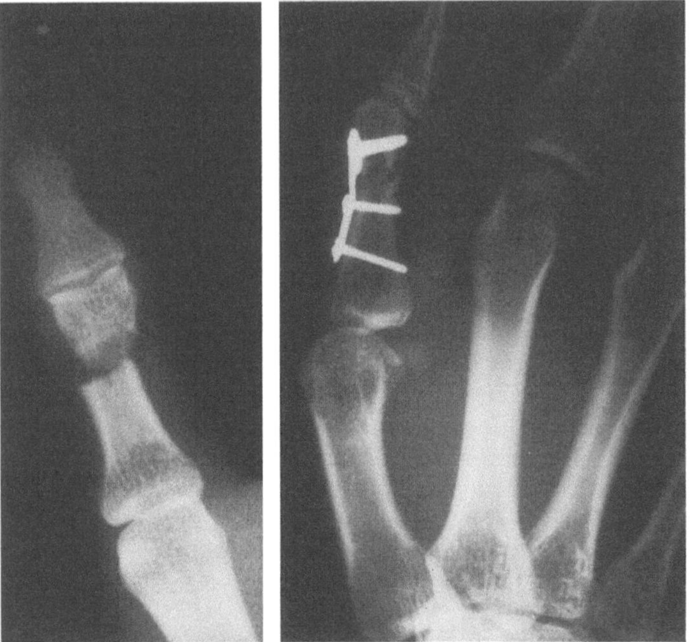

a   b

Fig. 19. a,b Fracture of the proximal phalanx of the thumb, fixed with a dorsally placed mini-plate. **c,d** Oblique fracture of the neck of the proximal phalanx, fixed by two interfragmentary screws of 1.5 mm diameter

hands, a mini-plate with four holes and 1.5-mm screws or interfragmentary screws alone can be placed on the lateral aspect of the bone. Bone exposure is limited to one side of the phalanx, and better stability is achieved (Fig. 19) [79–82].

Special consideration should be given to fractures at the base of the proximal phalanx (Fig. 20) [83]. These are usually transverse with a short oblique element and are usually the results of direct trauma. A mini-plate and screw system provides the best stability here. This can be placed on the dorsolateral aspect of the bone, and meticulous care is required to repair the extensor retinaculum. When the fracture is too close to the articular surface, one must resort to intraosseous wire loop supplemented with biodegradable implants or adhesives (Fig. 21).

The management of avulsion fractures depends on the sizes and locations. When they are on the lateral aspects of the joints and are small, they are minor avulsions of the collateral ligaments and can be treated conservatively with cross-finger taping and early mobilisation. When they are associated with gross instability of the joint, they should be fixed with a small tension wire loop [84]. Avulsion of the anterior lip of the base of the middle phalanx occurs in dorsal dislocation of the proximal phalangeal joint

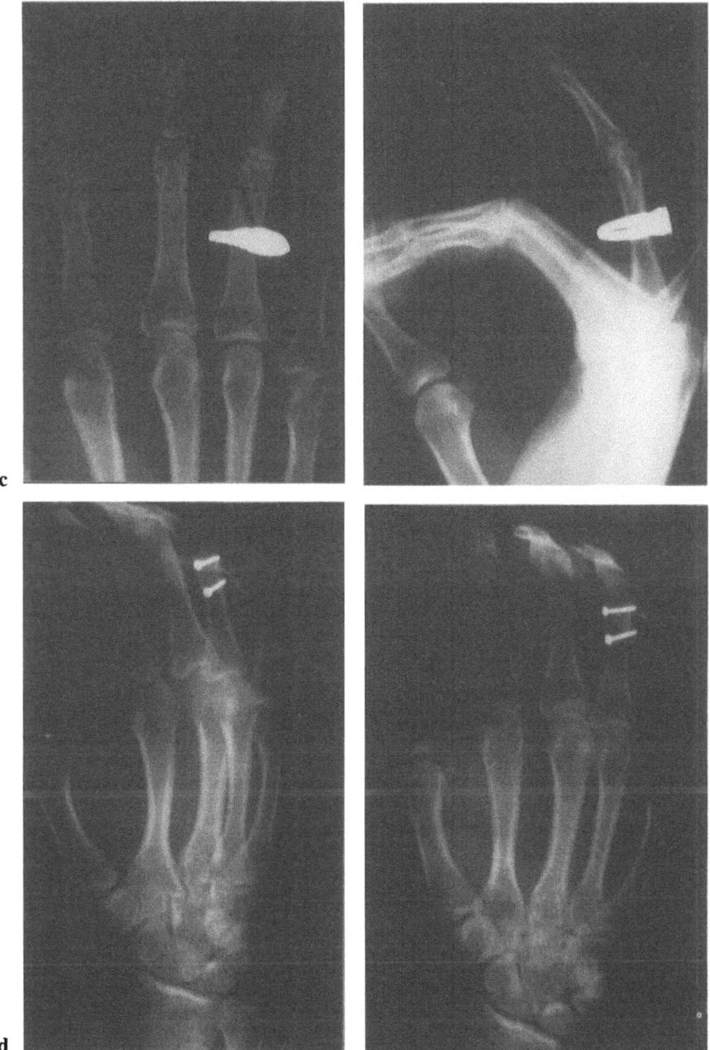

Fig. 19c,d.

and volar plate avulsion. Management depends on the size of the fragment [85,86]. We follow the rule of the "thirds". When the fragment is less than one-third of the width of the base of proximal phalanx, early mobilisation can be started after a closed reduction. The joint is prevented from extension to more than 30°, and full flexion is allowed [87]. To achieve this a dorsal kissing splint is the most effective and biomechanically sound one. This can be easily adjusted later to allow more extension (Fig. 1). Alternatively, a dynamic extension splint with a traction and downward force on the

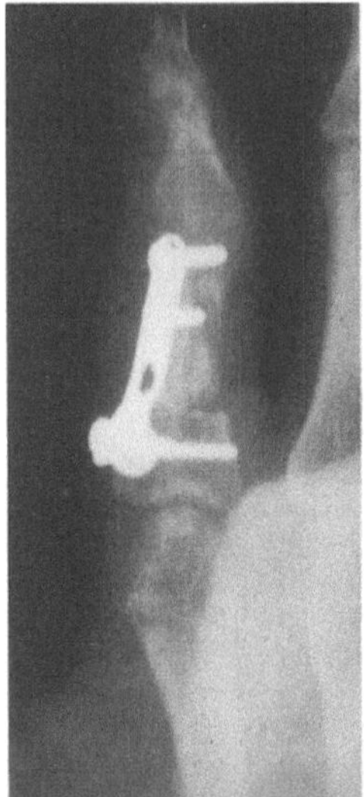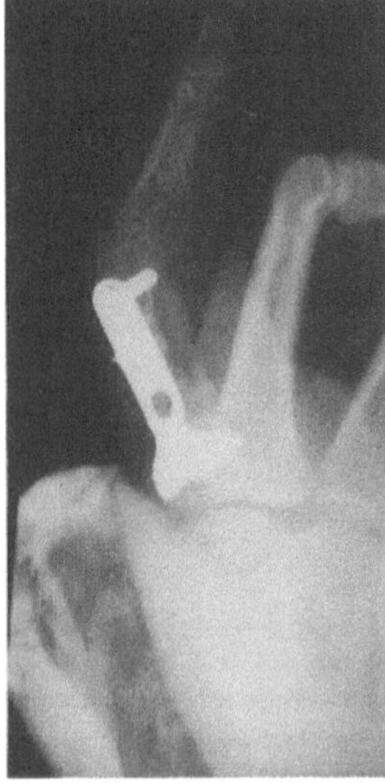

Fig. 20. Comminuted fracture of the shaft and base of the proximal phalanx, fixed by a T-shaped mini-plate and bone graft

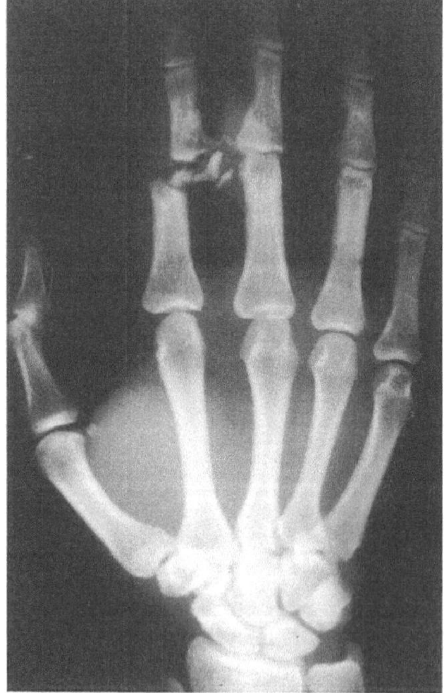

Fig. 21. Markedly comminuted fracture of the head of the proximal phalanx. The best fixation method for such a fracture may be biodegradable implants or tissue adhesives

joint can be constructed [85]. This "force couple splint" can be applied to more severe types of injuries (Fig. 22). Another design employs "serpentine" wires in holding external pins. This provides distraction and is also slightly flexible to allow some joint movement (Fig. 23) [50].

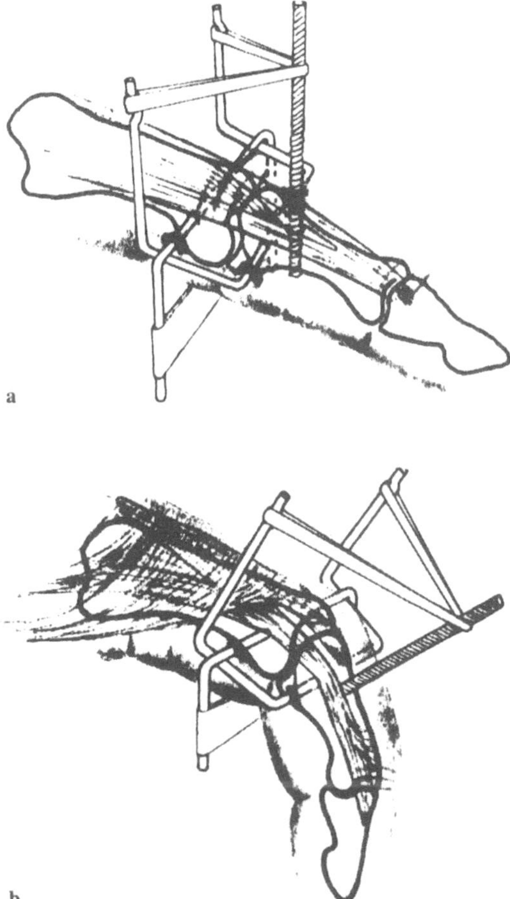

Fig. 22a,b. The "force couple splint" designed by Agee. (From [85]). Splint in extension (**a**) and flexion (**b**)

When the fragment is more than one-third of the width of the base of proximal phallanx, the joint is unstable after reduction, and open fixation is required. This does not mean fixation of the fragment, which is difficult and fraught with complications. It means repair of the collateral ligaments and to the volar capsule as well. This is achieved by bilateral lateral incisions. One incision is deepened to permit access to the front of the volar plate to aid reduction of the fragment. The joint is also stabilised at 30° flexion with a K-wire. Once the joint is stabilised in the reduced position, the fragment is naturally reduced. The K-wire can be removed after 1 week and dorsal blocking splint applied to allow early mobilisation in flexion.

Avulsion fracture of the dorsal part of the base of the middle phalanx, in a traumatic button-hole deformity, is treated similarly. The bone fragment is disregarded, and attention is directed to reattachment of the tendon and plication of the retinacular tendons, which are spread apart. The joint is

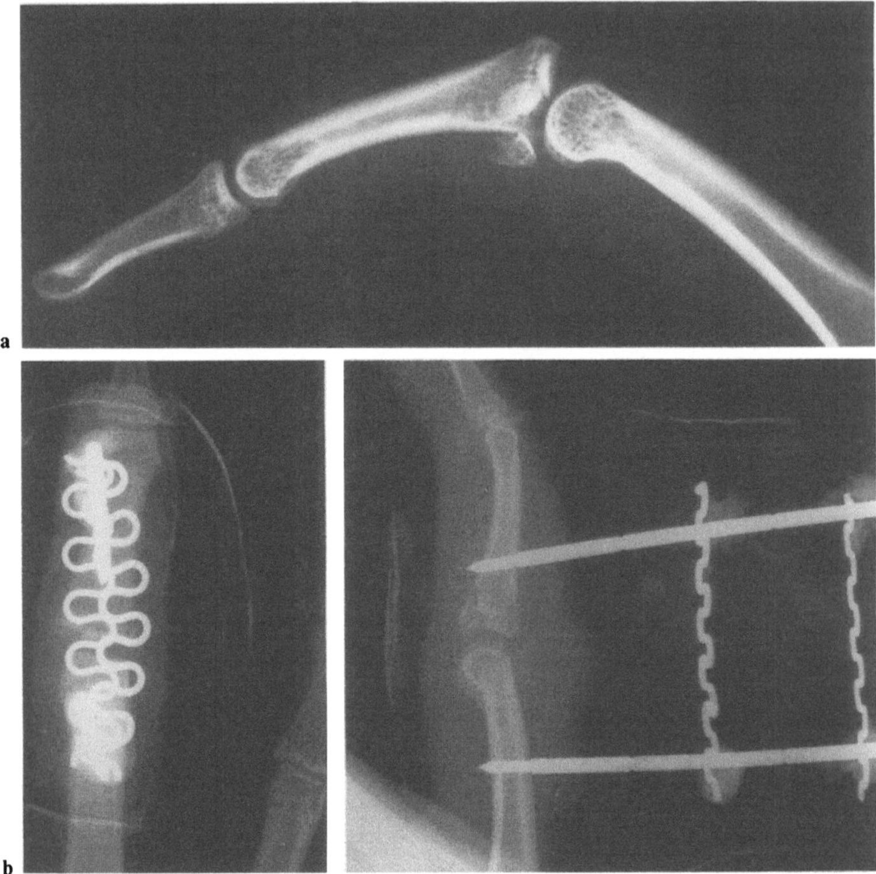

Fig. 23a,b. The "Stockport serpentine spring system". Fracture of base of middle phalanx reduced and fixed with the system. (Courtesy Dr. N.R.M. Fahmy, Stockport, U.K.)

stabilised in extension with a K-wire. Under favourable situations the K-wire may be removed after 1 week and a dynamic extension splint applied. This allows controlled mobilisation of the joint at an early stage [88].

A distinction must be made between condylar fractures and avulsion fractures, although the two may be associated. Condylar fractures are actually depression fractures of part of the condyle. They are best fixed with mini-screws (1.5 mm) which may be incorporated in a mini-plate or a mini-condylar plate (Fig. 24). The mini-condylar plates from the AO group [89] come in two sizes (2 and 1.5 mm) and have a small stylet at the distal part. The small stylet is meant to provide rotational stability to the fixation of the condyles. However, the stylet does not always match the drill hole well, may be too long and during insertion may distract the fragments in an inter-

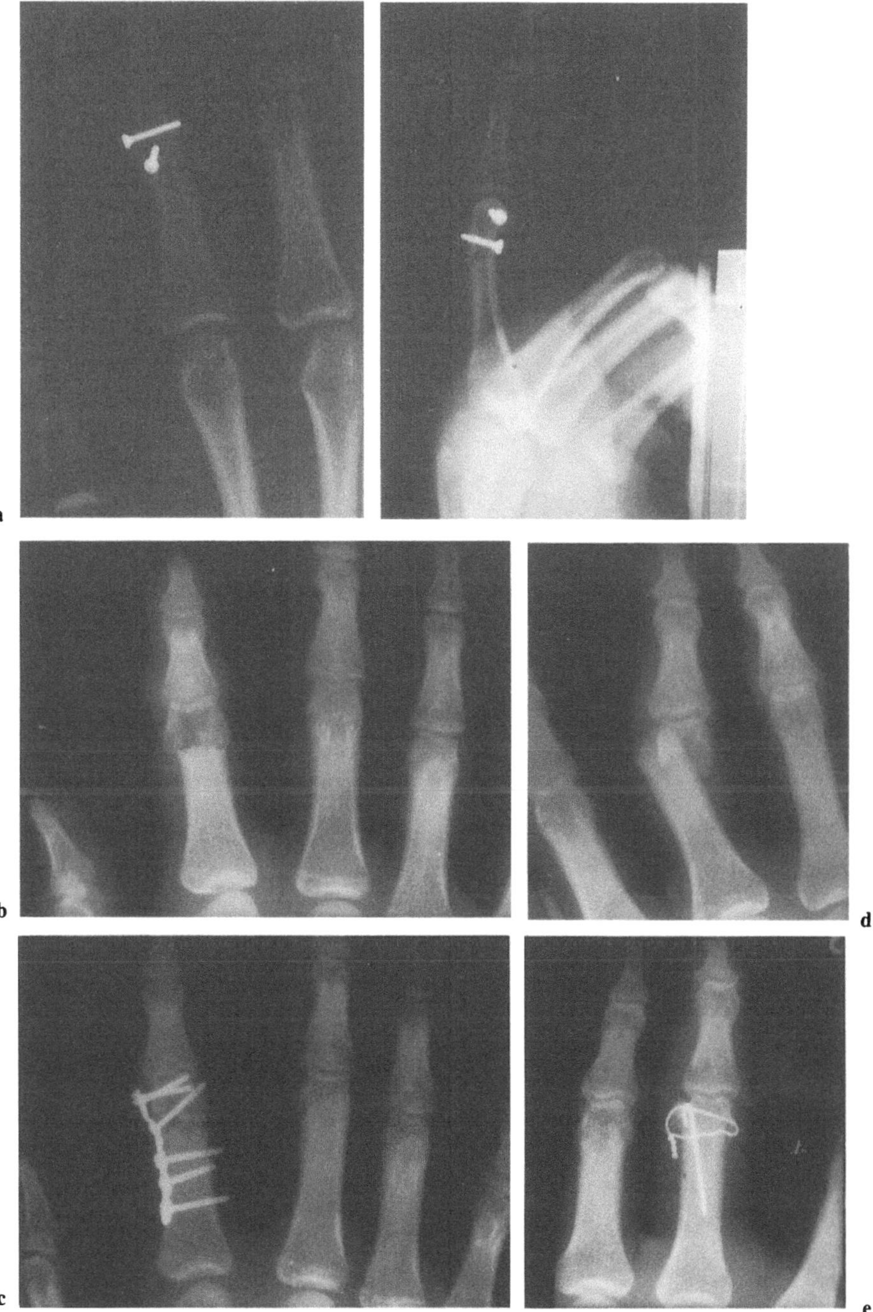

Fig. 24a–e. Condylar fractures of the proximal phalanx. **a** Fixation by interfragmentary screws of 1.5 mm diameter. **b,c** Fixation by AO minicondylar plate of 1.5 mm. **d,e** Fixation by wire loop and an intramedullary buttressing Kirschner wire

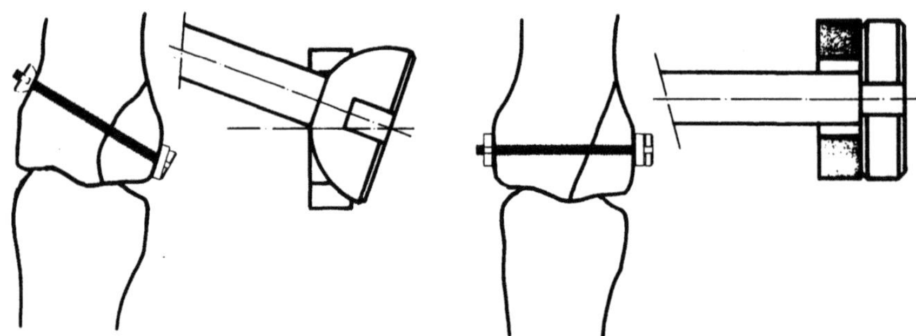

Fig. 25. Schematic drawings of the mini-pin and bolt. (Courtesy Osteo, Switzerland)

condylar fracture or may even shatter the fragments. They must be used with caution in small bones and in those with comminutions. A mini-plate is usually good enough. When there is good purchase by the screw, and when there is good contact between the condylar part and the metaphysis of the bone, rotational stability is usually achieved even when there is only one screw through the fragment. A threated mini-pin and bolt system has also been developed from Osteo (Switzerland). The pin is only 0.8 mm in size and is certainly ideal for small condylar fractures and with comminution. The pin can be incorporated to a mini-plate to fix the shaft (Fig. 25). When there is severe comminution, a mini-external fixator may be used, or one can consider the use of biodegradable implants or adhesives. It must be remembered that when comminution is severe, especially in situations of co-existing soft-tissue injuries, internal fixation and joint reconstruction becomes technically impossible. This is particularly true when both proximal and distal sides of the joint are involved (Fig. 13). Under such circumstances no hesitation should delay a compromising, "sacrifice" choice of fusing the joint in functional position. This allows early healing and gives a defective but functional finger. On the other hand, insistence on joint preservation may result in delayed healing, deformities, stiffness and multiple operations.

Fractures of the Metacarpals

There is substantial controversy surrounding metacarpal fractures. These are usually stable although even slight displacements are not tolerated since the effects are magnified at the finger tip. Fractures caused by direct trauma are unstable and are frequently associated with soft-tissue injuries.

Fracture of the metacarpal head occurs distal to the collateral ligaments and is usually comminuted; the fragments have few soft-tissue attachments and are therefore associated with a high risk of avascular necrosis (Fig. 26) [90,91]. If the fragments are not grossly displaced and can be readily reduced, it is preferable to attempt reduction and to maintain it by either

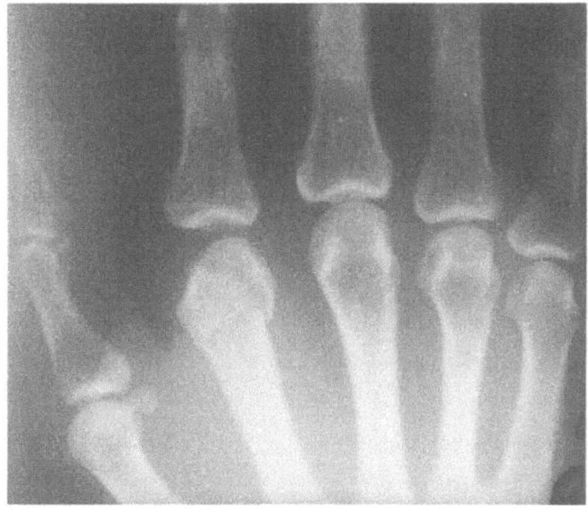

Fig. 26. Fracture of the head of the metacarpal, which was not grossly displaced and was treated conservatively

skeletal traction or external fixation. Traction or distraction is necessary to reduce loading on the fragments and at the same time to preserve the joint space. The collaterals are prevented from contracture, and future movement of the joint is preserved. A specially designed traction splint can be used to maintain traction and at the same time permit movement and therefore preserve joint function [49]. Alternatively, an external fixator may be used to maintain distraction of the joint and alignment of the fragments. The distraction is maintained for 2 weeks.

Open reduction for metacarpal head fractures may be required if they are grossly displaced, and reduction cannot be achieved by closed means. An ulnar-dorsal incision is made and the extensor retinaculum opened through the ulnar side. The joint capsule is identified and opened longitudinally on the ulnar side. This may be extended into the shaft of the metacarpal and with the periosteum stripped off in continuity from the bone. The fragments are identified and reduced. They may be held in place by biogegradable pins or adhesives. Once again, adhesives are preferred. The joint should also be distracted by external fixator or skeletal traction for 2 weeks.

If the fragments are too comminuted to be reduced, they should be removed. The fracture surface should be débrided and smoothened, and the defect can be replaced by various means. A tendon ball may be fashioned from a rolled-up slip of the extensor tendon and placed into the joint, or a small nonvascularised osteochondral graft obtained from a toe joint which is secured with either adhesives or wire. However, the overall result of osteochondral grafts is unsatisfactory. The graft frequently collapses or displaces, with degeneration of the joint and loss of range of movement. After such spacers, the joint, again, should be maintained in distraction by external fixator or skeletal traction for 2 weeks (Fig. 27).

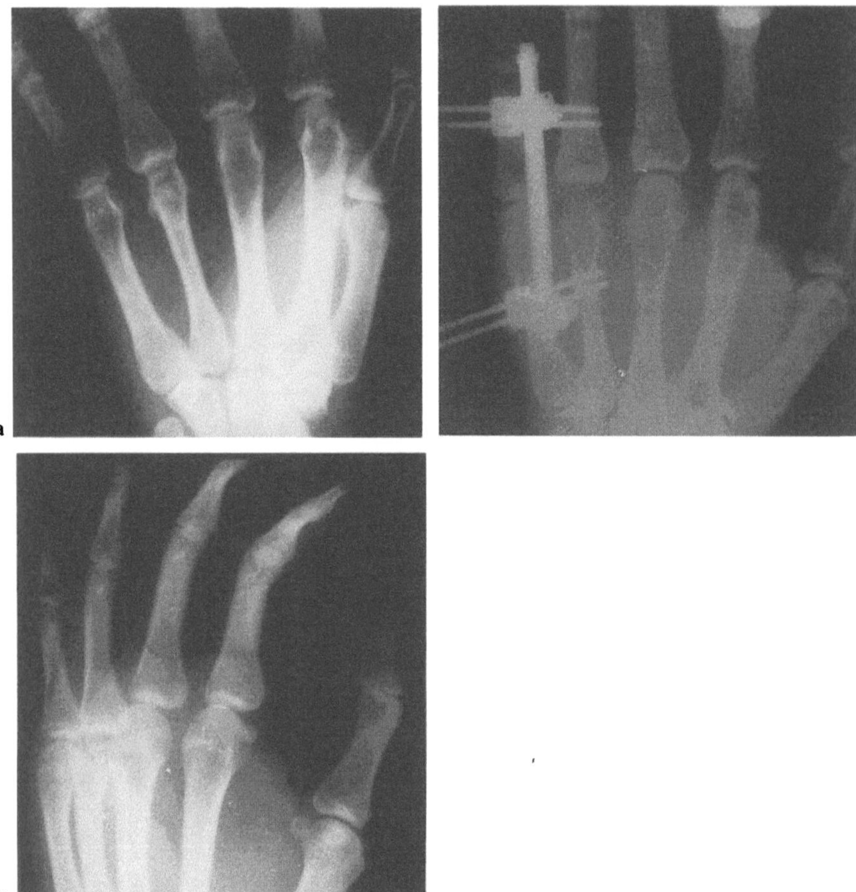

If there is residual joint degeneration with pain and loss of movement, a vascularised toe joint transplantation may be considered, allowing approximately a 40° range of movement [57,58]. Some advocate primary free vascularised joint transplantation.

Fractures of the metacarpal neck occur proximal to the attachments of the collaterals (Fig. 28) [92]. These are usually impacted and flexed with a dorsal angulation. They rarely occur in the thumb, where treatment is usually not required because of the degree of mobility of the first metacarpal. When they occur in the index or the middle finger, they must be reduced. When they occur in the ring or the little finger, one can accept a certain degree of deformity. For the ring finger up to 15° flexion is accepted and for the little finger up to 30° [92].

Reduction of the fracture is not difficult. Correction of the flexion can be readily achieved by flexion of the metacarpophalangeal joint and then pushing up of the proximal phalanx. Since the collaterals are attached to the

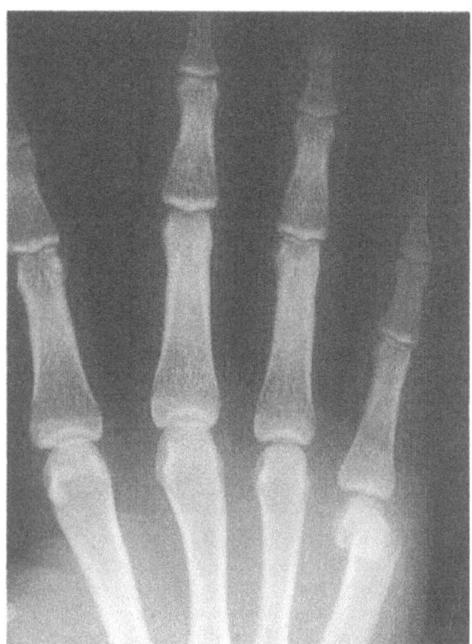

Fig. 28. Fracture neck of the fifth metacarpal

fragment, stacking the proximal phalanx to the adjacent fingers naturally aligns it to the other fingers. The problem with this fracture is in maintaining the reduction and allowing early mobilisation. The mini-plate and screw system is singularly unsuitable in this situation because when placed on the dorsum of the metacarpal it impedes the extensor tendon, which is closely applied to the joint. Placing the mini-plate on the lateral aspect of the bone is usually not feasible since this means either stripping of one collateral ligament or impeding its function. The approach is also limited by the adjacent metacarpals. However, it may be considered under special circumstances for the second and fifth metacarpals (Fig. 29).

Biodegradable pins driven through the joint surface into the medullary cavity is a viable alternative. This requires more time to be fully actualised because at the moment the pins are either too large (too traumatic to the joint) or too flexible (too weak). An intramedullary K-wire (1.6 or 2 mm) can be driven in retrograde fashion through the base of the metacarpal to be impacted into the metacarpal head to maintain the reduction (Fig. 30) [35,36]. The wire follows the curvature of the metacarpal and therefore provides three-point fixation and prevents backing out of the pin. The pin may be impacted into the base of the metacarpal and left there, or it can be removed after 3 weeks. To provide additional rotational stability the involved finger is taped to an adjacent finger.

Fracture of the shaft of the metacarpal may be treated merely expectantly, with a closed reduction and then braced with a well-moulded

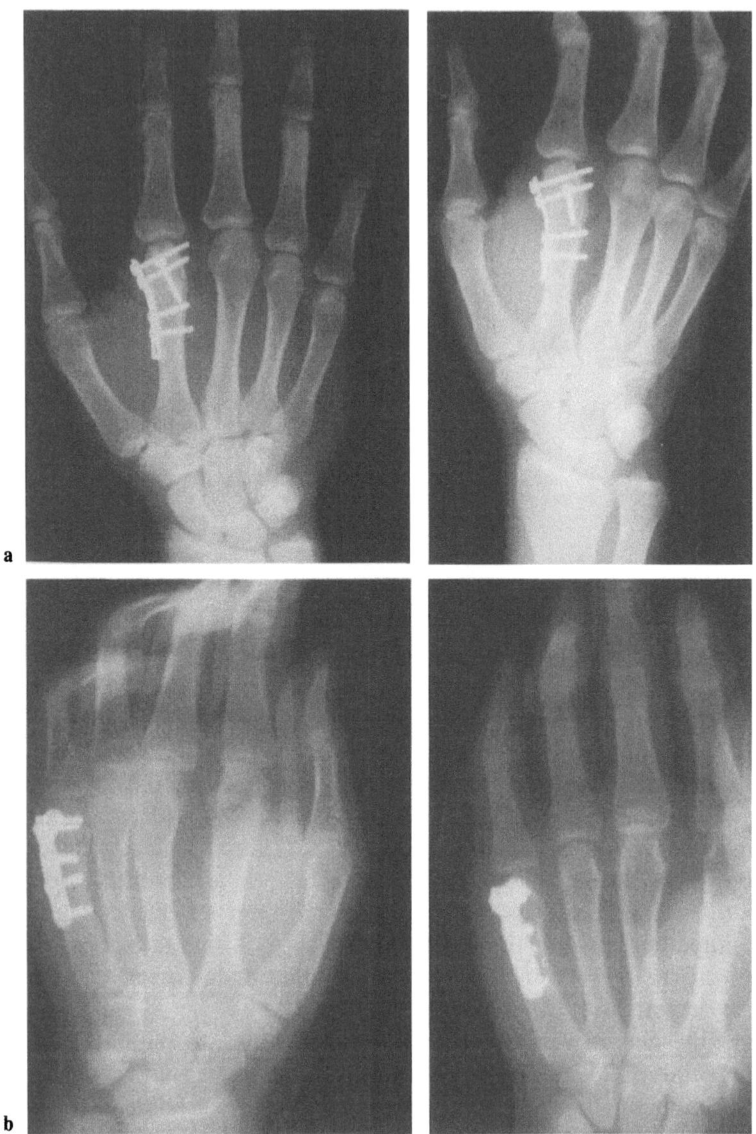

Fig. 29. a Fracture neck of the second metacarpal, fixed with a mini-plate and interfragmentary screw. **b** Fracture neck of the fifth metacarpal, fixed with a miniplate

plaster spica without immobilisation of the wrist, or by the use of functional braces. Open reduction may be required when there is irreducible rotation or an open wound. Mini-plate and screws is the most direct method of fixation since it can be applied to the dorsal aspect of the bone with little

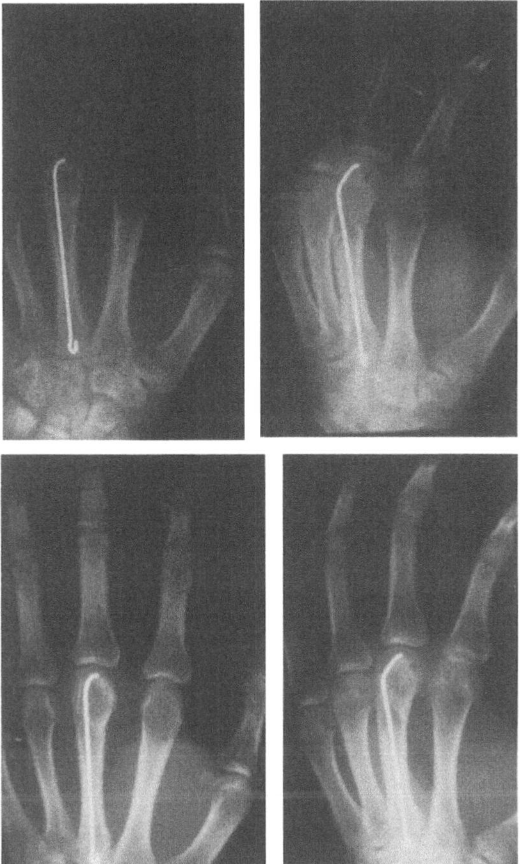

Fig. 30. Fracture neck of the third metacarpal, which was well reduced and buttressed by an intramedullary Kirschner wire driven through its base

stripping of the intrinsic muscles. Depending on the configuration of the fracture and the degree of comminution various other forms of fixation can be used with good results: screws or cerclage wire loops for long spiral fractures, special clamp-on plate for transverse or spiral fractures, and intraosseous wire loop with an intramedullary pin for transverse fractures. It appears, however, that the mini-plate and screw system meets all different demands (Fig. 31) [93,94].

Fractures of the base of the metacarpals require special attention [95]. These are joint injuries and are associated with subluxation of the metacarpals from the carpal bones. Bennette's fracture at the base of the thumb is a classical example (Fig. 32). Although there are many ways of treating this fracture [96,97], we favour open reduction and fixation of the avulsion fragment with either screws or screws and plate or with wire loop. An

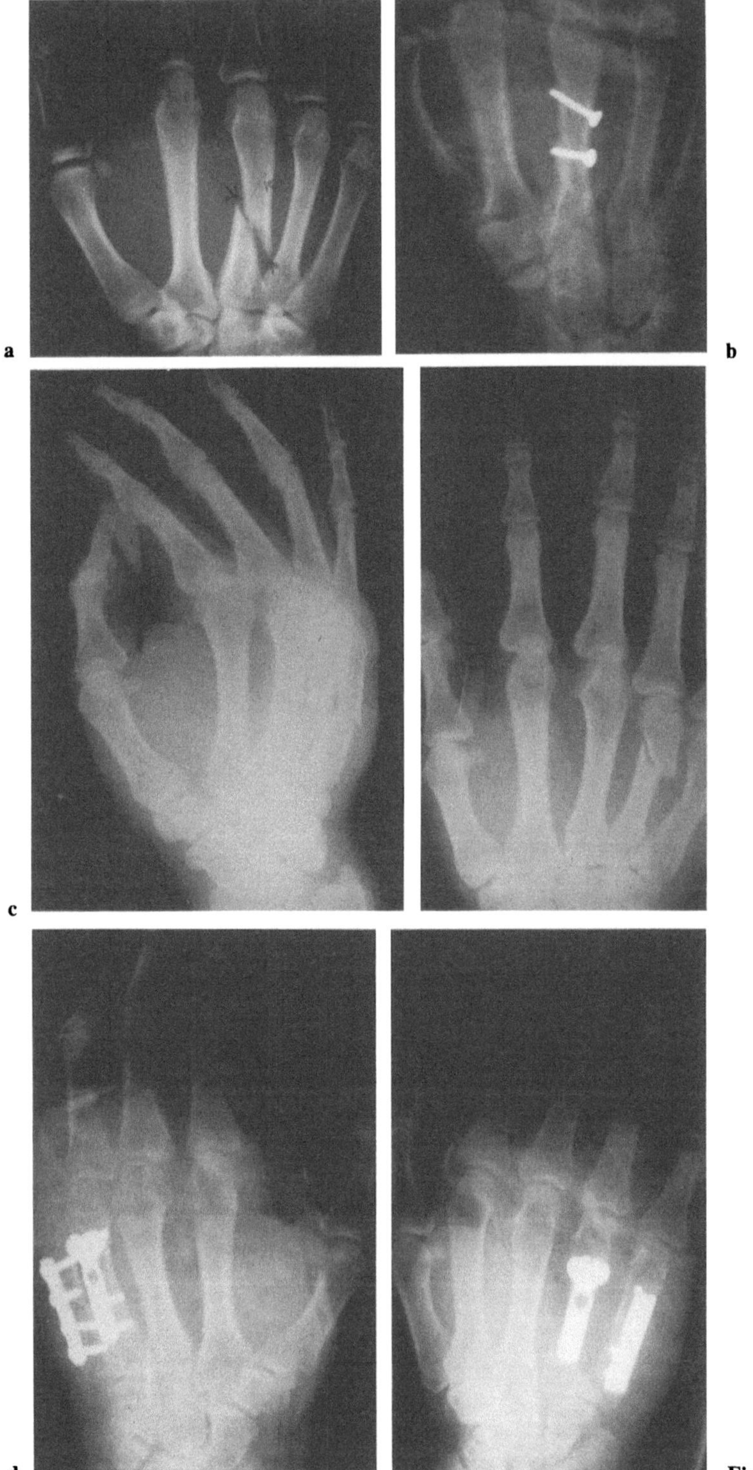

Fig. 31a–d.

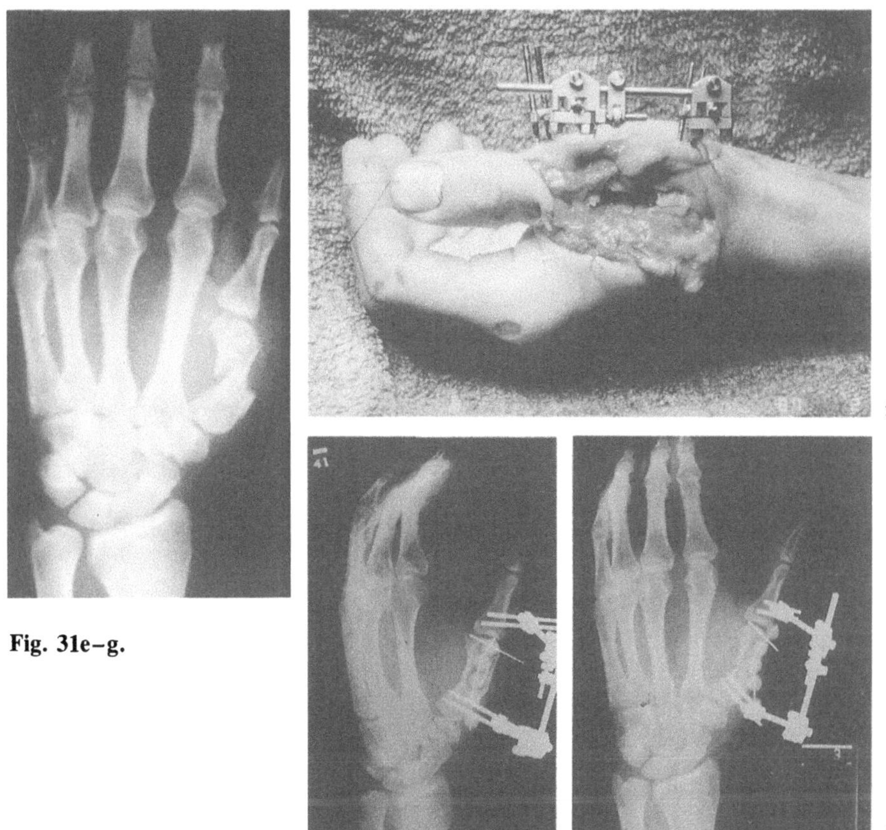

Fig. 31e–g.

Fig. 31. a,b Oblique fracture of the third metacarpal, fixed with interfragmentary screws. c,d Fractures of the fourth and fifth metacarpals, fixed with miniplates. e,f,g Severe open comminuted fracture of the first metacarpal, stabilised by a mini-Hoffmann external fixator. The gentamycin beads are inserted for local wound infection control

incision appearing curved as hockey stick is made on the radial aspect of the first metacarpal, just dorsal to the abductor pollicis brevis muscle, with the horizontal part of the incision curving towards the palm along the distal wrist crease. The plane between the abductor pollicis brevis and bone is developed and the muscle retracted. Part of the origin of the muscle may be detached from the flexor retinaculum. The fracture fragment is readily identified and fixed with the appropriate implant. If necessary, the extensor pollicis brevis tendon is freed from the dorsal aspect of the first metacarpal so that the dorsal aspect of the bone can be exposed. After the operation the thumb is bandaged in a bulky compressive dressing which serves some immobilisation, and mobilisation can be started as soon as pain becomes tolerable.

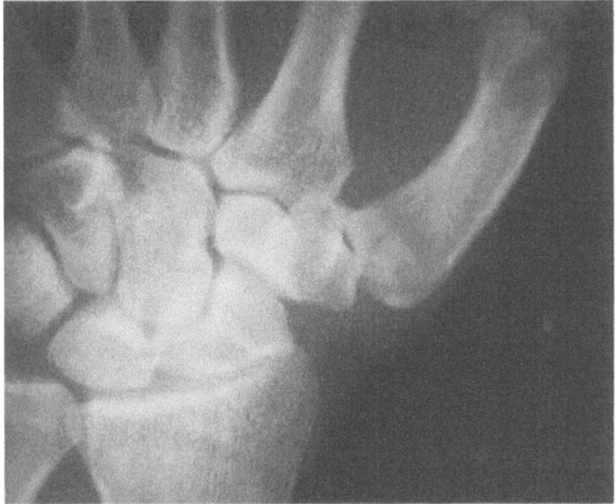

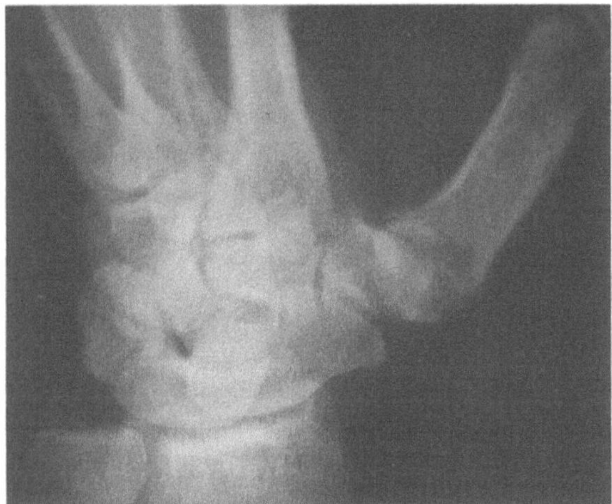

Fig. 32. a,b Bennett's fracture of the thumb

For fractures occurring at the base of other metacarpals the management is similar. Simple K-wire fixation is generally used, but occasionally the mini-plate is appropriate, and one can accept temporary violation of the carpometacarpal joint, with the implants removed by 6 weeks (Fig. 33). However, these are unusual injuries, and the nature of the injury is frequently severe compression or crushing, with substantial soft-tissue damage. Priority of attention is given to detecting and treating any associated compartment syndrome in the palm and the interosseous compartments. For fractures occurring at the base of the fourth or fifth metacarpal one must examine the deep branch of the ulnar nerve carefully to evaluate whether there is an associated injury of this nerve.

Common Carpal Injuries

Injury of the carpal bones is a special category of its own. The fractures are intra-articular, and they may result in carpal instabilities or disruption of stability of the finger rays [98]. There is no general rule of management, but the concensus is that most of these fractures are better treated with operative reduction and fixation by some form of devices. However, in the past fixation was usually achieved by K-wires. These are not entirely satisfactory (perhaps also because of the lack of good fluoroscopic machines for radiologically guided pinning), and additional, usually prolonged casting is required and mobilisation delayed. With the increasing demands by patients for earlier and better functional recovery of their injured limb this approach certainly needs to be reviewed and new treatment modalities explored.

Scaphoid fracture is the commonest carpal injury, and it exemplifies this situation well. Scaphoid has long been recognised as the key bone linking the two carpal rows. It is put under tremenduous stress during the extremes of wrist movements. Immobilisation of the bone inside a plaster cast is difficult, and some physicians even practise immobilisation of the whole forearm from the fingers up to and including the elbow in a long cast [99–101]. It would be logical to think that given a means of stabilising the fracture, wrist movement may be restored earlier and better. In the past this was not possible, and conservative treatment remained as the only widely practised treatment modality.

With the advent of the Herbert screw, the situation has been changing rapidly [102–104]. The Herbert screw affords a relatively atraumatic and sufficiently stable fixation of the scaphoid, and early mobilisation can be implemented. Although criticisms have been raised regarding the disturbance to the trapezioscaphoid joint and articular cartilage during the placement of the jig, this has been largely overcome by inserting the screw without the placement of the jig [105]. Another criticism is the lack of rotational stability with the screw, although in most fractures with little comminution the fixation is usually sufficiently stable. Until recently the screw was used only for delayed scaphoid unions or established nonunions together with bone grafting, but it is now being used increasingly for acute scaphoid fractures [105]. By slightly modifying the technique, the screw may be placed with radiological guidance through a small transverse volar incision over the trapezium. This causes the least insult to the joint capsule and carpal ligaments (Fig. 34). In acute fractures good fixation can usually be achieved. The indications for this procedure are for young and active adults who do not prefer prolonged cast immobilisation, and who might benefit from earlier return of the range of movement of the wrist and grip strength. When multiple fractures occur in the same limb involving the scaphoid, fixation of the scaphoid with the Herbert screw also permits earlier mobilisation of the whole limb. However, the long-term effect of early screw fixation on the

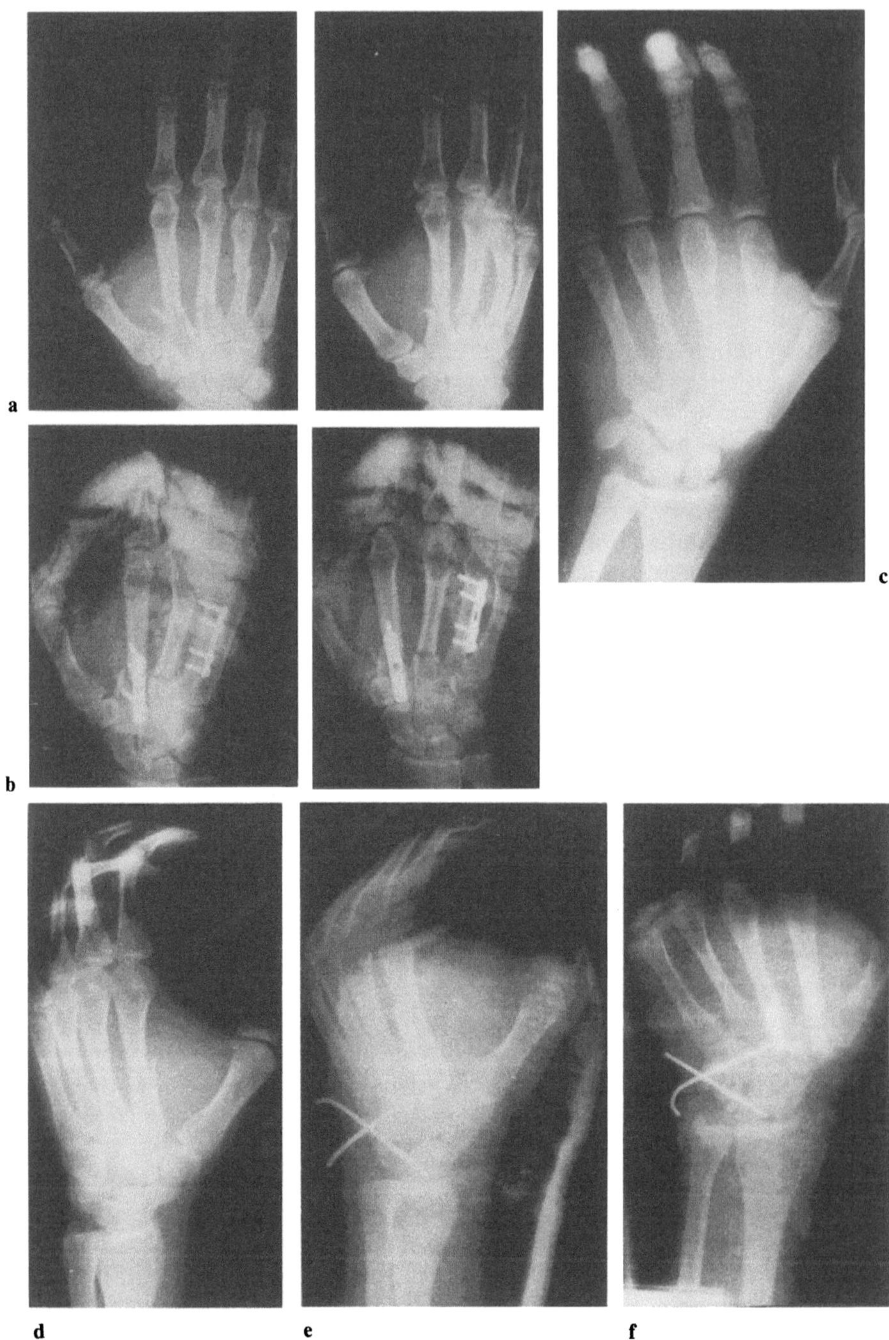

union rate of the scaphoid and whether it makes any difference in terms of the rate of return to work remains to be seen.

For other carpal fractures the management is individualised. The Herbert screw can provide temporary fixation between carpal bones, although removal is necessary.

Hand Fractures in Children

Although hand fractures present technical challenges to surgeons because of the small size of the bone and the anatomical complexity, such fractures occurring in children, whose hand bones are still of smaller dimensions, may be technically impossible [106–111]. Fortunately, hand fractures do not occur commonly among children. Domestic injuries commonly produce epiphyseal injuries.

Epiphyseal plates in the hand of children close at around 13 years of age. Most fractures in children under the age of 11 years are type II epiphyseal injuries around the joint, usually the base of the phalanges [112,113]. Closed reduction can usually be attempted, but good reduction is often difficult to achieve. When this occurs, we favour open reduction and fixing the fractures with 0.9-mm nonthreaded K-wires, which are removed after 3 weeks. If the child is under 6 years of age, a long-arm plaster cast may be necessary in addition. The wrist is kept extended, the metacarpophalangeal joints flexed and the interphalangeal joints extended, and all fingers supported. Fractures affecting other regions of the bones in the hand are managed by the same principles of fracture treatment, and indeed, in children aged over 13 years, the bone dimensions approach those of the adult, and wire loops and other devices may be used.

A few points are worth emphasising again: (a) Alignment and closed reduction of shaft fractures are usually sufficient means of treatment because such fractures are usually solitary, simple and not associated with soft-tissue damages. Moreover, the child's hand tolerates 3 weeks of immobilisation well, and stiffness does not normally develop. (b) Cross K-wire fixation for a shaft fracture in the hand of a child is technically very difficult, and multiple attempts may damage the epiphyseal plate. (c) Large implants should be avoided more often than in adults. (d) Additional attention should be given to dressings and plasters, as described above. (e) All implants must be removed. (f) Corrective splints with the aim of maintaining proper alignment do not work in the child because of poor compliance. It is therefore appro-

Fig. 33. a,b Multiple fractures of the metacarpals, with the second and fourth fixed with mini-plates. The plate on the second metacarpal has fixed the basal fracture and overlaid the trapezoid. This was removed at 6 weeks. **c,d,e,f** Fractures of the bases of the second and third metacarpals, with separation of the ulnar column and fracture of the triquetrum. The metacarpal fractures were fixed with mini-plates and the ulnar column stabilised by Kirschner wires

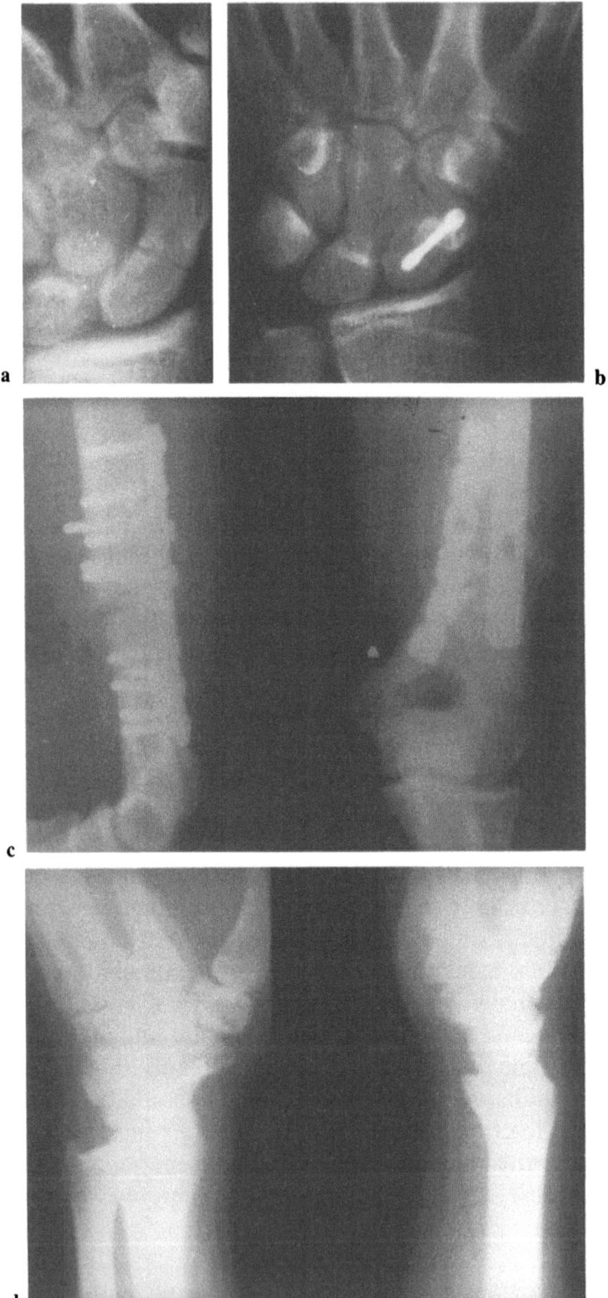

Fig. 34. a,b Undisplaced fracture of the scaphoid, fixed with fluoroscopy-guided insertion of the Herbert screw. **c,d** Comminuted fracture of the humerus and scaphoid in the same limb. The humerus was openly reduced and plated whereas the scaphoid was fixed with a Herbert screw inserted with fluoroscopy guidance

priate to conclude that treatment of hand fractures in the child should follow a conservative nonaggressive approach. Particular attention, however, should be paid to the potential of growth hazards. An angular or rotational deformity is much more harmful than a volar-dorsal one and needs to be corrected at an early stage.

Complications of Hand Fractures

Complications are common to fracture management, including infection, problems in union, deformities and loss of function (Fig. 35). The complexity of hand function and the multiplicity of structures involved in hand fractures predispose to a significant loss of hand function after injuries, especially when complications occur. It is therefore important to prevent complications. Hand fractures are very often associated with soft-tissue injuries and open wounds. Prophylactic antibiotics are advisable under those circumstances. Finger stiffness is the most significant factor limiting hand function. When fracture fixation is solid and sound, immediate motion can be encouraged to promote mobility. However, fixation is not always reliable. Motion in such situations need to be limited or prevented. The finger joints should then be immobilised in positions of maximal capsular and ligamental stretch so that adhesions and fibrosis, if occurring in the joints, are least likely to cause permanent stiffness. Therefore, the hand is dressed in the so-called "boxing glove" style: the metacarpophalangeal joints of fingers are flexed at 90°, the interphallangeal joints at full extension and the thumb opposed and extended. Keeping the "boxing glove" dressing for a period of 3–4 weeks rarely leaves stiffness which is difficult to correct. Additional plaster slab to extend the wrist is also necessary.

Rehabilitation Issues in Hand Fractures

No discussion on hand surgery is complete without considering rehabilitation. Stiffness always develops after fracture, even after the most successful rigid fixation and when mobilisation is started immediately. Stiffness occurs mainly as a result of tissue oedema and pain which prevents adequate motion. Patients should be warned of stiffness and the necessity to start joint mobilisation as soon as possible. At the same time, as soon as reasonable wound healing occurs, fitting a pressure glove helps to control oedema and allows a more active mobilisation programme. While joint stiffness persists, gentle, continuous stretches, either manually or through the use of splints are useful. Soft-tissue scarring and capsular contractures are causes of resistant stiffness. These may need to be injected with corticosteroid, or, if they are persistent, timely surgical release is necessary.

Rehabilitation after hand fractures is a long procedure that requires active participation from the patient and patience and perseverance from the rehabilitation therapists. Recovery is expected to be slow and takes weeks or months. There is no place for over-optimism or for a negative outlook.

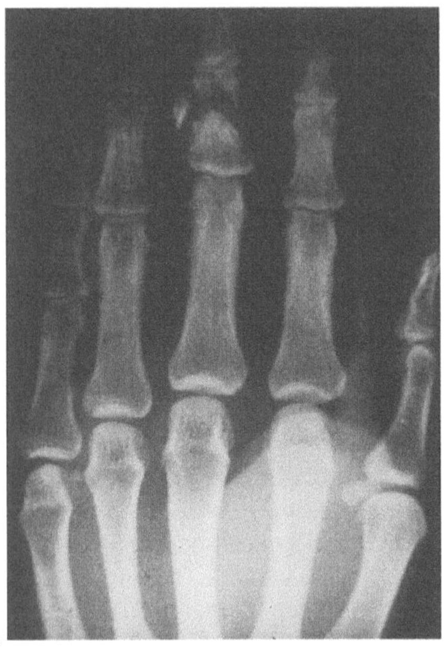

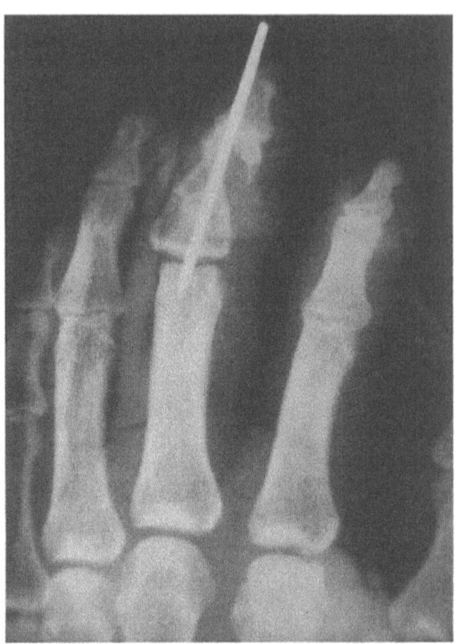

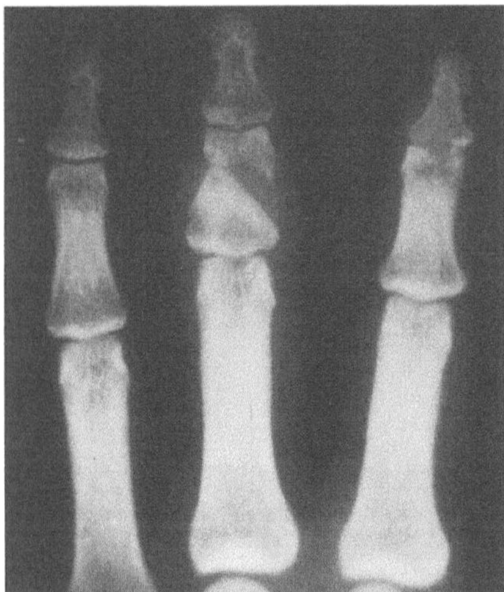

Fig. 35a–l. Examples of complications of inappropriate fracture fixation and management. **a,b,c** Comminuted fracture of the middle phalanx. This was simply splinted by an axial Kirschner wire, which resulted in fibrous nonunion. This was due partly to ischaemia. This fracture should have received bone graft primarily and would probably have best been stabilised by an external fixator. **d,e** Comminuted fracture of the proximal interphalangeal joint, which was fused primarily by crossed Kirschner wires. There is ulnar deviation, and flexion is inadequate. A mini-plate should have been used. **f,g** Multiple fractures in the ring finger. Poor application of the mini-plate

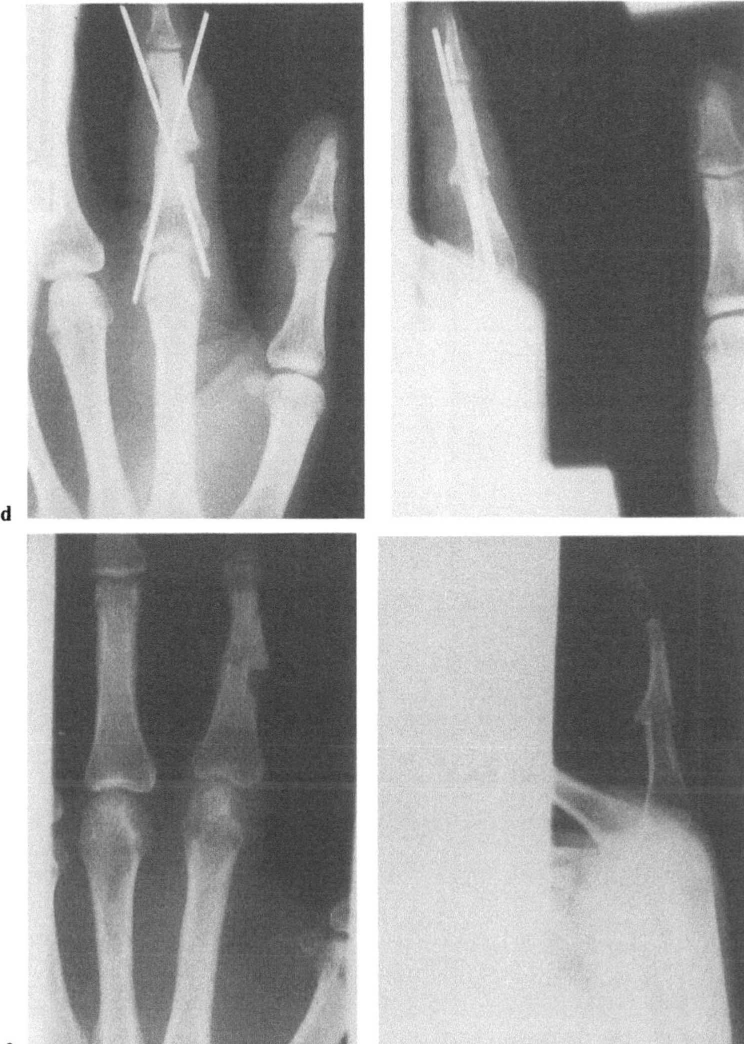

and screws, resulting in malalignment and impedance to movement and marked stiffness. **h,i,j** Open comminuted fracture of the second metacarpal, which was aligned only with Kirschner wires. Subluxation of the metacarpophalangeal joint persisted, and early mobilisation was not feasible. **k,l** Comminuted fracture of the metacarpal head. A mini-plate fixation was attempted (notice the screw holes) but failed, making the fracture more comminuted. A compromised form of fixation using Kirschner wire was used. The fracture could have been aligned and stabilised by a mini-external fixator

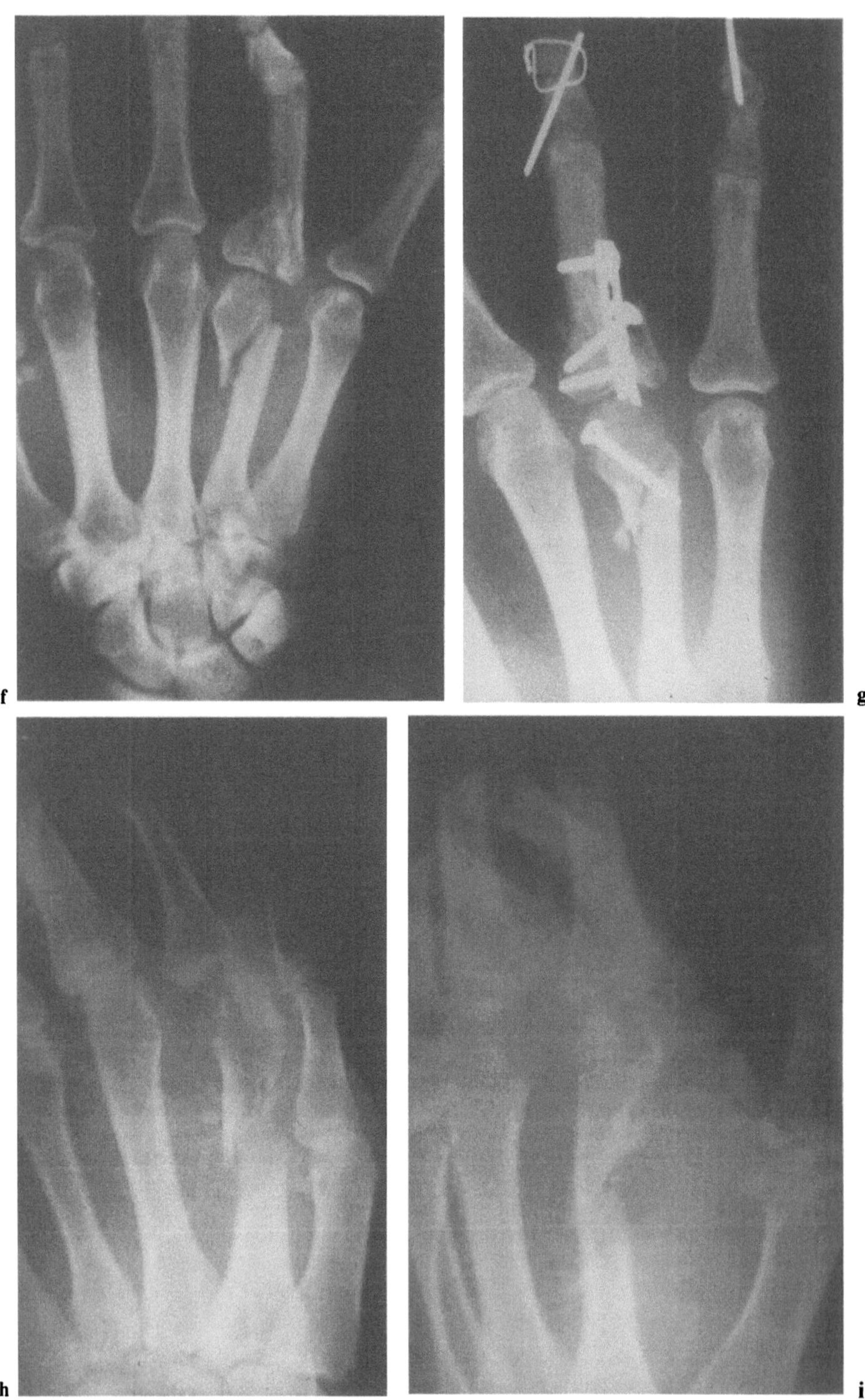

Fig. 35f–i.

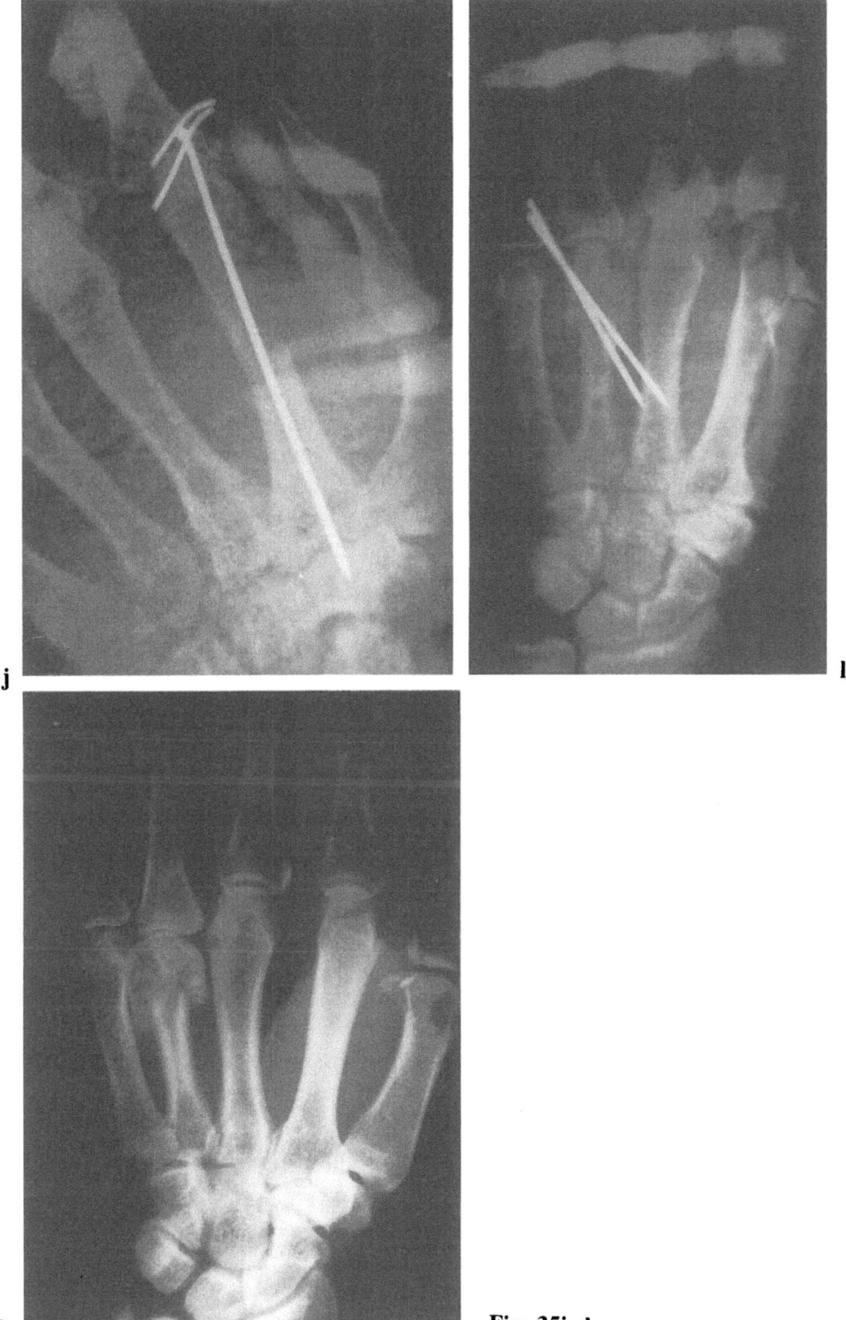

Fig. 35j–l.

Conclusion

Modern fracture treatment emphasizes achieving the best functional results within the least possible time. The Swiss AO school has revolutionised the old practice of fracture treatment and introduced the concept of anatomic reduction, rigid fixation and atraumatic technique. Although the early concept of the AO group – primary bone healing – has been shown to be overoptimistic and simplistic, rigid fixation to permit immediate mobilisation of the joints is still a very logical principle. The operative techniques of this group are used, not routinely, but when closed means are not expected to provide perfect reduction, rigid fixation and above all, immediate mobilisation. Such considerations are now standards in the planning of fracture treatment.

If this concept is accepted for fractures of long bones, it should also be applied to hand fractures. Since the hand has complicated functions, immediate motion to achieve the best possible functional return should be as important as (if not more important than) any other region of the body. If, on the other hand, mobility and functional restoration are not achieved, stiffness of the hand would be disastrous.

Hand fractures are frequent emergencies treated at the accident and emergency departments. As pure Hand Units are rare, such fractures are usually handled by inexperienced physicians. Aligning the fractures after reduction is easily achieved using external splintage or simply K-wire fixation. However, such procedures do not allow immediate finger mobilisation since the fixation which they provide is not rigid. They are often guilty of producing post-operative deformities and finger stiffness in spite of their popularity.

Operative treatment using more sophisticated implants, on the other hand, demands higher skill. Open fixation of hand fractures may therefore not yield the expected outcome of rigid fixation and may not allow immediate mobilisation.

This dilemma of operative versus nonoperative treatment clearly illustrates the difficulties involved in the choice of approach. It is true that operative fixation has much to offer, but if after operative fixation of a hand fracture mobilisation still cannot be started immediately, the surgery may have caused more harm than good. The choice of operative treatment therefore depends on the surgeon's competence in achieving rigid fixation which can allow immediate mobilisation.

References

1. Strickland JW, Steichen JB, Kleinman WB, Flynn N (1982) Factors influencing digital performance after phalangeal fracture. In: Strickland JW, Steichen JB (eds) Difficult problems in hand surgery. Mosby, St Louis, pp 126–139
2. Barton NJ (1988) Complications. In: Barton NJ (ed) Fractures of the hand and wrist. Churchill Livingstone, Edinburgh, pp 319–342
3. Pun WK, Chow S, So YC, Luk KDK, Ip FK, Chan KC, Ngai WK, Crosby C, Ng C (1989) A prospective study on 284 digital fractures of the hand. J Hand Surg [Am] 14(3):474–481
4. Wright TA (1968) Early mobilisation of the metacarpals and phalanges. Can J Surg 11:491–498
5. Widgerow AD, Edinburg M, Biddulph SL (1987) An analysis of proximal phalangeal fractures. J Hand Surg [Am] 12(1):134
6. Melone CP (1986) Rigid fixation of phalangeal and metacarpal fractures. Orthop Clin North Am 17(3):421–435
7. James JIP (1962) Fractures of the proximal and middle phalanges of the finger. Acta Orthop Scand 32:401–420
8. Barton NJ (1984) Fractures of the hand. J Bone Joint Surg [Br] 66(2):159
9. Belsole R (1980) Physiological fixation of displaced and unstable fracture of the hand. Orthop Clin North Am 11:393
10. Black D, Mann RJ, Constine R, Daniels AU (1985) Comparison of internal fixation techniques in metacarpal fractures. J Hand Surg [Am] 10:466
11. Mann RJ, Black D, Constine R, Daniels AU (1985) A quantitative comparison of metacarpal fracture stability with five different methods of internal fixation. J Hand Surg [Am] 10:1024
12. Hung LK, So WS, Leung PC (1989) Combined intramedullary Kirschner wire and intra-osseores wire loop for fixation of finger fractures. J Hand Surg [Br] 14(2):171
13. Massengill JB, Alexander H, Langrana N, Mylod A (1982) A phalangeal fracture model – quantitative analysis of rigidity and failure. J Hand Surg 7(3):264
14. Rayhack JM, Belsole RJ, Skelton WH (1984) A strain-recording model: analysis of transverse osteotomy fixation in small bones. J Hand Surg [Am] 9(3):383
15. Vanik RK, Weber RC, Matcloub HS, Sanger JR, Gingrass RP (1984) The comparative strengths of internal fixation techniques. J Hand Surg [Am] 9(2):216
16. Viegas SF, Ferren EL, Self J, Tencer AF (1988) Comparative mechanical properties of various Kirschner wire configurations in transverse and oblique phalangeal fractures. J Hand Surg [Am] 13(2):246
17. Fyfe IS, Mason S (1979) The mechanical stability of internal fixation of fractured phalanges. Hand 11(1):50
18. Stuchin SA, Kummer FJ (1984) Stiffness of small bone external fixation methods: an experimental study. J Hand Surg [Am] 9:718
19. Black D, Mann RJ, Constine R, Daniels AU (1985) Comparison of internal fixation techniques in metacarpal fractures. J Hand Surg [Am] 10(4):466
20. Alexander H, Langrana N, Massengill JB, Weiss AB (1981) Development of new methods for phalangeal fracture fixation. J Biomech 14:377
21. Heim U, Pfeiffer KM (1982) Small fragment set manual. Springer, Berlin Heidelberg New York
22. Steel WM (1978) The AO small fragment set in hand fractures. Hand 10:246
23. Simonetta C (1970) The use of AO plates in the hand. Hand 2:43
24. Dabezies EJ, Schutte JP (1986) Fixation of metacarpal and phalangeal fractures with minature plates and screws. J Hand Surg [Am] 11(2):283
25. Fambrough RA, Green DP (1979) Tendon rupture as a complication of screw fixation in fracture in the hand. A case report. J Bone Joint Surg [Am] 61(5):781

26. Stern PJ, Wieser MJ, Reilly DG (1987) Complications of plate fixation in the hand skeleton. Clin Orthop 214:59
27. Mullingan PJ (1988) Comminuted fractures. In: Barton NJ (ed) Fractures of the hand and wrist. Churchill Livingstone, Edinburgh, pp 74–86
28. Segmuller G (1988) Severe fractures, including those with loss of bone. In: Barton NJ (ed) Fractures of the hand and wrist. Churchill Livingstone, Edinburgh, pp 173–190
29. Hogh J, Jensen PO (1982) Compression-arthrodesis of finger joints using Kirschner wires and cerclage. Hand 14(2):149
30. Lister G (1978) Intra-osseous wiring of the digital skeleton. J Hand Surg 3(5):427
31. Vom Seal FH (1953) Intramedullary fixation in fractures of the hand and fingers. J Bone Joint Surg [Am] 35:5
32. Leung PC (1981) Use of intramedullary bone peg in digital replantations, revasculaization and toe-transfers. J Hand Surg 6(3):281
33. Lewis RC, Nordyke M, Duncan K (1987) Expandable intramedullary device for treatment of fractures in the hand. Clin Orthop 214:85
34. Grundberg AB (1981) Intramedullary fixation for fractures of the hand. J Hand Surg 6(6):568
35. Joshi BB (1976) Percutaneous internal fixation of fracture of the proximal phalanges. Hand 8:86
36. Belsky MR, Eaton RG (1988) Fractures of the shafts of the phalanges: percutaneous wire fixation. In: Barton NJ (ed) Fractures of the hand and wrist. Churchill Livingstone, Edinburgh, pp 41–46
37. Edwards GS, O'Brien ET, Heckman MM (1982) Retrograde cross-pinning of transverse metacarpal and phalangeal fractures. Hand 14(2):141
38. Hastings H II (1988) Open fractures and those with soft-tissue damage: treatment by external fixation. In: Barton NJ (ed) Fractures of the hand and wrist. Churchill Livingstone, Edinburgh, pp 145–172
39. Allieu Y (1985) External fixation in osteoarticular fracture of the hand. In: Tubiana R (ed) The hand, vol 2. Saunders, Philadelphia, p 525
40. Mulligan PJ, Scott MM (1985) Multiple compound comminuted phalangeal fractures. In: Tubiana R (ed) The hand, vol 2. Saunders, Philadelphia, pp 801–805
41. Riggs GA, Gooney WP (1983) External fixation of complex hand and wrist fractures. J Trauma 23:332
42. Rousso M (1985) Multipurpose unilateral external fixator for hand surgery. In: Tubiana R (ed) The hand, vol 2. Saunders, Philadelphia, p 550
43. Burny F, Moermans JP, Quintin J (1980) Use of minifixator in hand surgery. Acta Orthop Belg 46:251
44. Jenkin E (1983) The treatment of intra-articular metacarpal and phalangeal fractures with the small external fixation device. Handchirurgie 15:198
45. Freeland AE (1987) External fixation for skeletal stabilization of severe open fractures of the hand. Clin Orthop 214:93
46. Shehadi SI (1991) External fixation of metacarpal and phalangeal fractures. J Hand Surg [Am] 16:544
47. Barton N (1986) Conservative treatment of articular fractures in the hand. J Hand Surg [Am] 14:386
48. Fitzgerald JAW, Khan MA (1984) The conservative management of fractures of the shafts of the phalanges of the fingers by combined traction-splintage. J Hand Surg [Br] 9:303
49. Schenck RR (1986) Dynamic traction and early passive movement for fracture of the proximal phalangeal joint. J Hand Surg [Am] 11:850
50. Fahmy NRM (1990) The stockport serpentine spring system for the treatment of displaced comminuted intra-articular phalangeal fractures. J Hand Surg [Br] 15:303

51. Weber SC, Chapman MW (1984) Adhesives in orthopaedic surgery. A review of the literature and in-vitro bonding strengths of bone bonding agents. Clin Orthop 191:249
52. Scapinelli R (1990) Treatment of fractures of the humeral capitellum using fibrin sealant. Arch Orthop Trauma Surg 109:235
53. Bostrom OM (1991) Absorbable implants for the fixation of fractures (current concepts review). J Bone Joint Surg [Am] 73:148
54. McCarthy JA, Lesker PA, Peterson WW, Manske PR (1986) Continuous passive motion as an adjunct therapy for tenolysis. J Hand Surg [Br] 11:88
55. Bunker TD, Potter B, Barton NJ (1989) Continuous passive motion following flexor tendon repair. J Hand Surg [Br] 14:406
56. Ellis PR, Hanna D, Tsai TM (1991) Vascularised single toe joint transfer to the hand. J Hand Surg [Am] 16:160
57. Ellis PR, Tsai TM (1989) Management of the traumatised joint of the finger. Clin Plast Surg 16(3):457
58. Foucher G (1988) Vascularized joint transfers. In: Green DP (ed) Operative hand surgery, 2nd edn. Churchill Livingstone, New York, pp 1271–1293
59. Strickland JW (1982) A rationale for digital salvage. In: Strickland JW, Steichen JB (eds) Difficult problems in hand surgery. Mosby, St Louis, pp 243–252
60. Blomgren I, Blomqvist G, Ejeskar A, Fogdestam I, Volkman R, Edshage S (1988) Hand function after replantation or revascularisation of upper extremity injuries. Scand J Plast Reconstr Surg 22:93
61. Jones JM, Schenck RR, Chesney RB (1982) Digital replantation and amputation, comparison of function. J Hand Surg 7:183
62. Steichen JB, Idler RS (1986) Results of central ray resection without bony transposition. J Hand Surg [Am] 11:466
63. DeBoer A, Robinson PH (1989) Ray transposition by intercarpal osteotomy after loss of the fourth digit. J Hand Surg [Am] 14(2):379
64. Chow SP, Pun WK, So YC, Luk KDK, Chui Ky, Ng KH, Ng C, Crosby C (1991) A proplective study of 245 open digital fractures of the hand. J Hand Surg [Br] 16:137
65. McLain RF, Steyers C, Stoddard M (1991) Infections in open fractures of the hand. J Hand Surg [Am] 16:108
66. Swanson TV, Szabo RM, Anderson DD (1991) Open hand fractures: prognosis and classification. J Hand Surg [Am] 16(1):101
67. Nunley JA, Goldner RD, Urbaniak JR (1987) Skeletal fixation in digital replantation. Use of the "H" plate. Clin Orthop 214:66
68. Hung LK, Chang A, Chang J, Tsang A, Leung PC (1990) Early controlled active mobilisation with dynamic splintage for treatment of extensor tendon injuries. J Hand Surg [Am] 14:251
69. Seymour N (1966) Juxta-epihypeal fracture of the terminal phalanx of the finger. J Bone Joint Surg [Br] 48:347
70. DaCruz DJ, Slade RJ, Malone W (1988) Fractures of the distal phalanges. J Hand Surg [Br] 13:350
71. Smith FL, Rider DL (1935) A study of the healing of one hundred consecutive phalangeal fractures. J Bone Joint Surg 17:91
72. Read L (1982) Nonunion in a fracture of the shaft of the distal phalanx. Hand 14:85
73. Bildulph SL (1988) Fingertip fractures. In: Barton NJ (ed) Fractures of the hand and wrist. Churchill Livingstone, Edinburgh, pp 4–9
74. Hamas R, Horrell E, Pierret GP (1978) Treatment of Mallet finger due to intra-articular fracture of the distal phalanx. J Hand Surg 3:363
75. James JIP (1988) Fractures of the shafts of the phalanges: conservative treatment. In: Barton NJ (ed) Fractures of the hand and wrist. Churchill Livingstone, Edinburgh, pp 22–31

76. Thomine JM, Milliez PY (1988) Fractures of the shafts of the phalanges: treatment by functional bracing. In: Barton NJ (ed) Fractures of the hand and wrist. Churchill Livingstone, Edinburgh, pp 32–40
77. Kutz JE, Ruff ME (1988) Fractures of the shafts of the phalanges: open reduction and internal fixation. In: Barton NJ (ed) Fractures of the hand and wrist. Churchill Livingstone, Edinburgh, pp 47–54
78. Diwaker HN, Stothard J (1986) The role of internal fixation in closed fractures of the proximal phalanges and metacarpals in adults. J Hand Surg [Br] 11:1103
79. Crawford GP (1976) Screw fixation for certain fractures of the phalanges and metacarpals. J Bone Joint Surg [Am] 58:487
80. Ford DJ, El-Hadidi S, Lunn PG, Burke FD (1987) Fractures of the phalanges: results of internal fixation using 1.5 mm and 2 mm AO screws. J Hand Surg [Br] 12:28
81. Ikuta Y, Tsuge K (1974) Micro-bolts and microscrews for fixation of small bones in the hand. Hand 6:261
82. Pun WK, Chow SP, So YC, Luk KDK, Ngai WK, Ip FK, Peng WH, NG C, Crosby C (1991) Unstable phalangeal fractures: treatment by AO screw and plate fixation. J Hand Surg [Am] 16:113
83. Steel WM (1988) Articular fractures. In: Barton NJ (ed) Fractures of the hand and wrist. Churchill Livingstone, Edinburgh, pp 55–73
84. Jupiter JB, Sheppard JE (1987) Tension wire fixation of avulsion fractures in the hand. Clin Orthop 214:113
85. Agee JM (1987) Unstable fracture dislocations of the proximal interphalangeal joint. Clin Orthop 214:101
86. Robertson RC, Cawley JJ, Faris AM (1946) Treatment of fracture dislocation of the interphalangeal joints of the hand. J Bone Joint Surg [Am] 28:68
87. McElfresh EC, Dobyns JH, O'Brien ET (1972) Management of fracture dislocation of the proximal interphalangeal joint by extension-block splinting. J Bone Joint Surg [Am] 54:1705
88. O'Dwyer FG, Quinton DN (1990) Early mobilisation of acute middle slip injuries. J Hand Surg [Br] 15:404
89. Buchler U, Fischer T (1987) Use of a minicondylar plate for metacarpal and phalangeal periarticular injuries. Clin Orthop 214:53
90. McElfresoh EC (1988) Metacarpal head fractures. In: Barton NJ (ed) Fractures of the hand and wrist. Churchill Livingstone, Edinburgh, pp 88–107
91. McElfresh EC, Dobyns JH (1983) Intra-articular metacarpal head fractures. J Hand Surg 8:383
92. Lamb DW (1988) Fractures of the neck and shaft of the metacarpals. In: Barton NJ (ed) Fractures of the hand and wrist. Churchill Livingstone, Edinburgh, pp 108–119
93. Ford DJ, EL-Hadidi S, Lunn PG, Burke FD (1987) Fractures of the metacarpals: treatment by AO screw and plate fixation. J Hand Surg [Br] 12:34
94. Hastings H (1987) Unstable metacarpal and phalangeal fracture treatment with screw and plates. Clin Orthop 214:37
95. Dobyns JH (1988) Fractures and dislocations at the base of the metacarpals. In: Barton NJ (ed) Fractures of the hand and wrist. Churchill Livingstone, Edinburgh, pp 120–134
96. Howard FM (1987) Fractures of the basal joint of the thumb. Clin Orthop 220:46
97. Foster RJ, Hastings H (1987) Treatment of Bennett, Rolando, and vertical intra-articular trapezial fractures. Clin Orthop 214:121
98. Buterbaugh GA, Palmer AK (1988) Other carpal fractures. In: Barton NJ (ed) Fractures of the hand and wrist. Churchill Livingstone, Edinburgh, pp 236–250
99. Dickson RA (1988) Scaphoid fractures: conservative management. In: Barton NJ (ed) Fractures of the hand and wrist. Churchill Livingstone, Edinburgh, pp 210–219

100. Gellman H, Caputo RJ, Carter V, Aboulafia A, McKay M (1989) Comparison of short and long thumb spica casts for nondisplaced fractures of the carpal scaphoid. J Bone Joint Surg [Am] 71:354
101. Dias JJ, Brenkel IJ, Finlay DBL (1989) Patterns of union in fractures of the waist of the scaphoid. J Bone Joint Surg [Br] 71:307
102. Herbert TJ (1988) Scaphoid fractures: operative treatment. In: Barton NJ (ed) Fractures of the hand and wrist. Churchill Livingstone, Edinburgh, pp 220–235
103. Radford PJ, Mathewson MH, Meggitt BF (1990) The Herbert screw for delayed and nonunion of scaphoid fractures: a review of fifty cases. J Hand Surg [Br] 15:455
104. Chun S, Wicks BP, Meyerdierks E, Werner F, Mosher JF (1990) Two modifications for insertion of the herbert screw in the fractured scaphoid. J Hand Surg [Am] 15:669
105. Toh S, Harata S, Nakamura R, Inoue S, Tsubo K (1991) The treatment of scaphoid fracture using free hand insertion of Herbert screw. International Symposium on the Wrist, March 6–8, Nagoya
106. Barton NJ (1979) Fractures of the phalanges of the hand in children. Hand 11(2):134
107. Wood VE (1976) Fractures of the hand in children. Orthop Clin North Am 7:527
108. Hastings H, Simmons BP (1984) Hand fractures in children. Clin Orthop 188:120
109. Green DP (1977) Hand injuries in children. Paediatr Clin North Am 24:903
110. Leonard MH, Dubravcik P (1970) Management of fractured fingers in the child. Clin Orthop 73:160
111. O'Brien ET (1984) Fracture of the hand and wrist region. In: Rockwood CA, Wilkins KE, King RE (eds) Fractures in children. Lippincott, Philadelphia, pp 229–300
112. Weiland AJ, White GM, Moore JR (1988) Epiphyseal fractures. In: Barton NJ (ed) Fractures of the hand and wrist. Churchill Livingstone, Edinburgh, pp 10–21
113. Bora FW, Ignatius P, Nissenbaum M (1976) The treatment of epiphyseal fractures of the hand. J Bone Joint Surg [Am] 58:286
114. Harkess JW (1975) Principles of fractures and dislocations. In: Rockwood CA, Green DP (eds) Fractures, vol 1. Lippincott, Philadelphia, p 4

9 Fractures of the Distal Radius and Ulna

K.S. Leung and P.C. Leung

Introduction

Fractures of the distal radius and ulna are common fractures. The classical description of these fractures by Abraham Colles has remained unchanged for the past 180 years [1]. However, what would no longer find agreement today is his comment on treatment results for these fractures: "One consolation only remains, that the limb will at some remote period again enjoy perfect freedom in all it motions, and be completely exempt from pain: the deformity, however, will remain undiminished through life." Indeed, distal radius fractures have previously been accepted as a simple and easy fracture for treatment. Indeed, almost every intern and junior trainee in orthopaedics and traumatology departments starts his professional career by treating these presumably simple and easy fractures. Times have changed, and distal radial fractures are now approached with a better understanding of the pathoanatomy and pathomechanics involved and with an improvement in the treatment modalities. These fractures are classified today not only into volar Barton's fracture-dislocation, volar Smith's fracture and Chauffeur's radial styloid fracture (the classical Colles' fractures), but intra-articular fractures of the distal radius, fracture dislocation of the distal radio-ulnar joint and ulnar wrist fibro-cartilage complex injuries are also identified as distinct entities in the management of the complex injury problems around this region. As a result, more aggressive approaches are taken to recognise and treat these fractures. The oversimplified consideration that all fractures affecting the distal radius may be treated as the classical Colles' fracture may be criticised as negligence since significant functional losses so very often result.

Distal Radial Fractures

Pathoanatomy and Pathomechanics

The most common mechanism of injury is a fall on the outstretched hand. The force that produces the fracture is transmitted from the palm to the distal radius with the wrist in dorsiflexion. The characteristic fracture pattern, with the sharp and clear-cut fracture edges on the palmar side of the distal radial metaphysis and various degrees of comminution in the dorsal cortex, indicates that the volar cortex failed under tension. The fracture propagates dorsally, where the cortex failed under compressive force [2]. Comminution in the dorsal cortex is common because considerably larger force is absorbed and then dissipated when bone fails under compression. The relatively thin dorsal cortex also accounts for the comminution. The fractures are therefore unstable in the dorsal direction. Fracture under compression also leads to impaction of the cancellous bone in the metaphysis. This results in further loss of trabeculae, and after the fracture is reduced, a considerable gap is produced. It is therefore common to see fracture collapse even after satisfactory reduction and immobilisation. The residual deformities in the form of shortening, radial displacement and dorsal angulation are inevitable. The degree of instability of the fracture is determined by the fracture line orientation, the degree of initial displacement and the degree of comminution.

With the increasing incidence of high-energy injuries, distal radial fractures are no longer confined to the elderly. When they occur in young and active individuals, extensive comminutions and intra-articular involvements are common among these fractures. The final results of treating these fractures are not only affected by the extreme instability; the long-term effect of intra-articular fractures is reflected in protracted weakness of the wrists, stiffness and early post-traumatic arthrosis. Treatment for this group of fractures is extremely difficult [3–9].

Classifications

Several attempts have been made to classify the distal radial fractures. The following classification put forward by Frykman in 1967 [10] is the most widely accepted [11]:

   I. Extra-articular, no fracture of ulna
  II. Extra-articular, fracture of ulna
 III. Intra-articular radio-carpal, no fracture of ulna
 IV. Intra-articular radio-carpal, fracture of ulna
  V. Intra-articular radio-ulnar, no fracture of ulna
 VI. Intra-articular radio-ulnar, fracture of ulna
VII. Intra-articular radio-carpal and radio-ulnar, no fracture of ulna
VIII. Intra-articular radio-carpal and radio-ulnar, fracture of ulna

This classification is based on the extent of involvement of the radio-carpal joint and the distal radio-ulnar joint. It also takes into account the involvement of fractures in the ulnar styloid, which indicates a destabilising condition of the triangular fibro-cartilage complex. However, this classification does not take into consideration the initial degree of comminution and displacement of the fractures. One must therefore be careful in assessing the results of any treatment modalities for these very complex fractures. Nevertheless, Frykman's classification is the most widely accepted and is still pable to address the unsolved problems of the fracture-dislocation involving the ulnar wrist complex.

Apart from the patterns of the distal radial fractures, isolated articular involvement should also be considered in the classification. These fractures include the radial styloid fracture involving the scaphoid fossa, the die punch fracture of the lunate fossa and the fracture involving the sigmoid fossa.

The prognosis of distal radial fractures certainly depends on the fracture pattern, initial displacement, comminutions and extent of intra-articular involvement. The other factors of prognostic importance include the results of reductions. The restoration of the radial length and the volar angle have also proven to be important factors in determining the prognosis after treatment [12–16].

Treatment of Comminuted Distal Radial Fractures

While most of noncomminuted extra-articular fractures of the distal radius can be treated with closed manipulation and casting, with excellent anatomical and functional results, comminuted fractures represent a completely different category because of the degree of instability and intra-articular involvement. To tackle these problems different approaches have been taken to reestablish the stability and restore the congruity of articular surfaces. The technique introduced by Bohler in 1929 using pin and plaster to treat these fractures was the first attempt to provide stability [17]. While the length of the radius can be satisfactorily maintained, the volar tilt and intra-articular fragments remain unreduced. Complications were common with the use of prolonged casting and pins [4,8,18–22]. This technique also lacks versatility because adjustment of the cast and pins is difficult. The reoperation rate was as high as 16%.

Use of the external fixator in the treatment of these unstable fractures represents another approach to providing immediate stability. The external fixator, if properly applied, can certainly provide the best stability for these fractures [23–28]. Maintenance of the reduction depends on the intact soft tissues, particularly the ligaments around the wrists, by the principle of ligamentotaxis. This technique, however, is critizised for failing to reduce the palmar tilt of the comminuted fragments [6], failing to reduce the depressed intra-articular fragments, particularly the die punch fragments [29], and the complications resulting from prolonged application [7]. In these comminuted fractures most workers recommend 8–12 weeks of external fixation before considerable healing and stability is regained [4,23,25,30]. Common complications of prolonged immobilisations include stiffness, Sudek's dystrophy, pin tract infection and loosening. As a result, modification of the external fixator to allow control motion during the initial period of fixation has been introduced. The Clyburn external fixator [31] and recently the Pennig fixator [32] are typical examples. One of the unsolved problems is the difficulty in exactly aligning the axis of the flexion and extension of the radiocarpal joint during application of these external fixators. Failure results in the early loss of volar tilt due to the common dorsal cortex comminutions in these fractures. Furthermore, the duration of application of the external fixator is not shortened. The other approach is to limit the external fixation to the distal radius without crossing the wrist joint [33]. This may be possible in selected cases with moderate comminutions.

The problems of displaced intra-articular fractures remain unsolved with the use of the external fixator. Many advocate the combined use of the external fixator and limited open reduction and fixation of the intra-articular fregments with implants such as Kirschner wires, plates and screws. It is extremely difficult, however, if not impossible to fix the numerous tiny osteochondral fragments with implants. Furthermore open reduction may lead to a loss of the effect of ligamentotaxis due the surgical trauma to the soft tissue around the wrist.

Since 1987 we have been using the concept of ligamentotaxis and primary bone grafting in treating all of these fractures [34]. The treatment protocol also includes use of the functional brace, which allows the wrist flexion and not extension in the latter half of the treatment. The principle of such combinations is the full exploitation of the stability provided by the external

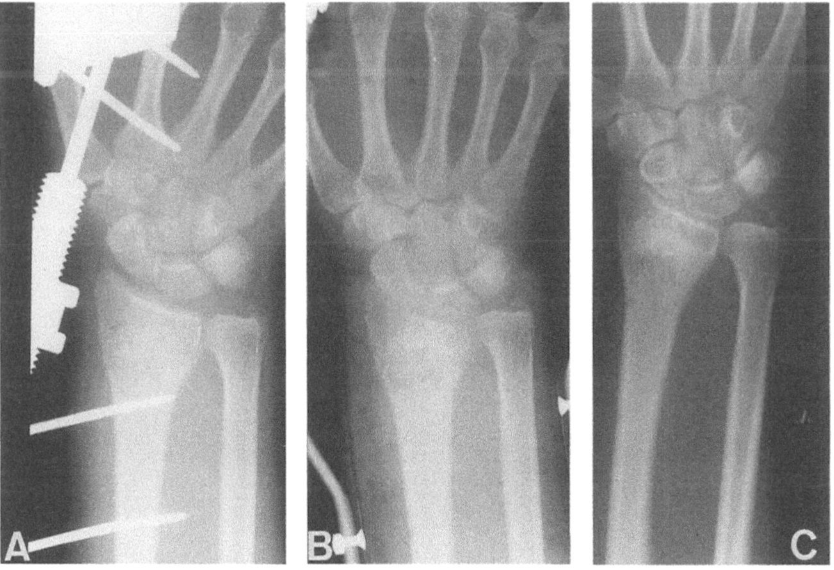

Fig. 1A–C. Serial X-ray films of a comminuted distal radial fractures treated by ligamentotaxis, bone graft and functional bracing. **A** Fracture is well reduced with the external fixator. Bone graft is packed into the fracture site. **B** Fracture alignment maintained with the short-arm brace. **C** Fracture well consolidated after 6 months fixator, while cancellous bone graft not only provides early mechanical stability [34] but also helps to reduce and support the depressed intra-articular fragments and enhance fracture healing (Fig. 1). Biomechanical tests carried out on the cadaveric model show a four-fold increase in the compression strength in fractures of the distal radius which were reduced and packed with cancellous bone chips. The biological effects of the autogenous bone graft in healing of fractures are also well established. This treatment protocol thus shortens the period of external fixator application dramatically and helps to decrease the numerous complications resulting from the prolonged use of the external fixators, such as pin tract infection and pin loosening. Use of the functional bracing helps to restore early motion and facilitate rehabilitations.

Operation Technique

The operation is simple and relatively atraumatic in that no major dissections are required. With the patient under general anaesthesia, the external fixator is constructed across the wrist. We have found the Hoffmann external fixator ("small C") configuration very suitable for this purpose. The 3-mm half pins are inserted with limited exposure. Predrilling with 2.5-mm drill bit is recommended even with the self-tapping 3-mm half pins. Predrilling ensures a more accurate positioning of the pin in the bone and avoids the complications caused by multiple attempts at insertion with the self-tapping half pins. For those pins purchasing the second metacarpal (Fig. 2), the proximal one should be purchasing the base of the second and third metacarpals while the distal should purchase as distal as possible. The first dorsal interosseus and the extensor tendon of the index finger should be free from the pins. For the half pins in the radius, the distal pin should be at least 5 cm from the tip of the radial styloid to avoid the superficial branch of the sensory branch of the radial nerve [25]. The pins are connected with the small ball joint and the 5-mm adjustable rod. The fracture is then manipulated and reduced under X-ray control. All the joints in the external fixator are tightened, and the reduction is completed with distraction by turning the knob on the adjustable rod.

While the external fixator is being constructed, another surgeon harvests the cancellous graft from the opposite iliac crest with a small wound. The two tables of the ilium are split, and only the cancellous bone is removed. The wound can usually be closed without drainage. With the popularisation of artificial bone substitutes, there is no reason why these cannot be used as graft in future.

A small longitudinal incision is made on the dorsum of the distal radius. The fracture site is approached by splitting the soft tissue transversely. Care should be taken to preserve all the longitudinal structures so that the effect of ligamentotaxis is not affected. The cancellous grafts are packed into the fracture site through the dorsal comminutions. The graft should be tightly

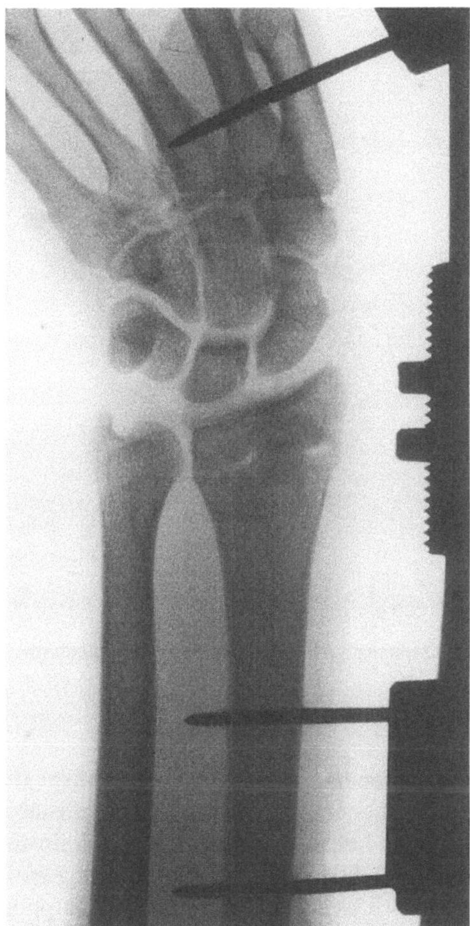

Fig. 2. Comminuted fracture of the distal radius treated with ligamentotaxis. Note the purchase of the proximal pin in the distal clamp onto the base of the second and third metacarpals

packed towards the distal fragment with the aim of aligning the comminuted fragments to reform the smooth articular surface. In most cases, a substantial amount of graft must be used to fill the space created after reduction of the fractures. The wound is then closed without drainage.

Postoperatively, the injured limb is elevated with elastic bandage for 48 h to decrease swelling. Thereafter active and passive exercises are started. Special attention is given to rotation of the forearm and to finger movements. The patient is then discharged with the instructions for pin tract care and physiotherapy programme. At the end of 3 weeks, the external fixator is removed in the clinic, and a forearm brace is applied. The brace allows wrist flexion and blocks extension at neutral wrist position (Fig. 3). More energetic exercise is started. The brace is removed at the end of 6 weeks after the operation. Free mobilisation and strengthening exercise are allowed.

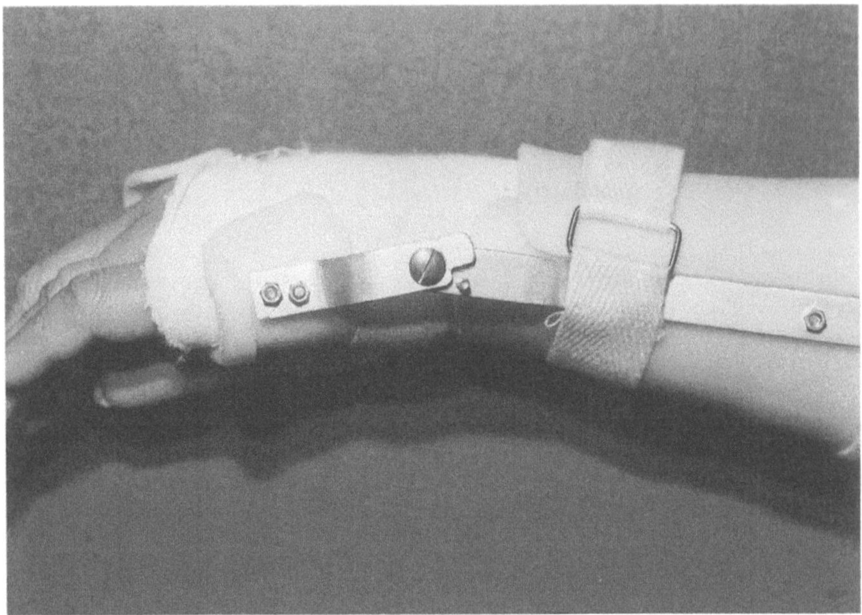

Fig. 3. Short-arm brace to control the extension of the wrist with the mechanical block in the hinge

The results of treating comminuted distal radial fractures confirm the effectiveness of the external fixator in the management of these unstable fractures. The principle of ligamentotaxis helps to reduce and maintain the fractures. The addition of cancellous graft fills the bone gap resulting from the comminuted injury since it works both as mechanical expansile support and as a biological spacer. It significantly shortens the duration of external fixation. The functional return of the wrist is very satisfactory. The unique treatment with the addition of primary cancellous graft in all these fractures is the key to good results. As in all metaphyseal fractures, impaction of the cancellous bone during injuries is common. The relative bone loss is even more obvious in high-energy injuries which cause marked impaction and comminutions. Without the addition of the bone graft, most authors recommend the external fixator to be kept for 8–12 weeks. This long period of application leads to many complications. However, the iliac incision for autogenous bone graft is additional trauma and induces another potential complication. The availability of bone substitutes such as tricalcium phosphates, hydroxyapatite and coral should be seriously considered as alternatives. The physical properties of the granule form are particularly suitable for this purpose. The effect of these substitutes is currently under investigation.

In long-term follow-up of these groups of patients [35] minimal arthritic changes have been detected in the radiocarpal joint. Most patients enjoy

Table 1. Comparative results in the treatment of comminuted distal radial fractures by various methods

	Gartland and Werley [56]	Cole and Obletz [21]	Sarmiento et al. [57]	Conney et al. [4]	Knirk and Jupiter [29]	Leung et al. [34]
n	60	33	44	60		4354
Mean age (years)	53	18–81	40s	63	27.6	40.9
Percentage intraarticular	88	NA	100	88	100	96.4
Method	Plaster cast	Pins and plaster	Functional brace	External fixator	Varied	Fixator and brace
Average follow-up (years)	1.5	1.5–5.0	0.5	2.4	6.7	2.65
Percentage arthritis	22	NA	NA	2	65	9.2
Percentage finger stiffness	18	0	12	0	0	0
Final result (%)						
Excellent	22	51	42	32	26	3
	>69	>84	>81	>87	>61	>90.4
Good	47	43	39	55	35	57.4
Fair	28	6	18	13	33	9.6
Poor	3	0	0	0	6	0

NA, not applicable.

pain-free and functional wrists. Assessment with the demerit point system of Gartland and Werley shows 90.4% good and 9.6% fair results. The results are very comparable with other series (Table 1). Arthritic changes and joint incongruity are rare. However, the residual problems of the ulnar wrist complex are obvious in patients with Frykman's type VI and VIII fractures. The intraoperative finding of displacement of the fracture in the distal radio-ulnar joint during pronation (Fig. 4) prompted us to immobilise these fractures by adding an accessory component to the external fixator (Fig. 5). With two additional half pins inserted into the shaft of the ulna, a cross-bar can be connected to the external fixator on the radius. This ensures that the volar ligaments of the distal radio-ulnar joint are rendered taut when the forearm is supinated and helps to reduce the fractures in the distal radio-ulnar joint. After the radial fractures are reduced and immobilised with the external fixator, the forearm is kept supinated, and the additional pins are introduced into the ulna for construction of the cross-bar to immobilise the forearm. Again, the external fixator is kept for 3 weeks. The wrist and forearm are then maintained in an long-arm brace which allows wrist flexion and forearm in supination. Graduated supination and pronation is allowed by using a specially designed lock (Fig. 6). The recognition of problems in treating Frykman VI and VIII fractures has led to other designs to tackle these controversial fractures [32,35].

The use of distraction and external fixator is not totally successful in the treatment of fractures with volar comminution and instability due the

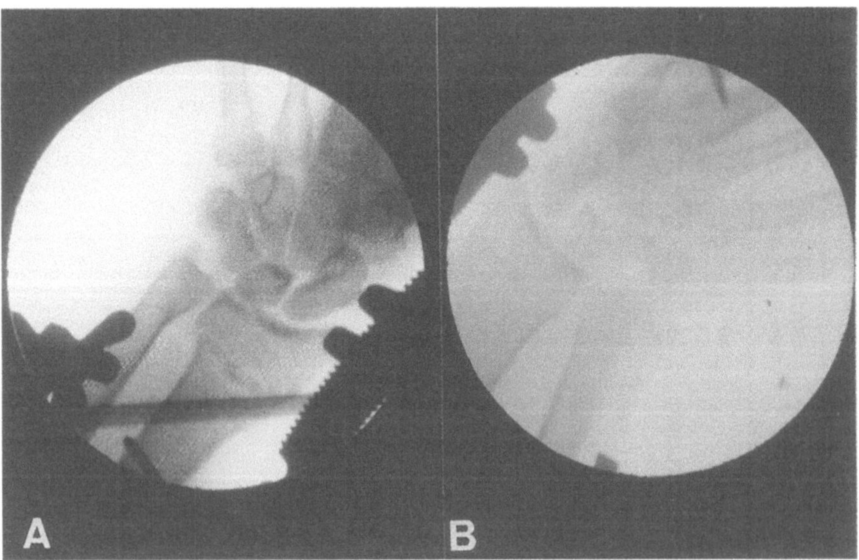

Fig. 4A–B. Intraoperative radiological screening of the distal radial fracture. **A** In pronated position, the distal radio-ulnar joint is unreduced. **B** In supinated position, the distal radio-ulnar joint is reduced

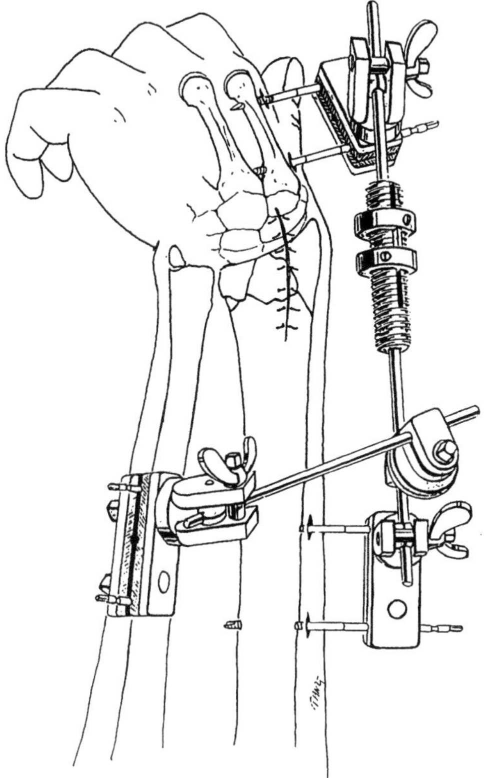

Fig. 5. Schematic drawing of the configuration of the external fixator used in the ligamentotaxis and control of forearm rotational movement

difficulty in realigning the floating fragments on the volar side of the fracture. Therefore for comminuted fractures and large volar fragments it is recommended to put the graft through the volar side. With this approach the large volar fragment can be reduced satisfactorily and the bone gaps effectively filled. The fixation may have to be augmented with Kirschner wires either temporarily during the operative procedures or throughout the external fixator period.

With the exception of elderly patients (over 65) who do not require active use of their wrists, we find this method of treatment should be recommended. We accept that in the best hands multiple options and combination of treatment protocols could be recommended. Nevertheless, the use of plates and screws in this region for communicated fracture is extremely demanding technically, and the amount of tissue trauma could leave tremendous problems of stiffness. The use of external fixator alone is much easier, but the empty gaps within the comminution tend to collapse even after long periods of distraction, not to speak of pin tract infections. Deformities and stiffness are still not uncommon with prolonged external fixator application. The addition of bone grafts maintains the reduction form within

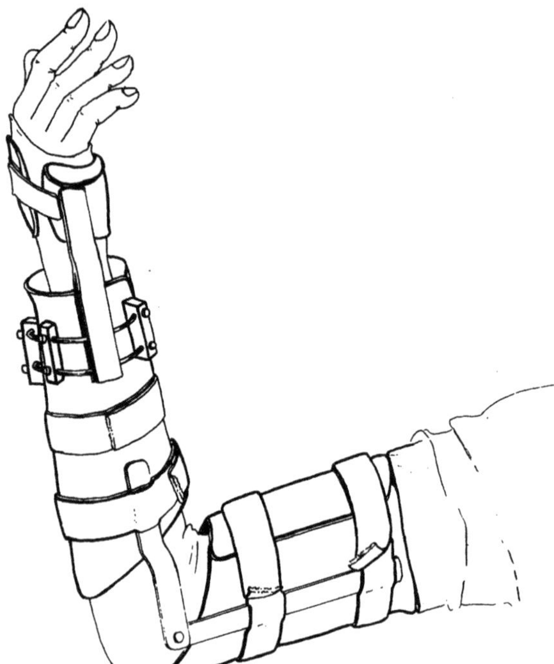

Fig. 6. A long-arm brace to control wrist extension as well as forearm rotation

and significantly minimises the late complication of radial shortening and deformities. The relative simplicity of the operation allows this operation to be performed by even a junior, who requires only very basic training for the application of the external fixator and bone grafting.

The management of other fractures involving the distal radius are less controversial. Volar Barton's fractures are known to be unstable both volarly and proximally. Anatomical reduction should be the aim, but fixation is difficult to achieve and maintain. Most Barton's fractures should be treated with open reduction and internal fixation [36]. The use of a volar T-plate as a antiglide buttressing device restores stability and allows early mobilisation (Fig. 7), which is of prime importance with fractures involving the articular surface. Other fractures involving the isolated articular surface of the distal radius should be treated with the same principles, i.e. those for treating intra-articular fractures in general.

Combined Radial Carpal Fractures

Simultaneous fractures of the distal radius and the scaphoid usually result from severe trauma [37,38]. Distal radial fractures are unstable and com-

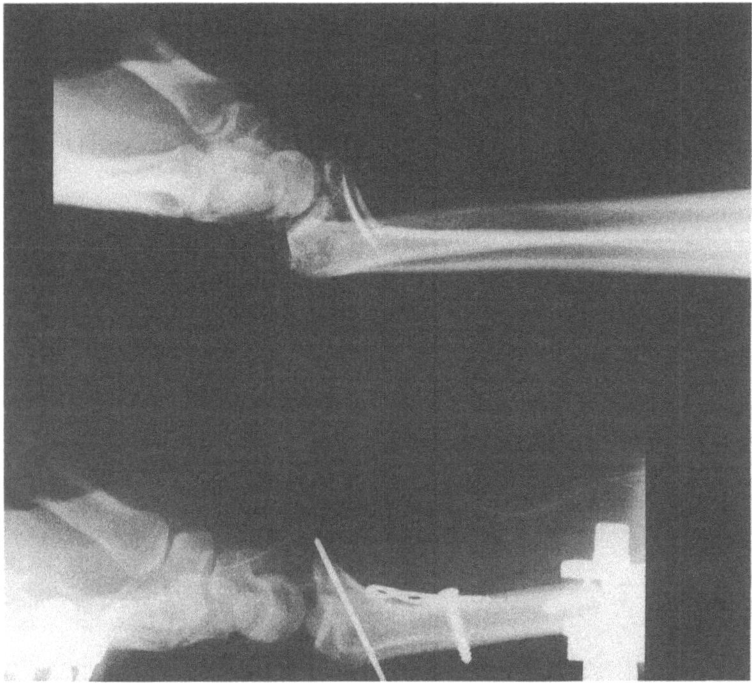

Fig. 7. A comminuted volar Barton's fracture treated with volar buttress plate and external fixator

minuted. Opinions differ concerning the treatment of scaphoid fractures. As in the other unstable distal radial fractures, the external fixator and bone graft should be used for the radial component. The scaphoid fracture should then be treated at the same time with internal fixation. Fixation of the scaphoid not only allows distraction on the distal radius but also facilitate rehabilitation in the later stage. Either a single 4-mm cancellous lag screw or the Herbert screw gives good results [39]. The percutaneous cannulated screw [40], usually through a dorsal approach for fixation of the scaphoid, is another alternative since most scaphoid fractures are minimally displaced. Percutaneous fixation of the scaphoid fracture minimises surgical trauma and thus maximises the effects of ligamentotaxis.

Other, more complicated combined radio-carpal fractures are the result of severe trauma associated invariably with soft tissue injuries. The principle of management should therefore be a combination of open fixation, soft tissue management and infection control with the aim of preserving as much wrist formation as possible. A compromise approach of temporary wrist fusion aiming at early healing and subsequent painless fibrous ankylosis might be desirable in the most devastating damages if proper wrist function is not considered a realistic outlook. A half-hearted, indecisive staged approach to such problems may eventually be harmful.

Injuries of the Distal Ulnar Wrist Complex

The distal ulnar wrist complex is composed of the distal radio-ulnar articulation, triangular fibro-cartilage, ulnar styloid and ulnar collateral ligament. The stability of the distal radio-ulnar joint depends on the volar and dorsal radio-ulnar ligaments. The volar ligament becomes taut when the forearm is supinated and is usually torn when the distal radio-ulnar joint is dislocated. The dorsal ligament is taut when the forearm is in pronated position [41]. The triangular fibro-cartilage is defined as the stabiliser of the distal radio-ulnar joint and the axial load bearing structure on the ulnar side of the wrist [42,43]. It sweeps across the distal surface of the ulnar head during rotational movement of the forearm. The close anatomical proximity and functional integration among these structures lead to the complexity of the injury pattern. Considerable attention has been paid to injuries of the ulnar wrist complex in recent years [43–47]. These injuries may be isolated or combined with distal radius fracture. The association of the distal radial fractures and the distal radio-ulnar complex are discussed in the previous section, and isolated injuries are discussed below. Although the actual significance of the individual involvement of the different components in injury is still controversial, observations have shown that isolated ulnar styloid fracture and distal radio-ulnar joint separation may remain symptom free, whereas the occurrence and complaints about ulnar wrist pain as a result of past injuries have been increasing. Injuries of this region therefore deserve closer scrutiny.

Fracture of the Distal Ulna

Isolated fracture of the ulnar styloid can be at the tip or at the base. Since the triangular fibro-cartilage is attached to the base of the ulnar styloid, the stability of the distal radio-ulnar joint depends on a good reduction of these basal ulnar styloid fractures. Instability of the distal radio-ulnar joint may result if these fractures are not properly treated. Treatment for undisplaced fractures uses a long-arm plaster slab to keep the forearm in supination and mild ulnar deviation. Displaced fractures should be treated with closed or open reduction and joint stabilisation. The technique of using temporary Kirschner wire transfixing the ulna to the radius is a simple and effective means of stabilising the distal radio-ulnar joint (Fig. 8) and hence the styloid process. A similar protocol should be used with the isolated fracture of the ulnar head. With demonstratable instability of the distal radio-ulnar joint, the fracture should be reduced and fixed early with a short one-third tubular plate to achieve early stability.

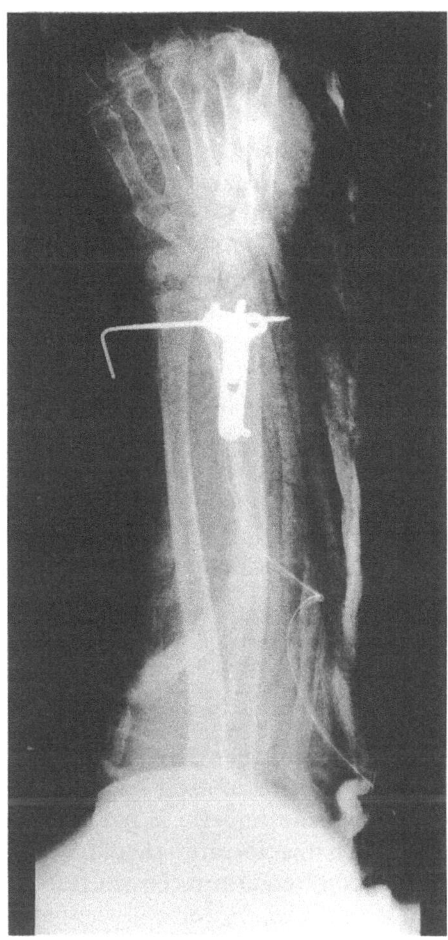

Fig. 8. Fracture of the distal radius with dislocation of the distal radio-ulnar joint. The radial fracture was fixed with T-plate and the distal radio-ulnar joint temporarily with the trans-ulna K-wire

Triangular Fibrocartilage, Complex Damages

With fractures occurring in the distal ulna the association of triangular fibro-cartilage injuries is common. The following classification of the injury pattern based on the anatomy and biomechanics of the distal radio-ulnar joint has been advocated [43]:

A. Central perforation
B. Ulnar avulsion with distal ulnar fracture without distal ulnar fracture
C. Distal avulsion
D. Radial avulsion with sigmoid notch fracture without sigmoid notch fracture

The lesions are thus classified according to anatomical site. Class 1A is central perforation; 1B is avulsion of the complex from the distal ulna either with or without bone; 1C is avulsion from the insertion onto the lunate or triquetrum; and the 1D is avulsion from the distal aspect of the sigmoid notch of the radius. As the meniscus in the knee, the central part of the triangular fibrocartilage complex is avascular. Injury of this part often leads to late symptoms because of the failure of healing. Displaced peripheral injury is often associated with instability of the distal radio-ulnar joint. Arthroscopic evaluation has been advocated to delineate the extent of the injury so that the treatment protocol can be formulated [45,46]. The distal radio-ulnar instability associated with the peripheral lesion can be treated by immobilisation since healing is no problem. Surgical repair may be indicated in persistently displaced complete tear associated with gross instability.

With the advent of arthroscopic surgery interest in arthroscopic examination and treatment through the arthroscope has been mounting. Different modes of acute traumatic tears have been described and arthroscopic repair attempted (Palmer). These new endeavours have been exciting and enlightening; however, it is still doubtful whether complicated repairs are technically feasible. Moreover, the ultimate results of such treatment should await more time for a proper evaluation of the indications and therapeutic approaches.

Dislocation of Distal Radio-Ulnar Joint

The dislocation may be in the volar or dorsal direction. By far the commonest is the dorsal dislocation, in which the volar radio-ulnar ligaments are torn. The dislocation is readily reduced whent he forearm is put into full supination, and this is the position in which the forearm should be immobilised after injury. Ligamental laxity seldom requires reconstruction.

Volar dislocation is much rarer and is produced by forceful supination or direct injury to the dorso-ulnar side of the wrist. It is a mechanism similar to that by which the triangular fibro-cartilage is injured. The reduction is carried out with direct pressure over the ulna volarly and forearm pronation. The forearm is immobilised in pronation for 3 weeks with or without temporary K-pin fixation.

Chronic Distal Radio-Ulnar Subluxation

Less frequently, severe maltreated distal radioulnar joint dislocation is the cause of ulnar wrist pain, and the ulnar head subluxates dorsally on full pronation. Many passive sling procedures have been described [48–51] although they are all technically demanding, and the results are not guaranteed [52–54].

A new technique has been described by our group for the treatment of post-traumatic dislocation of this joint, which produces symptoms of pain and unsightliness [55]. In this technique, the long, distally attached palmaris tendon is used. The tendon is passed through a drill hole at the base of the ulna styloid to the medial side. After wrapping around the medial border of the ulna, it is then passed through another drill hole in the radius at the level of the distal radio-ulnar joint and turned back on the volar and sutured to the tendon on the ulnar side. The long-term clinical results of this technique have been excellent. Its simplicity and the long-term effectiveness in maintaining the tension have made this a useful method.

Conclusion

Straightforward distal radial fractures are simple and easy to treat. Problems of fractures in this region arise when the fractures are grossly unstable, and when they have intra-articular involvements. Our philosophy of anatomical reconstruction followed by stable immobilisation and early motion follows closely the modern principles of fracture treatment principles. In the situation of comminuted intra-articular distal radial fracture, the provision of immediate stability with external fixator distraction, rebuilding the bone stock with primary bone grafts and early functional rehabilitation represent one of the most aggressive treatment protocols for these fractures [9]. The results of this treatment protocol have proven comfortably predictable and satisfactory. All these components of treatment, namely distraction reduction, bone graft gap filling and functional bracing, need to be emphasised equally. Omitting any of the reconstructive procedures would lead to defective functional results. Nevertheless, in terms of bone healing and prevention of deformity and shortening, bone grafting justifies more emphasis.

Injuries in the ulnar wrist complex are less frequent and are often associated with distal radial fractures, and the long-term results are affected by chronic instability and incongruity of the distal radio-ulnar joint. It is therefore important to assess the ulnar wrist complex routinely in treating distal radial fractures. Early joint stabilisation and reconstruction of congruity must be attained in the initial stage to prevent late, chronic problems of either disabling pain or mild ulnar wrist ailment.

References

1. Colles A (1814) On the fracture of the carpal extremity of the radius. Edinb Med Surg J 10:182
2. Short WH, Palmer AK, Werner FW, Murphy DJ (1987) A biomechanical study of distal radial fractures. J Hand Surg [Am] 12(4):529
3. Bassett RL (1987) Displaced intraarticular fractures of the distal radius. Clin Orthop 214:148
4. Cooney WP, Linscheid RL, Dobyns JH (1979) External pin fixation for unstable Colles' fractures. J Bone Joint Surg [Am] 61(6):840

5. Depalma AF (1952) Comminuted fractures of the distal end of the radius treated by ulnar pinning. J Bone Joint Surg [Am] 34(3):651
6. Szabo RM, Weber SC (1988) Comminuted intraarticular fractures of the distal radius. Clin Orthop 230:39
7. Solgaard S, Borg L, Bunger C (1988) Displaced distal radius fractures – a comparative study of treatment by external fixation, dorsal plaster immobilisation and functional bracing in supination. Rev Chir Orthop 74[Suppl]
8. Weber SC, Szabo RM (1986) Severely comminuted distal radial fracture as an unsolved problem: complications associated with external fixation and pins and plaster techniques. J Hand Surg [Am] 11(2):157
9. Sledge CB, Poss R, Cofield RH, Frymoyer JW, Griffin PP, Hansen ST, Johnson KA et al. (1990) 1990. The year book of orthopaedics. Mosby, St Louis
10. Frykman G (1967) Fracture of the distal radius including sequelae – shoulder-hand-finger syndrome, disturbance in the distal radio-ulnar joint, and impairment of nerve function: a clinical and experimental study. Acta Orthop Scand Suppl 108:1
11. Cooney WP (1987) Correspondence newsletter 1988–4, Nov 11, 1987. Mayo Clinic, Rochester
12. Porter M, Stockley I (1987) Fractures of the distal radius – intermediate and end results in relation to radiologic parameters. Clin Orthop 220:241
13. De Bruijn HP (1987) Functional treatment of colles fractures. Acta Orthop Scand 58[Suppl]223
14. Villar RN, Marsh D, Rushton N, Greatorex RA (1987) Three years after Colles' fracture – a prospective review. J Bone Joint Surg [Br] 69(4):635
15. Kaukonen JP, Karaharju EO, Porras M, Luthje P, Jakobsson A (1988) Functional recovery after fractures of the distal forearm – analysis of radiographic and other factors affecting the outcome. Ann Chir Gynaecol 77:27
16. Kaukonen JP, Porras M, Karaharju E (1988) Anatomical results after distal forearm fractures. Ann Chir Gynaecol 77:21
17. Bohler L (1932) The treatment of fractures. Grune and Stratton, New York, pp 90–96
18. Chapman DR, Bennett JB, Bryan WJ, Tullos HS (1982) Complication of distal radial fractures: pins and plaster treatment. J Hand Surg [Am] 7:509
19. Green DP (1975) Pins and plaster treatment of comminuted fractures of the distal end of the radius. J Bone Joint Surg [Am] 57:304
20. Scheck M (1962) Long term follow-up of treatment of comminuted fractures of the distal end of the radius by transfixation with Kirschner wires and cast. J Bone Joint Surg [Am] 44:337
21. Cole JM, Obletz NE (1966) Comminuted fractures of the distal end of the radius treated by skeletal transfixion in plaster cast. J Bone Joint Surg [Am] 48(5):931
22. Carrozzella J, Stern PJ (1988) Treatment of comminuted distal radius fractures with pins and plaster. Hand Clin 4(3):391
23. Jakob RP, Fernandex DL (1982) The treatment of wirst fractures with the small AO external fixation device. In: Uhthoff HK (ed) Current concepts of external fixation of fractures. Springer, Berlin Heidelberg New York, pp 307–314
24. Conney WP III (1983) External fixation of fractures of the distal radius. In: Brooker AF Jr, Cooney WP, Chao EXS (eds) Principles of external fixation. Williams and Wilkins, Baltimore, pp 103–121
25. Schuind F, Donkerwolcke M, Burny F (1984) External fixation of wrist fractures. Orthopaedics 7:841
26. Grana WA (1982) External fixation for comminuted fractures of the distal radius. In: Seligson D, Pope M (eds) Concepts in external fixation. Grune and Stratton, New York, pp 171–182
27. Seitz WH, Froimsom AI, Brooks BD, Postak PD, Parker RD, Laporte JM, Greenwald AS (1990) Biomechanical analysis of pin placement and pin size for external fixation of distal radius fractures. Clin Orthop 251:207

28. Seitz WH, Putnam MD, Dick HM (1990) Limited open surgical approach for external fixation of distal radius fractures. J Hand Surg [Am] 15(2):288
29. Knirk JL, Jupiter JB (1986) Intra-articular fractures of the distal end of the radius in young adults. J Bone Joint Surg [Am] 68(5):647
30. Vidal J, Buscayret C, Paran M, Melka J (1983) Ligamentotaxis. In: Mears DC (ed) External skeletal fixation. Williams and Wilkins, Baltimore, pp 493–496
31. Clyburn TA (1987) Dynamic external fixation for comminuted intra-articular fractures of the distal end of the radius. J Bone Joint Surg [Am] 69(2):248
32. Pennig D (1991) Operative manual – the Pennig dynamic wrist fixator. Orthofix Publication, Bussolengo
33. Jenkins NH, Jones DG, Johnson SR, Mintowt-Czyz WJ (1987) External fixation of Colles' fractures – an anatomical study. J Bone Joint Surg [Br] 69(2):207
34. Leung KS, Shen WY, Leung PC, Kinninmonth AWG, Chang JCW, Chan GPY (1989) Ligamentotaxis and bone grafting for comminuted fractures of the distal radius. J Bone Joint Surg [Br] 71(5):838
35. Leung KS, So WS, Chiu VDF, Leung PC (1991) Ligamentotaxis treatment for comminuted distal radial fractures modified by primary cancellous grafting and functional bracing – long term results. J Orthop Trauma 5(3):265
36. Smith RS, Crick JC, Alonso J, Horowitz M (1988) Open reduction and internal fixation of volar lip fractures of the distal radius. J Orthop Trauma 2(3):181
37. Vukov V, Ristic K, Stevanovic M, Bumbasirevic M (1988) Simultaneous fractures of the distal end of the radius and the scaphoid bone. J Orthop Trauma 2(2):120
38. Tountas AA, Waddell JP (1988) Simultaneous fractures of the distal radius and scaphoid. J Orthop Trauma 1(14):312
39. Herbert TJ (1986) Use of the Herbert bone screw in surgery of the wrist. Clin Orthop 202:79
40. Wozasek GE, Moser K (1991) Percutaneous screw fixation for fractures of the scaphoid. J Bone Joint Surg [Br] 73:138
41. Kapandji IA (1970) The physiology of the joints. Churchill Livingstone, New York
42. Palmer AK, Werner FW (1984) Biomechanics of the distal radioulnar joint. Clin Orthop 187:26
43. Palmer AK (1990) Triangular fibrocartilage disorders: injury patterns and treatment. Arthroscopy 6(2):125
44. Boulas HJ, Milek MA (1990) Ulnar shortening for tears of the triangular fibrocatilaginous complex. J Hand Surg [Am] 15(3):415
45. Osterman AL (1990) Arthroscopic debridement of triangular fibrocartilage complex tears. Arthroscopy 6(2):120
46. Frahm R, Saul O, Mannerfelt L (1989) Diagnostic applications of wrist arthrography. Arch Orthop Trauma Surg 109:39
47. Buterbaugh GA, Palmer AK (1988) Fractures and dislocations of the distal radioulnar joint. Hand Clin 4(3):361
48. Liebolt FL (1950) A new method for repair of the distal radio-ulnar ligaments. NY J Med 50:2817
49. Tsai T, Stillwell JH (1984) Repair of chronic subluxation of the distal radio-ulnar joint using flexor carpi ulnar is tendon. J Hand Surg [Br] 9:289
50. Liebolt FL (1982) A new procedure for the treatment of luxation of the distal end of the ulna. J Bone Joint Surg [Am] 35:261
51. Hui FC, Linschield RL (1982) Ulnotriquetral augmentation tendodesis – a reconstructive procedure for dorsal subluxation of the distal radio-ulnar joint. J Hand Surg 7:230
52. Hui FC, Linschield RL (1982) Ulnotriquetral angmentation tenodesis – a reconstructive procedure for dorsal subluxation of the distal radio-ulnar joint. J Hand Surg 7:230
53. Johnson RK (1985) Muscle tendon transfer for stabilization of the distal radio-ulnar joint. J Hand Surg [Am] 10:439

54. Johnson RK, Shrewsbury MM (1976) The pronator quadratus in motions and in stabilization of the radius and ulna at the distal radio-ulnar joint. J Hand Surg 1:205
55. Leung PC, Hung LK (1990) An effective method of reconstructing posttraumatic dorsal dislocated distal radioulnar joints. J Hand Surg [Am] 15(6):925
56. Gartland JJ Jr, Werley CW (1951) Evaluation of healed Colles' fractures. J Bone Joint Surg [Am] 33:895–907
57. Sarmiento A, Pratt GW, Berry NC, Sinclair WF (1975) Colles' fractures functional bracing in supination. J Bone Joint Surg [Am] 57:311–317

10 Problems in Elbow Fractures

W.Y. SHEN and J.C.Y. CHENG

Distal Humeral Fractures in Children

This section discusses only fractures of the distal end of the humerus; fractures of the proximal radius and ulna are discussed in the chapter for children fractures. For all practical purposes, only three types of fractures occur in the distal end of the humerus in children under the age of 12 years. They are, in order of prevalence, supracondylar fracture, fracture of the lateral condyle and fracture of the medial epicondyle.

General Considerations

Diagnosis. Growth plates around the elbow cause much confusion. Memorisation of the ossification charts is difficult and indeed not necessary if the opposite elbow is radiographed for comparison. More often than not, the painful elbow of an uncooperative child is malpositioned when the X-ray is taken. It is in these occasions that fractures are missed or their severity underestimated. Small-sized films including only the metaphyseal region of the distal humerus often lead to an underestimation of the degree of varus angulation in a supracondylar fracture. A painful elbow in a crying toddler, often with "normal" X-ray findings, poses a difficult problem even for the experienced trauma surgeon. It is only with patience and repeated, careful examinations that these problems are identified.

Quality of Reduction. As much as pre-operative films are confusing, post-reduction films can also be difficult to interpret. In supracondylar fractures, various methods have been described for the measurement of varus-valgus angulation: the Baumann's angle, the metaphyseal-diaphyseal angle and the humeral-ulnar angle. The latter has been shown to correlate best with clinical carrying angle [1]. However, in practice it is impossible for two reasons to take a long intra-operative film of a fully extended elbow: (a) reduced fractures not fixed with wires lose reduction on full extension and (b) intra-operative films are generally taken with the C-arm image intensifier, which is not capable of taking long films. A radiograph of the lower third to half of the humerus is often the only practical procedure. In this situation a comparison should be made of the Baumann's angle on both sides. Because that films of opposite elbows are usually not taken in strictly comparable positions, it is often difficult to draw comparable lines along the capitellar growth plates on either side, giving rise to error in the measurement of Baumann's angle. We have found that the most practical method is to overlap, against a strong light, the medial and lateral condyles on films of opposite elbows, and to measure the degree of divergence between the two humeral shafts. Alternatively, a tracing of the distal humerus on the un-injured side can be used as a template and overlapped onto the X-ray of the injured side. There should be no deviation at all if there is no varus or valgus tilt. As most of the fracture line goes through radiolucent cartilage, the quality of reduction of lateral condylar fractures is best assessed intra-operatively by the operating surgeon. As there may be differential growth disturbance at the lateral condyle with respect to the medial condyle, the carrying angle of the elbow can be assessed only by measurement of the humeral-ulnar angle.

Supracondylar Fractures

The extension type supracondylar fracture of the humerus is the most common fracture in children. The fracture may be complicated by acute vascular embarrassment and other nerve injuries. Although associated vascular injuries are not common, increased awareness has reduced the risks of ischaemic contractures [2]. Associated neural injuries are more common, but these rarely lead to permanent disability [3–7]. Many methods of treatment have been described, including: (a) closed reduction and plaster im-mobilisation in aculte flexion, (b) reduction by continuous skin or skeletal traction, (c) closed reduction followed by percutaneous insertion of Kirschner wires, crossed or unilateral, and (d) open reduction and internal fixation with Kirschner wires. Experimental evidence from cadaveric studies by Smith in 1894 [8] showed that extension-type fractures are reduced most stably with the elbow in acute flexion and full pronation. However, this position often leads to embarrassment of circulation in a grossly swollen elbow. McLaughlin termed this the "supracondylar dilemma" [9]. Con-tinuous skin or skeletal traction avoids the need to flex the elbow at an acute angle but necessitates prolonged hospitalisation [10–13].
    Swenson [14] was one of the first to describe "blind pinning" of supra-condylar fractures in the English literature. Flynn et al. [15] reported 72 patients treated over 16 years using a method of closed reduction and percutaneous pins inserted from both the lateral and medial condyles. He employed a special bracket in the shape of an inverted U for stabilisation of the upper arm during the reduction and fixation. Fowles and Kassab [16], also reported that supracondylar fractures can be fixed adequately using two Kirschner wires inserted from the lateral condyle only, avoiding injury to the ulnar nerve in a grossly swollen elbow. Flynn cut his wires subcutaneously and buried the ends, thus requiring another procedure to remove the pins.

Fowles, however, bent the pins and exposed the ends so that removal is much easier. Subsequently, many authors have reported on various modifications of the technique [17–20].

Open reduction and internal fixation is the choice for irreducible fractures [21–27].

Treatment. Since April 1986 we have adopted the following protocol.

1. In all children with suspected or frank supracondylar fractures of the humerus an X-ray is taken of the lower end of the injured humerus for comparison and accurate assessment of deformity. The X-ray is also used for assessment of the quality of reduction.

2. The fractures are then classified as follows: (a) minimally displaced: no varus or valgus angulation, no rotational deformity, no translational displacement and posterior angulation of less than 30°; (b) moderately displaced: more deformation than minimally displaced fractures while the two fragments are still in contact with each other (Fig. 1); (c) grossly displaced: complete separation of the two fragments from each other (Fig. 2).

3. *Minimally displaced fractures* are treated with the application of an above-elbow plaster made of radiolucent synthetic material (conventional plaster of paris obstructs clear visualisation of the distal humerus on X-rays and is therefore not recommended). The forearms are maintained in full pronation to prevent varus deformity. X-rays are checked after the application of plaster to make sure that the displacement is not disturbed. The plaster is maintained for 4 weeks. All children with *moderately or grossly displaced fractures* are put under general anaesthesia for closed reduction under X-ray screening. Fractures that are stable after reduction are immobilised by an above-elbow plaster of radiolucent material for 4 weeks; those that are not stable are fixed with percutaneous wires and the elbows protected by an above-elbow plaster. The plaster and wires are removed without anaesthesia at the end of 4 weeks. *Irreducible fractures* are treated with open reduction via a posterior approach through the triceps aponeurosis, Kirschner wire fixation and above-elbow plaster immobilisation applied only when the swelling subsides after a period of elevation. Plasters and wires are removed at the end of 6 weeks in this group.

4. Circulation to the hand is closely monitored, with the aid of a pulse oximeter if necessary, during the early post-operative period [28].

5. Children with minimally displaced fractures do not need supervised mobilisation exercises when the plasters are taken off. Those with displaced fractures and aged over 4 years are referred for a course of mobilisation exercises while those under age 4 are left to play and use the limbs by themselves. Mobilisation exercises are continued on a twice-or thrice-weekly programme until the total loss of range of motion is less than 20°, i.e. regaining about 85% of full range.

6. X-rays are rechecked when the total loss in range of motion is less than 20° to assess accurately the humeral-ulnar angle.

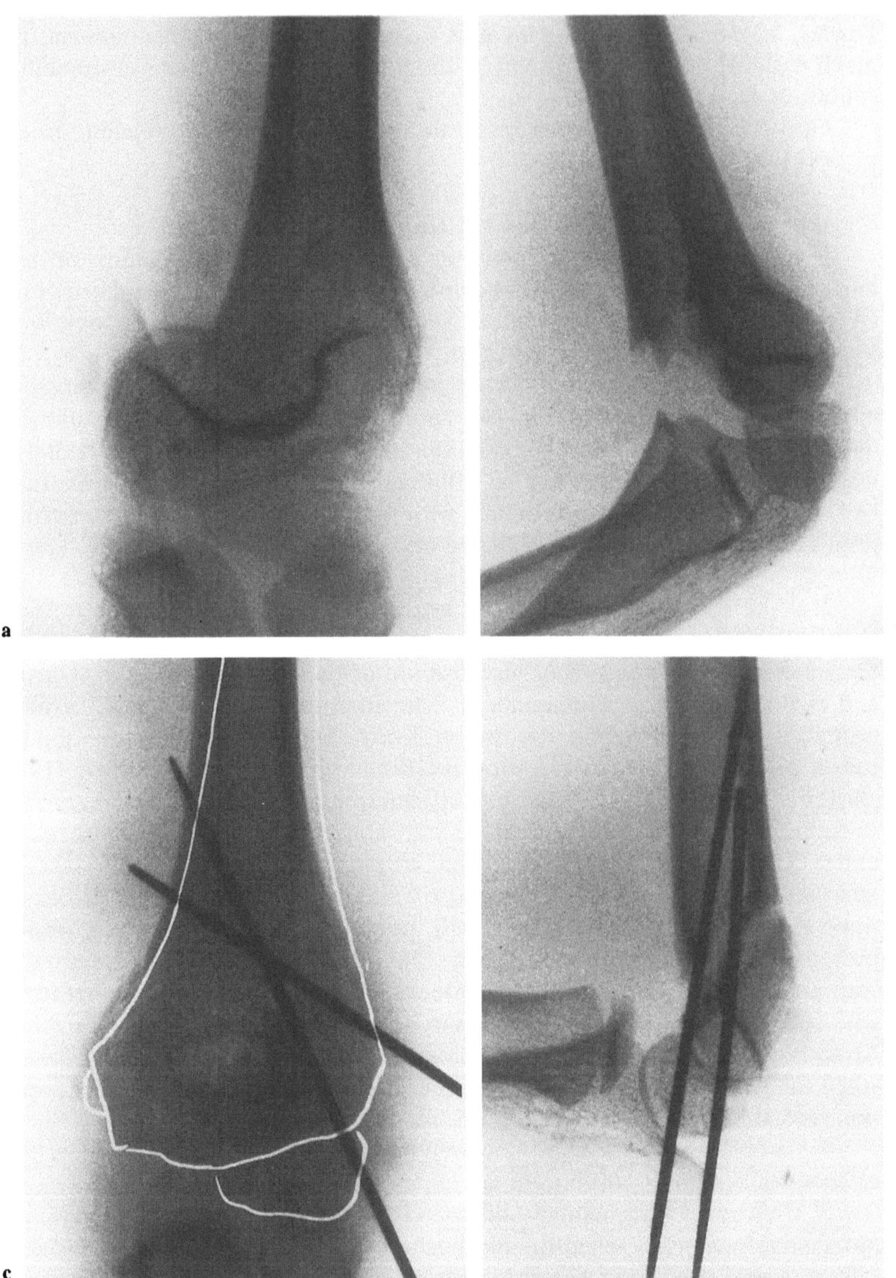

Fig. 1a–d. Moderately displaced supracondylar fracture of the humerus treated by closed reduction and percutaneous Kirschner wire fixation. **a** Antero-posterior view. **b** Lateral view. **c,d** After closed reduction and percutaneous Kirschner wire fixation. **c** Antero-posterior view (*line drawing*, superimposed outline of the opposite humerus). **d** Lateral view

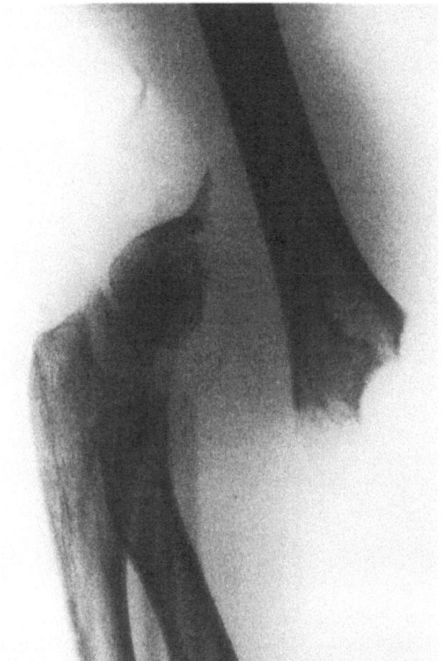

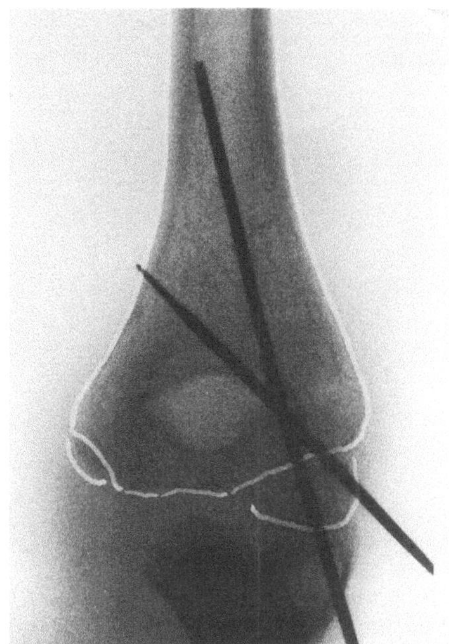

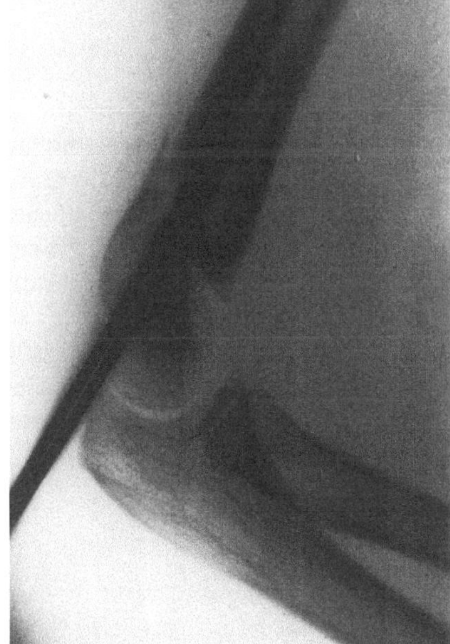

Fig. 2a–c. Grossly displaced supracondylar fracture of the humerus treated by closed reduction and percutaneous Kirschner wire fixation. **a** Pre-operative X-ray. **b,c** After closed reduction and percutaneous Kirschner wire fixation. **b** Anteroposterior view (*line drawing*, superimposed outline of the opposite humerus). **c** Lateral view

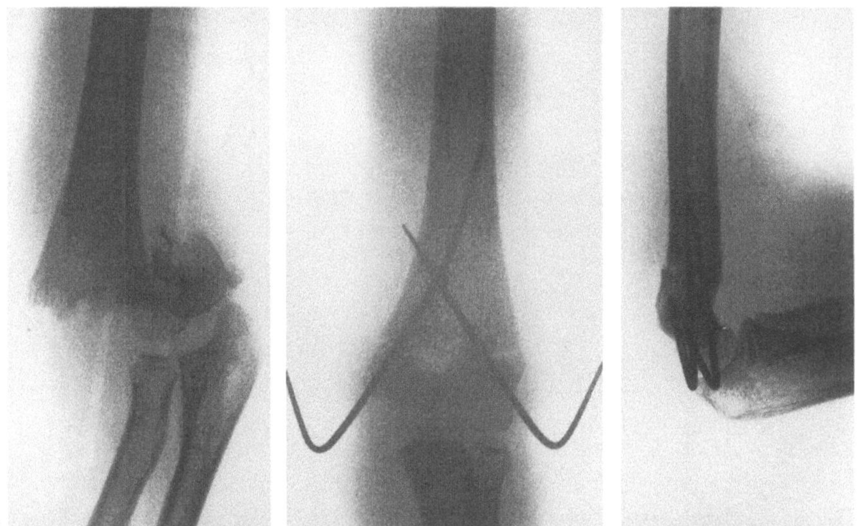

Fig. 3a–c. Grossly displaced supracondylar fracture of the humerus treated by open reduction and Kirschner wire fixation. **a** Pre-operative X-ray. **b,c** After open reduction and Kirschner wire fixation. **b** Antero-posterior view. **c** Lateral view

Results. During a period of 30 months, 224 children under the age of 12 years were treated in our Department for extension-type supracondylar fracture of the humerus, following the protocol outlined above. Of these, 82 fractures (36.6%) were minimally displaced and were treated with plaster only; 91 (40.6%) were moderately displaced, and 51 (22.7%) were grossly displaced. Closed reduction was successful in 73 (80.2%) of the moderately displaced (Fig. 1) and 39 (76.4%) of the grossly displaced fractures (Fig. 2), these being fixed with percutaneous wires. Closed reduction was unsuccessful in 11 (12.0%) moderately displaced and in 12 (23.5%) grossly displaced fractures; these were subsequently treated with open reduction and Kirschner wire fixation (Fig. 3).

Nerve Palsies

Nerve palsies should be carefully checked before manipulation. In our experience, these have included five (2.23%) radial nerve, three (1.34%) median nerve, and three (1.34%) ulnar nerve palsies. There have also been five (2.23%) ulnar nerve palsies detected only after closed reduction and bilateral percutaneous pinning. One ulnar nerve palsy was detected after open reduction and bilateral pinning. In contrast to the report of Culp et al. [29], all nerve palsies, whether detected before or after manipulation, recovered completely within 6 months. Only two of the cases of ulnar nerve palsies occurred after bilateral percutaneous pinning. These nerves were explored, and neurolysis was performed after a period of unsatisfactory recovery in very much the same fashion as described by Royce et al. [30].

Plaster Alone

Reduced fractures are considered stable if reduction can be maintained without acute flexion of the elbow to more than 90°. These, and the minimally displaced fractures, as described above, are treated with plaster alone. All children should have an uncomplicated course. As soft tissue and periosteal damage is minimal, these elbows recover their full ranges of motion rapidly.

Results. In our series, of the 82 elbows treated by plaster alone and 7 treated by closed reduction and plaster, all recovered functional range of movement within 4 weeks after removal of the plaster. None developed varus or valgus deformity of more than 5°. Ten had an initial loss of flexion range coupled with a corresponding increase in hyperextension. These were related to unreduced extension angulation at the fracture site. All of these gradually had recovered their flexion range completely on subsequent follow-up, but the full restoration may take up to 1 year to reach the normal flexion range. There were no nerve palsies in this group.

Closed Reduction and Percutaneous Kirschner Wire Fixation

We have modified the techniques described by Flynn et al. [15] and Fowles and Kassab [16]. We used a specially made radiolucent arm table instead of Flynn's inverted U-shaped bracket because we find that it is awkward to position the image intensifier with the arm flexed in front of the chest. With this arm table, the upper arm is fixed to the table by means of bandages. The arm is abducted to 90° and can be easily screened in both the antero-posterior and lateral projections (Fig. 4). The bandages serve to immobilise the upper arm during the manoeuvre to reduce the fracture, to counter-tract and to immobilise the reduced fracture during the insertion of pins. Throughout the reduction and pinning the image intensifier can be positioned comfortably for antero-posterior and lateral projections. Initially we inserted the Kirschner wires as described by Flynn et al. [15], from both the lateral and medial condyles (Fig. 5). After 40 cases in which 5 ulnar nerve palsies occurred, we changed our policy. Most fractures are now fixed with lateral wires only, as described by Fowles and Kassab [16] (Figs. 1, 2). Bilateral wires are used in comminuted fractures in which the stability provided by unilateral wires may be doubtful. All Kirschner wires were bent and cut outside the skin. The entry holes on the skin are enlarged to prevent impingement. Intra-operative X-rays of the lower humerus before the application of plaster are necessary to ensure good quality of reduction.

Results. In our series all children regained their functional range of motion. None lost more than 10° of motion. In 85% the normal range was regained

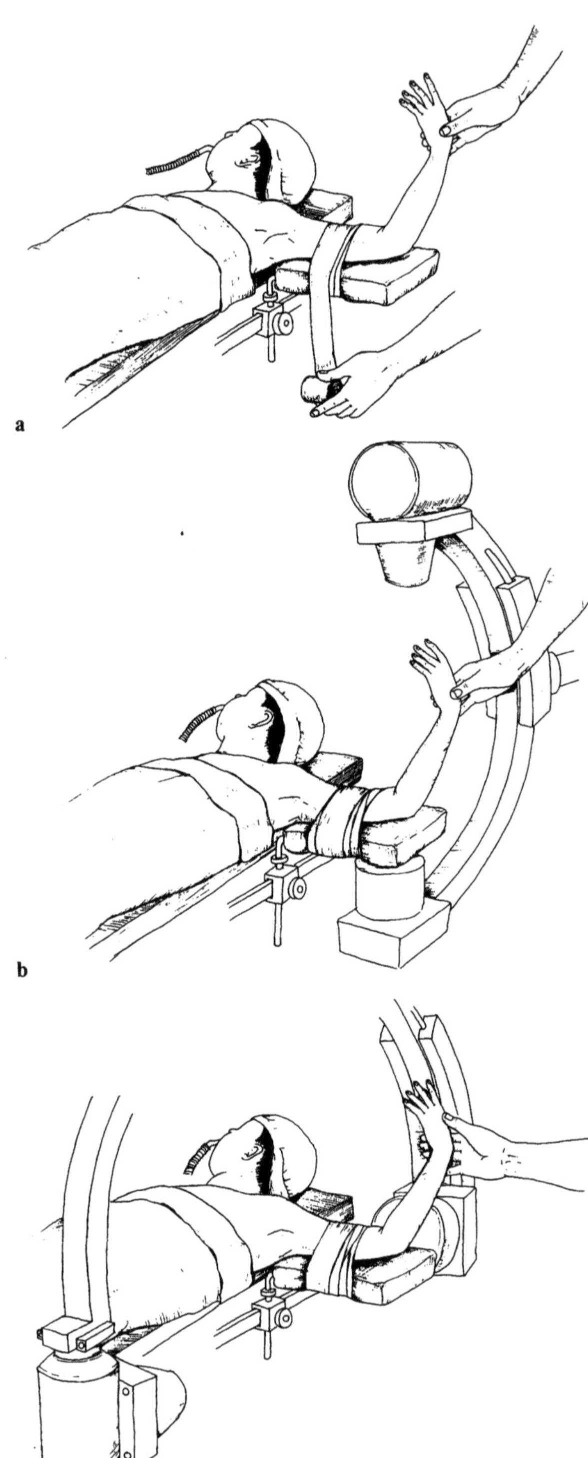

Fig. 4a–c. Positioning for closed reduction and percutaneous Kirschner wire fixation of supracondylar fractures of the humerus. **a** Immobilisation of the upper arm onto the radiolucent arm board by crepe bandage. **b** Positioning of the C-arm for anteroposterior projection. **c** Positioning of the C-arm for lateral projection

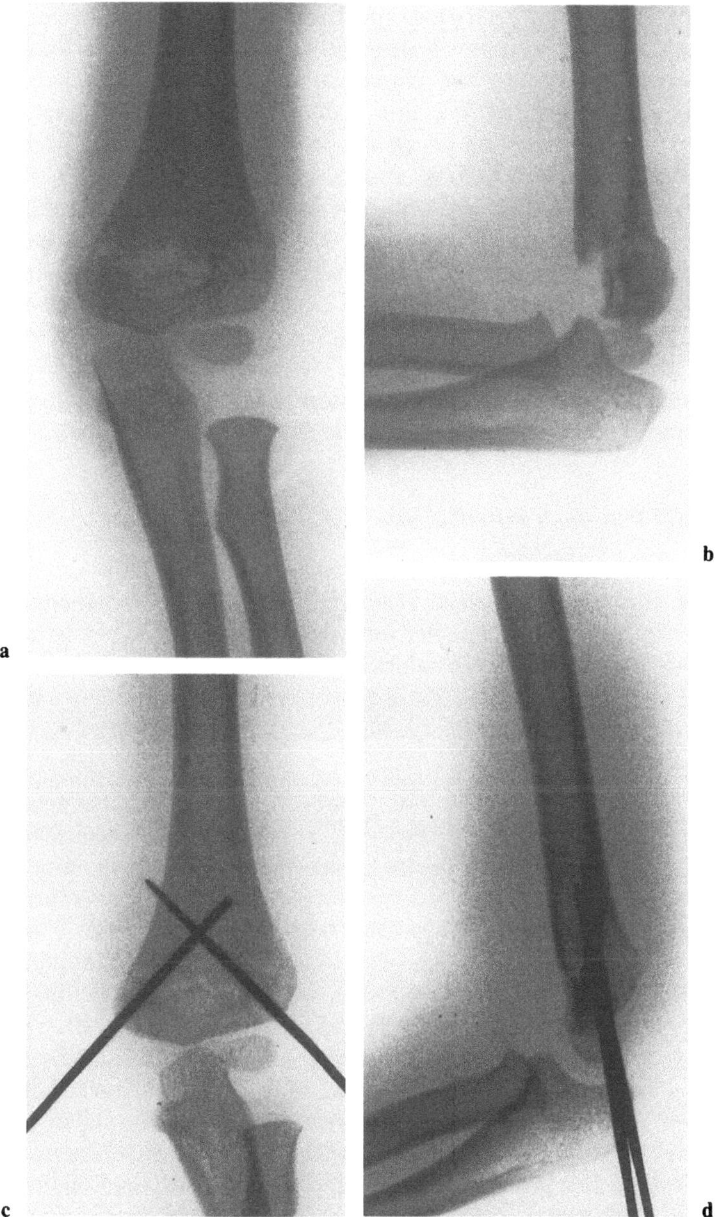

Fig. 5a–d. Moderately displaced supracondylar fracture of the humerus treated by closed reduction and bilateral percutaneous Kirschner wire fixation. **a** Antero-posterior view. **b** Lateral view. **c,d** After closed reduction and bilateral percutaneous Kirschner wire fixation. **c** Antero-posterior view. **d** Lateral view

at an average of 10.73 weeks from operation. Eight cases had varus deformities ranging from 5° to 15° compared with the uninjured side. Five were the result of imperfect reductions; the imperfect reductions were accepted because the elbows were so swollen that open reduction was contra-indicated at the acute stage. Three were the result of poor intra-operative X-rays leading to misjudgment. As described above, there were five cases of transient ulnar nerve palsies associated with bilateral pinning. Two of these required exploration and neurolysis because of slow recovery. All five cases recovered completely by 6 months. There were no ulnar nerve problems associated with lateral pinning. There were two cases of superficial pin tract infection; both subsided with the use of antibiotics. There was no loss of fixation in either the bilateral pinning or the lateral pinning group. The position of the fragments was successfully maintained, as shown in the intra-operative X-rays and those taken about 10 weeks later.

Open Reduction and Kirschner Wire Fixation

All open reductions were performed via a posterior triceps splitting exposure. Kirschner wires were inserted from both the lateral and medial condyles under direct vision after safeguarding the ulnar nerve. Wires were bent and cut outside the skin to enable removal without another anaesthesia. Open reduction is contra-indicated in the grossly swollen elbow. Control of swelling by elevation for a few days makes the operation much easier.

Results. We have treated 23 elbows with open reduction and Kirschner wire fixation. Of these, seven moderately displaced and five grossly displaced fractures were presented more than 5 days after the injury, having been treated by bone setters or other practitioners. The other four moderately displaced and seven grossly displaced fractures were truly irreducible. This set of patients consists of a mixed group who received definitive treatment after a delay of 0–20 days for various reasons. A few patients had open reduction immediately after unsuccessful closed reduction. Some elbows were elevated for a few days for control of swelling after unsuccessful closed reduction. Some elbows were stained with herbs and complicated with dermatitis on presentation; these were operated on after a few days of treatment for the skin condition. Some cases set by bone setters presented after periods as long as 20 days. As expected, the outcome has been highly variable. Recovery of motion to the range of 85% of normal took 15–50 weeks. Varus deformity ranged from 0° to 15°.

Summary. We recommend (a) the application of an above-elbow plaster with the elbow at 90° in minimally displaced fractures, (b) closed reduction and plaster for displaced fractures that are stable after closed reduction, (c) closed reduction and percutaneous lateral pinning for displaced fractures that are not stable after reduction, and (d) open reduction and Kirschner wire fixation for irreducible fractures.

Lateral Condylar Fractures

Lateral condylar fractures are type IV (Salter-Harris) trans-epiphyseal intra-articular fractures. The fracture line extends from the metaphyseal bone on the lateral side to the physeal plate of the capitellar epiphysis and then into the middle of the trochlear articular surface. By virtue of the intra-articular extension, displaced lateral condylar fractrues require accurate open reduction to reconstruct a congruent articular surface. However, about 50% of lateral condylar fractures are very minimally displaced (<2 mm in any direction). These can be treated conservatively with an above-elbow radiolucent plaster but must be watched closely for further displacement [31–33]. Displaced lateral condylar fractures are prone to nonunion or malunion if treated conservatively [34]. They should be reduced accurately by open reduction via an antero-lateral approach and fixed with unthreaded Kirschner wires (Fig. 6). The most important step is the restoration of congruity of the trochlear articular surface. Therefore it is essential to expose the whole of the anterior aspect of the capitellum and trochlear.

Occasionally, a type II (Salter-Harris) epiphyseal fracture is found on exploration. The tell-tale sign on X-rays is that the relationship between the radial head, olecranon and capitellar epiphysis is maintained while the proximal radius and ulna are shifted backwards with respect to the humerus as in a dislocation (Fig. 7). Occasionally these appear the same as the more common type IV injury on radiographs, only that the swelling on the medial aspect of the elbow is more pronounced. Although type II injuries are neither trans-epiphyseal nor intra-articular in the usual sense, they have a worse prognosis. This is probably related to the fact that any callus formation at the epiphyseal-metaphyseal junction of the trochlear epiphysis is indeed intra-articular and thus obstructs the humero-ulnar joint.

Results. Within a period of 3 years, 67 fresh lateral condylar fractures in children under the age of 12 were treated. Of these, 34 were minimally displaced and were treated by cast alone, while 33 were displaced and were treated by open reduction, Kirschner wire fixation and cast. In both situations, the casts and Kirschner wires are maintained for 6 weeks. After a minimal follow up of 2 years, all patients enjoyed full range of movement. Three who had open reduction developed cubitus varus, as measured by comparison of the humero-ulnar angle between the two elbows, of 10°. Two patients treated conservatively developed cubitus varus of 10° and 5°, respectively. Clinically, the occurrence of cubitus varus is indicated by comparison of the arm-forearm angles between the normal and affected sides rather than radiological evidence. A possible explanation is that the lateral condyle usually appears more prominent laterally at the elbow after such

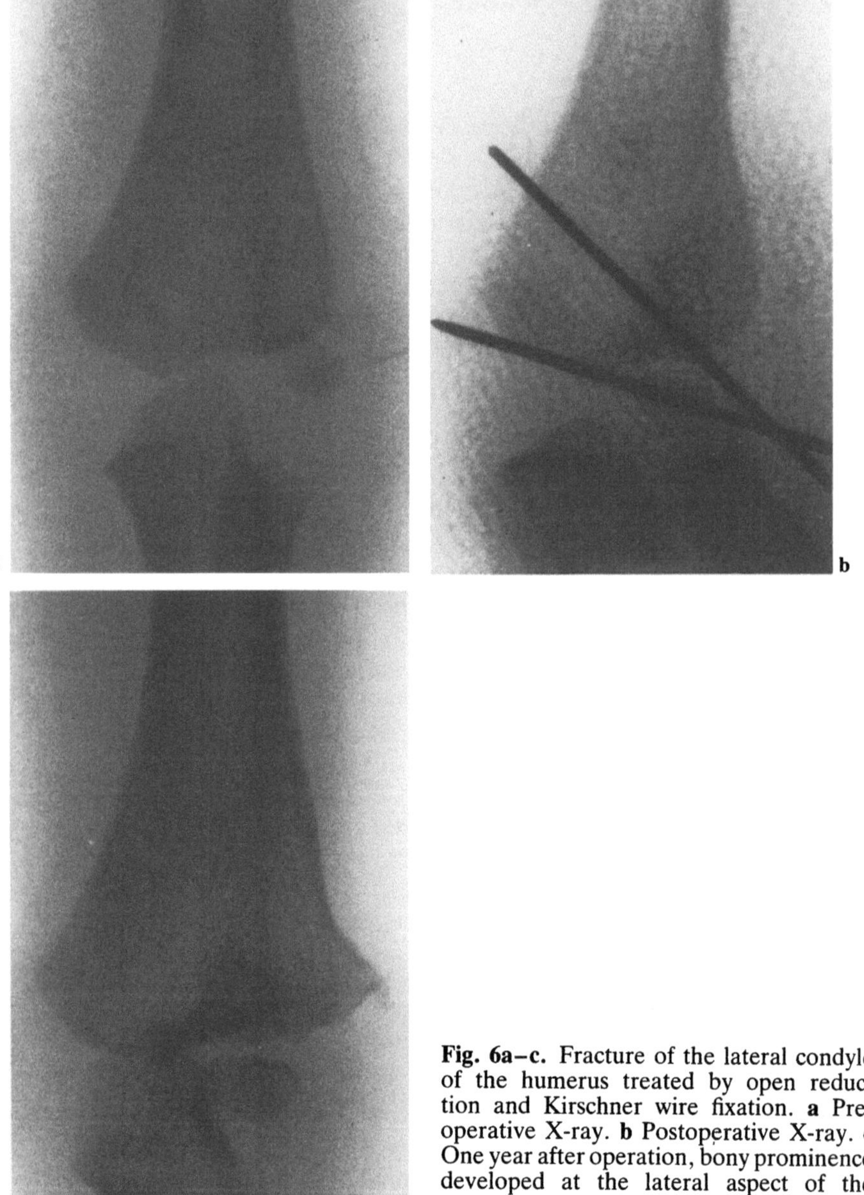

Fig. 6a–c. Fracture of the lateral condyle of the humerus treated by open reduction and Kirschner wire fixation. **a** Preoperative X-ray. **b** Postoperative X-ray. **c** One year after operation, bony prominence developed at the lateral aspect of the healed fracture

fractures (Fig. 7). The lateral prominence at the elbow gives an apparent loss of carrying angle on clinical measurement. Although our follow-up period is relatively short, we concur with previous reports that clinical loss of carrying angle is a common sequela of lateral condylar fractures, but we

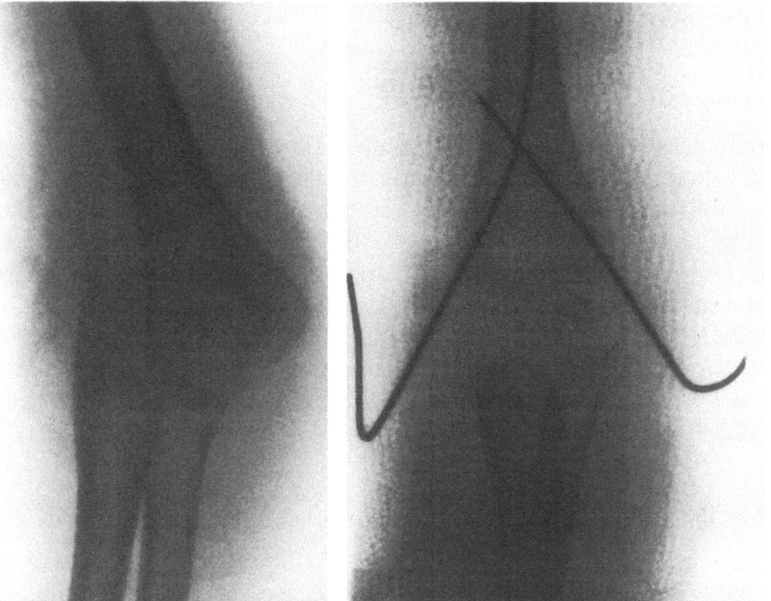

Fig. 7a–b. Type II epiphyseal fracture of the distal humerus. **a** Pre-operative X-ray. Note that, grossly, it appears as a simple dislocated elbow, but that the capitellar epiphysis is displaced together with the proximal radius and ulna, while the relationship among these three structures remain intact. **b** X-ray after open reduction and Kirschner wire fixation

would add that the incidence of a varus change in the humero-ulnar angle is not common [35]. Bone healing complications should not occur. There was neither nonunion nor delayed union among our 67 fractures.

Summary. We recommend the following. (a) Displaced fractures of the lateral condyle should be treated with open reduction and Kirschner wire fixation. The fixation is further augmented and protected by application of an above-elbow plaster for 6 weeks. (b) Fractures with displacement of less than 2 mm can be treated with an above-elbow plaster of radiolucent material and be monitored closely with X-ray checks.

Medial Epicondylar Fractures

Fracture of the medial epicondyle is common in teenagers. The treatment modalities are basically those described for elbow fractures in adults. However, for these younger patients Kirschner wire fixation is employed instead of screw fixation to facilitate removal and to minimise epiphyseal damage.

Elbow Fractures in Adults

Special Anatomical Considerations

The distal humerus has a very complex shape. The lateral column is a bar of bone that extends from the lateral aspect of the lower shaft down to the capitellum and the lateral edge of the trochlear. On an antero-posterior projection this column is relatively straight, but curves anteriorly on a lateral projection. The medial column extends from the medial aspect of the lower shaft to end at the medial epicondyle and medial edge of the trochlear. On antero-posterior projection this column is curved while on lateral projection it is rather straight. Between the two columns is the articular part of the trochlear and a thin piece of bone separating the olecranon fossa at the back from the coronoid fossa in front. (Fig. 8)

Fractures of the Distal Humerus

Recently the AO classification proposed by Muller et al. [36] has become the most widely adopted. This classification has the virtue of being part of the system that applies to all fractures; therefore the complexity and thus prognosis are reflected simply by the alpha-numeric value of the type. In our experience, only type A1, C1 and C2 fractures are common, and we describe only these below.

Fractures of the Medial Epicondyle

Fractures of the medial epicondyle are type A1 fractures and result from dislocation of the elbow in adolescents. The fracture is easily missed because the medial epicondylar fragment is often hidden within the dislocated joint. The fracture is easily managed by closed reduction of the dislocated elbow, followed by open lag screw fixation of the fracture (Fig. 9). Care must be taken that the screw does not violate the olecranon or coronoid fossae; otherwise the range of movement is seriously affected. Because of the ligamentous injuries associated with dislocation of the elbow, we routinely protect these elbows with a hinged brace, the allowed arc of movement of which is gradually increased over 6 weeks. Contrary to common belief, associated ulnar nerve injury is rare.

Inter-condylar Fractures of the Humerus

Inter-condylar fractures of the humerus belong to types C1, C2 and C3 in the AO classification. Being intra-articular fractures of a joint with a great range of movement, these fractures pose the most difficult problem. Charnley in 1961 [37] observed that "The elbow almost invariably does badly after operative treatment. Particularly disappointing is open reduction and

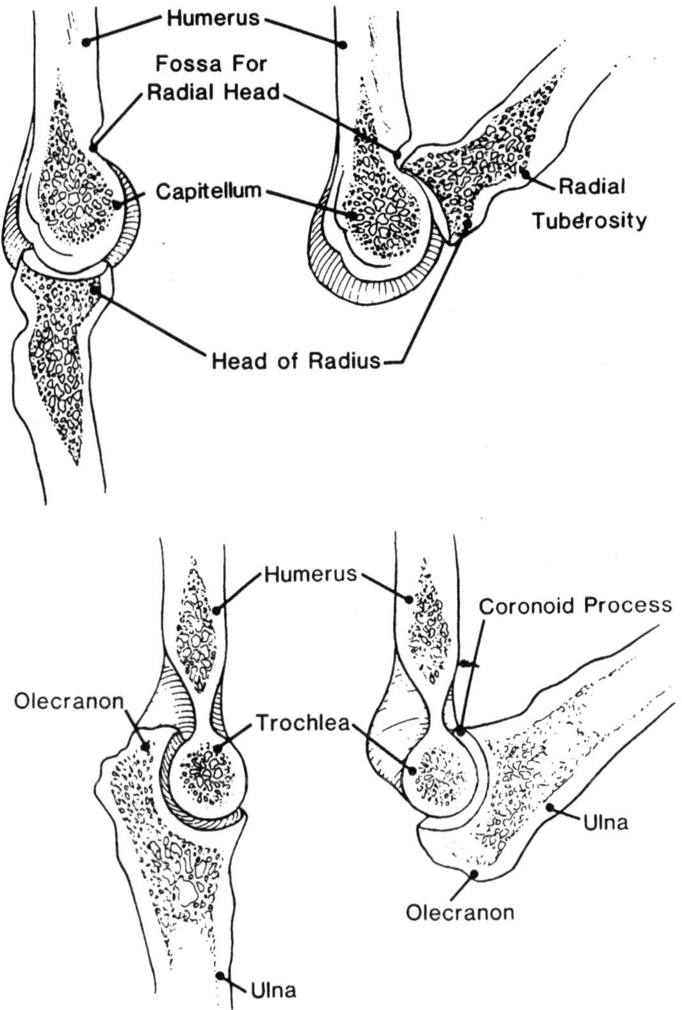

Fig. 8. Anatomy of the distal humerus. (From [44])

internal fixation for Y fractures in the adult." We cannot agree more with view of Jupiter et al. in 1985 [38]: "The problem of management has been made more difficult by the fact that the fracture is relatively uncommon, which prevents the individual surgeon from accumulating sufficient personal experience to critically evaluate the results of treatment."

Treatment. Recommendations have ranged widely, from "conscientious neglect", to closed reduction and immobilisation in a functional position, to open reduction and internal fixation. Even among those who advocate internal fixation, the modes of fixation range widely, from multiple pinning

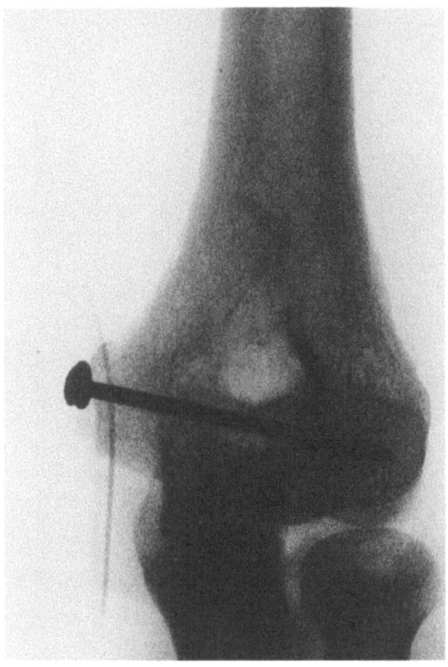

Fig. 9. Dislocation of the elbow with avulsion fracture of the medial epicondyle treated with open reduction and screw fixation

to stable plate and screw fixation. The rehabilitative programme also varies widely from centre to centre.

The recent trend, however, is heading towards stable internal fixation and early mobilisation, except for fractures that occur in osteoporotic bone [38–41].

During internal fixation, four areas must not be trespassed: the articular surfaces of the capitellum and the trochlear and the olecranon and coronoid fossae. The fixation of an intercondylar fracture of the humerus can be subdivided into three elements. (a) The intercondylar element: this can be fixed by a transverse lag screw, usually one of 6.5 mm diameter. Small intercondylar comminuted fragments should be discarded and the space filled with cancellous bone graft. (b) The lateral supracondylar element: this can be fixed with a plate placed along the posterior surface of the lateral column. This is usually a 3.5-mm dynamic compression plate and is bent to take up the curvature. It should be placed as far distally as the lowermost tip of the capitellum in order that two screws can be inserted through the plate into the capitellum. The more proximal screws are inserted in "compression" mode. Some authors prefer the use of a 3.5-mm reconstruction plate in this region, but we consider this not to be strong enough to provide inter-fragmentary compression and thus stability. (c) The medial supracondylar element: a one-third tubular plate can be bent and placed along the medial edge of the medial column (Fig. 10). However, inter-fragmentary compression may not be achieved. In the series described below, five fractures were

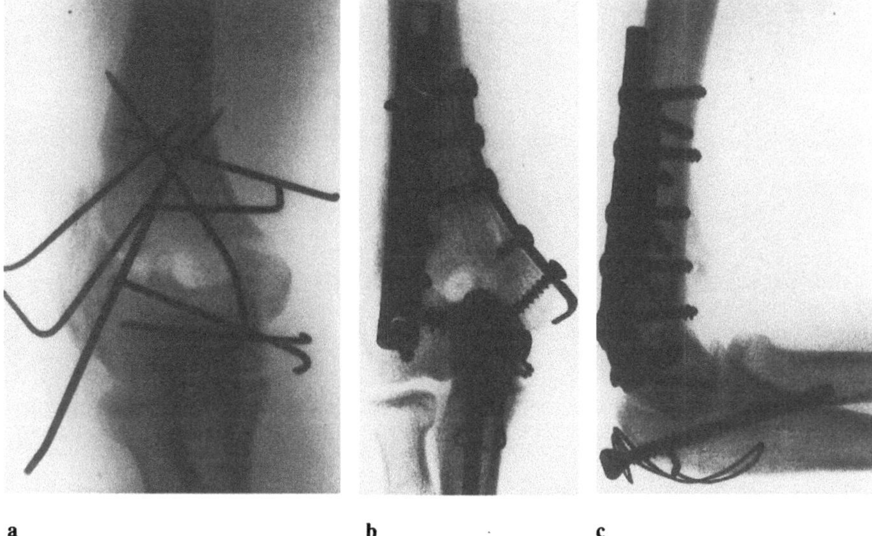

Fig. 10a–c. C2 fracture of the distal humerus. **a** X-ray after unsuccessful open reduction and fixation with multiple Kirschner wires. **b,c** Second operation performed with olecranon osteotomy to achieve a more stable internal fixation with 6.5-mm lag screw for the intercondylar fracture, 3.5-mm dynamic compression plate on the lateral column and one-third tubular plate on the medial column. **b** Antero-posterior view. **c** Lateral view

fixed with a screw inserted through the inferior aspect of the medial epicondyle obliquely towards the lower shaft of the humerus, along the substance of the medial column. This affords inter-fragmentary compression and thus improved stability of fixation (Fig. 11).

We recommend early open reduction of these fractures by an experienced surgeon. Stable internal fixation to enable early mobilisation should be the aim. To achieve this, a more extensile exposure using an olecranon osteotomy is necessary. The inter-condylar element should be fixed with one or two lag screws, discarding any small fragments. A contoured 3.5-mm dynamic compression plate should be applied to the posterior surface of the lateral column as far distally as possible to secure a good grip into the capitellar fragment. A lag screw or a contoured one-third tubular plate should then be applied to fix the medial column. The ulnar nerve is routinely transposed anteriorly in the subcutaneous plane for all type C2 and type C3 fractures. The olecranon osteotomy is repaired by a lag screw protected further with a figure-of-eight tension band wire. (Fig. 12) Depending on the quality of the fixation, early protected movement is encouraged. For complex fractures which cannot be effectively and perfectly fixed, elbow movement must be deferred for 1–2 weeks during which immobilisation is achieved with a brace.

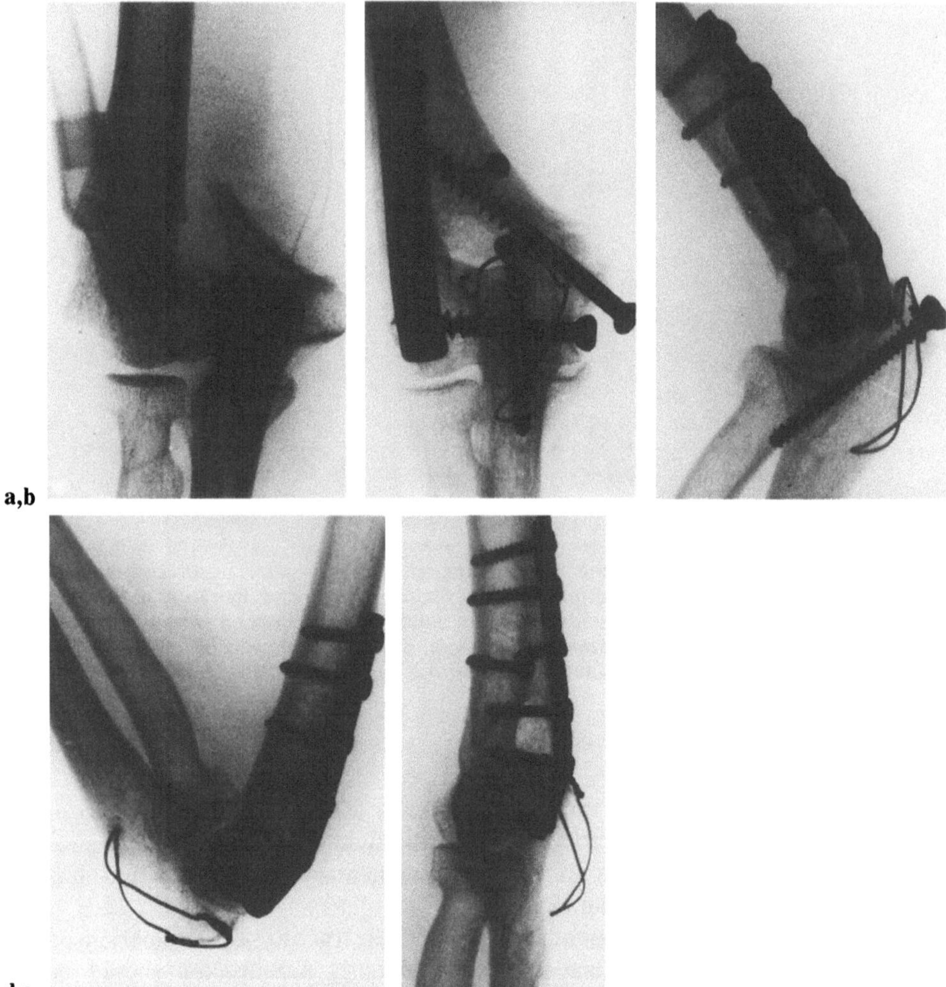

Fig. 11a–e. C2 fracture of the distal humerus treated with open reduction performed with olecranon osteotomy and internal fixation with 6.5-mm lag screw for the intercondylar fracture, 3.5-mm dynamic compression plate on the lateral column and 6.5-mm lag screw in the medial column. **a** Antero-posterior view. **b** Post-operative antero-posterior view. **c** Post-operative lateral view. **d,e** One year after operation, the olecranon repair screw was removed. **d** Lateral view with elbow in extension. **e** Lateral view with elbow in flexion. Range of movement achieved was 10°–135°

Results. Over the past 5 years, ten type C fractures of the distal humerus (two C1, seven C2, one C3) have been treated by the first author with open reduction and internal fixation. The patients were 15–64 years of age (mean 31.8). The follow-up period ranged from 6 to 55 months (mean 27.7). All

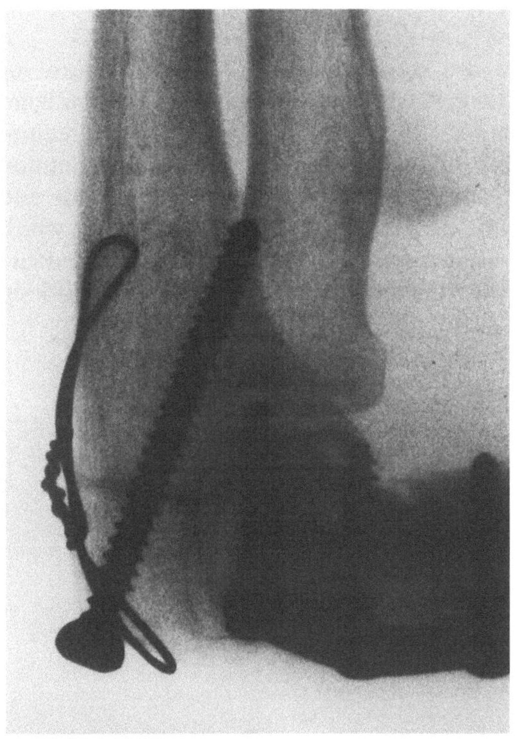

Fig. 12. Repair of olecranon osteotomy using 4.5-mm cortical screw (proximal sliding hole) and figure-of eight wire

the fractures were operated on via a posterior incision. The simpler fractures were exposed by the bilatero-tricipital exposure [42] while more complex fractures were exposed with olecranon osteotomies. In this series, there were three ulnar nerve palsies, one radial nerve palsy and one combined median and ulnar nerve palsy. Ulnar nerve palsy apparently cannot be reduced effectively by the later practice of prophylactic transposition of the ulnar nerve. All palsies recovered completely. None of the patients experienced pain requiring analgesics. None of the elbows were significantly weak. The elbow with type C3 fracture showed narrowing of joint space but no significant symptoms. There were no cases of nonunion, infection or broken implants. One olecranon repair loosened, but the osteotomy healed well without intervention. There were no varus or valgus deformities, no limitation of pronation or supination, and no myositis ossificans. The arc of movement for the two type C1 fractures were 110° and 120°, respectively; the average arc of movement for the type C2 fractures was 122° (range 110°–135°); and the single type C3 fracture achieved 95°. These results compare favourably with those from Holdsworth and Mossad [41], who achieved, respectively, 120°, 95° and 100° in type C1, C2 and C3 fractures.

Fractures of the Olecranon

Almost all olecranon fractures are intra-articular. Simple transverse or oblique fractures are adequately treated by the Weber type of tension band wiring or bicortical screw fixation. More comminuted fractures require fixation by plate and screws. In the latter cases, severity of comminution may hinder the effective use of screws. Under such circumstances, the end of a one-third tubular plate may be cut at its hole and bent into hooks which anchor into the cortical bone at the tip of the olecranon process. Plate fixation can be further protected by the application of a figure-of-eight loop of stainless steel wire. (Fig. 13)

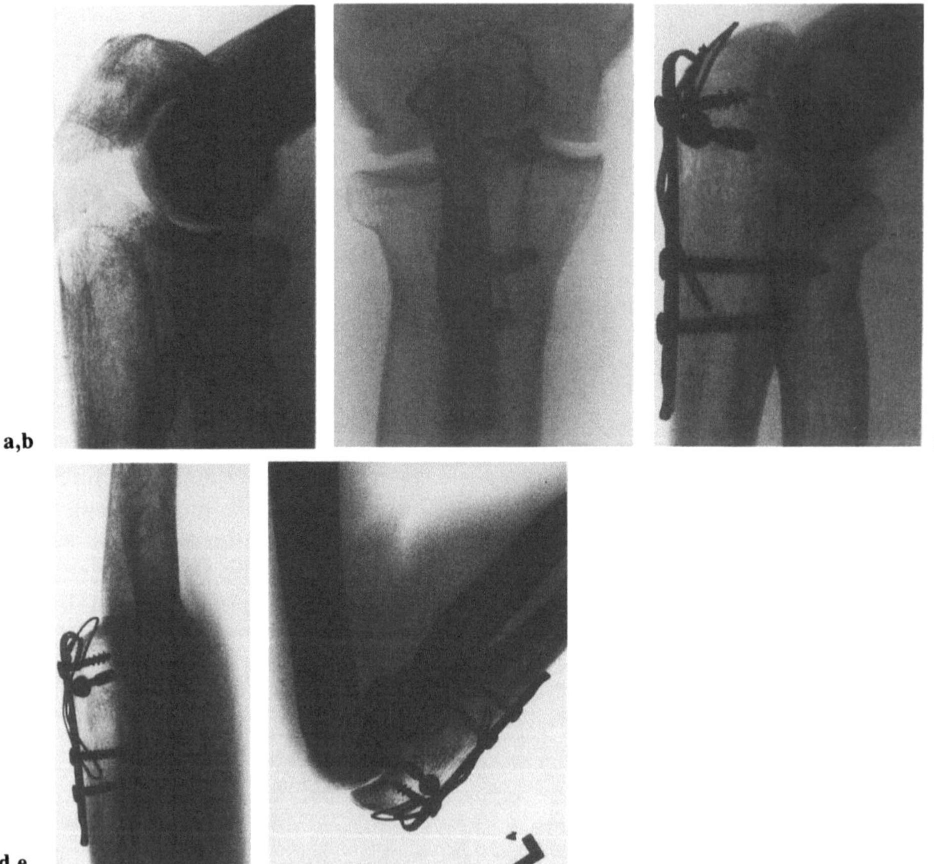

Fig. 13a–e. Comminuted fracture of olecranon treated with open reduction and internal fixation with hook plate and wire. **a** Pre-operative X-ray. **b** Post-operative antero-posterior view. **c** Post-operative lateral view. **d,e** One year after operation. **d** Lateral view with elbow in extension. **e** Lateral view with elbow in flexion. Range of movement achieved was 5°–135°

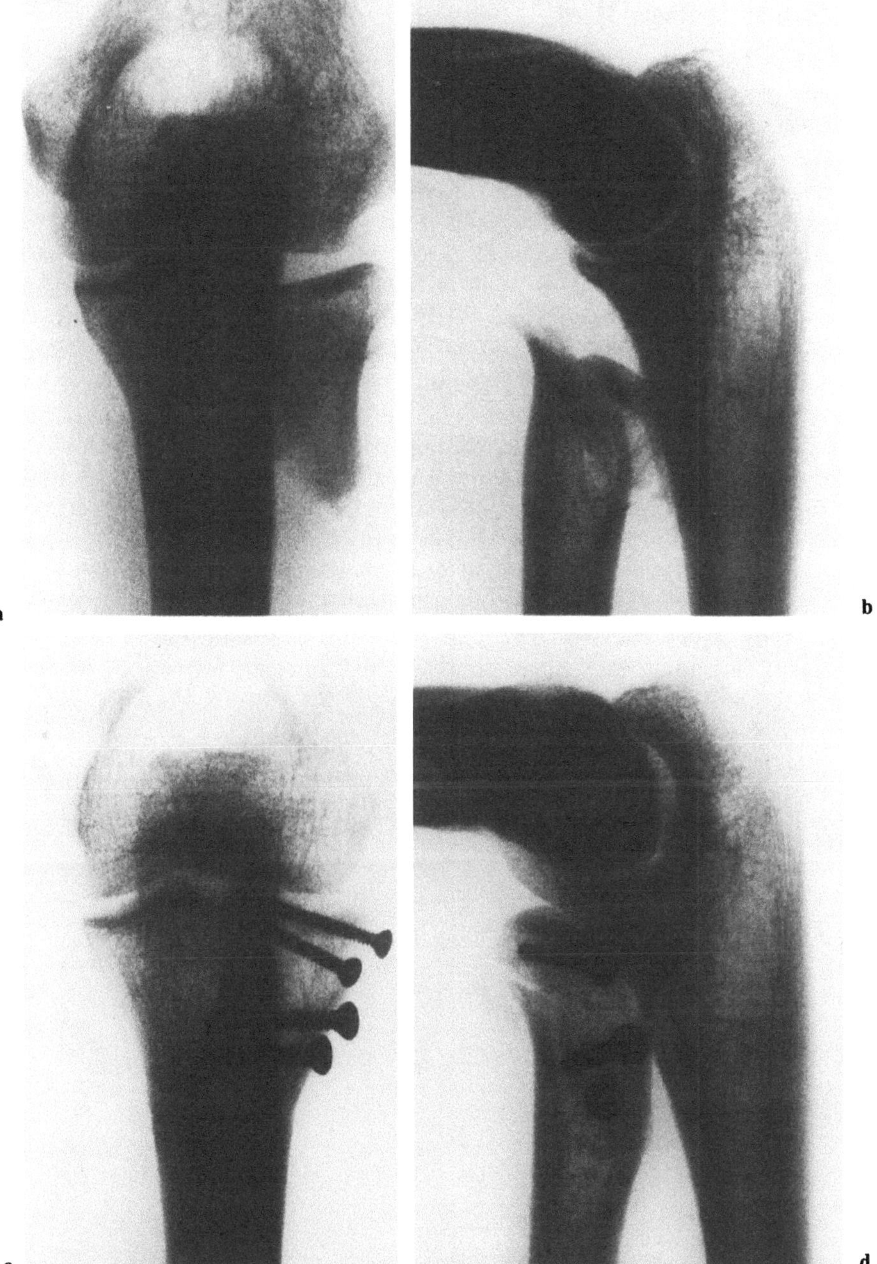

Fig. 14a–d. Fracture of radial head and neck treated with open reduction and fixation with multiple lag screws. **a** Pre-operative antero-posterior view. **b** Pre-operative lateral view. **c** Post-operative antero-posterior view. **d** Post-operative lateral view

Fractures of the Radial Head

In fractures of the radial head biplanar radiography is most essential for an accurate diagnosis and assessment of the degree of displacement. Simple undisplaced fractures are treated by a brief period of cast application followed by early mobilisation. Single-fragment displaced fractures are treated by open reduction and lag screw fixation (Fig. 14); if this fails, the fragment is discarded and the elbow mobilised (Fig. 15). Comminuted fractures are extremely difficult to reduce and fix. Even in those that are apparently well fixed, rotation of the forearm may be severely jeopardised by a minimal amount of incongruity together with the fibrosis associated with extensive surgical exposure. These comminuted fractures are best treated by early excision of the radial head. The complications of radial head excision are not common and not severe even when present; these include significant proximal migration of the radius causing wrist symptoms, valgus deformity of the elbow, loss of strength, degenerative arthritis, heterotopic calcification and myositis ossificans. The possibility of these complications per se do not out-balance the benefits of radial head sacrifice for comminuted fractures. Prosthetic replacement of the radial head should be reserved for the very few cases of gross instability resulting after radial head excision when severe ligamentous injury coexists. The late problems of silastic radial head replacement, including loosening, breakage and silicoma formation, further narrow the indications.

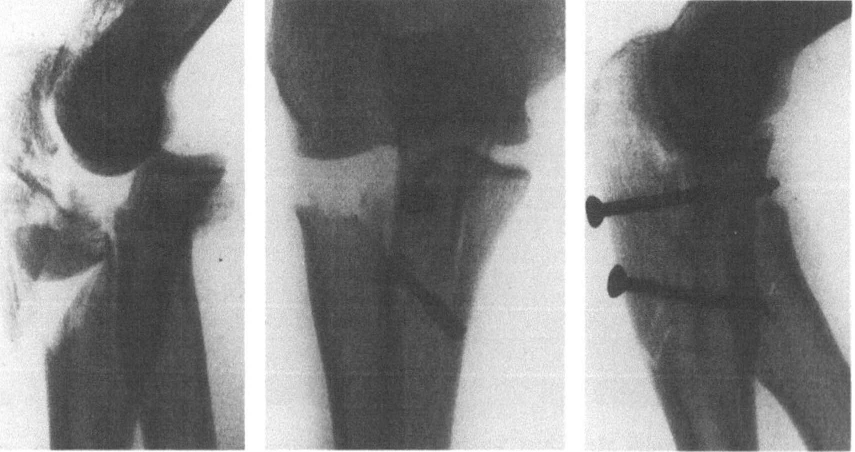

a,b   c

Fig. 15a–c. Comminuted fracture of the radial head associated with fracture of the proximal ulna treated with excision of the radial head and fixation of the ulna. **a** Pre-operative X-ray. **b** Post-operative antero-posterior view. **c** Post-operative lateral view

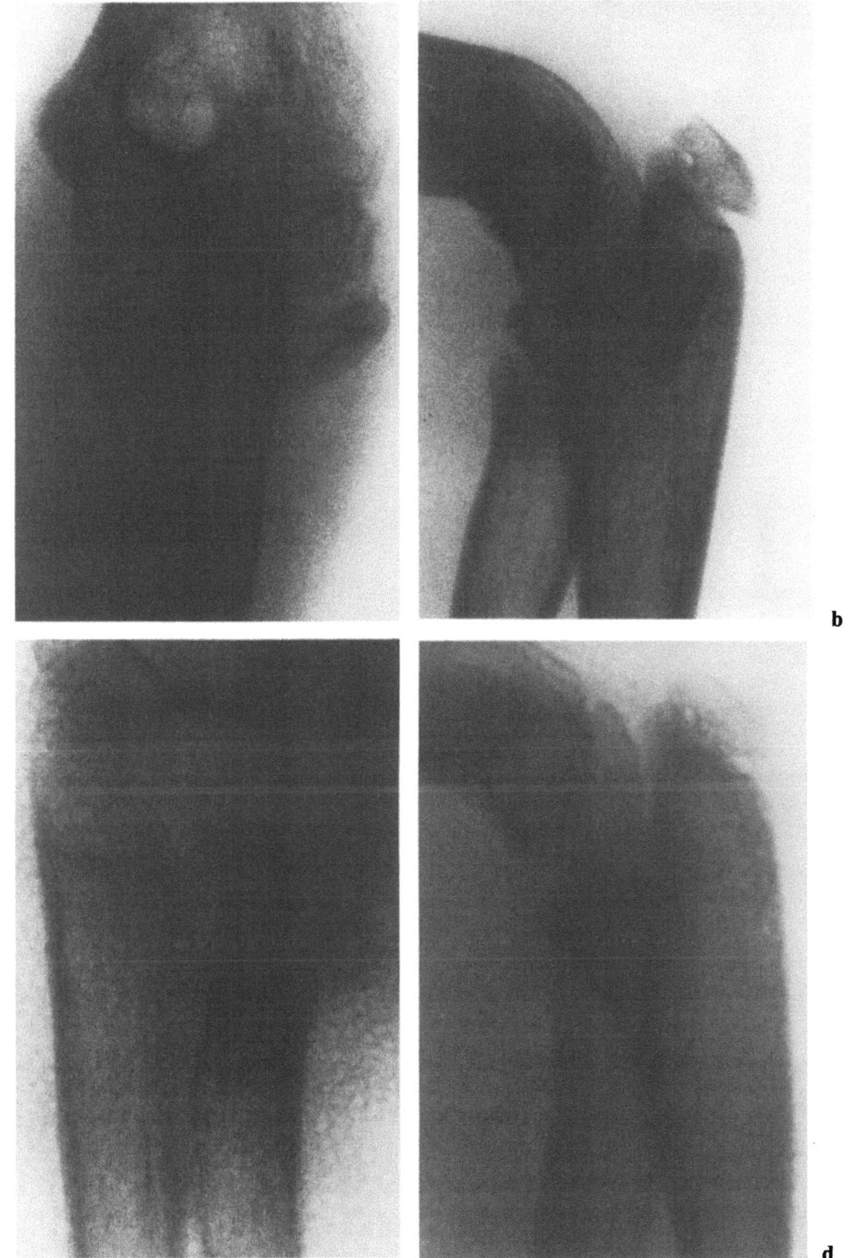

Fig. 16a–d. Fracture neck of the radius treated with open reduction and plaster immobilisation without internal fixation. **a** Pre-operative antero-posterior view. **b** Pre-operative lateral view. **c** Post-reduction antero-posterior view. **d** Post-reduction lateral view

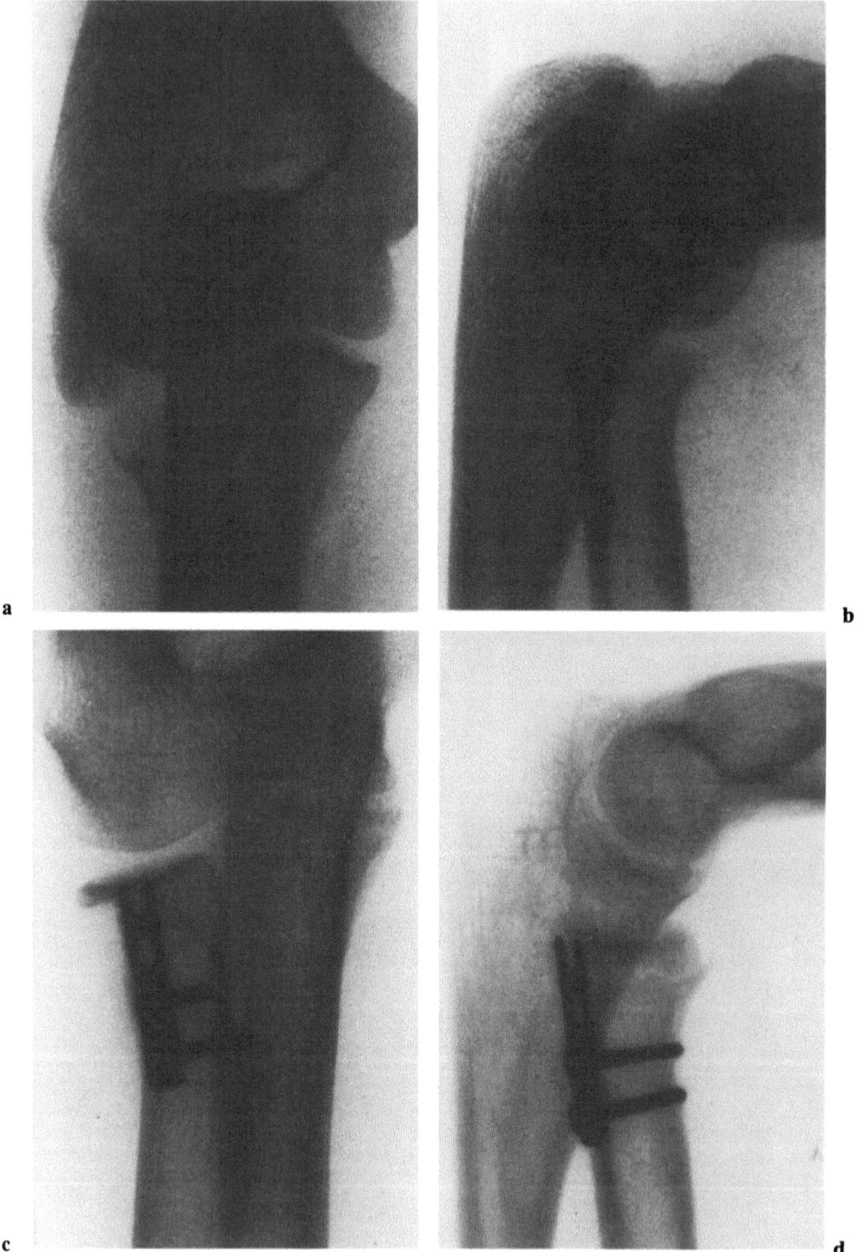

Fig. 17a–d. Fracture neck of the radius treated with open reduction and internal fixation using "fork" plate. **a** Pre-operative antero-posterior view. **b** Pre-operative lateral view. **c** Post-operative antero-posterior view. **d** Post-operative lateral view

Fractures of the Radial Neck

Completely separated fractures and those with translational displacement are treated by open reduction (Fig. 16). Internal fixation is indicated for those that are not stable after reduction. For oblique fractures one or two 2.7-mm mini-screws are sufficient to fix the fracture. For subcapital transverse fractures our recommended mode of fixation is that described by Leung and Tse [43]. A four-hole straight mini-plate is cut at one end hole to create a fork which is pushed firmly to anchor into the radial head while the rest of the plate is fixed to the radial shaft with 2-mm-diameter screws (Fig. 17). The annular ligament is repaired. Protected elbow and forearm mobilisation is achieved with the help of a hinged brace. We object to fixation using trans-capitellar Kirschner wire, which neither fixes nor aligns properly but, on the contrary, damages the articular surfaces. For those that are not completely separated, the angulation should be measured on a film taken at right angles to the plane of maximal angulation and compared with that on a film of the normal side taken in the same position. Screening under fluoroscopy is the most reliable method to determine the plane of maximal angulation. In general, angulations of less than 30° can be accepted while open reduction is indicated in those of more than 60°. With intermediate angulations the treatment modality becomes controversial.

References

1. Webb AJ, Sherman FC (1989) Supracondylar fractures of the humerus in children. J Pediatr Orthop 9:315
2. Clement DA (1990) Assessment of a treatment plan for managing acute vascular complications associated with supracondylar fractures of the humerus in children. J Pediatr Orthop 10:97
3. Lalanandham T, Laurence WN (1984) Entrapment of the ulnar nerve in the callus of a supracondylar fracture of the humerus. Injury 16:129
4. McGraw JJ, Akbarnia BA, Hanel DP, Keppler L, Burdge RE (1986) Neurological complications resulting from supracondylar fractures of the humerus in children. J Pediatr Orthop 6:647
5. Thorleifsson R, Karlsson J, Thorsteinsson T (1988) Median nerve entrapment in bone after supracondylar fracture of the humerus. Arch Orthop Trauma Surg 107:183
6. Bamford DJ, Stanley D (1989) Anterior interosseous nerve paralysis: an underdiagnosed complication of supracondylar fracture of the humerus in children. Injury 20:294
7. Martin DF, Tolo VT, Sellers DS, Weiland AJ (1989) Radial nerve laceration and retraction associated with a supracondylar fracture of the humerus. J Hand Surg [Am] 14:542
8. Smith HC (1894) Position in the treatment of elbow joint fractures: an experimental study. Boston Med Surg J 131:386
9. McLaughlin HL (1959) Trauma. Saunders, Philadelphia
10. D'Ambrosia RD (1972) Supracondylar fractures of humerus – prevention of cubitus varus. J Bone Joint Surg [Am] 54:60
11. Lund-Kristensen J, Vibild O (1976) Supracondylar fractures of the humerus in children. A follow-up with particular reference to late results after severely displaced fractures. Acta Orthop Scand 47:375

12. Worlock PH, Colton C (1987) Severely displaced supracondylar fractures of the humerus in children: a simple method of treatment. J Pediatr Orthop 7:49
13. Pirone AM, Graham HK, Krajbich JI (1988) Management of displaced extension-type supracondylar fractures of the humerus in children. J Bone Joint Surg [Am] 70:641
14. Swenson AL (1948) The treatment of supracondylar fractures of the humerus by Kirschner-wire transfixion. J Bone Joint Surg [Am] 30:993
15. Flynn JC, Matthews JG, Benoit RL (1974) Blind pinning of displaced supracondylar fractures of the humerus in children. Sixteen years' experience with long-term follow-up. J Bone Joint Surg [Am] 56:263
16. Fowles JV, Kassab MT (1974) Displaced supracondylar fractures of the elbow in children. A report on the fixation of extension and flexion fractures by two lateral percutaneous pins. J Bone Joint Surg [Br] 56:490
17. Jones KG (1967) Percutaneous pin fixation of fractures of the lower end of the humerus. Clin Orthop 50:53
18. Nacht JL, Ecker ML, Chung SMK, Lotke PA, Das M (1983) Supracondylar fractures of the humerus in children treated by closed reduction and percutaneous pinning. Clin Orthop 177:203
19. Aronson DD, Prager BI (1987) Supracondylar fractures of the humerus in children. A modified Technique for closed pinning. Clin Orthop 219:174
20. Thometz JG (1990) Techniques for direct radiographic visualization during closed pinning of supracondylar humerus fractures in children. J Pediatr Orthop 10:555
21. Gruber MA, Hudson OC (1964) Supracondylar fracture of the humerus in childhood. J Bone Joint Surg [Am] 46:1245
22. Carcassonne M, Bergoin M, Hornung H (1972) Results of operative treatment of severe supracondylar fractures of the elbow in children. J Pediatr Surg 7:676
23. Ramsey RH, Griz J (1973) Immediate open reduction and internal fixation of severely displaced supracondylar fractures of the humerus in children. Clin Orthop 90:130
24. Hart GM, Wilson DW, Arden GP (1977) The operative management of the difficult supracondylar fracture of the humerus in children. Injury 9:30
25. Weiland AJ, Meyer S, Tolo VT, Berg HL, Mueller J (1978) Surgical treatment of displaced supracondylar fractures of the humerus in children. J Bone Joint Surg [Am] 60:657
26. Danielsson L, Pettersson H (1980) Open reduction and pin fixation of severely displaced supracondylar fractures of the humerus in children. Acta Orthop Scand 51:249
27. Kekomaki M, Luoma R, Rikalainen H, Vilkki P (1984) Operative reduction and fixation of a difficult supracondylar extension fracture of the humerus. J Pediatr Orthop 4:13
28. Best CJ, Woods KR (1989) An aid to the treatment of supracondylar fracture of the humerus: brief report. J Bone Joint Surg [Br] 71:141
29. Culp RW, Osterman AL, Davidson RS, Skirven T, Bora W (1990) Neural injuries associated with supracondylar fractures of the humerus in children. J Bone Joint Surg [Am] 72:1211
30. Royce RO, Dutkowsky JP, Kasser JR, Rand FR (1991) Neurologic complications after K-wire fixation of supracondylar humerus fractures in children. J Pediatr Orthop 11:191
31. Flynn JC, Richards JF, Saltzman RI (1975) Prevention and treatment of non-union of slightly displaced fractures of the lateral humeral condyle in children. J Bone Joint Surg [Am] 57:1087
32. Van Vugt AB, Severijnen RVSM, Festen C (1988) Fractures of the lateral humeral condyle in children: late results. Arch Orthop Trauma Surg 107:206
33. Flynn JC (1989) Nonunion of slightly displaced fractures of the lateral humeral condyle in children: an update. J Pediatr Orthop 9:691
34. Herring JA (1986) Lateral condylar fracture of the elbow. J Pediatr Orthop 6:724

35. So YC, Fang D, Leong JCY, Bong SC (1985) Varus deformity following lateral humeral condylar fractures in children. J Pediatr Orthop 5:569
36. Muller ME, Nazarian S, Koch P (1988) The AO classification of fractures. Springer, Berlin Heidelberg New York
37. Charnley J (1961) The closed treatment of common fractures, 3rd edn. Churchill Livingstone, Edinburgh, p 71
38. Jupiter JB, Neff U, Holzach P, Allgöwer M (1985) Intercondylar fractures of the humerus. An operative approach. J Bone Joint Surg [Am] 67:226
39. Waddell JP, Hatch J, Richards R (1988) Supracondylar fractures of the humerus – results of surgical treatment. J Trauma 28:1615
40. Letsch R, Schmidt-Neuerburg KP, Sturmer KM, Walz M (1989) Intraarticular fractures of the distal humerus. Surgical treatment and results. Clin Orthop 241:238
41. Holdsworth BJ, Mossad MM (1990) Fractures of the adult distal humerus. Elbow function after internal fixation. J Bone Joint Surg [Br] 72:362
42. Alonso-Llames M (1972) Bilaterotricipital approach to the elbow. Its application in the osteosynthesis of supracondylar fractures of the humerus in children. Acta Orthop Scand 43:479
43. Leung KS, Tse PYT (1989) A new method of fixing radial neck fractures: brief report. J Bone Joint Surg [Br] 71:326
44. Morrey BF (1985) The elbow and its disorders. Saunders, Philadelphia

11 Problems in Shoulder Fractures

S.Y.C. Hsu

The gleno-humeral joint is the most mobile joint of the body. Its pivotal role in the motion of the upper limb makes it particularly vulnerable to direct and indirect trauma. Fracture around the shoulder poses many problems to orthopaedic surgeons, and the incidence of proximal humeral fractures is increasing. Because of the three-dimensional nature of the fracture in this region, plain radiographs cannot always depict fully the true picture. Although consensus has been reached for the treatment of most fractures around the shoulder, unsatisfactory results are encountered both in fractures treated conservatively and in those treated operatively. Complications arising from the trauma itself and from the treatment given can be avoided only if the clinician is fully aware of their causative factors.

Proximal Humeral Fracture

Introduction

Fracture of the proximal humerus in the adult has been rightly considered an unsolved problem [1] because of the high incidence of unsatisfactory results after treatment. This is particularly true for displaced fractures, 50% of which cases involve complications of some sort. These range from the almost inevitable pain and stiffness to the not infrequent problems of nonunion, malunion, impingement syndrome and avascular necrosis of the humeral head to the rare but catastrophic occurrence of brachial plexus and axillary vessel damage. A better understanding of this fracture would definitely help in improving the management of the injury: its incidence, the difficulty in defining the fracture character, the problem of fracture reduction and fixation, and the potential complications involved.

Epidemiology

Fracture of the proximal humerus accounts for around 5% of all the fractures, but the incidence is on the rise. In a Swedish study of more than 2000 cases over more than 30 years, Bengner and Johnell [2] noted a progressive rise in the age-related incidence of this fracture in elderly women (Fig. 1).

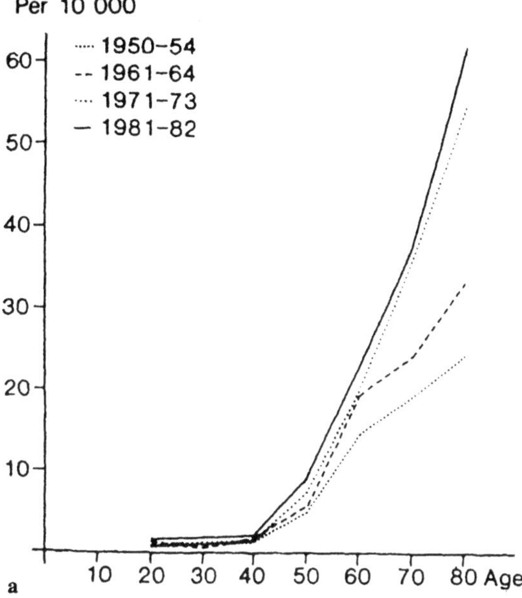

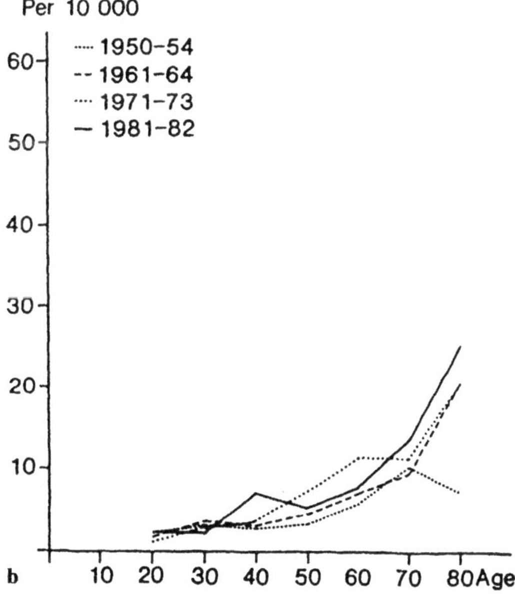

Fig. 1a–b. Age-specific annual incidence of fracture of the upper end of the humerus per 10 000 patients in the 1950s, 1960s, 1970s, and 1980s. **a** Women. **b** Men. (From [2])

This increase in incidence was found not to be an isolated one but to apply also to fractures related to osteoporosis such as the hip and the distal radius. They also found an increase in the percentage of fractures classified as severe. They postulated that the rise is related to a reduction in bone mineral content, leading to a more vulnerable skeleton. Other possibilities include a declining frequency of physical activities and a change in life-style that makes persons more prone to geriatric trauma. In a Danish study [3] 75% of cases occurred in patients 60 years of age or older, and the majority of these patients sustained their injury by a fall on level ground or at home. Although it is a common belief that 85% of proximal humeral fractures are minimally or nondisplaced [4], the authors reported 71% two-part and 17% three-part fractures.

Although no age group is immune from these fractures, the elderly are particularly at risk because of their more osteoporotic skeleton and their poorer body coordination. Coupled with the difficulty in fixing these fractures because of the poor bone stock and the inferior rehabilitation potential, it is not surprising that the end results are less than desirable overall.

Problems with Identification of Pathology

A good classification of fractures should serve a number of functions. First, it should depict the direction or mode of displacement of bone fragments; second, it should have a directive role in deciding the form of management; and, third, it should have a predictive value for the occurrence of complications, as a result both of the injury and of the treatment itself.

It has long been recognised that proximal humeral fractures tend to occur along previous epiphyseal lines [5,6]. Neer [7] developed upon this and proposed a classification based on the pattern of displacement and on the key segments that are displaced (Fig. 2). This classification has stood the test of time both in its wide acceptance in the orthopaedic field and its prognostic value. Neer's classification, which has now become a classic [8] is based upon the definition of displacement as being more than 10 mm separation or angulation of more than 45° between the fragments. However, this classification rests heavily if not entirely on radiology, which is dependent upon operator, technique, patient and examiner.

Because the shoulder joint lies at an oblique plane to the body and because of the superimposition of shadows, a single antero-posterior radiographic projection cannot reveal the fracture pattern in its totality. Neer [7] and Hawkins and Angelo [9] have suggested a trauma series of three roentgenographic views: one perpendicular and one parallel to the scapular plane, together with an axillary view by putting the arm in 20°–40° of abduction. The latter view is thought essential because it is perpendicular to the two previous views and can reveal the easily missed pathologies of shoulder dislocation and glenoid rim fractures. However, this axillary view

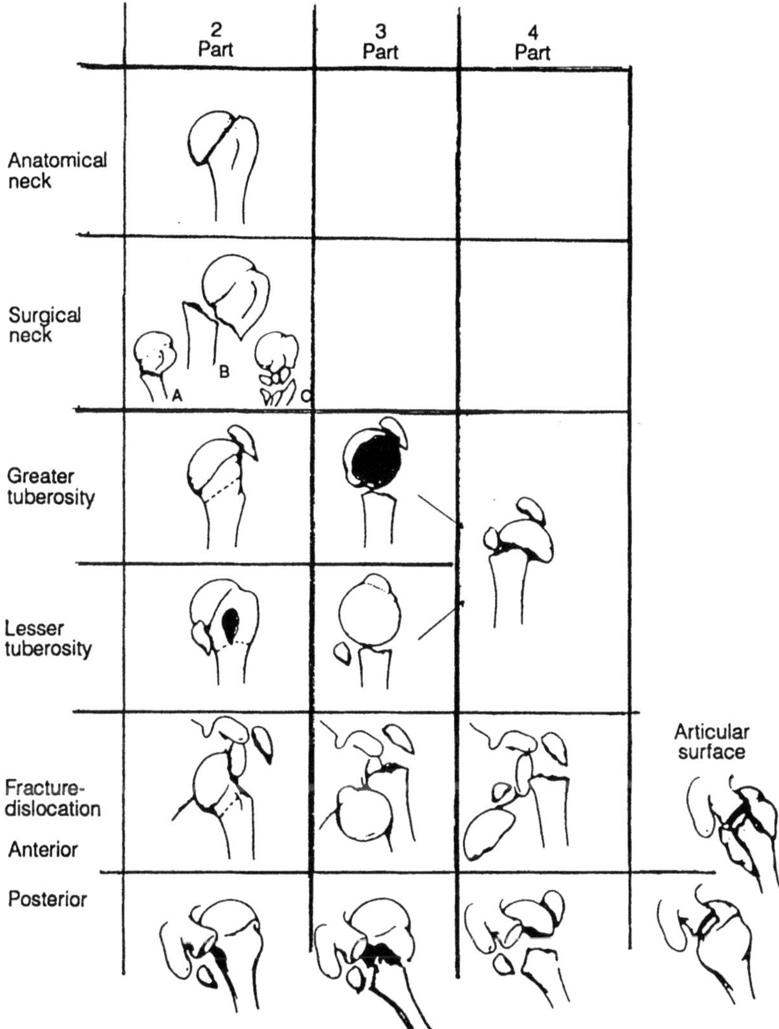

Fig. 2. Neer's classification of proximal humeral fractures

may at times pose a problem when it induces pain or discomfort by abducting the patient's arm.

The apical oblique projection has been suggested by Garth et al. [10] to be included in cases of trauma around the shoulder because it can easily be mastered by the radiographer and is entirely pain free to the patient (Fig. 3). It is taken by placing the injured shoulder in a 45° posterior oblique position while angulating the central ray 45° caudad. Although the apical oblique view is less sensitive than the routine antero-posterior view, it is

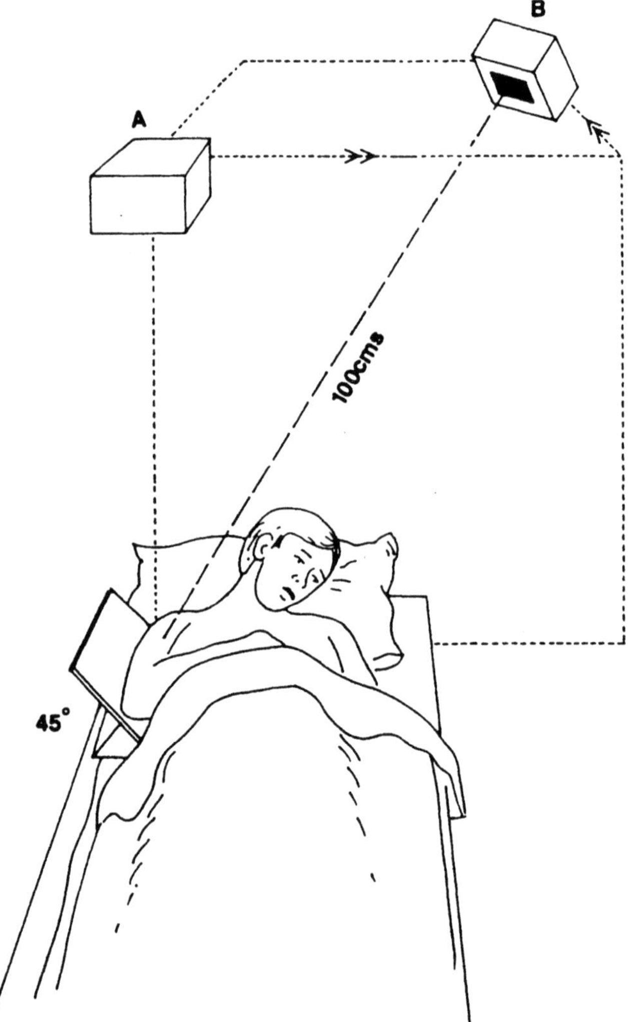

Fig. 3. Method for obtaining an apical oblique projection in a supine patient: (a) take antero-posterior view as usual from *A* at 100 cm; (b) imagine a cube of 100 cm on each side and move tube to opposite corner, *B*; (c) centre on glenoid; (d) check that the anode-to-film distance is 100 cm

sensitive in identifying Hill-Sachs lesion, glenoid rim fracture, posterior dislocation, intra-articular extension of scapular fracture and occult clavicular fracture [11].

Kristiansen et al. [12] studied 100 cases of surgical neck fractures on the basis of both antero-posterior and lateral radiographs and found good agreement among examiners in the minimally displaced fractures. However, the inter-observer variation was high regarding displaced fractures. This may be due to the fact that it is inherently difficult to judge the distance and rotation of displaced fractures in a two-dimensional projection shadow. This is particularly significant because the optimal mode of treatment of displaced fractures depends heavily on the correct classification. Thus, it was suggested that radiographs of proximal humeral fractures should be examined by experienced orthopaedic surgeons or radiologists, and that there should be no hesitation in requesting for more views if in doubt.

Castagno et al. [13] evaluated the role of computed tomography (CT) in depicting the pathology of complex proximal humeral fractures. In each of their 17 patients, CT provided new information that helped the surgeons decide the correct mode of treatment. They found CT particularly good in defining the existence of fracture lines, amount of displacement of fracture fragments, degree of rotation of these fragments, and status of the head and articular surface – factors which are absolutely essential for correct classification. They also found that in healed fractures, CT may provide a clue as to the cause of limitation of movement. They therefore recommended CT as a valuable complement when the fracture pattern is hard to define by plain radiology alone. Other authors [14] have also reported CT to be helpful in evaluating complex and comminuted fracture-dislocation of the proximal humerus.

Problems with Management

Because of the complexity of the fracture and the many factors to be considered, management of proximal humeral fractures must be individualised. The best and most appropriate treatment cannot be offered until due consideration is given to: (a) accurate and correct definition of the fracture pattern; (b) patient's physiological condition, including physiological age, medical health, degree of osteoporosis and pre-morbid activity level; (c) patient's cooperation and expectation; and (d) surgeon's experience and the availability of a good rehabilitation team. A decision-making algorithm such as that proposed by Tile [15] (Fig. 4) is very helpful in deciding the treatment programme; nevertheless, one must be aware of the many problems associated with each and every choice.

Closed Treatment

Closed treatment for proximal humeral fractures has always had its advocates [4,16,17]. Although Mills [17] did not categorise his cases on the basis of Neer's classification, he nevertheless found that closed treatment of comminuted proximal humeral fractures yields results that are similar to if not better than those of open treatment. Leyshon [18] conducted a retrospective review of 42 patients suffering from three- or four-part fractures of the proximal humerus treated by rest in a broad arm sling for 4 weeks followed

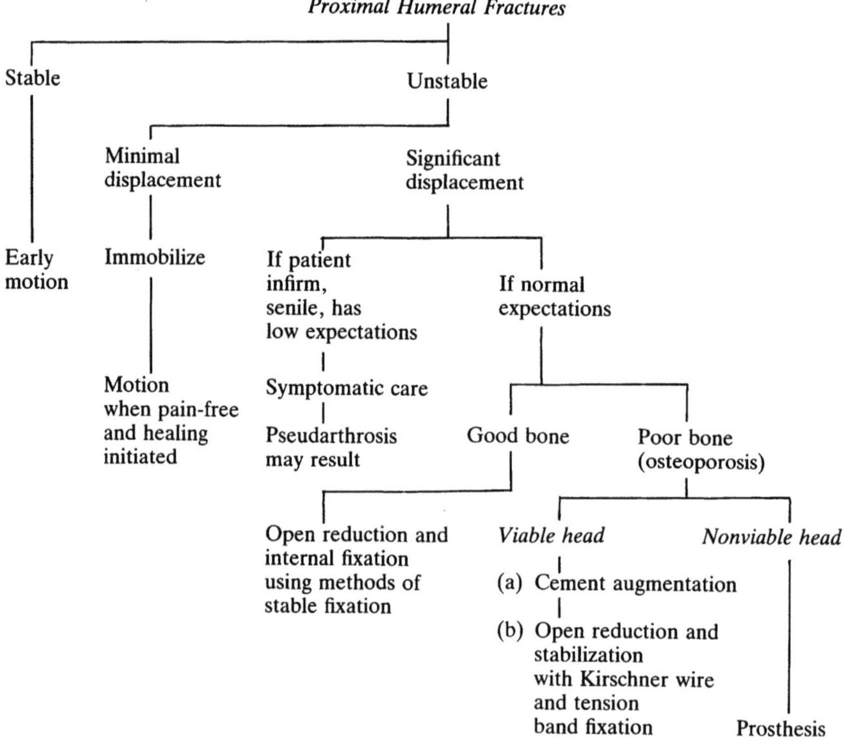

Fig. 4. Decision-making algorithm for proximal humeral fractures. (From [15])

by physiotherapy for 10 weeks. He found that outcome was quite satisfactory in the three-part fractures, especially in elderly patients. This finding was confirmed by another study by Young and Wallace [19] who found that 94% of patients treated by conservative means had either good or satisfactory results. However, the results for four-part fractures in Leyshon's series were poor as a result of the high incidence of avascular necrosis and failure of remodelling. This was confirmed in Stableforth's [20] retrospective study on 32 patients treated by nonoperative means who had persistent pain, stiffness and dysfunction of the shoulder.

It is not too surprising that closed treatment can provide acceptable results especially in the elderly (Fig. 5). First of all, although closed treatment does not yield the initial stability of internal fixation, it avoids the surgical trauma to soft tissue and thus allows rather early rehabilitation. Secondly, it diminishes the chance of further disrupting the blood supply to the bone fragments and lessens the propensity to avascular necrosis. Thirdly, pain is not found to be disabling in these patients even when the fracture is severe [17,21]. Fourthly, Miller [17] observed in 1940 that incom-

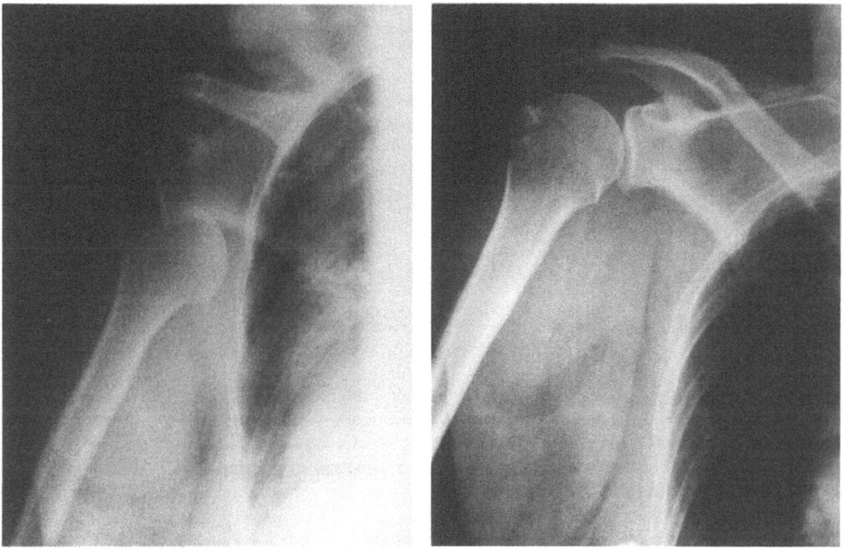

Fig. 5. a Fracture-dislocation in an 80-year-old woman. **b** Successful closed treatment, after 8 weeks

plete reduction of fractures in the upper fourth of the humerus was compatible with good results. Lastly, DePalmar and Cautilli [22] Mills [17] and Young and Wallace [19] have observed that the roentgenographic appearance does not correlate with the clinical results.

However, closed treatment is not entirely free of problems. The proximal humerus is notoriously difficult to immobilise because it is so near the trunk. Because of the actions of the different muscle groups on the separated bone fragments, various forms of malpositioning are possible, especially varus angulation between the head and shaft, medial displacement of the shaft and external or internal rotation of the humeral head. At times, soft-tissue interposition is inevitable due to periosteum, biceps tendon, deltoid muscle or pectoralis major, which may lead to nonunion.

Open Treatment

Increasing numbers of authors [9,23–25] now agree that operative treatment is the treatment of choice for high-grade unstable, displaced and comminuted fractures. Open reduction and internal fixation is not indicated in minimally displaced fractures, occasionally indicated in two-part fractures such as in avulsion fracture of the greater tuberosity giving rise to a mechanical block under the acromion (Fig. 6), frequently indicated in three-part fractures, and not infrequently indicated in four-part fractures especially if the patient is young.

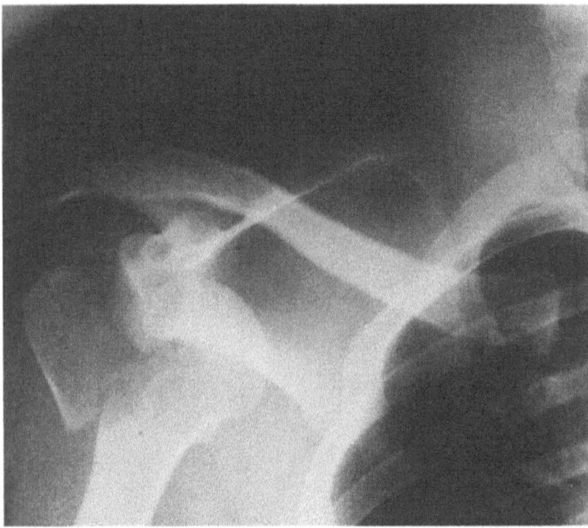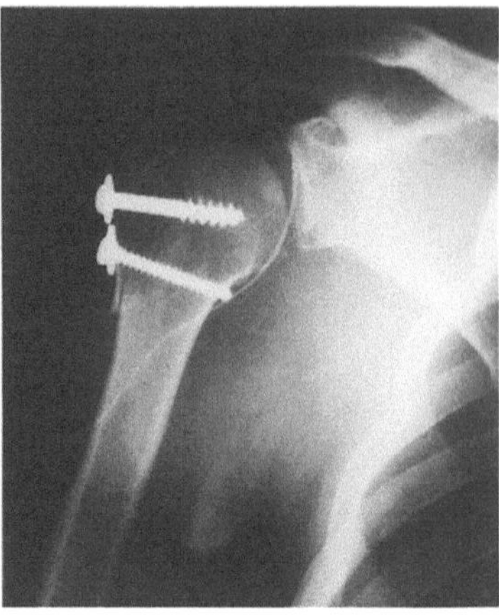

a   b

Fig. 6. a Avulsion fracture-dislocation in a 45-year-old man. **b** Treated by open reduction and AO screw fixation

There is better consensus concerning the technical details of the surgical approach of open reduction and internal fixation but more dispute over the best methods of fixation. The salient features in the technique of open reduction and internal fixation can be summarised as follows:

1. Delto-pectoral approach
2. Detachment or subperiosteal elevation of deltoid insertion to widen exposure
3. Release of pectoralis major tendon if further widening of the exposure is required
4. Preservation of the ascending branch of the anterior humeral circumflex artery at the bicipital groove
5. Secure fixation of the bone fragment at least to allow passive mobilisation without dislodgement
6. Use of intra-operative X-ray to confirm reduction and exclude penetration of implant into the joint
7. Evaluation of all ranges of shoulder motion and attention to the possibility of impingement syndrome
8. Determination of whether excision of the coraco-acromial ligament and acromioplasty is required
9. Inspection and repair of tears of the rotator cuff
10. Careful closure of all layers with suction drainage

There is a wide diversity of opinion as to the most appropriate fixative device for proximal humeral fractures. Obviously, each case must be decided on its own merits. Most of the time it is determined by both the surgeon's preference and the demand of the circumstances. Hawkins et al. [26] have strongly recommended the use of tension band wiring. They maintain that this technique requires less soft-tissue dissection, and that theoretically there should therefore be less chance of avascular necrosis. Savoie et al. [23] used the T or L buttress plate but cautioned that the top of the plate should be placed at the mid-part of the humeral head to avoid impingement syndrome. Kristiansen and Christensen [27] also used a buttress plate but encountered significant complications, including infection, impingement, loosening and avascular necrosis of the humeral head. Other authors have used percutaneous pinning, hook plate, Rush pin with sutures, transcutaneous reduction and Hoffman external fixator, and improvised plate (Fig. 7).

Hemi-Arthroplasty Replacement

Neer's hemi-arthroplasty (Fig. 8) has become an indispensible item in the armamentarium of implants for the surgical treatment of comminuted fracture of the proximal humerus. Its indications have been extended to:

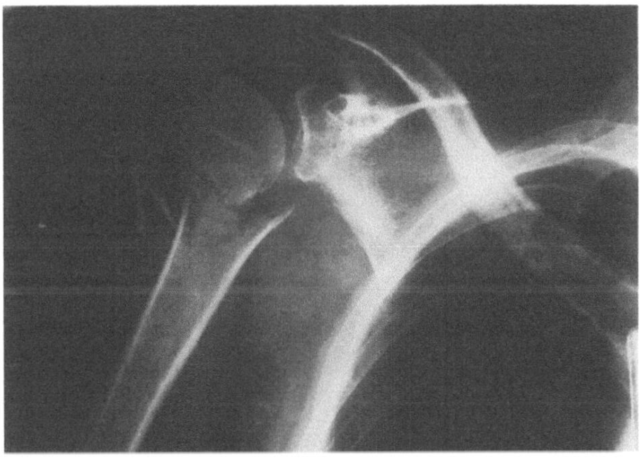

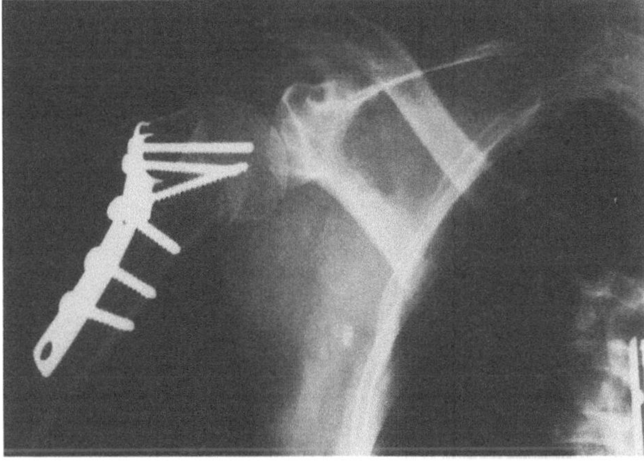

Fig. 7. a Three-part fracture in a 58-year-old woman. **b** Treated by open reduction and internal fixation with an improvised plate

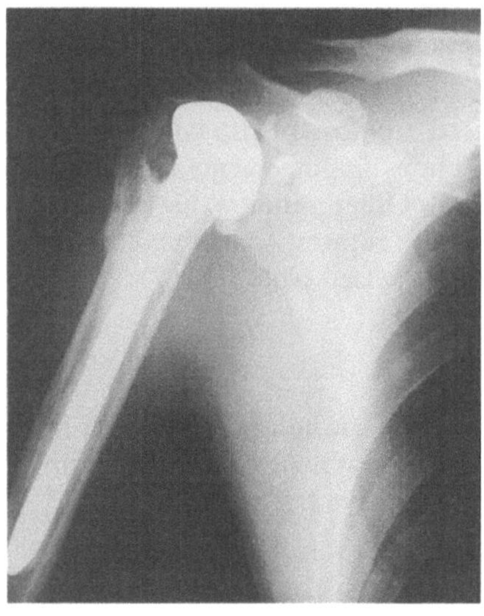

Fig. 8. Neer's hemi-arthroplasty

1. Four-part fractures or fracture-dislocation
2. Three-part fractures in the elderly, especially those with severe osteoporosis and comminution
3. Humeral head denuded of all soft-tissue attachment
4. Humeral head suffering from more than 50% impaction
5. Old, untreated fracture with nonunion, malunion or avascular necrosis

Various authors have spelled out the technical details that must be
adhered to in order to achieve the best clnical results [7,28,29]. These
include:

1. Improvement of exposure by detaching part of the deltoid and osteoto-
   mising the coracoid process
2. Identification and protection of the axillary nerve deep to the deltoid
3. Placement of the prosthesis at 30° of retroversion
4. Maintaining the humeral length by not pushing the prosthesis too deep
   into the shaft
5. Use of cement whenever required
6. Secure fixation of the tuberosities using both horizontal and vertical
   sutures
7. Bone-grafting (harvested from humeral head) between tuberosities and
   shaft whenever necessary
8. Repair of the rotator cuff
9. Post-operative arm support putting the arm between neutal and 45° of
   abduction depending on the tension of the tuberosity sutures
10. Excellent compliance to post-operative rehabilitative programme

Despite the awareness of the possible problems and complications of the Neer's arthroplasty in the past two to three decades, the clinical results have been inconsistent and variable [28]. This is due largely to the relatively high complication rate associated with this procedure, some of which are inherent while others are avoidable.

Stiffness. In most series, the abduction range was at best 90°–110° after hemi-arthroplasty for acute fracture. This was found to be inferior to a similar procedure carried out for chronic fracture problems [28] or avascular necrosis of the humeral head [29]. The reason for this not entirely clear, but it has been suggested to be due to damage or scarring of the rotator cuff [28]. Willems and Lim [30] used video-fluoroscopy to study the movement after Neer's arthroplasties and found that gleno-humeral movement is minimal in most cases. In fact, they stated that the prosthesis acted more as a spacer than as an arthroplasty. However, in spite of this finding most of their patients enjoyed good mastering of the activities of daily life.

Transient Inferior Subluxation. This has been found to be quite a common problem especially in the first 3–4 weeks [20]. Provided that this is not due to a decrease in arm length or paralysis of the deltoid, it usually resolves spontaneously when the muscle tone returns.

Nonunion or Malunion of Tuberosities. This is due to failure of contact of the tuberosities to the parent shaft. The causes are multiple. It may be due to a technical failure to secure good bone contact or to excessive bone removal from the fracture fragments. Sometimes it is a result of the pulling off of the bone fragments from the shaft due to excessive tension in the repair of tuberosities or inappropriate, premature, active and resistive exercises.

Shortened Arm Length. Unduly deep insertion of the prosthesis into the shaft causes weakness of the deltoid and possible instability.

Dislocation. This usually results from a technical failure to put the prosthesis in 20°–40° of retroversion with respect to the two humeral epicondyles.

Pericapsular Calcification

Impingement Syndrome

Loosening. This has not been found to be a common problem provided the right size of prosthesis has been press-fit into the shaft. Some authors [29] routinely cement their Neer's hemi-athroplasties.

Problems with Rehabilitation

Rehabilitation always involves an unending battle between stability of the fracture and early mobilisation. This cannot be more true than in the case of proximal humeral fractures. All authors agree that an early and aggressive mobilisation programme is of the utmost importance in achieving functional recovery.

As a general rule, passive mobilisation is started very early. Depending on the initial stability of the fracture, gentle passive abduction and external mobilisation should be started between the first and fourth weeks. This is followed by active assisted exercises and isometric strengthening at around the sixth week, when considerable stability is established. Isotonic strengthening can generally be started after around 3 months, when clinical union occurs.

It is well known that shoulder rehabilitation after proximal humeral fracture is time consuming. Hawkins et al. [26] have warned that maximal recovery is seldom realised earlier than 1 year following injury. In some cases it may take as long as 18 months.

Problems with Complications

The possible complications are many. These may result from the injury itself or from the treatment offered, but is often a consequence of both.

Stiffness. Joint stiffness is usually due to bursal adhesion and capsular contracture [26]. Delayed mobilisation is often the culprit and should be avoided at all cost. However, when joint stiffness sets in, prolonged and persistent stretching is required. Hawkins et al. [26] have advised against manipulation under anaesthesia lest it result in refracture.

Nonunion. This is not an infrequent complication of fracture of surgical neck of humerus [26]. This is thought to be due to one of the following: excessive distraction, inadequate immobilisation, soft-tissue interposition or poor blood supply. Various types of rigid internal fixation and bone grafting procedures have been suggested.

Malunion. Malunion of the greater tuberosity may give rise to impingement syndrome and result in limitation of abduction. On the other hand, malunion of the surgical neck of the humerus may give rise to an anterior angulation and result in limitation of flexion [26].

Avascular Necrosis. Ischaemic necrosis of the humeral head is a very common and well-known sequela of four-part fractures. Leyshon [18] reported an incidence as high as 75% following closed treatment. Sturzenegger et al. [31] believed that the chance of avascular necrosis increases with the complexity of osteosynthesis and suggested that atraumatic open reduction and simple internal fixation should be used when retention of the head is deemed feasible. Since avascular necrosis invariably gives rise to severe pain and limitation of motion, prosthetic replacement is a reasonable prophylaxis and choice of treatment for such a condition.

Axillary Artery Damage. Although axillary artery damage is a rare complication of proximal humeral fracture, it is a real surgical emergency when it occurs. Weile and Fjeldborg [32] believed that the proneness of the axillary artery to damage is due to its proximal fixation by the thoraco-acromial artery and distally by the humeral circumflex arteries. The axillary artery may be damaged by spasm from kinking, thrombosis from intimal damage or actual transection from jagged ends of the fracture. Because of the preservation of the collateral circulation, axillary artery damage may be masked initially, and the diagnosis may rest on vigilance and the use of Doppler ultrasound. Prompt confirmation by arteriogram and immediate exploration has been recommended to avoid the dreaded complication of distal gangrene [33].

Brachial Plexus Injury. It is not uncommon to miss a brachial plexus injury after proximal humeral fracture dislocation. Detailed motor and sensory examination is mandatory. When doubt arises, electro-myographic study may be undertaken after around 2–3 weeks to better define the neurological injury [26]. Leffert and Seddon [34], with one of the largest series of brachial plexus injuries after shoulder fracture dislocations, found that although infra-clavicular injuries have a better prognosis than the supra-clavicular counterpart, functional recovery is often affected by pain, stiffness and weakness. Damage to the axillary nerve invariably results in poor prognosis. Parsons and Rowley [35] suggested that early reduction is absolutely essential because the trauma is usually a traction injury. Gentle reduction through operative means under full muscle-relaxing anaesthetic is often preferred.

Impingement Syndrome. The best time for the evaluation of impingement after open reduction and internal fixation or prosthetic replacement is during the operation. The shoulder should be brought through all the ranges, and prophylactic acromioplasty should be performed when the need arises.

Heterotopic Ossification. Neer [7] thought that heterotopic ossification is related to repeated, forceful closed reduction or to a delay of open reduction for more than 1 week. Management is similar to that in myositis ossificans in that excision and releases should be considered only when the lesion is no longer active.

Scapular Fracture

Scapular fracture is not uncommon in multi-injured patients. The energy involved in such injuries is usually very high. Despite the fact that it is usually clinically obvious, it is often missed in the acute stage. There is little controversy over the management of this type of fracture, but consideration should also be given to the associated injuries.

Energy Involved in Scapular Fractures

Since the scapula is enveloped by muscles, it is well known that significant energy is needed in order to fracture it. Most cases of scapular fractures result from direct high-energy trauma such as road-traffic accidents and falling from heights. Although scapular fractures are rare [36], the mortality rate in this group of patients is high. Armstrong and Van der Spuy [36] in their prospective review of 62 patients with 64 fractures of the scapula found a mortality rate of 9.7% while Thompson et al. [37] in their study of 56 patients with 58 fractures reported a mortality rate of 14.3%.

Because of the severe nature of the injury involved, patients suffering from scapular fractures stand a high chance of multiple associated injuries [36,38]. Thompson et al. [37] found that their patients had an average of 3.9 major injuries in addition to their scapular fractures. Fracture rib and pulmonary contusion were the most frequent associated injuries. They also found that pulmonary contusion has a poor prognosis in that half of the mortality resulted from pulmonary sepsis as a consequence of pulmonary contusion. They also noted a high association of fracture of the body of the scapula with brachial plexus injuries and arterial injuries.

Diagnosis of Scapular Fractures

Since most scapular fractures result from blunt trauma, it is not surprising that they are commonly overlooked [36]. Another reason for delaying or missing the diagnosis is probably the fact that the examiner is usually overwhelmed by the gravity of other associated injuries. Therefore, numerous authors [36,39] have suggested that it is essential to be alert to fracture of the scapula in multi-injured patients and vice versa.

Scapula fracture per se is not life threatening, and there is no absolute necessity to call for a complete evaluation in the acute stage. Nevertheless, subsequent detailed examination of the X-rays is essential to decide on the most appropriate treatment. Hardegger et al. [39] have suggested the use of three views: an antero-posterior view perpendicular to the plane of the scapula, a lateral view parallel to the scapular plane and an axillary view. Fracture of the scapula is best classified into eight types, although combinations do occur (Fig. 9).

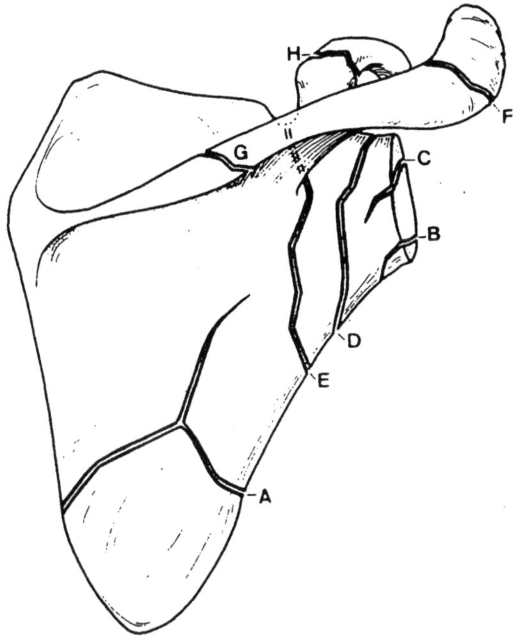

Fig. 9. Fracture types: *A*, body; *B*, glenoid rim; *C*, glenoid fossa; *D*, anatomical neck; *E*, surgical neck; *F*, acromion; *G*, spine; *H*, coracoid process. (From [39])

The site of scapular fracture is most commonly in the body, followed by the neck and glenoid process, while fractures of the spine, coracoid or acrominon are relatively uncommon.

Treatment of Scapular Fracture

McGahan et al. [40] described the treatment of scapular fractures as depending on the age of the patient, his occupation and his clinical presentation. Hardegger et al. [39] suggested that treatment of scapular fracture should be dictated by the site of the fracture and the amount of displacement. They divided scapular fractures into two groups: (a) those with fracture of the body, neck or apophyses (coracoid, acromion and spine) with minimal displacement and (b) those with fracture-dislocation of the glenoid, unstable fracture of the scapular neck or significant displacement of the apophyses. They recommended that conservative treatment should be sufficient for the former while open anatomical reduction and internal fixation should be performed for the latter to avoid prolonged immobilisation, stiffness and osteoarthritis. Specifically, they recommend surgical intervention in the following circumstances:

- Fracture of the body of the scapula with a large sharp spike that enters the joint
- Fracture of the glenoid rim associated with traumatic dislocation of the humeral head
- Fracture of the glenoid fossa with significant displacement
- Fracture of the anatomical neck with significant displacement by the pull of the long head of triceps
- Fracture of the surgical neck of scapula associated with concomitant fracture of the clavicle or disruption of the coraco-clavicular ligaments or both
- Fracture of the acromion with significant displacement leading to impingement syndrome
- Fracture of the coracoid process with compression of the neuro-vascular bundle

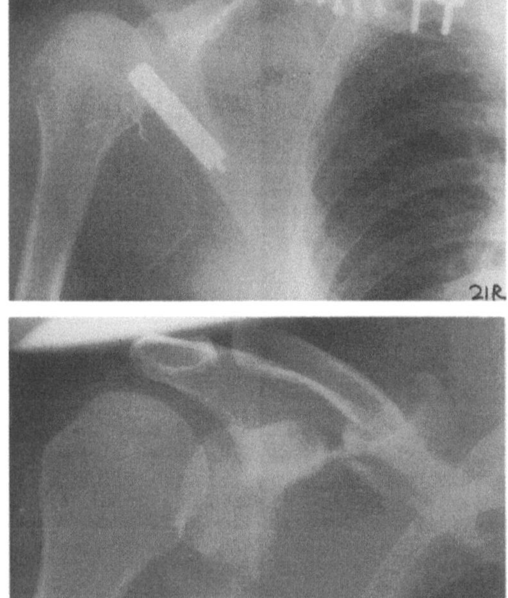

Fig. 10. a Fracture of the neck of scapular together with fracture of the clavicle. **b** Post-operative radiograph after open reduction and internal fixation

Of all the suggested indications for operative treatment, fracture of the anatomical or surgical neck of the scapula when combined with fracture of the clavicle may lead to loss of continuity between the upper limb and the shoulder girdle, giving rise to a "floating shoulder" situation. This demands open reduction and internal fixation to restore such a continuity (Fig. 10).

Early mobilisation can be started within the first week if surgical fixation is performed. Healing is expected to occur within 6–8 weeks because of the excellent muscular envelope around the fracture. Optimal function can be expected after 12 weeks.

Conclusion

Despite what had been said, fracture of the proximal humerus remains an unsolved problem, and fracture of the scapula often continues to be missed. However, through the inquiring nature and vigilent care of orthopaedic surgeons, many of the potential problems associated with these fractures will hopefully be eradicated or minimised in the future.

References

1. Mills HJ, Horne G (1985) Fractures of the proximal humerus in adults. J Trauma 25:801
2. Bengner U, Johnell O (1988) Changes in the incidence of fracture of the upper end of the humerus during a 30-year period. Clin Orthop 231:179
3. Lind T, Kroner K, Jensen J (1989) The epidemiology of fractures of the proximal humerus. Arch Orthop Trauma Surg 108:285
4. Neer CS, Rockwood CA (1984) Fractures and dislocations of the shoulder. In: Rockwood CA, Green DP (eds) Fractures in adults, vol 1. Lippincott, Philadelphia, p 675
5. Codman FA (1934) The shoulder. Todd, Boston
6. Clifford PC (1980) Fractures of the neck of the humerus: a review of the late results. Injury 12:91
7. Neer CS (1987) Displaced proximal humeral fractures. Clin Orthop 223:3
8. Neer CS II (1987) The classic displaced proximal humeral fractures. Clin Orthop 223:3
9. Hawkins RJ, Angelo RL (1987) Displaced proximal humeral factures. Orthop Clin North Am 18:421
10. Garth WP, Slappey CE, Ochs CW (1984) Roentgenographic demonstration of instability of the shoulder: the apical obligues projection. J Bone Joint Surg [Am] 66:1450
11. Kornguth PJ, Salazar AM (1987) The apical oblique view of the shoulder: its usefulness in acute trauma. Am J Roentgenol 149:113
12. Kristiansen B, Andersen ULS, Olsen CA, Varmarken JE (1988) The Neer classification of fractures of the proximal humerus. Skeletal Radiol 17:420
13. Castagno AA, Shuman WP, Kilcoyne RF, Haynor DR, Morris ME, Matsen FA (1987) Complex fractures of the proximal humerus: role of CT in treatment. Radiology 165:759
14. Blasier RB, Burkus JK (1988) Management of posterior fracture-dislocations of the shoulder. Clin Orthop 232:197

15. Tile M (1987) Fracture of the proximal humerus. In: Schatzker J, Tile M (eds) The rationale of operative fracture care. Springer, Berlin Heidelberg New York, p 31
16. Einarsson F (1958) Fractures of the upper end of the humerus. Discussion based on the follow up of 302 cases. Acta Orthop Scand Suppl 32:131
17. Mills KLG (1974) Severe injuries of the upper end of the humerus. Injury 6:13
18. Leyshon RL (1984) Closed treatment of fractures of the proximal humerus. Acta Orthop Scand 55:48
19. Young TB, Wallace WA (1985) Conservative treatment of fractures and fracture-dislocations of the upper end of the humerus. J Bone Joint Surg [Br] 67:373
20. Stableforth PG (1984) Four-part fractures of the neck of the humerus. J Bone Joint Surg [Br] 66:105
21. Knight RA, Mayne JA (1957) Comminuted fractures and fracture-dislocations involving the articular surface of the humeral head. J Bone Joint Surg [Am] 39:1343
22. Depalma AF, Cantilli RA (1961) Fractures of the upper end of the humerus. Clin Orthop 20:73
23. Savoie FH, Geissler WB, Vander Griend RA (1989) Open reduction and internal fixation of three-part fractures of the proximal humerus. Orthopedics 12:65
24. Kristiansen B, Christensen SW (1986) Plate fixation of proximal humeral fractures. Acta Orthop Scand 57:320
25. Cofield RH (1988) Comminuted fractures of the proximal humerus. Clin Orthop 230:49
26. Hawkins RJ, Bell RH, Gurr K (1986) The three-part fracture of the proximal part of the humerus. J Bone Joint Surg [Am] 68:1410
27. Kristiansen B, Christensen SW (1987) Proximal humeral fractures. Acta Orthop Scand 58:124
28. Tanner MW, Cofield RH (1983) Prosthetic arthroplasty for fractures and fracture-dislocations of the proximal humerus. Clin Orthop 179:116
29. Kay SP, Amstutz HC (1988) Shoulder hemiarthroplasty at UCLA. Clin Orthop 228:42
30. Willems WJ, Lim TEA (1985) Neer arthroplasty for humeral fracture. Acta Orthop Scand 56:394
31. Sturgenegger ME, Fornaro E, Jakob RP (1982) Results of surgical treatment of multifragmented fractures of the humeral head. Arch Orthop Trauma Surg 100:249
32. Weile F, Fjeldborg O (1971) Lesions of the axillary artery associated with dislocation of the shoulder. Acta Chir Scand 137:279
33. Lim EVA, Day LJ (1987) Thrombosis of the axillary artery complicating proximal humeral fractures. J Bone Joint Surg [Am] 69:778
34. Leffert RD, Seddon HJ (1965) Intra claricular brachial plexus injuries. J Bone Joint Surg [Br] 34:72
35. Parsons SW, Rowley DI (1986) Brachial plexus lesions in dislocation and fracture dislocation of the shoulder. J R Coll Surg Edinb 31:85
36. Armstrong CP, van der Spuy J (1984) The fractured scapula: importance and management based on a series of 62 patients. Injury 15:324
37. Thompson DA, Flynn TC, Miller PW, Fischer RP (1985) The significance of scapular fractures. J Trauma 25:974
38. McGinnis M, Denton JR (1989) Fractures of the scapula: a retrospective study of 40 fractured scapulae. J Trauma 29:1488
39. Hardegger FH, Simpson LA, Weber BG (1984) The operative treatment of scapular fractures. J Bone Joint Surg [Br] 66:725
40. McGahan JP, Rab GT, Dublin A (1980) Fracture of the scapula. J Trauma 20:880

12 Fractures Around the Hip

K.S. LEUNG

Introduction

The hip is a major weight-bearing joint at the mid-point of the body. By virtue of its position, the structural architecture and the anatomical arrangements, injuries are common and the sequelae of such trauma are serious.

The unique position of the hip in the human body makes it particularly susceptible to mechanical trauma. As the most proximal weight-bearing joint, it supports the weight of the proximal segment of the body. Biomechanical analyses [1–7] and in vivo telemetric studies [8–11] have shown that the hip joint is constantly subjected to a load 3–4 times that of human body weight in slow walking, and 10–15 times the body weight in vigorous exercise. The fact that the hip joint is loaded significantly during muscle contractions even under circumstances in which weight bearing is eliminated indicates that this joint is very much under constant wear and tear. The neck shaft angle configurations further exaggerate the mechanical effects working on the joint by increasing the moment arm. This angle leads to a further concentration of force acting on the femoral neck and trochanteric region. Koch's [12] computed lines of maximal stress in the proximal femur clearly illustrate this phenomenon (Fig. 1) of eccentric load application. The much higher compressive stress on the medial cortex compared with the tensile stress on the lateral cortex significantly affects the results of treating fractures with implants in this region.

As the most distant weight-bearing joint counting from the ground, the hip is again subjected to the effect of a long lever arm with the ground reaction force. This is particularly serious in unexpected circumstances (such as a sudden slip and fall) in which the magnitude and direction of the ground reaction force are unguarded. The deleterious effect of these forces is significantly magnified. Mathematical calculation readily demonstrates the effect of the long moment arm which easily exceeds the threshold of fracture in the proximal femur [13]. Fracture at the proximal femur is therefore a common injury especially among those with suboptimal bone quality, such as in osteoporosis, which prevails among the elderly.

Indeed, osteoporosis is one of the major factors that contribute to proximal femoral fractures among the elderly. Ostcoporosis is a common finding in this part of the hip among these patients. The characteristic loss of

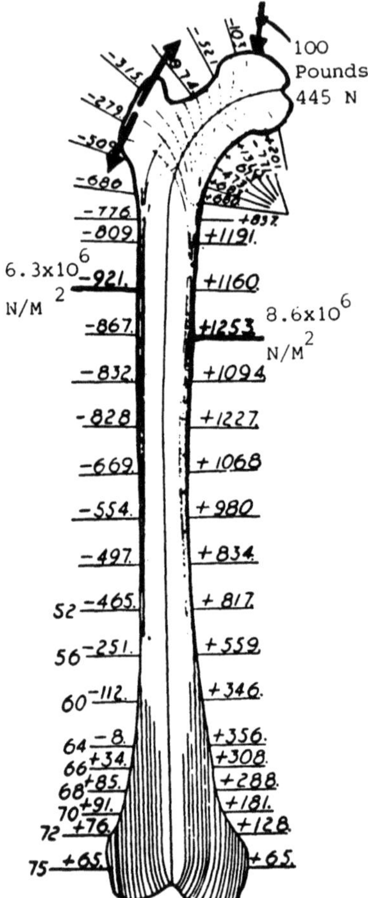

Fig. 1. Koch's diagram of computed lines of stress in the femur

calcium within the trabeculae in the peritrochanteric regions is universal among elderly persons [13–18]. This accounts for the high incidence of fracture in this region. The high risks related to osteoporotic bone, the lack of realistic hope of preventing osteoporosis in the near future and the increase in the aging population in the world have all led to the ever-increasing incidence of hip fractures. These fractures not only present a major challenge to the orthopaedic surgeons but create special health care problems which are likely to continue in the coming decades.

Anatomically, the femoral head is more or less a vascular end organ. The vascular supply of the femoral head has been studied extensively [19–26]. There are three sources of blood supply to the femoral head: (a) the intra-osseous vessels from the intra-medullary branches of the superior nutrient artery system, (b) the artery of the ligamentum teres, and (c) the most important system, deriving from the retinacular vessels and the branches of the extra-capsular arterial ring, which run along the base of the femoral neck beyond the synovium. The femoral head is particularly susceptible to ischaemia after fracture: the intra-osseous system is disrupted, and the blood supply from the ligamentum teres is unreliable [27,28] while the retinacular system is also interrupted by the fracture displacements. The risk of ischaemia is further increased by the tamponade effects of intra-capsular bleeding [29–31] which damages the already tenuous circulation.

Healing of the femoral neck fracture is also unique because this is the only site in the skeleton that is devoid of periosteum [32]. The marrow stroma and the endosteum provide the sole source of the osteogenic cells responsible for fracture repair. Therefore healing is achieved through the formation of endosteal callus and subsequently by creeping substitution. The endosteum healing is relatively slow and weak. It is not readily observable in X-ray films and hence poses practical problems in clinical monitoring.

The structure of the hip as a ball-and-socket joint allows a wide range of movements while at the same time granting perfect stability. Injuries to the hip are usually caused by high-energy trauma which produces extensive tissue damage. Fracture comminutions and multiple trauma are other common occurrences. In fact, 5%–10% of hip fractures are missed in the initial management of polytrauma patients [33–35]. It therefore needs to be stressed that for polytrauma patients, routine X-ray examination of the pelvis should be performed to detect fractures around the hips. The early and stable fixation of hip fracture-dislocations forms an integral part of the total management of polytrauma patients.

Fractures of the Femoral Head

Fractures of the femoral head are rare and are produced only by severe trauma. The fracture is usually associated with posterior dislocations of the hip with or without fractures of the posterior wall of the acetabulum. As a result, the hip is dislocated, and the fragment remains in the acetabulum. Pipkin's classification is the commonly accepted one [36]:

Type I: fracture of femoral head caudal to fovea
Type II: fracture of femoral head cephalad to fovea
Type III: fracture of femoral head in association with a femoral neck fracture
Type IV: Type 1, 2 or 3 fracture with associated fracture of the acetabulum

The difficulties in treating these fracture-dislocations include the decision-making, operative technique and long-term uncertainty of fracture healing. The existing literature on this problem is scanty, and the general lack of long-term prospective studies makes the choice of optimal treatment modality difficult. Nevertheless, the general principles of treating intra-articular fractures should form guidelines for their management. The results of treatment depend on the possibility of reconstructing the femoral head so as to maintain the congruity of the articular surfaces, particularly in fractures that involve the weight-bearing part of the femoral head. The fixation, bone fragment viability and healing of the fracture fragments affect the outcome of the treatment. As most of the fragments are either ischaemic or retain only very feeble blood supply from the ligamentum teres, healing and revascularisation are slow, probably going through a slow process of creeping substitution. Since the dislocation of the hip should be treated as an emergency, the availability of urgent computed tomography (CT) scan helps in determining the size and number of fracture fragments, so that the choice of treatment may be predetermined before the actual operative procedures. CT scanning also helps greatly in assessing the post-reduction joint congruity of the femoral head after closed reduction is chosen as the treatment method.

In type I fracture dislocation, the fracture fragment is usually small and does not involve the weight-bearing part of the femoral head (Fig. 2); closed reduction should be performed. The post-reduction congruity is then assessed with CT scan. If the congruity is acceptable, and there are no loose fragments apart from the major fragment while joint motion is smooth and unhindered, the hip is treated as a case of simple dislocation. Skeletal traction is maintained for 3 weeks, followed by non-weight-bearing ambulation within a hip brace which keeps the hip at 10° abduction and allows 90° of hip flexion (Fig. 3). However, if the congruity is unacceptable (Fig. 4), arthrotomy through the posterior capsular tear is recommended. The frag-

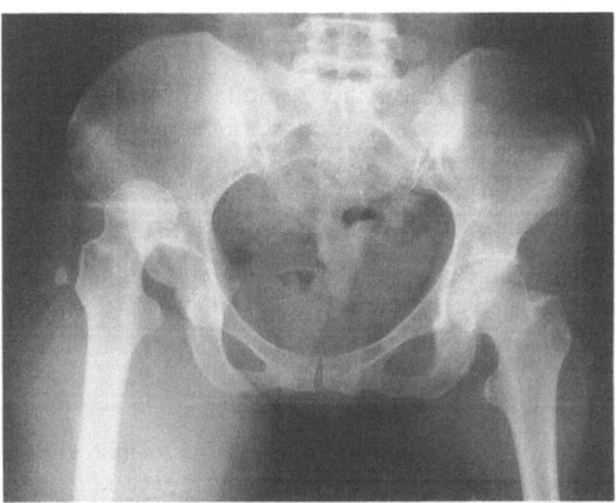

Fig. 2. X-ray of the pelvis showing fracture dislocation of the right hip. The femoral head fracture involves the non-weight-bearing part of the head, and the fragment remains inside the acetabulum

ment is excised and the joint lavaged. Anatomical reduction of the fragment is not essential, if not impossible. Excision of the fragment usually does not compromise the stability of the hip joint since the fragment comes from the infero-medial part of the femoral head.

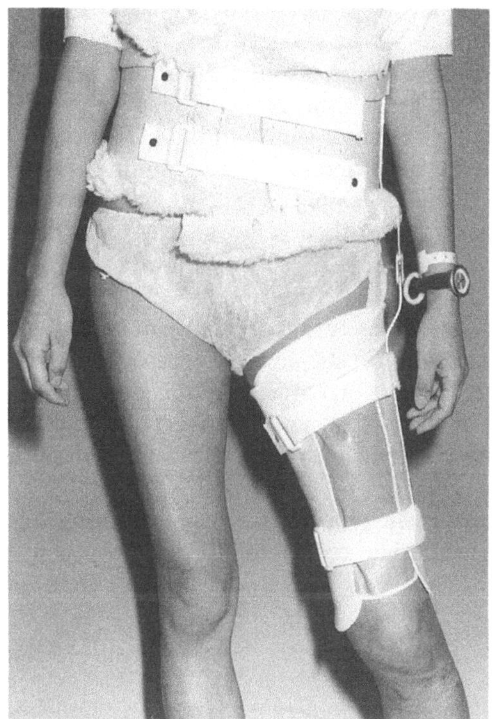

Fig. 3. Post-reduction hip brace to control hip motion. The hip is kept in 10° abduction and allows 90° flexion

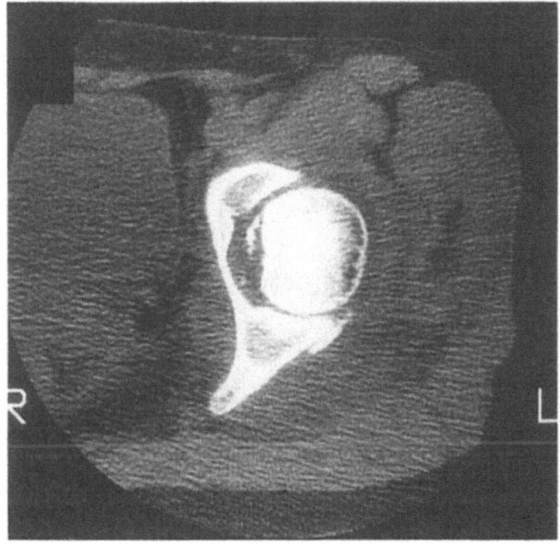

Fig. 4. Post-reduction CT of the hip showing fracture of the femoral head with reasonable congruity

The fragment in type II fracture dislocation is usually large and involves part of the weight-bearing surface of the femoral head. Open reduction and internal fixation is recommended. Operative reduction and fixation are exceedingly difficult surgical procedures, more so if the fragment is left attached to the acetabulum with the ligamentum teres. Detaching the fragment facilitates the fixation, but, on the other hand, if the fragment is left attached, blood supply may be enhanced. If open reduction and internal fixation is decided on, the hip should not be reduced before exploration. Locating the fragment is much easier with the hip in a dislocated position. The operation should be carried out as an emergency. The most reliable method of fixation is the use of two counter-sunk 4-mm AO cancellous screws which act as lag screws to fix the fragment. Late resorption of the fragment may occur even after fracture healing (Fig. 5). The protruded screw heads cause irritation to the hip, and their removal may be difficult. To avoid this late complicated procedure, the use of a newly developed absorbable screw may be desirable.

Type III fractures are rarer, sometimes resulting from complication of brutal closed reduction for dislocations of the hip. The associated neck fracture dominates the choice of treatment. Treatment of the neck fracture is very much affected by the age of the patient and the degree of displacement (see next section). Treatment of the head fractures should then follow the principles outlined above.

The associated acetabular fracture in type IV fracture-dislocation dictates the choice of treatment protocol. The commonly associated posterior

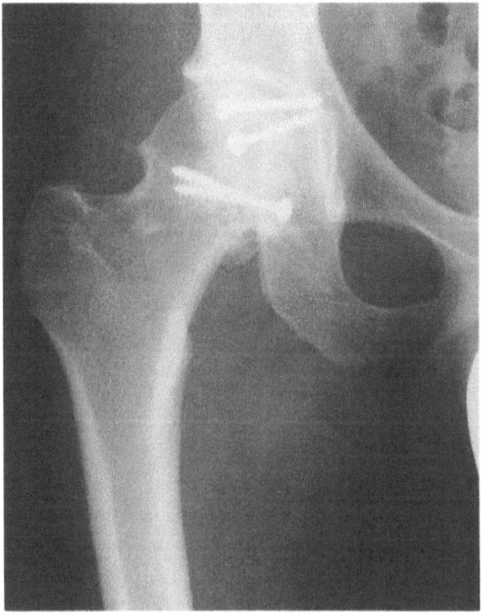

Fig. 5. Type IV fracture dislocation of the hip. The fractures of both the femoral head and the acetabulum were fixed with the 4-mm screws. Note the resorption of the femoral head fragment; the screws appear very prominent inside the acetabulum

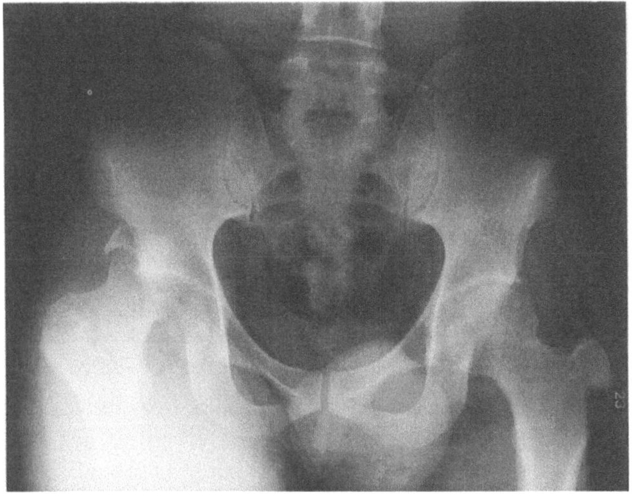

Fig. 6. Type IV fracture dislocation of the hip. The fracture of the femoral head is cephalad to the fovea

wall fractures sometimes facilitate the fixation of the femoral head fractures because of the increased exposure through the fracture (Fig. 6). Fixation of the acetabular wall guarantees the congruity and stability of the hip joint, particularly when the fragment is large. Fixing the posterior wall fragment also allows earlier rehabilitation. Motion restriction is not necessary since bone-to-bone union is much more predictable than fibrous healing of the capsular structures. The high incidence of loose fragments [37] inside the acetabulum further supports the choice of open reduction, during which the loose fragments can be adequately removed. During the operation the joint is lavaged. Head fractures are reduced and fixed with 4-mm AO cancellous screws. After relocating the hip, the acetabular wall with the capsular attachment is fixed with two or three 4-mm AO cancellous lag screws.

The post-operative management of all these fracture-dislocations follows the same protocol as in the pure dislocation of hip. X-ray examination and bone scan (particularly marrow scan) [38,39] at regular intervals are indicated for the early detection of avascular necrosis.

Fractures of Femoral Neck

Fractures of the femoral neck continue to be a common problem, and the incidence among the elderly population is ever increasing. These present a special challenge to the orthopaedic surgeon because of the serious complications of avascular necrosis after fixation. The prognosis of fractures of the femoral neck differs significantly according to the age of the patients; therefore the treatment protocols are different for different age groups.

The prognosis of these fractures also depends on the initial displacement of the fractures. Garden's classification is the most commonly used one:

Type I: incomplete or impacted fracture
Type II: complete fracture without displacement
Type III: complete fracture with partial displacement
Type IV: complete fracture with total displacement

Clinically, it is difficult to identify a good correlation between the prognosis and the four types of fractures. Therefore it may be more practical to classify the fractures simply as displaced and non-displaced types. It is generally agreed that even undisplaced fractures should be treated with internal fixation. The non-operative treatment for these fractures has been shown to be inferior as a large proportion of them become displaced during the so-called bed-rest period [40]. The use of multiple parallel lag screws is a well-accepted method. The availability of cannulated screws (Fig. 7) greatly facilitates the procedure. Biomechanical studies show that there are no additional advantages with the use of more than three screws, and that the results are more related to the bone quality of the proximal femur. Study of the mechanical property of the femoral head has shown that the weakest part is the supero-medial quadrant [17]. Hence, it is recommended that the lag screws should be placed well to the inferior half of the neck and head

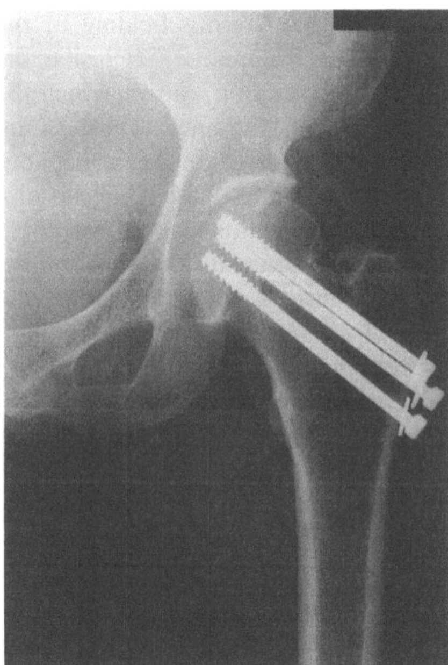

Fig. 7. Fracture neck of the femur was treated by closed reduction and screw fixation. Note the parallel arrangement of the screws and excellent healing of the fracture

region. Two lag screws should be inserted into the inferior half of the femoral head and neck first to fix the fracture with compression. The third additional screw inserted more superior improves the stability of fixation. Parallel placement of the lag screws is essential for the fixation and late impaction.

Fixation is followed by anterior arthrotomy to release the pressure inside the hip. A few studies [29,30,41] have reported the increase in intra-capsular pressure after hip fracture, and this is expected to further jeopardises the tenuous blood flow after the fracture. Arthrotomy leads to a decrease in intra-capsular pressure and improves blood flow [31].

The treatment protocol for undisplaced fractures is applicable in different age groups. Non-union and avascular necrosis are uncommon. For this group of fractures, most series report less than 8% avascular necroses and less than 5% non-unions [42].

For displaced fractures, controversy remains in the choice of the best operation for different age groups. In the elderly, who constitute the largest proportion of patients with these fractures, the aim of the treatment is to achieve early mobilisation and to regain independent walking. The choice of treatment lies between closed reduction with screw fixation and prosthetic replacement. Compared with prosthetic replacement, screw fixation after closed reduction has the advantage of causing a lesser degree of surgical trauma, which results in lower infection rate [43], and early mobilisation after operation. However, the result of screw fixation depends on the quality of reduction. The post-reduction alignment index of Garden [44] is one of the practical guidelines for assessing the reduction, although anatomical reduction should always be the primary aim. By achieving a post-reduction alignment index within the range of 155°–180° on both the frontal and lateral views, a higher rate of union and a lower rate of late segment collapse can be assured. However, the alignment index assessment depends on good-quality post-reduction X-ray films to demonstrate the trabeculae. This may be difficult to obtain intra-operatively. The alternative method is to measure the centring line in the centre of the femoral head and neck and align it with the centring line of the shaft [45]. The acceptable reduction with this method is to have the post-reduction alignment of 130°–150° in the frontal view and 0°–15° of anteversion in the lateral view. The reduction in the lateral view is most critical to ensure good results.

The potential complications of screw fixation include the risk of avascular necrosis. This risk is enhanced by the difficulty in obtaining satisfactory reduction, especially in fractures with severe posterior comminutions and among geriatric patients with osteoporotic bone. It is logical to look for methods of revascularising the proximal fragment during the time of fixation. This is even more important in young patients who are not candidates for prosthetic replacement. The posterior muscle pedicle graft based on the quadrator femoris is one of the procedures advocated [46]. The results, however, are not favourable. The use of the pedicle vascularised bone graft

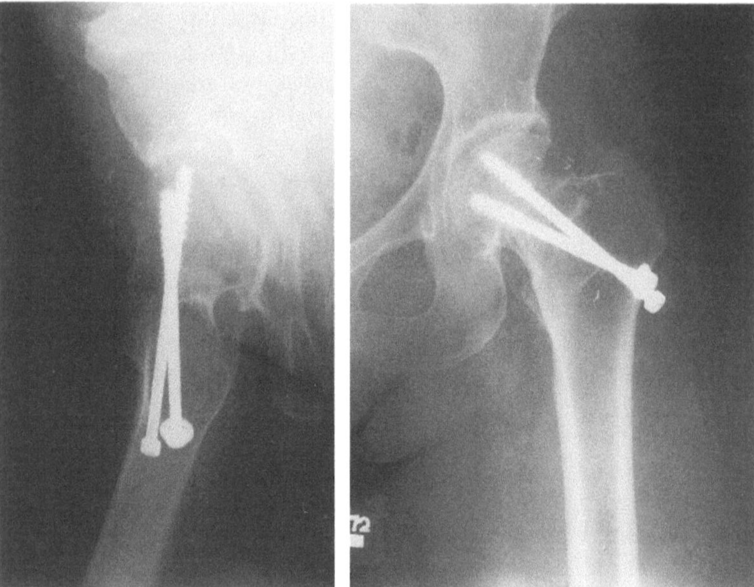

Fig. 8. Fracture neck of femur treated with screw fixation and vascularised pedicle iliac crest graft

is recently reported [47]. The fractures are exposed through an anterior approach and reduced under direct vision. The fractures are fixed with two or three cannulated lag screws. Vascularised iliac crest bone based on the deep circumflex iliac vessels is used as a pedicle inlay graft through a trough on the anterior surface of the neck into the head (Fig. 8). Some 95% of the fractures are successfully revascularised. As simple bone grafting does not improve the rate of healing, vascularised bone graft serves the purposes of enhancing new vascularity as well as osteogenic cells. This seem to be the right direction in which to tackle the problem and may be useful as a salvage procedure for established vascular necrosis. However, these revascularisation procedures involve major dissections and considerably lengthen the operation. It may not be applicable for older patients, particularly those with compromised physiological reserves.

Primary prosthetic replacement is reserved in general for patients aged over 75 years with a lower level of mobility. The relative indications for younger patients include failed closed reduction, pathological fractures and those with neurological diseases, for example, Parkinson's disease. The inherent complications of the hemi-prosthesis can be reduced if more accurate sizing of the prosthesis to the acetabulum is achieved. Telemetric study has shown that with accurate sizing the pressure from the prosthesis can be evenly distributed to the acetabulam, decreasing the friction between the prosthesis and the articular surface of the acetabulum. The problems of prosthesis wear and tear and protrusion are thus minimised [9]. The availability of the bipolar hemiprosthesis also improves the result of treating fracture femoral neck with primary prosthetic replacement [48–51]. Mechanical enhancement of the joint action through an improved friction mechanism is achieved with a primary articulation of a polyethylene bearing part and a secondary articulation with the articular surface of the acetabulum. The improvement in results with the newer designs with or without cement fixation is encouraging. Primary prosthetic replacement with improved designs remains the treatment of choice for femoral neck fractures in elderly persons for whom immediate stability and early mobilisation are vital.

Femoral neck fractures among young adults usually result from high-energy trauma. Careful evaluation of the other systems is essential to exclude concomitant injuries. Ipsilateral fracture in the femoral shaft may coexist. The treatment is difficult, although various options have been proposed [33–35,52]. The use of the sliding hip screw with a long plate fixation of the femoral fractures is commonly advocated. As the general principle of treating femoral neck fractures with lag screws should also be followed in these fractures, the choice of fixation of femoral shaft fractures remains controversial. The use of the long plate requires lengthy incision and extensive dissections. In some cases, even double plating may be required. The disadvantages of such an approach are obvious with regard to the modern concept of fracture treatment and healing. The use of locked intra-medullary nails in the treatment of diaphyseal femoral fractures is one of the major advances in musculo-skeletal trauma. The combination of lag screw fixation of femoral neck fractures and the locked nail in diaphyseal fractures provides stable fixations in these fractures.

During the operation the diaphyseal fracture is fixed by closed intra-medullary nailing first. The use of the locking screws is indicated in unstable diaphyseal fractures. The femoral neck fracture is then reduced by closed method, and the lag screws are inserted anterior and posterior to the proximal end of the nail. Due to the size of the nail only two lag screws can be inserted in most cases (Fig. 9). In a series of 16 cases there was no avascular necrosis. One patient developed non-union in the femoral neck fracture due to varus displacement of the femoral head and subsequently required bone graft for healing. All fractures in the femoral diaphyses healed. The function of the hip and the involved lower limb was restored. The other implant available for these fractures is the newly designed long gamma nail (Fig. 10). The proximal sliding lag screw design provides adequate stability and at the same time allows control impaction of femoral neck fractures. In comminuted diaphyseal fractures distal locking screws can be inserted as in the use of the other locked intramedullary nails. However, caution is necessary in the use of this implant due to its rigidity, and the clinical results need further evaluation.

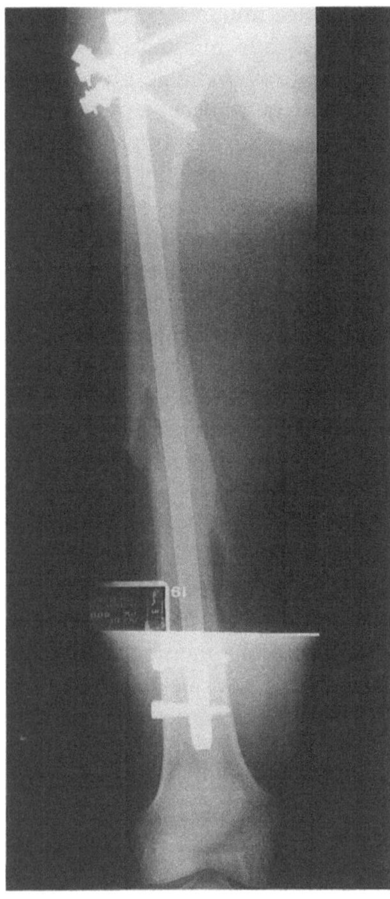

Fig. 9. Ipsilateral fracture of the femoral neck and shaft treated with intra-medullary locked nail and cannulated hip screws

Trochanteric Fractures

Trochanteric fractures are common among geriatric patients. These constitute approximately 40%–50% of all proximal femoral fractures in the elderly [53–58]. As in all geriatric fractures, one of the problems in dealing with these fractures is, again, related to the increasing incidence of fractures in the aging world population. The other problem is poor bone quality in the trochanteric region. The trochanteric region is most commonly affected by senile osteoporosis [18,59]. Biomechanically the tremendous bending moment across this region is obvious: the neck-shaft arrangement of the trochanter increases the moment arm of the varus force of the hip, and this is particularly important in fractures with no medial bony support [60–63]. The fractures are rendered more unstable when there is associated subtrochanteric extension.

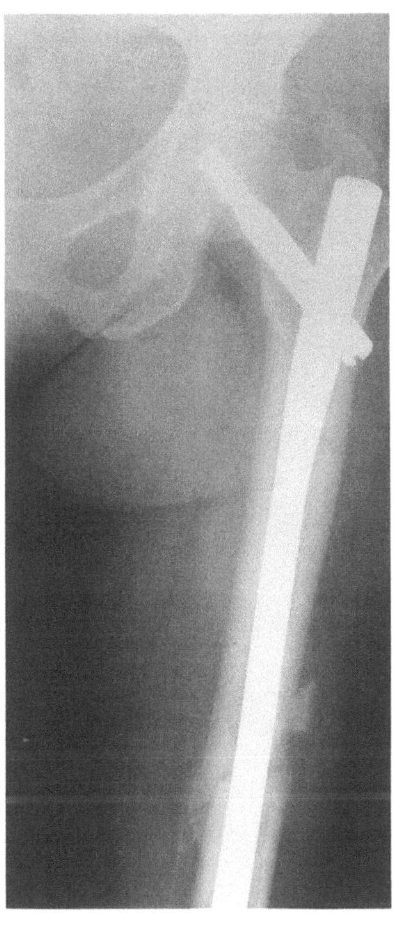

Fig. 10. Ipsilateral fracture of the femoral shaft and trochanter treated with a long gamma nail

The anatomical arrangement of the soft tissue around this region dictates the unique features of the fractures. The relative lack of soft-tissue attachment of the posterior cortex leads to common posterior comminution. Bone failure under tension of the lateral cortex leads to the typical oblique fracture line and loss of medial cortical support in a certain percentage of fractures. These result in a characteristic deformity of external rotation and varus deformity of the hip when the fractures are allowed to heal in a natural way. It is therefore clear that the problems related to the treatment of peritrochanteric fractures are not those related to healing but rather those related to bone failure and implant failure. However, the final outcome of the treatment for these fractures is also affected by the general well-being of the patients as these fractures commonly occur in an older age group compared with those of femoral neck fractures, and a large proportion of the patients have concomitant medical diseases. Nevertheless, operative fixation of the fractures has been shown to be the best means to help the

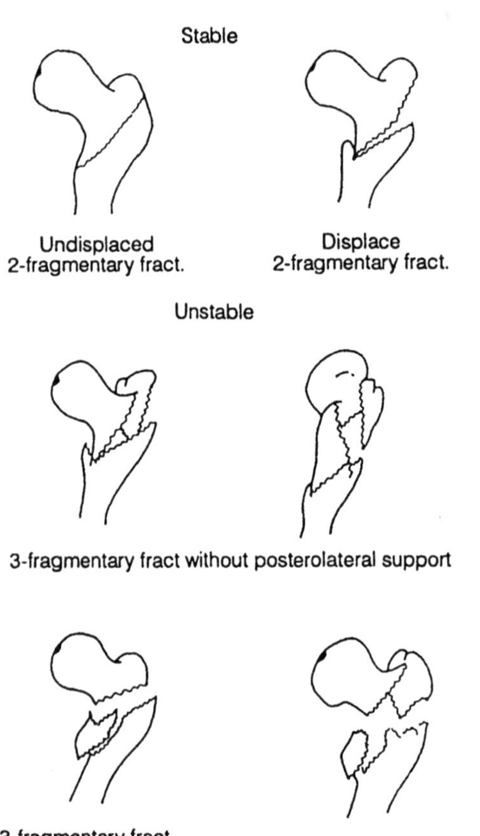

Fig. 11. Classification of trochanteric fractures according to Evans [71] as modified by Jensen and Michaelsen [94]

patients regain mobility early and avoid numerous complications resulting from the fractures [64–70].

Evans' [71,72] concept of fracture stability (Fig. 11) is the most widely accepted. The importance of the medial bony support has been confirmed both biomechanically and clinically [73–75]. In stable fractures as much as 75% of load is borne by bone-to-bone contact, and in unstable fractures the implant must bear most of the transmitted load. Implant failure is therefore common in unstable fractures. The result is further complicated by comminution in the fracture sites, the natural tendency of the fracture impaction in the metaphyseal region and the poor mechanical property of the osteoporotic bone. All these factors cause a high rate of bone failure [60,76–78]. It is well documented that the results of treating stable and unstable fractures differ significantly. The complication rate of treating unstable fractures can be ten times higher than that of stable fractures [55,60,76,79,80].

By considering all the above factors, it is possible to establish the criteria for an ideal implant for these common fractures. (a) It must allow a guided collapse of the fracture during healing. This prevents the penetration of the implant into the acetabulum during the healing process, particularly in unstable fractures. The guided collapse of the fractures improves the bony contact and at the same time decreases the moment arm of the varus force of the hip joint. (b) It should be strong enough to allow early weight bearing even in unstable fractures. Biomechanical studies have shown that the hip is under constant load even when the patient is not walking [8]. The force created by muscle contraction can be as high as that during weight-bearing walking. The modern concept of early post-operative mobilisation in geriatric patients makes this requirement even more important. (c) The instrument must be simple and easily handled at all levels of surgical experience. The ever-increasing incidence makes this operation the commonest in any orthopaedic unit. User-friendly instrumentation would certainly decrease the complications due to technical error [81–84]. (d) The surgical procedures involved should be as atraumatic as possible. The common association of medical abnormalities and compromised physiological reserves among geriatric patients make them poor candidates for surgery. The avoidance of major dissection and lengthy operation will certainly decrease complications such as excessive bleeding, wound infection and the delay in mobilisation.

The surgical treatment of trochanteric fractures has gone through several changes [53,77]. Rigid and non-telescoping implants do not fulfil the criteria of an ideal implant, and as a result their complication rate unacceptably high [78,85]. The older designs such as the Jewette and the Mclaughlin nail-plate systems gave rise to implant failure in the form of bending or bone failure in the form of penetrations (Fig. 12). The less traumatic designs such as Ender's multiple flexible nails or Küntscher's condylo-cephalad nails fail in unstable fractures due to the lack of guided collapse. Complications, including back-out and penetrations, are common. The other approaches of surgically converting an unstable trochanteric fracture into a stable one are best illustrated by Dimon-Hughston's medial displacement osteotomy [79] and Sarmiento's valgus osteostomy [86]. The need of major dissection and the technically demanding procedure also make these procedures less favourable. The late complications of shortening and valgus deformity of the knees [80,87,88] are common.

The telescoping nail-plate system originally designed by Pohl is perhaps the most widely used implant nowadays. Numerous systems with improvement in instrumentation and minor modifications are available. The reported complication rate of such implants is around 10%–15% [57,78,89–91]. Most of the complications are due to technical errors. Placement of the lag screw in the superomedial segment of the femoral head leads to superior cut-out (Fig. 13). Jamming of the lag screw in the barrel and the lack of sliding due to the unexpectedly lengthy impaction might change this system to a rigid one, and hence the complications of penetration occur as in those fixed with

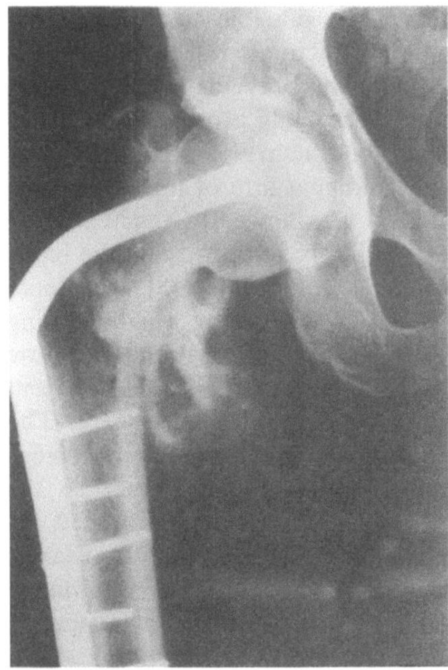

Fig. 12. Implant failure in the form of bending in a trochanteric fracture fixed with a Jewette plate

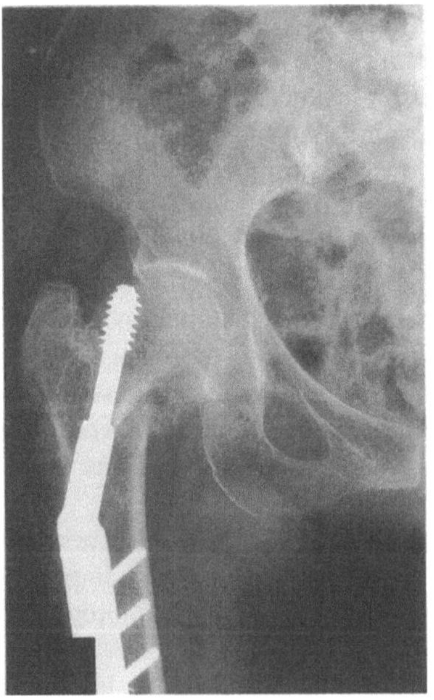

Fig. 13. Superior cut-out of the lag screw of the sliding screw plate system due to the screw was placed in the supero-medial quadrant of the femoral head

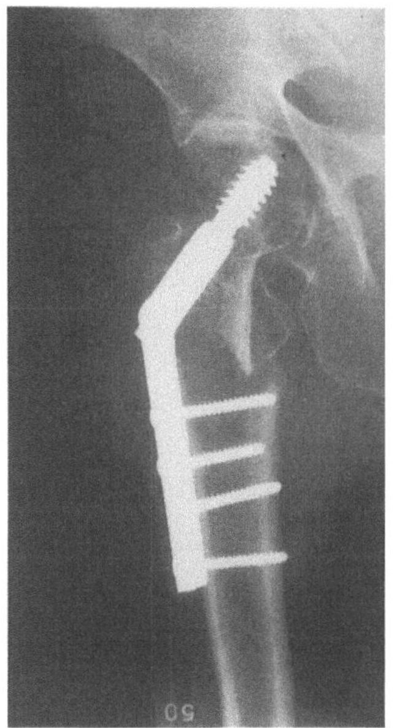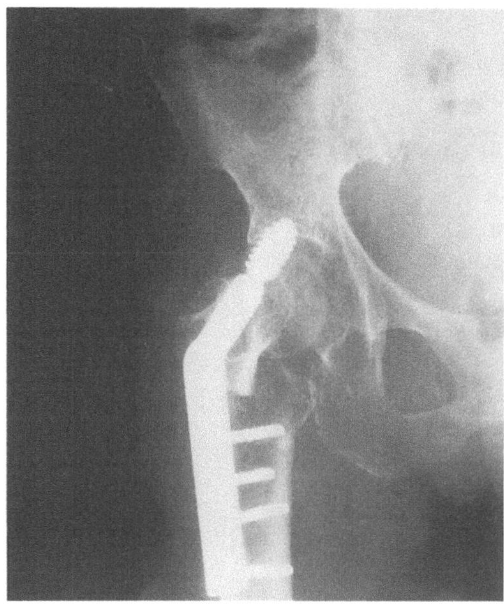

Fig. 14. Penetration of the lag screw into the acetabulum due to the lack of sliding with the lag screw

the rigid implants (Fig. 14). The femoral component requires certain dissection for fixation, and the lateralisation of this part also makes this system biomechanically less ideal. The tendency of lateral pull-off due the varus bending force on the hip is substantial. All these factors leave room for further improvement.

The gamma nail was introduced in 1988. The major difference from the sliding nail-plate system is the intra-medullary fixation of the femoral component (Fig. 15). The intra-medullary fixation of the femoral component enables the implant to be fixed by a closed procedure. It inherits all the theoretical advantages of closed treatment of fractures. The medial displacement of the femoral component decreases the moment arm of the hip joint force (Fig. 16) and may entail fewer problems of implant failure.

The operative procedure is very similar to that of the locked intra-medullary nails. With the patient supine on the traction table, closed reduction is performed with fluoroscopic control. The reduction is maintained by traction with boot. The trunk is flexed laterally towards the opposite side of the fracture. After scrubbing and draping, the image intensifier is positioned to give a lateral view of the head and neck. A 2-mm Kirschner wire is passed percutaneously anterior to the femur and parallel to the femoral neck in the coronal plane (Fig. 17). This Kirschner wire helps to define the anteversion angle and is very important for the accurate position of the lag screw in the neck and head. An incision of 6–8 cm is made in the trochanteric region.

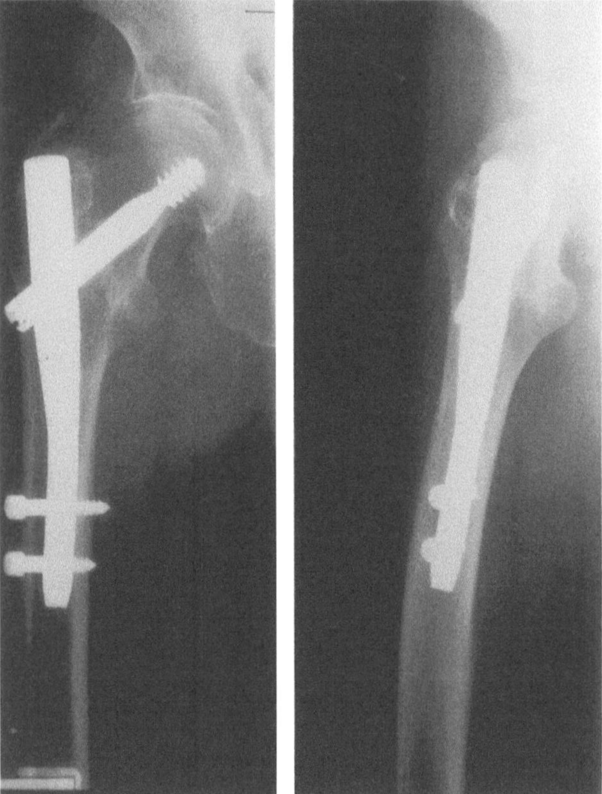

Fig. 15. Trochanteric fracture fixed with gamma nail

The medullary cavity is entered through the tip of the greater trochanter. The medullary cavity is reamed to 1 mm larger than the diameter of the nail to be inserted. The appropriate nail is attached on the nail mount and inserted into the medullary cavity manually without hammering to the correct depth. The handle of the nail mount should be kept parallel to the anteversion Kirschner wire in the coronal plane (Fig. 18) during insertion. The corresponding targetting device is assembled onto the nail mount. The lateral cortex of the proximal femur is perforated with the awl, and the lag screw guide is inserted through the centring sleeve until the tip reaches the subchondral line. The position of the guide wire should be in the inferior half of the head and neck in the frontal plane and central in the lateral plane. The lag screw track in the femoral head and neck is prepared with the triple reamer. The lag screw of the correct length is inserted to 5 mm from the subchondral line. The set screw is inserted through the nail-holding bolt. Distal locking is indicated in unstable fractures. The locking screws can be

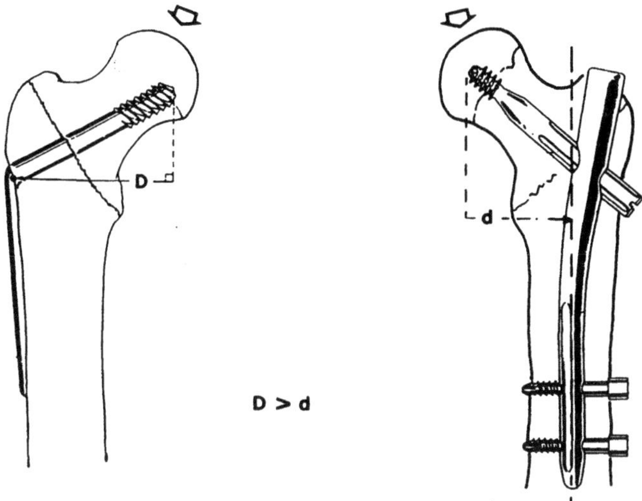

Fig. 16. The intramedullary fixation of the femoral component of the gamma nail decreases the moment arm of the hip joint force and hence the lateral pull-out force on the implant

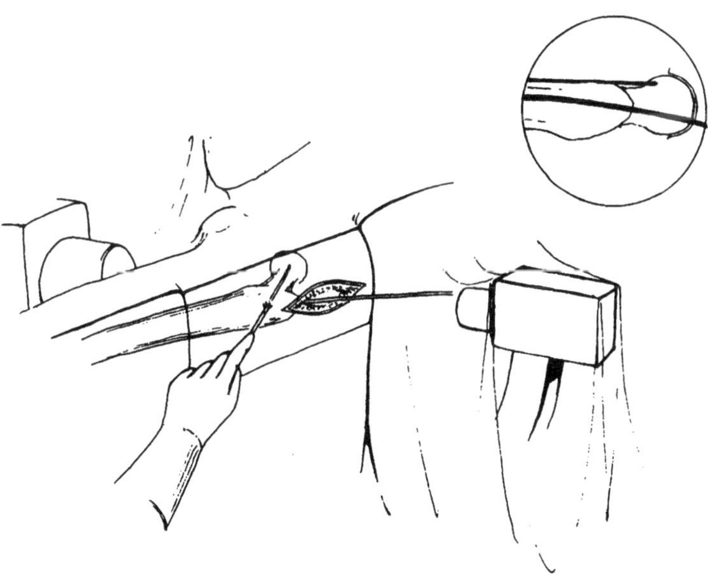

Fig. 17. The anteversion angle is determined with the percutaneous Kirschner wire inserted parallel to the axis of the femoral head and neck

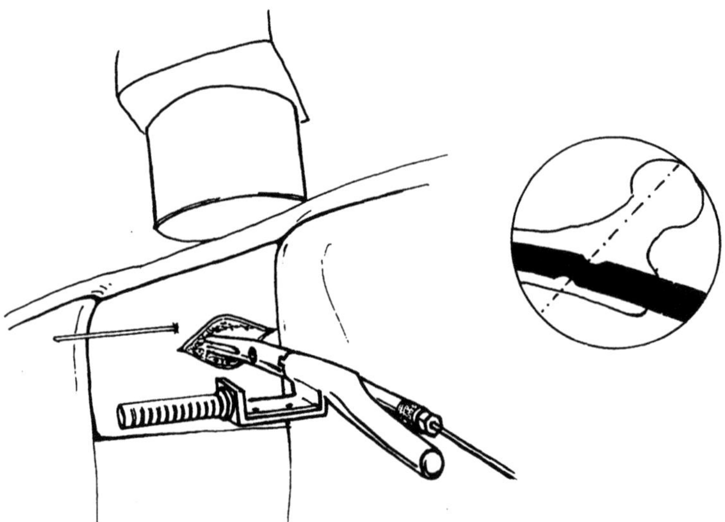

Fig. 18. During the insertion of the gamma nail, the handle of the nail mount is kept parallel to the anteversion Kirschner wire in the coronal plane. This facilitates the insertion of the lag screw targetting

inserted with the same targeting device. The fixation is then screened with the image intensifier, and the wound is closed with drainage.

We carried out a randomised prospective comparative study of dynamic hip screw and the gamma nail in the treatment of geriatric trochanteric fractures [92], with similar patient characteristics and fracture patterns in the two groups. We found the significant differences (Table 1) to be: in the gamma nail group, the operation could be done with shorter intra-operative X-ray screening time, less blood loss and smaller incisions. Post-operatively, shorter convalescent hospital stay and earlier weight bearing could be commenced in gamma nail group. However, we could not demonstrate any significant differences in the duration of operation, fracture healing, post-operative hip function or mobility between patients treated with the two fixation methods. Operative mortality and complications were similar. The unique patterns of complications between the two groups reflect the differences of the designs (Table 2). Intra-operative complications were higher in the gamma nail group. Most of these occurred during insertion of the femoral component and were amendable during the same operation. Modifications of the femoral component resulted in dramatic decrease in these complications [93]. The study showed that the gamma nail can be implanted with considerable less surgical trauma and with the modification of the femoral component and attention to the operative procedure; complications are also minimised. It can be concluded that the gamma nail represents a recent advance in the treatment of trochanteric fractures.

Table 1. Results of the prospective trial on the use of the dynamic hip screw and gamma nail in the treatment of geriatric trochanteric fractures

	Gamma nail	Dynamic hip screw	Significance
Radiation duration (s)			
Stable	30.41 ± 2.87	48.47 ± 5.02	$p < 0.0377$
Unstable	41.90 ± 10.39	71.91 ± 15.22	$p < 0.0009$
Blood loss (ml)			
Stable	765.2 ± 644.78	1157.86 ± 609.66	$p = 0.069$
Unstable	837.85 ± 497.17	1012.29 ± 477.18	$p = 0.047$
Length of incision (cm)			
Stable	8.9 ± 1.63	15.9 ± 1.63	$p = 0.0001$
Unstable	8.9 ± 1.01	15.5 ± 1.68	$p = 0.0001$
Time in convalescent hospital			
Stable	17.7 ± 11.97	15.4 ± 10.86	$p > 0.05$
Unstable	15.9 ± 8.2	19.1 ± 10.34	$p = 0.06$
Time of full weight-bearing walking started (weeks)			
Stable	1.3 ± 0.88	1.9 ± 0.89	$p = 0.0453$
Unstable	1.2 ± 0.64	1.7 ± 0.76	$p = 0.0009$
Intra-operative complications	14.0%	10.8%	$p = 0.048$

Table 2. Intra-operative complications with the use of the dynamic hip screw and gamma nail in the treatment of geriatric trochanteric fractures

	Gamma nail	Dynamic hip screw
Failure of reduction	1	2
Fracturing of lateral cortex	3	2
Breakage of drill	1	2
Jamming of nail	3	0
Displacement of fracture during operation	2	4
Failure of distal locking	3	0
	14.0%	10.8%

$p = 0.048$ (χ^2 test).

The indications for use the gamma nail may be further extended to trochanteric fractures with subtrochanteric extension and those of pure subtrochanteric fractures. These fractures are more common in younger age groups. The conventional treatment for these fractures is a long side plate with combination of one of the designs for fixing trochanteric fractures: the 95° angle-blade plate or the dynamic condylar screw. The disadvantages of these methods are obvious. They require lengthy incision and extensive dissection. The risk of devitalisation of bony fragments and infection are substantial. The need for additional bone grafting is frequent. Complications such as delayed union, non-union and implant failure are common. The use of intra-medullary fixation for these difficult fractures can avoid all these complications. By a closed procedure, major dissections are avoided; the morselised bony material serves as autogenous graft. The patients can be mobilised much earlier due to the smaller would and dissection. Nevertheless, the use of the long Gamma nail is still in the trial period. Its wide clinical application needs further evaluation.

Conclusion

The management of hip fractures remains a challenge to orthopaedic surgeons. With better understanding of fracture physiology, progress in biomechanical application in implant designs and the accumulation of clinical experience with these difficult fractures, definite guidelines can be established for the general management of fractures around the hip. As the trend for the treatment of fractures tends towards a more atraumatic approach, fixation of fractures by closed means dominates the recent advances in the management of fractures. The use of cannulated screws for fixation of femoral neck fractures and the use of gamma nails in the treatment of trochanteric fractures reflect such an approach. Future advances in the fractures around the hips will depend on breakthroughs in research on the prevention and the treatment of senile osteoporosis.

References

1. Rydell NW (1966) Forces acting on the femoral head-prosthesis – a study on strain gauge supplied prostheses in living persons. Munksgaard, Copenhagen
2. Hirsch C (1965) Forces in the hip-joint. In: Kenedi RM (ed) Biomechanics and related bio-engineering topics. Pergamon, Oxford, pp 341–350
3. Paul JP (1971) Load actions on the human femur in walking and some resultant stresses. Exp Mech 11:121–125
4. McLeish RD, Charnley J (1970) Abduction forces in the one-legged stance. J Biomech 3:191
5. Indong OH, Harris WH (1978) Proximal strain distribution in the loaded femur – an in vitro comparison of the distributions in the intact femur and after insertion of different hip-femoral components. J Bone Joint Surg [Am] 60(1):75
6. Rydell N (1972) Biomechanics of the hip-joint. Clin Orthop 92:6
7. Williams JF, Svensson NL (1968) A force analysis of the hip joint. Biomed Eng:365
8. Bergmann G, Rohlmann A, Graichen F (1990) Hip joint forces during physical therapy after joint replacement. In: Orthopaedic Research Society (ed) Transactions of the 36th annual meeting, Feb 5–8, 1990. Orthopaedic Research Society New Orleans, p2
9. Harris WH, Rushfeldt PD, Carlson CE, Scholler JM, Mann RW (1975) Pressure distribution in the hip and selection of hemiarthroplasty. In: Proceedings of the 3rd Annual Open Scientific Meeting of the Hip Society, Mosby, St Louis, pp 93–98
10. Davy DT, Kotzar GM, Brown RH, Heiple KG, Goldberg VM, Heiple KG Jr, Berilla J, Burstein AH (1988) Telemetric force measurements across the hip after total arthroplasty. J Bone Joint Surg [Am] 70(1):45

11. Hodge WA, Carlson KL, Fijan RS, Burgess RG, Riley PO, Harris WH, Mann RW (1989) Contact pressures from an instrumented hip endoprosthesis. J Bone Joint Surg [Am] 71(9):1378
12. Koch JC (1917) The laws of bone architecture. Am J Anat 21(2):177
13. Riggs BL, Wahner HW, Dunn WL, Mazess RB, Offord KP, Melton LJ (1981) Differential changes in bone mineral density of the appendicular and axial skeleton with aging. J Clin Invest 67:328
14. Lindsay R (1985) Prevention of osteoporosis. In: MuirGray JA (ed) Prevention of disease in the elderly. Churchill Livingstone, Edinburgh, pp 95–113
15. Meier D (1990) Disorders of skeletal aging. In: Cassel CK, Sorensen LB, Riesenberg DE, Walsh JR (eds) Geriatric medicine, 2nd edn. Springer, Berlin Heidelberg New York, pp 164–183
16. Lau EMC, Donnan SPB (1990) Falls and hip fracture in Hong Kong Chinese. Public Health 104:117
17. Brown TD, Ferguson AB Jr (1980) Mechanical property distributions in the cancellous bone of the human proximal femur. Acta Orthop Scand 51:429
18. Cornell CN, Schwartz S, Bansal M, Lane JM Bullough P (1987) Quantification of osteopenia in hip fracture patients. J Orthop Trauma 2(3):212
19. Crock HV (1965) A revision of the anatomy of the arteries supplying the upper end of the human femur. J Anat 99:77
20. Crock HV (1980) An atlas of the arterial supply of the head and neck of the femur in man. Clin Orthop 152:17
21. Mussbichler H (1970) Arteriographic findings in necrosis of the head of the femur after medial neck fracture. Acta Orthop Scand 41:77
22. Mussbichler H (1970) Arteriographic investigation of the hip in adult human subjects. Acta Orthop Scand Suppl 132:4
23. Trueta J, Harrison MHM (1953) The normal vascular anatomy of the femoral head in adult man. J Bone Joint Surg [Br] 35:442
24. Wolcott WE (1933) Circulation of the head and neck of the femur. JAMA 100:27
25. Marty M (1953) Blood supply of the femoral head. Br Med J 2:1236
26. Trueta J (1957) The normal vascular anatomy of the human femoral head during growth. J Bone Joint Surg [Br] 39:358
27. Sevitt S (1964) Avascular necrosis and revascularization of the femoral head after intracapsular fractures. J Bone Joint Surg [Br] 46:270
28. Sevitt S, Thompson RG (1965) The distribution and anastomoses of arteries supplying the head and neck of the femur. J Bone Joint Surg [Br] 47:560
29. Soto-Hall R, Johnson LK, Johnson R (1963) Alterations of the intra-articular pressure in transcervical fractures of the hip. J Bone Joint Surg [Am] 45:662
30. Crawfurd EJP, Emery RJH, Hansell DH et al. (1988) Capsular distension and intracapsular pressure in subcapital fractures of the femur. J Bone Joint Surg [Br] 70:195
31. Stromqvit B, Nilsson LT, Egund N et al. (1988) Intracapsular pressure in undisplaced fractures of the femoral neck. J Bone Joint Surg [Br] 70:192
32. Urist MR (1980) Fundamental and clinical bone physiology. Lippincott, Philadelphia, pp 292–293
33. Swiontkowski MF, Hansen ST, Kellam J (1984) Ipsilateral fractures of the femoral neck and shaft. J Bone Joint Surg [Am] 66(2):260
34. Barquet A, Fernandez A, Leon H (1985) Simultaneous ipsilateral trochanteric and femoral shaft fracture. Acta Orthop Clin Scand 56:36
35. Swiontkowski MF (1987) Ipsilateral femoral shaft and hip fractures. Orthop Clin North Am 18(1):73
36. Pipkin G (1957) Treatment of grade IV fracture – dislocation of the hip. J Bone Joint Surg [Am] 39:1027
37. Epstein HC (1980) Traumatic dislocation of the hip. Williams and Wilkins, Baltimore

38. Meyers MH, Telfer N, Moore TM (1977) Determination of the vascularity of the femoral head with technetium 99 mm-sulfur-colloid: diagnostic and prognostic significance. J Bone Joint Surg [Am] 59:658
39. Fairclough J, Colhoun E, Johnston D et al. (1987) Bone scanning for suspected hip fractures: a prospective study in elderly patients. J Bone Joint Surg [Br] 69:251
40. Bentley G (1980) Treatment of non-displaced fractures of the femoral neck. Clin Orthop 153:93
41. Soto-Hall R, Johnson LH, Johnson R (1964) Variations in the intra-articular pressure of the hip joint in injury and disease. J Bone Joint Surg [Am] 46: 509
42. Tooke SM, Favero KJ (1985) Femoral neck fractures in skeletally mature patients, fifty years old or less. J Bone Joint Surg [Am] 67:1255
43. Arnold CC, Lempberg RK (1977) Fracture of the femoral neck. Clin Orthop 122:217
44. Garden RS (1974) Reduction and fixation of subcapital fractures of the femur. Orthop Clin North Am 5:683
45. Bray TJ, Chapman MW (1984) Percutaneous pinning of intracapsular hip fractures. Instr Course Lect 33:168–179
46. Meyers MH, Harvey JP, Moore TM (1973) Treatment of displaced subcapital and transcervical fractures of the femoral neck or muscle-pedicle-bone graft and internal fixation. J Bone Joint Surg [Am] 55:257
47. Leung PC (1989) Current trends in bone grafting. Springer, Berlin Heidelberg New York, pp 39–41
48. Bochner RM, Pellicci PM, Lyden JP (1988) Bipolar hemiarthroplasty for fracture of the femoral neck. J Bone Joint Surg [Am] 70:1001
49. Bray TJ, Smith-Hoefer E, Hooper A et al. (1988) The displaced femoral neck fracture: internal fixation versus bipolar endoprosthesis. Results of a prospective randomized comparison. Clin Orthop 230:127
50. Yamagata M, Chao EY, Ilstrup DM et al. (1987) Fixed-head and bipolar hip endoprostheses: a retrospective clinical and roentgenographic study. J Arthroplasty 2:327
51. Lestrange NR (1990) Bipolar arthroplasty for 496 hip fractures. Clin Orthop 251:7
52. Friedman RJ, Wyman ET et al. (1986) Ipsilateral hip and femoral shaft fractures. Clin Orthop 208:188
53. Leung KS (1989) Trochanteric fracture – evolution of fixation devices. 9th Annual Congress of Hong Kong Orthopaedic Association, Nov 19, Hong Kong
54. Hofeldt F (1987) Proximal femoral fractures. Clin Orthop 218:12
55. Bannister GC, Gibson AGF, Ackroyd CE, Newman JH (1990) The fixation and prognosis of trochanteric fractures – a randomized prospective controlled trial. Clin Orthop 254:242
56. Wolfgang GL, Bryant MH, O'Neill JP (1982) Treatment of intertrochanteric fracture of the femur using sliding screw plate fixation. Clin Orthop 163:148
57. Jacobs RR, Armstrong HJ, Whitaker JH, Pazell J (1976) Treatment of intertrochanteric hip fractures with a compression hip screw and a nail plate. J Trauma 16:599
58. Laros GS, Moore JF (1974) Complications of fixation in intertrochanteric fractures. Clin Orthop 101:110
59. Cummings SR, Kelsey JL, Nevitt MC, O'Dowd KJ (1985) Epidemiology of osteoporosis and osteoporotic fractures. Epidemiol Rev 7:178
60. Jensen JS, Sonne-Holm S, Tondevold E (1980) Unstable trochanteric fractures. A comparative analysis of four methods of internal fixation. Acta Orthop Scand 51:949
61. Kauffer H, Matthew L, Sonstegard D (1974) Stable fixation of intertrochanteric fractures: a biomechanical evaluation. J Bone Joint Surg [Am] 56:899

62. Sonstegard DA, Kaufer H, Matthews LS (1974) A biomechanical evaluation of implant, reduction, and prosthesis in the treatment of intertrochanteric hip fractures. Orthop Clin North Am 5(3):551
63. Larsson S, Elloy M, Hansson LI (1988) Stability of osteosynthesis in trochanteric fractures. Acta Orthop Scand 59(4):386
64. Laskin RS, Gruber MA, Zimmerman AJ (1979) Intertrochanteric fractures of the hip in the elderly – a retrospective analysis of 236 cases. Clin Orthop 141:188
65. Ceder L, Lindberg L, Odberg E (1980) Differentiated care of hip fracture in the elderly – mean hospital days and results of rehabilitation. Acta Orthop Scand 51:157
66. Nue Moller B, Lucht U, Grymer F, Bartholdy NJ (1985) Early rehabilitation following osteosynthesis with the sliding hip screw for trochanteric fractures. Scand J Rehabil Med 17(1):39
67. Sexson SB, Lehner JT (1987) Factors affecting hip fracture mortality. J Orthop Trauma 1(4):298
68. Foubister G, Hughes SPF (1989) Fractures of the femoral neck: a retrospective and prospective study. J R Coll Surg Edinb 34:249
69. Pillar T, Gaspar E, Poplingher AR, Dickstein R (1988) Operated versus non-operated hip fractures in a geriatric rehabilitation hospital. Int Disabil Stud 10(3):104
70. Larsson S, Friberg S, Hansson L (1990) Trochanteric fractures – mobility, complications, and mortality in 607 cases treated with the sliding-screw technique. Clin Orthop 260:232
71. Evans EM (1949) The treatment of trochanteric fractures of the femur. J Bone Joint Surg [Br] 31:190
72. Jensen JS (1980) Classification of trochanteric fractures. Acta Orthop Scand 51:803
73. Chang WS, Zuckerman JD, Kummer FJ, Frankel VH (1987) Biomechanical evaluation of anatomic reduction versus medial displacement osteotomy in unstable intertrochanteric fractures. Clin Orthop 225:141
74. Martinek H, Egkher E, Wielke B, Spingler H (1979) Experimental tests concerning the biomechanical behaviour of pertrochanteric osteosyntheses. Acta Orthop Scand 50:675
75. Apel DM, Patwardhan A, Pinzur MS, Dobozi WR (1989) Axial loading studies of unstable intertrochanteric fractures of the femur. Clin Orthop 246:156
76. Harrington KD, Johnston JO (1973) The management of comminuted unstable intertrochanteric fractures. J Bone Joint Surg [Am] 55:1367
77. Waddell JP (1980) Sliding screw fixation for proximal femoral fractures. Orthop Clin North Am 11(3):607
78. Herrlin K, Stromberg T, Pettersson H, Walloe A, Lidgren L (1989) Trochanteric fractures – a clinical and radiological evaluation of McLaughlin, Ender, and Richard's osteosynthesis. Arch Orthop Trauma Surg 108:36
79. Dimon JH, Hughston JC (1967) Unstable intertrochanteric fractures of the hip. J Bone Joint Surg [Am] 49(3):440
80. Hunter GA, Krajbrich IJ (1978) The results of medial displacement osteotomy for unstable intertrochanteric fractures of the femur. Clin Orthop 137:140
81. Altner PC (1978) How not to pin a hip. Int Surg 63(5):11
82. Simpson AHR, Varty K, Dodd CAF (1989) Sliding his screws: modes of failure. Injury 20(4):227
83. Manoli A (1986) Malassembly of the sliding screw-plate device. J Trauma 26(10):916
84. Davis TRC, Sher LJ, Horsman A, Simpson M, Porter BB, Checketts RG (1990) Intertrochanteric femoral fractures. J Bone Joint Surg [Br] 72(1):26
85. Jensen JS (1980) Mechanical strength of Jewett and McLaughlin hip nail plates manufactured from cobalt-chromium-molybdenum alloy – a biomechanical study of unstable trochanteric fractures IV. Acta Orthop Scand 51:145

86. Sarmiento S, Williams EM (1970) The unstable intertrochanteric fracture: treatment with a valgus osteotomy and I-beam nail-plate. A preliminary report of one hundred cases. J Bone Joint Surg [Am] 52:1309
87. Roberts A, Rooney T, Loupe J et al. (1972) A comparison of the functional results of anatomic and medial displacement valgus nailing of intertrochanteric fractures of the femur. J Trauma 12:341
88. Jacobs RR, McClain O, Armstrong HJ (1980) Internal fixation of intertrochanteric hip fractures: a clinical and biomechanical study. Clin Orthop 146:62
89. Doppelt SH (1980) The sliding compression screw – today's best answer for stabilization of intertrochanteric hip fractures. Orthop Clin North Am 11(3):507
90. Jensen JS (1980) Mechanical strength of sliding screw-plate hip implants. A biomechanical study of unstable trochanteric fractures VI. Acta Orthop Scand 51:625
91. Mulholland RC, Gunn DR (1972) Sliding screw plate fixation of intertrochanteric femoral fractures. J Trauma 12(7):581
92. Leung KS, So WS, Shen WY, Hui PW (1991) Treatment of peritrochanteric fractures with gamma nails and dynamic hip screws in geriatric patients – a randomised prospective study. J Bone Joint Surg [Br] 74:345
93. Leung KS (1991) The development of Asiatic gamma nail. 3rd Advance Course of Locked Nails, Jan 28–Feb 1, Courchevel
94. Jensen JS, Michaeldsen M (1975) Trochanteric femoral fractures treated with McLaughlin osteosynthesis. Acta Orthop Scand 46:795–803

13 Problem Fractures Around the Knee

K.M. CHAN

Introduction

Fractures around the knee present with a unique biomechanical feature to the entire function of the lower limb. The knee is the centre of two long lever arms of the lower limb and has a complicated structural arrangement with a number of important intra-articular components that determine the stability and afford weight bearing with wide range of motion. Five specific types of problematic fractures are discussed in this chapter as they all share a unique feature of juxta-articular fractures that may present a special problem to the restoration of normal function of the knee joint. These are tibial plateau, intercondylar eminence, femoral condyle, patellar and osteo-chondral fractures.

Principles of Management

The principle of management of juxta-articular fractures is well illustrated in some of the problematic fractures around the knee.

Main Objectives

Accurate anatomical reduction with restoration of anatomical continuity and normality of the soft tissues and intra-articular structures is the major objective. In this respect special attention must be paid to the collateral ligaments, cruciate ligaments and menisci. It is also important to appreciate that the knee is composed primarily of three distinct compartments: the patello-femoral, the medial tibial femoral, and the lateral femoral tibial femoral compartments. Disruption of the normal anatomy of one compartment may lead to mechanical irritation and destruction of articular cartilage. Degenerative arthritis can throw the other compartments into a biomechanically disadvantaged position in weight bearing and may thereby increase the risk of degeneration in the other compartments. It is therefore important in the decision making for treatment options that all three functional compartments be taken into consideration as a whole.

Stability of the knee joint depends very much on the associated soft-tissue structures as the bony configuration is primarily an unstable type. The stabilizing structures are: the capsule, medial and lateral collateral ligaments, anterior and posterior cruciate ligaments, and menisci. In fractures around the knee it is therefore important to delineate the exact nature and extent of the injury of both the bony and soft-tissue components. In this regard it may be necessary to extend the scope of investigation to another, more sophisticated imaging modality such as (a) tomography, to delineate the extent of articular cartilage damage; (b) stress radiography, to access the degree and extent of ligamental instability; and (c) computed tomography and magnetic resonance imaging, to assess the associated soft-tissue injuries.

Mobility around the knee is very important particularly after juxta-articular fractures. The ultimate aim is to restore full functional range of motion with special emphasis on attaining full extension of the knee. Any flexion contracture of the knee should be minimised as much as possible because it can produce most undesirable effects in the biomechanical function of the lower limbs, such as unequal leg length and additional stress on the patello-femoral joint. In recent years, the use of continuous passive motion after stable fixation of juxta-articular fracture around the knee has definitely improved the overall results.

Factors Affecting the Prognosis of Juxta-articular Fracture Around the Knee

The pattern of fracture is the key determining factor as it indicates the extent of the injury, degree of intra-articular involvement and associated in-stability. It is therefore important that a common classification be used when different series are compared for efficacy of various treatment modalities.

The extent of associated articular cartilage and soft-tissue injuries in relation to the juxta-articular fracture around the knee also provides a significant prognostic guide. In particular, the associated meniscal, cruciate or collateral ligament injury presents special problems in the consideration of stability of the knee. It is also important to design a plan of rehabilitation such that the knee can be mobilised at an early stage.

In compound fractures around the knee the first priority should be given to the management of skin and soft tissue. This may necessitate the need for adequate débridement and careful planning for resurfacing of both skin and soft tissue such that repair of the fractures and concomitant treatment of the ligamental structures can be carried out.

The status of bone stock, particularly in elderly patients with established osteoporosis, plays an important role in the prognosis of juxta-articular fractures around the knee. This is well illustrated particularly in supracondylar and tibial plateau fractures. In these weight-bearing situations a special need for bone grafting to build up the bone loss should be considered.

In high-energy trauma it is of vital importance from the very beginning to assess the presence and extent of possible neuro-vascular complications.

It should be emphasised that repeated examinations within the first 6 h is important. Prior to the surgical intervention for fracture and soft tissue, it must be absolutely certain that there is no significant neuro-vascular complication as this affects the choice of anaesthesia, positioning of the patient and selection of tourniquet control.

Tibial Plateau Fractures

Classification of Tibial Plateau Fractures

There are myriad opinions regarding the best treatment protocol for tibial plateau fractures [1–7]. To compare the efficacy of various treatment protocol objectively it is important to establish a common basis for presentation. There are two major classifications adopted for tibial condylar fractures. The commonly adopted one was introduced by Hohl in 1967 [8]. This has the following categories (Fig. 1): type A, undisplaced; type B, local compression; type C, split compression; type D, total condylar depression; type E, split; and type F, comminuted. In 1979 Shatzker et al. [9] introduced a slight modification of the classification and offered a scheme of treatment as follows (Fig. 2):

Type I: pure cleavage fracture. Usually fixed with lag screws.
Type II: cleavage combined with depression. Reduction is required with elevation of the fragment with bone grafting, and the lateral wedge is lagged onto the lateral cortex with a buttress plate.
Type III: pure central depression with no lateral wedge; the depression is usually anterior or posterior or involves the whole condyle. Elevation and bone grafting is necessary, and the lateral cortex is buttressed with a plate.
Type IV: medial condyle either split off as a wedge (subgroup A) or crumbled and depressed (subgroup B); it usually occurs in elderly patients with osteoporosis. Bone grafting and medial buttress plating are necessary.
Type V: plateau fracture with dissociation of the metaphysis and diaphysis. This type of fracture is not suitable for conservative treatment with traction and should be properly reduced and buttress plated on one or both sides depending on the extent of condylar involvement.
Type VI: bicondylar fracture with the metaphysis and diaphysis retaining continuity. Both condyles need to be fixed with the buttress plates and cancellous screw.

For extensive comminution of the tibial plateau with extension to the shaft, it is sometimes necessary to extend the fixation across the knee joint by means of an external fixator [10] (Fig. 3).

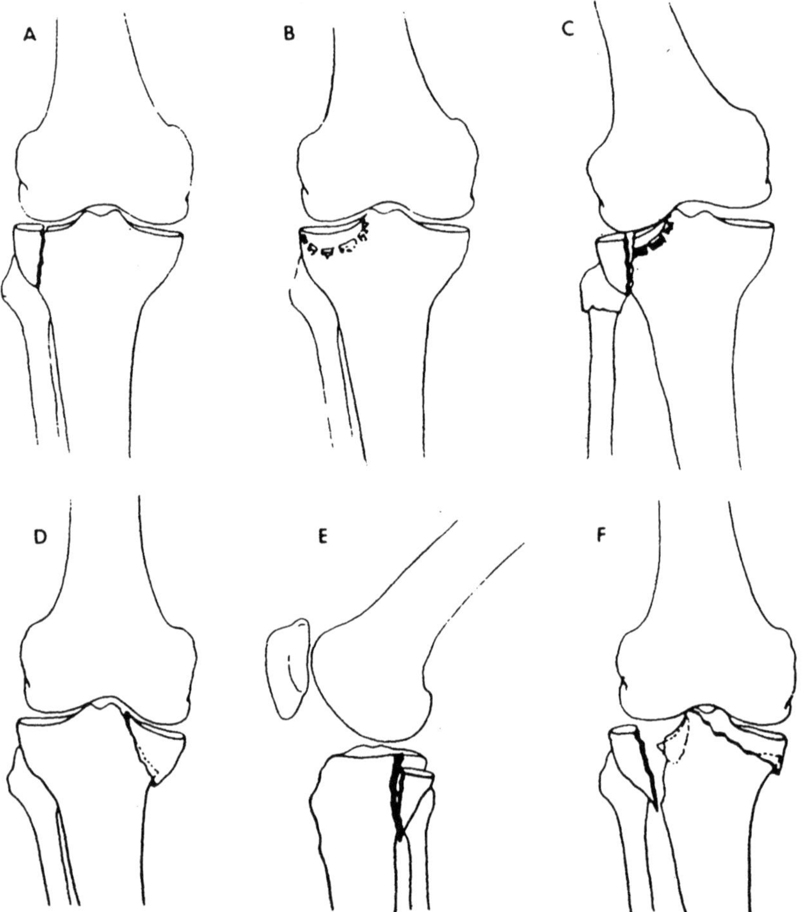

Fig. 1. Hohl's classification of tibial condylar fractures. *A* Undisplaced. *B* Local compression. *C* Split compression. *D* Total condylar compression. *E* Split. *F* Comminuted

Assessment of Tibial Plateau Fractures

It has been well documented in most series that the single most important factor in the long-term prognosis of tibial plateau fractures is the degree of displacement and depression of the fracture [11]. It is generally recognised that if the depression is less than 5–6 mm, non-operative treatment consisting of traction, early motion and late weight bearing is usually sufficient to provide good long-term results. When the depression is 6–8 mm, the decision for surgical intervention depends very much on the patient's age and his demand for activities. For example, in elderly patients with a relatively sedentary life-style, non-operative treatment may be indicated; otherwise

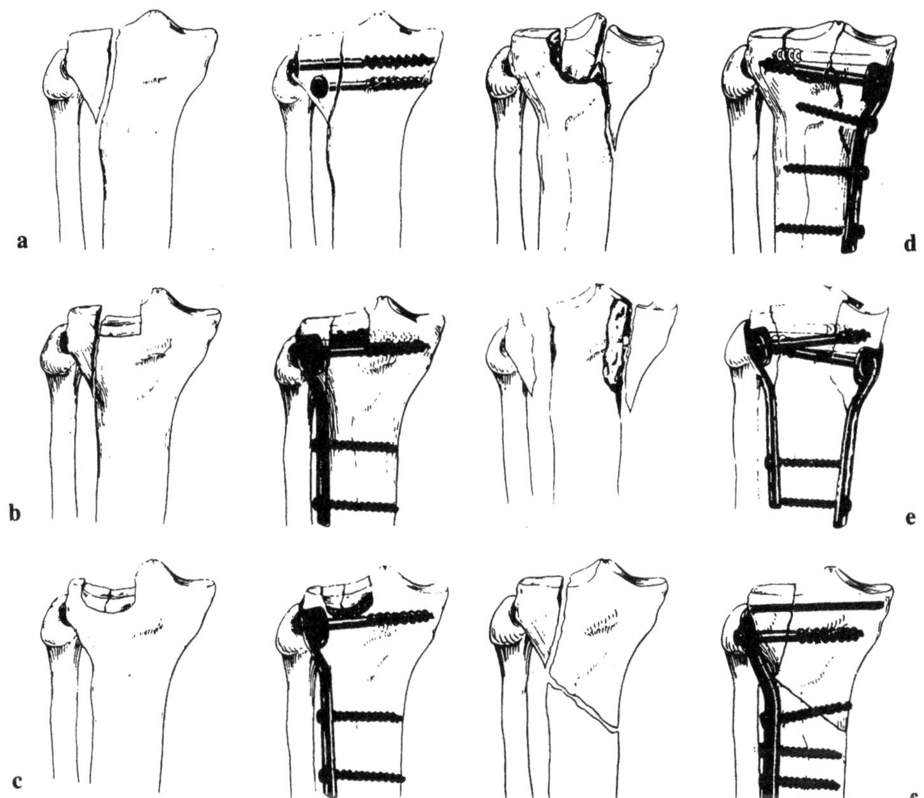

Fig. 2a–f. Shatzker et al.'s classification of tibial condylar fractures. **a** Type I. **b** Type II. **c** Type III. **d** Type IV. **e** Type V. **f** Type VI. (See text for descriptions)

there is a general preference in the younger and the more active individuals to aim for accurate surgical reconstruction of the joint surfaces. When the depression exceeds 10 mm, surgical intervention is always indicated, with the aim of elevating and restoring the joint surfaces, often with bone grafting and adequate fixation with buttress plating.

To delineate the extent of depression and displacement in all tibial plateau fractures a thorough assessment using radiological and imaging techniques is of paramount importance. (a) Standard antero-posterior and lateral views are necessary in all cases. It must be noted that the upper tibial articular surfaces are normally inclined to the posterior by 10°–15°, and an antero-posterior X-ray with the beam angled distally 10°–15° usually provides a much better view of the tibial plateau. (b) An oblique X-ray is sometimes necessary to assess the extent of displacement of the fragment. (c) Tomography is an important adjunct to assess the extent of depression, particularly in the posterior compartment. (d) Stress X-ray particularly in

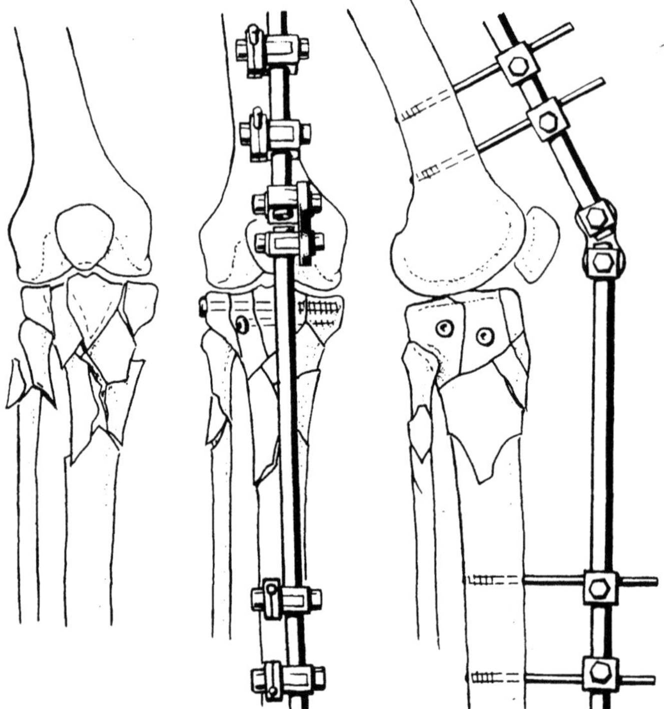

Fig. 3. External fixation for comminuted tibial plateau fracture

comparison with a normal knee provides valuable information on associated collateral ligament injuries, which are reported to occur in 10%–30% of cases. These have a very significant bearing on the final functional outcome.

Percutaneous Fixation with Arthroscopically Assisted Procedures

Some tibial plateau fractures are amenable to percutaneous or minimally invasive surgical fixation, with sufficient stability to allow early mobilisation. With the advent of arthroscopy, such fractures with intra-articular extension can be well visualised and assessed arthroscopically [12–14]. The extent of articular cartilage damage and other associative lesions such as meniscal tear or loose bodies is well delineated. Percutaneous screw fixation can be performed with arthroscopic monitor of the coaptation of the intra-articular fracture line thus allowing more accurate reduction (Fig. 4).

Intercondylar Eminence Fractures

The intercondylar eminence is the part of the proximal surface of the tibia that lies between the anterior tibial spine and the anterior pole of the medial

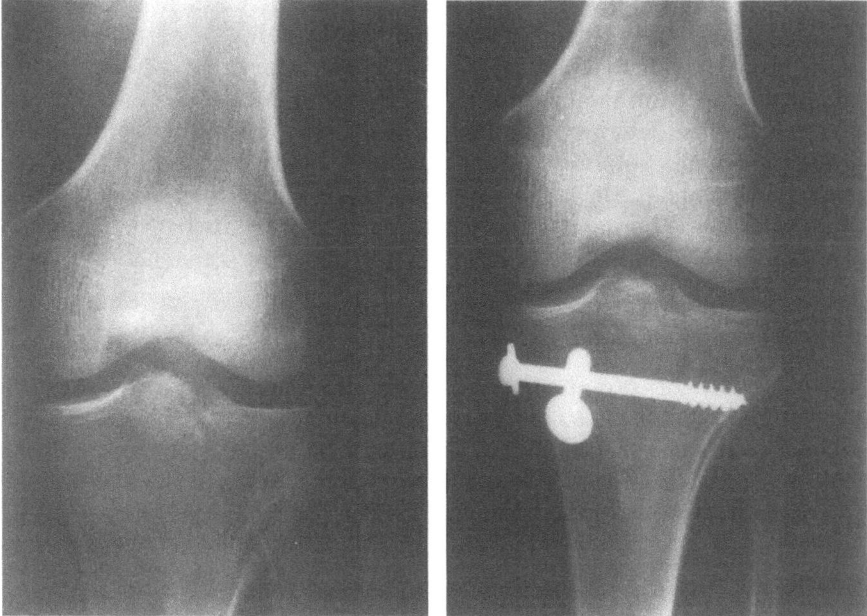

Fig. 4. Percutaneous fixation of tibial plateau fracture

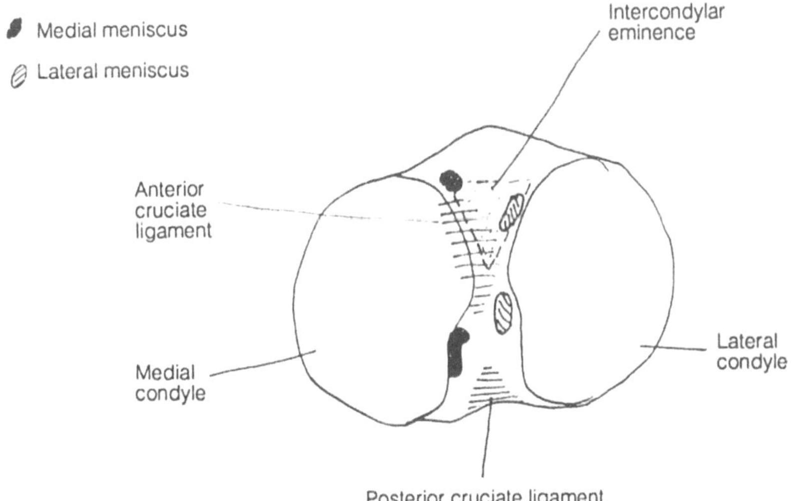

Fig. 5. Line diagram showing relationship of structures of the intercondylar eminence

menisci (Fig. 5). It is triangular in shape, with the apex pointing towards the tibial spine and sloping slightly upwards. Fractures of this region are considered childhood fractures comparable with anterior cruciate rupture in adults [15,16]. As with all avulsion fractures, these are said to occur more commonly when the epiphyses are open, the relative elasticity and strength of the ligament being greater than the physes. In adults they are more likely to be associated with concomitant soft-tissue injury. Of all tibial spine fractures reported in the literature, 60% occurred in children [17–19].

Since its first description by Poncet in 1875 as "a tearing off of the spine of the tibia by the anterior cruciate ligament", much has been written about these fractures [20]. Meyers and McKeever [21] classified the fractures into three types based on the degree of displacement of the fragment (Fig. 6). A fourth group was added by Zaricznyj [22] to allow for comminution.

Clinical Presentation

The characteristic presentation is of a child (8–15 years of age) with haemarthrosis following a fall from a bicycle, unable to bear weight and with a decreased range of movement. There may be no anterior cruciate laxity because of muscle spasm. An apriori suspicion is necessary as the fracture can easily be overlooked on radiographs. The mechanism of injury is either a direct blow on the lowermost part of the femur with the knee flexed or

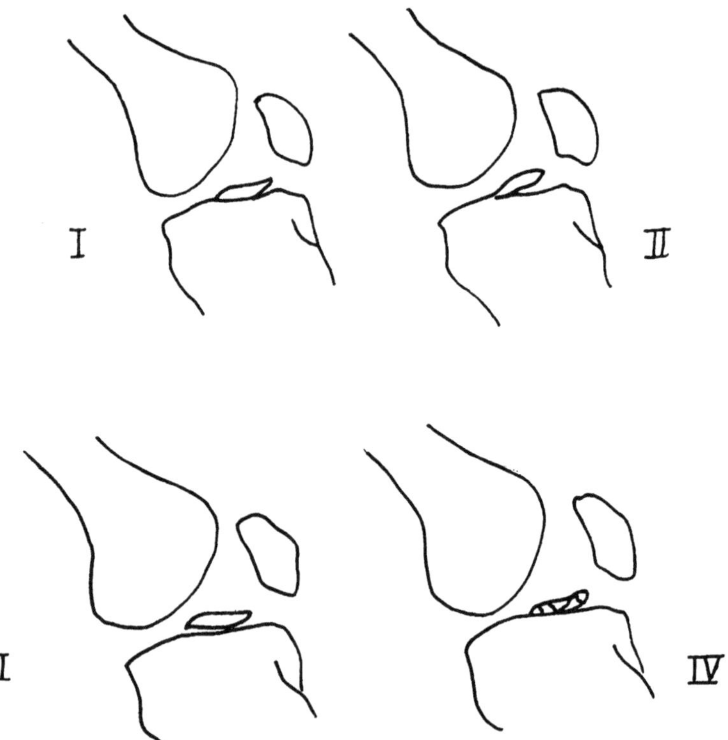

Fig. 6. Meyers and McKeever's classification of tibial eminence fracture

forceful hyperextension; both put a strain on the anterior cruciate ligament. Prior to avulsion the ligament is stretched. Associated injuries are rare in children. In adults they include meniscal lacerations and tears of the medial collateral ligament [23,24]. Chondral fractures may also be associated with the adult fracture. Diagnosis is best made on lateral views, although occasionally tunnel, oblique and stress views may all be required. In some instances arthroscopy may be required to make the diagnosis.

Treatment

Most authors recommend conservative treatment for undisplaced or minimally displaced fractures (type I). This involves immobilisation in a plaster of paris cast or brace for at least 4–6 weeks. Closed reduction can be attempted in a type II fracture, but if this fails, arthroscopic or open reduction with internal fixation is required. All type III and IV fractures require internal fixation. In children care must be taken to avoid the proximal growth plate with the fixation device. Some displaced fractures can now be adequately reduced and fixed arthroscopically by absorbable pins [25]. Post-operatively the limb should be immobilised for at least 3 weeks prior to allowing movement in a protective brace (Fig. 7).

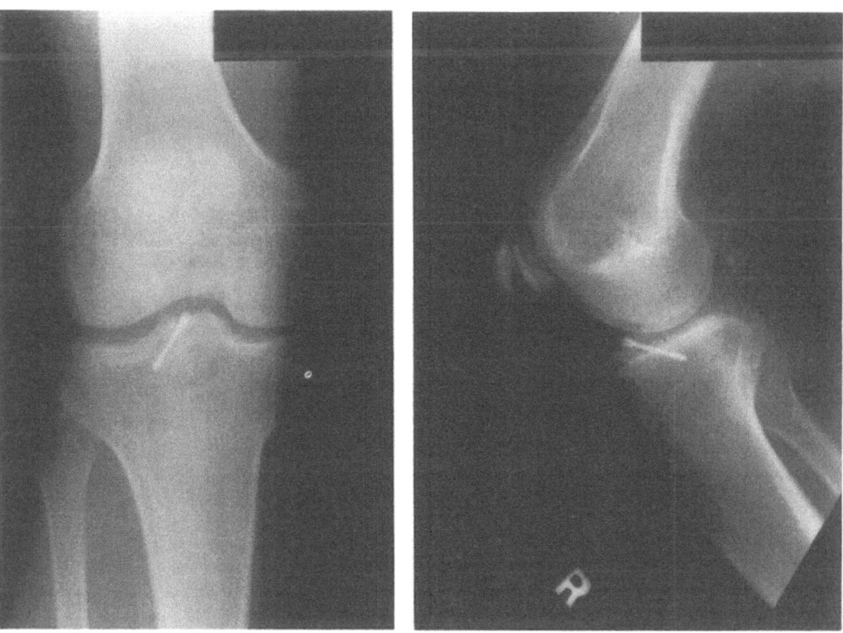

Fig. 7. Fixation of tibial eminence fracture

Prognosis and Complications

Children with avulsion fractures usually return to full function with little or no instability. One study suggests that this may be due to differential growth of the bone and ligament which takes up the slack caused by lengthening of the ligament during the injury. In adolescents and more so in adults the possibility of differential growth does not exist, and although instability may be demonstrated, the patient is usually asymptomatic. In adults poor outcome is associated with the presence of intra-articular fractures and medial collateral ligament tears.

Complications are fairly rare. These include non-union [26], mal-union, delayed arthritis (with associated intra-articular fractures) and quadriceps atrophy. One case of meniscal entrapment has been reported [27]. Occasionally extension lag is present, but this is small, a matter of 3°–8°, and related to mal-union. Diagnostic pitfalls include missed meniscal tears and chondral fractures.

Femoral-Condylar Fractures

The AO classification of supracondylar fracture is generally used to indicate the level of fracture, complexity of fracture and extent of intra-articular involvement (Fig. 8). Depression of the articular cartilage of the femoral condyle is rather uncommon compared to tibial plateau fractures. In the 1960s and 1970s most reports indicated only fair results with operative treatment [28]. The main reasons for a relatively negative attitude to internal fixation in this type of difficult fracture are that (a) a suitable implant to secure the fixation is lacking, (b) the extensiveness of surgical exposure often compromises the post-operative function of the soft tissue, and (c) insufficient bone stock particularly in elderly patients precludes the use of a suitable implant.

Technical Considerations

With the introduction of the AO principle, there are more encouraging reports indicating that a reasonably high level of achievement can be attained with strict adherence to the surgical principle [29]. Obviously, an experienced surgeon is required in many of these difficult fractures. Some of the current techniques are the following:

Lag screw and buttress plate: For a single condylar fracture with intra-articular extension (type B) the fracture should be accurately reduced and fixed with lag-screw with or without additional T-plate for buttressing (Fig. 9).

AO condylar plate: For a type C fracture the AO condylar plate provides stable fixation [29] (Fig. 10).

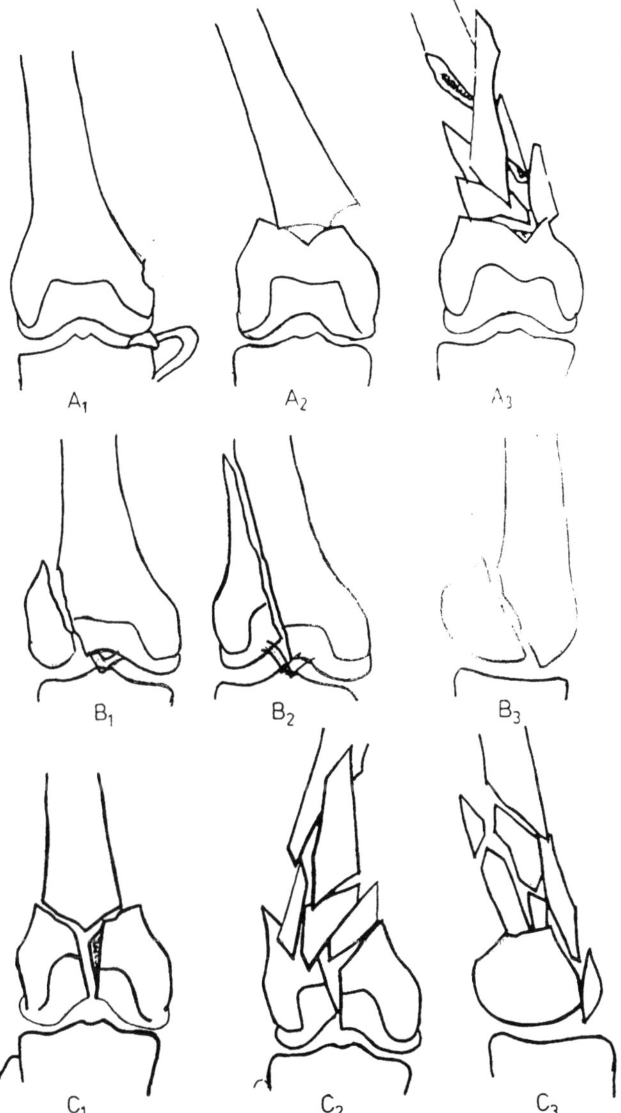

Fig. 8. The AO classification of supracondylar fracture

AO dynamic condylar screw: A recent introduction, this provides the further mechanical advantage of fixation of the supracondylar fragments [30]. It has the combined efficacy of compression screw fixation for the condylar element and dynamic axial compression of the condylar plate for the shaft (Fig. 11).

Interlocking nailing with percutaneous lag screw fixation under fluoroscopy: In certain situations of supracondylar fracture without extensive com-

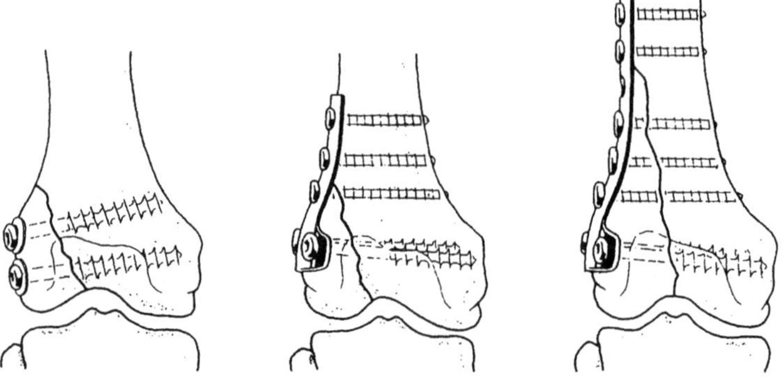

Fig. 9. Lag screw and buttress plate for type B fracture

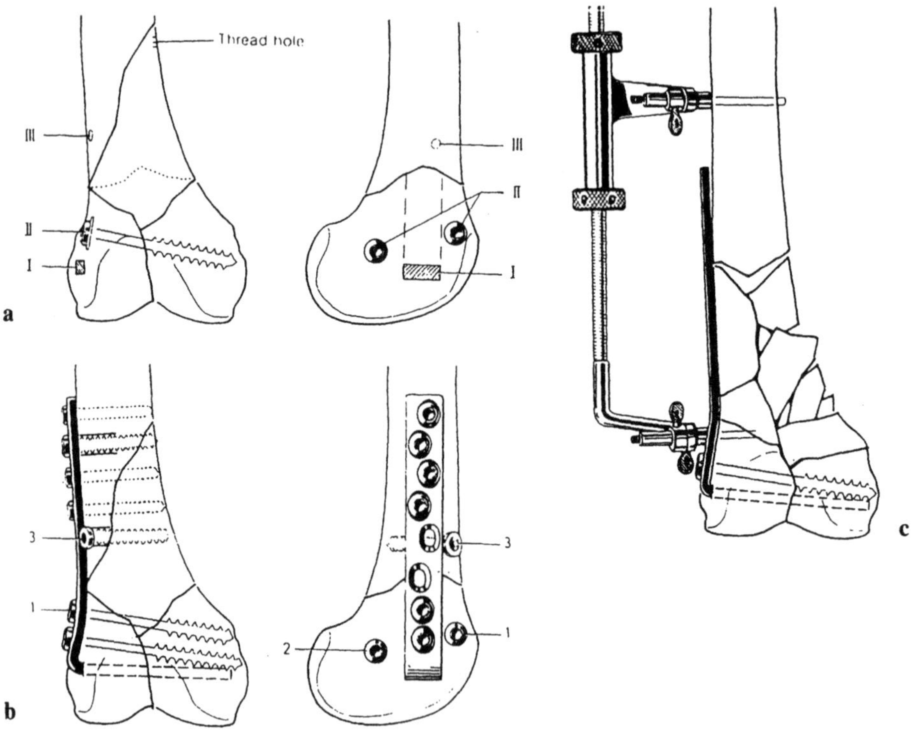

Fig. 10a–c. AO condylar plate for type C fracture. **a** Lag screw fixation for the condylar. **b** AO condylar plate for stabilisation of the entire supracondylar fracture. **c** For comminuted fracture the use of the distractor may facilitate reduction

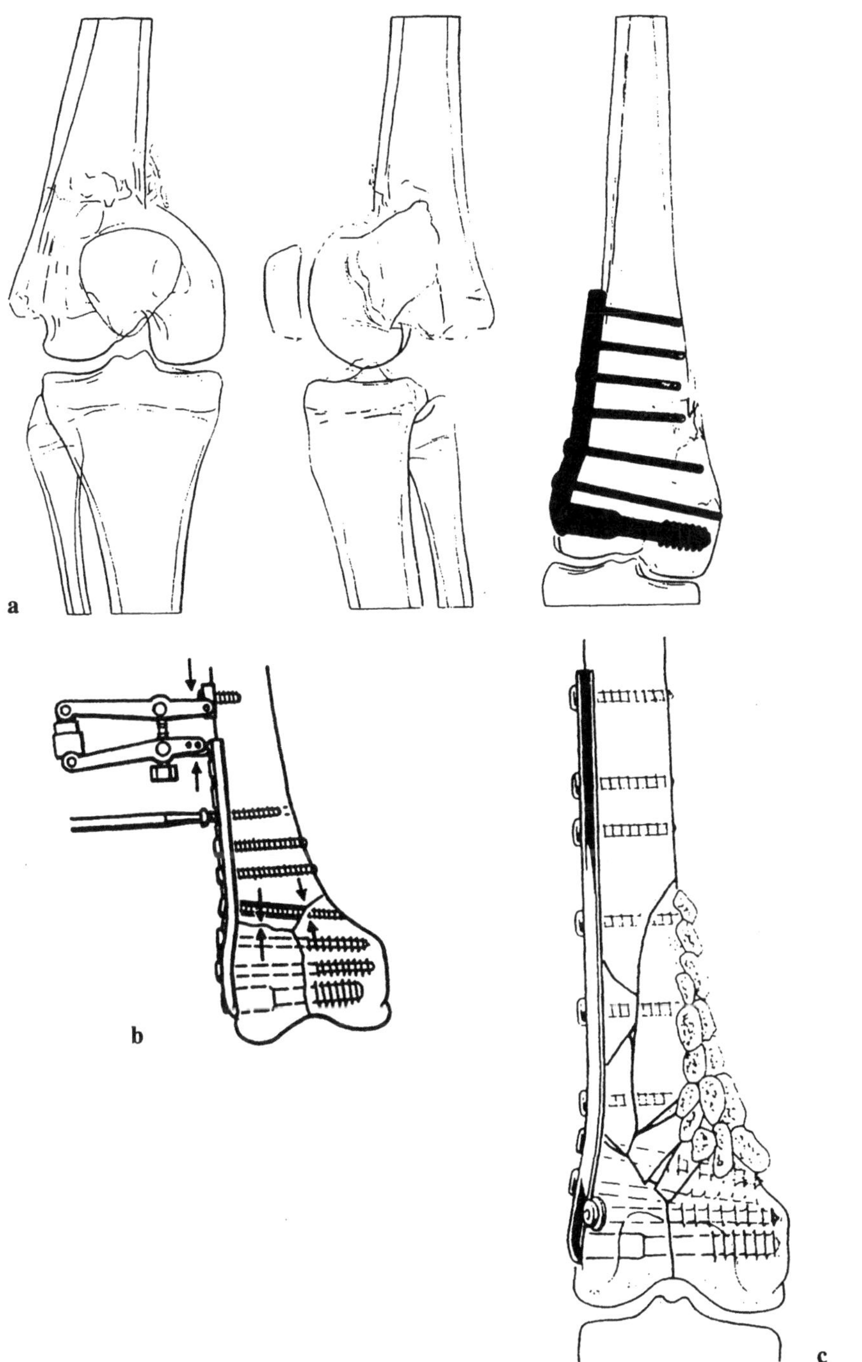

Fig. 11a–c. AO Dynamic condylar screw for type C fracture. **a** Supracondylar fracture with dynamic condylar screw fixation. **b** The use of compression device enhances axial stability. **c** For comminuted fracture the defect should be grafted in addition to the dynamic condylar screw system

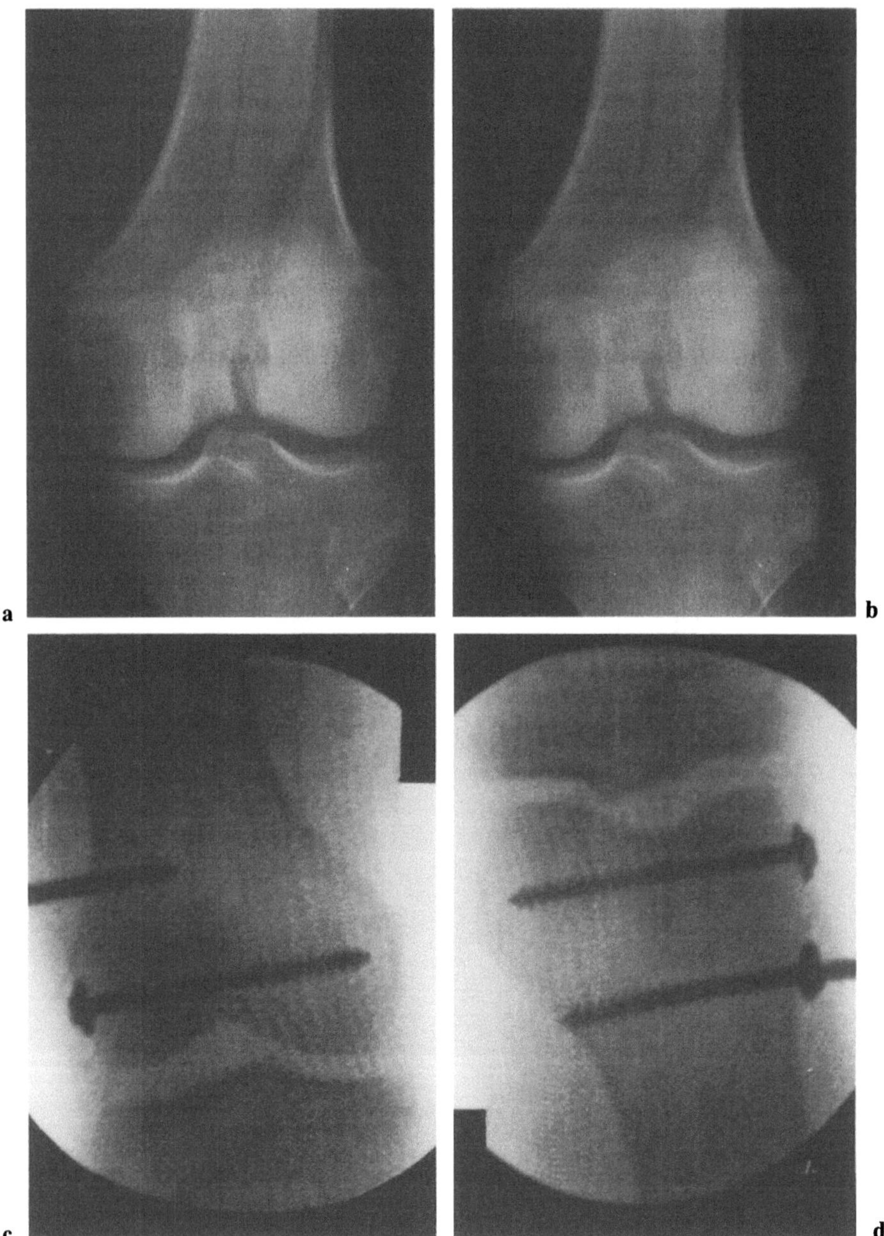

Fig. 12a–d. Interlocking nailing and percutaneous lag screw for type C fracture. **a** Antero-posterior radiograph showing a type C2[5] fracture. **b** Fluroscopic screw fixation. **c** Fluroscopic screw fixation. **d** Interlocking screw fixation

minutions and displacement, a relatively less traumatic approach uses intramedually fixation with a locked nail [31–33]. Distal screw fixation of the locked nail can furnish adequate fixation of the supracondylar element while an additional lag screw can be applied under fluoroscopic control to reinforce the fixation of the condylar (Fig. 12).

Patellar Fractures

Fracture of the patella is common in adults and usually occurs as a result of simple falls, traffic accidents or industrial accidents. Most fractures of the patella traverse the articular cartilage and hence pose an important element of intra-articular disruption of the patello-femoral articulation. The general principles of fixation and mobilisation of intra-articular fracture should be observed. The tension band principle has been widely applied, with outstanding results, and should be the treatment of choice (Fig. 13). Figure 14 illustrates the principle of tension band wiring and the variation of technique in different circumstances [34].

Osteochondral Fractures Around the Knee

The subject of osteochondral fractures around the knee has been discussed extensively by Rosenberg [35], Ahstrom [36], Kennedy [37], and Milgram [38]. The advent of magnetic resonance imaging and arthroscopy has greatly enhanced the diagnosis of osteochondral or chondral fractures. It is generally believed that osteochondral fractures are associated with dislocation of the

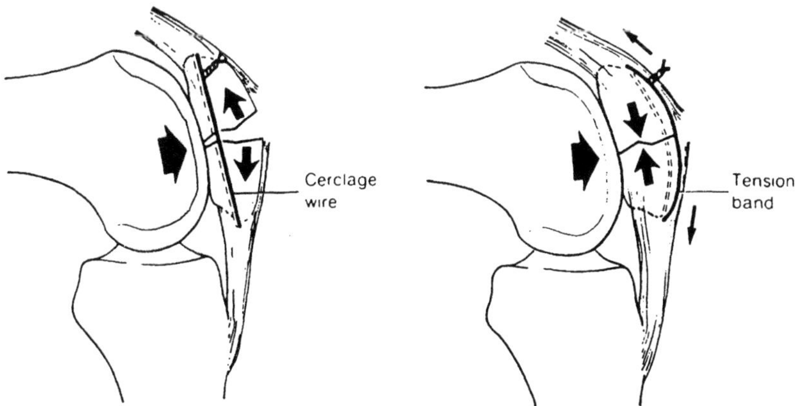

Fig. 13. The biomechanical advantage of tension band injury as compared with cerclage wiring is illustrated here as the knee is actively flexed to produce a coaptation force on the transverse fracture

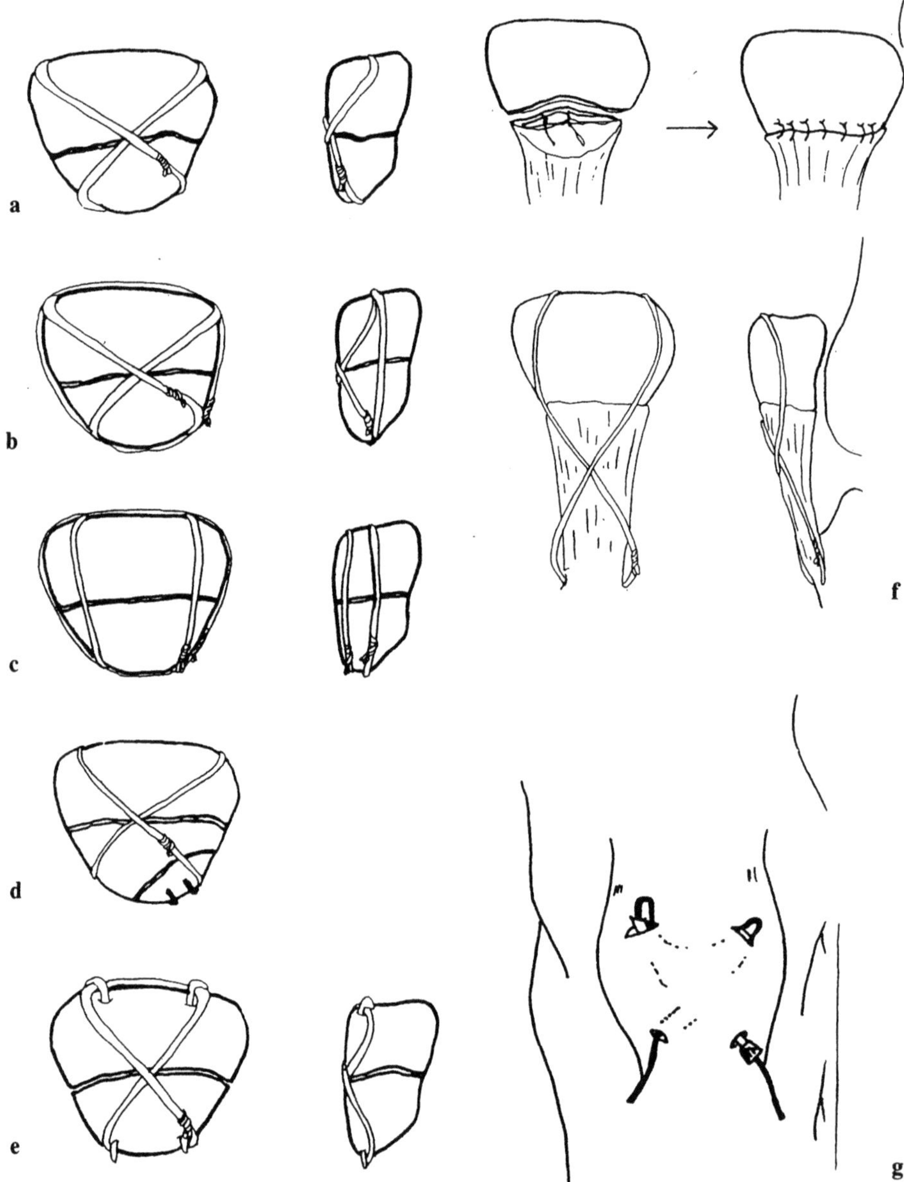

Fig. 14a–g. Tension band wiring technique for various types of patellar fracture. **a** A single figure-of-eight tension band is usually sufficient to provide adequate coaptation of a simple transverse fracture with minimum displacement. **b** A circumferential wire plus a figure-of-eight tension band is indicated if additional cerclage effect is required for fractures with significant displacement. **c** A circumferential wire plus a parallel tension band is a variation of the method in **c** and provides the same principle of fixation. **d** Additional local Kirschner wire fixation may be indicated for small polar fragments which are not well coapted by two circumferential wires. The use of a mini-screw may serve the same purpose. **e** A figure-of-eight tension band looped

patella which shears off a fragment of the condyle. Milgram [38] described the mechanism injury as follows:

"Probably the best documented mechanism for the production of osteochondral fractures from the articular surfaces of the knee joint is a momentary dislocation of the patella. As the quadriceps muscle contracts during relocation, the patella is driven into the lateral femoral condyle. This may shear off a portion of the joint surface of the lateral femoral condyle or the medial facet of the patella."

Management depends very much on the size and time of detection of the osteochondral fragment. Since this is an intra-articular disruption with the presence of a mechanical block, it should be dealt with as a matter of urgency. If it is a very small fragment, it is usually impossible to fix, and the fragment should be removed either arthroscopically (Fig. 15) or openly. For a sizable fragment every attempt should be made to reposition it with the use of various internal fixation devices. The recently introduced adsorbable

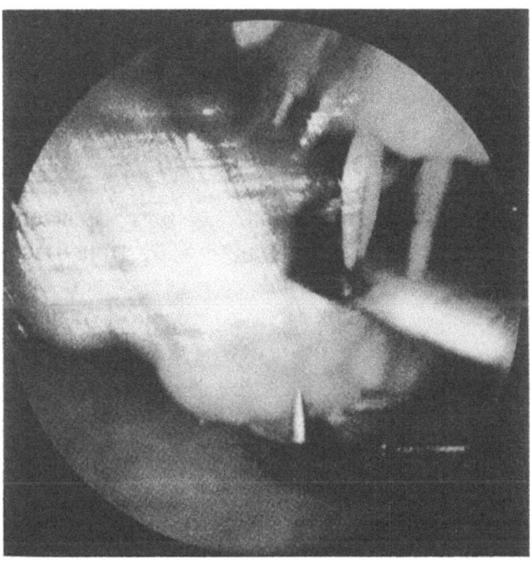

Fig. 15. Arthroscopic removal of loose osteochondral fragment

around two parallel Kirschner wires is a classical illustration of the tension band principle. This provides additional stability to axial rotation. f For comminuted lower pole fractures beyond salvage a partial patellectomy may be indicated to enhance the rehabilitation programme; the repair of the lower pole to the patellar tension may be further protected by an additional tension band wired to the tibial tuberosity, as shown. This reduces the stress across the bone tendon in the place. No further cast or brace protection is required, and the knee can be mobilised immediately. g For undisplaced fractures a special technique of percutaneous wiring is advocated [39,40]. The minimal surgical invasion offers good and stable fixation to allow immediate mobilisation pins provide an additional advantage. The main principle in the choice of implant is that there should not be any breach of the articular surface in order to minimise further damage to the articular cartilage.

Conclusion

The management of juxta-articular fractures around the knee has evolved through different stages in the past few decades. As illustrated here by the five problematic fractures, the major advance achieved is the recognition of restoration of normal anatomy and stable fixation to allow early mobilization. As a weight joint, the knee must be aligned in its proper position for the entire axis of the lower limb in order to stand the stress of motion. With the advent of the various new fixation devices together with the new technique of minimal surgical invasion, it is now possible to achieve the principle of stable fixation in many of these juxta-articular situations. However, a major gap in our understanding is the extent of damage to the articular cartilage. In some instances there is such extensive damage to the articular cartilage that the joint undergoes premature degeneration despite adequate fixation of the fracture. However, this limitation is beyond the scope of our objective in fracture management.

References

1. Blokker CP, Rorabeck CH, Bonrne RB (1984) Tibial plateau fractures – an analysis of the results of treatment in 60 patients. Clin Orthop 182:193–199
2. Drennan DB, Locher FG, Maylahn DJ (1979) Fracture of the tibial plateau – treatment by closed reduction and spica case. J Bone Joint Surg [Am] 61:989–995
3. Lansinger O, Bergman B, Korren L, Andersson GBJ (1986) Tibial condylar fractures – a twenty-year follow-up. J Bone Joint Surg [Am] 68:13–19
4. Rasmussen PS (1973) Tibial condylar fractures – impairment of knee joint stability as an indication for surgical treatment. J Bone Joint Surg [Am] 55:1331–1350
5. Gossling HR, Peterson CA (1979) A new surgical approach in the treatment of depressed lateral condylar fractures of the tibia. Clin Orthop 140:96
6. Apley A (1979) Fractures of the tibial plateau. Orthop Clin North Am 10:61
7. Waddell JP, Johnston DWC, Neidre A (1981) Fractures of the tibial plateau: a review of ninety-five patients and comparison of treatment methods. J Trauma 21:376
8. Hohn M (1967) Tibial condylar fractures. J Bone Joint Surg [Am] 49:1455
9. Shatzker J, McBroom R, Bruce D (1979) The tibial plateau fracture: the Toronto Experience 1968–1975. Clin Orthop 138:94–110
10. Muller ME, Allgöwer M, Schneider R, Willenegger H (1979) Manual of internal fixation, 2nd edn. Springer, Berlin Heidelberg New York
11. Shybut GT, Spiegel PG (1979) Tibial plateau fractures (Editorial comment). Clin Orthop 138:12
12. Lemon RA, Bautlett DH (1985) Arthroscopic assisted internal fixation of certain fractures about the knee. J Trauma 25:355–358

13. McLennan JG (1982) The role of arthroscopic surgery in the treatment of fractures of the intercondylar eminence of the tibia. J Bone Joint Surg [Br] 64:477–480
14. Reiner MJ (1982) The arthroscope in tibial plateau fractures: its use in evaluation of soft tissue and bony injury. J Am Osteopath Assoc 81:704–707
15. Rockwood CA Jr, Green DP (1984) Fractures, vol 2. Lippincott, Philadelphia, pp 1475–1478
16. Sharrard J (1959) The management of the tibial spine in children. Proc R Soc Med 51:905–906
17. Fyfe IS, Jackson JP (1913) Tibial intercondylar eminence fractures in children: a review of the classification and the treatment of malunion. Injury 13:165–169
18. Garcia A, Neer CS II (1958) Isolated fractures of the intercondylar eminence of the tibia. Am J Surg 95:593–598
19. Gronkvist H, Hirsch G, Johansson L (1984) Fractures of the anterior tibial spine in children. J Pediatr Orthop 4(4):465–468
20. Roth PB (1928) Fractures of the spine of the tibia. J Bone Joint Surg 10:509–518
21. Meyers MH, McKeever FM (1959) Fractures of the intercondylar eminence of the tibia. J Bone Joint Surg [Am] 41:209–222
22. Zaricznyj B (1977) Avulsion fractures of the tibial eminence treatment by open reduction and pinning. J Bone Joint Surg [Am] 59(8):1111–1114
23. Hayes JM, Masear VR (1984) Avulsion fractures of the tibial eminence associated with severe medial ligamentous injury. Am J Sports Med 12(4):330–333
24. Jones R, Smith SA (1913) On the rupture of the crucial ligament of the knee and on fractures of the spine of the tibia. Br J Surg 1:70–89
25. McLennan JG (1982) Role of arthroscopic surgery in treatment of fractures of the intercondylar eminence of the tibia. J Bone Joint Surg [Br] 64:477–480
26. Keys GW, Walters J (1988) Non-union of intercondylar eminence fractures of the tibia. J Trauma 28(6):870–871
27. Burstein DB, Viola A, Fulkerson JP (1988) Entrapment of the medial meniscus in a fracture of the tibial eminence. J Arthroscopic Related Surg 4(1):47–50.
28. Laros GS (1979) Supracondylar fractures of the femur: editorial comment and comparative results. Clin Orthop 138:9–12
29. Schatzker J, Tile M (1987) The rationale of operative fracture care. Springer, Berlin Heidelberg New York, pp 255–294
30. Sanders R, Regazzoni P, Ruedi TP (1989) Treatment of supracondylar-intracondylar fractures of the femur using the dynamic condylar screw. J Orthop Trauma 3:214–222
31. Leung KS, Shen WY, So WS, Mui LT, Groose A (1991) Interlocking intramedullary nailing for supracondylar and intercondylar fractures of the distal part of the femur. J Bone Joint Surg [Am] 73:332–340
32. Wiss DA, Felming CH, Matta JM, Clark Douglas (1986) Comminuted and rotationally unstable fractures of the femur treated with an interlocking nail. Clin Orthop 212:35–47
33. Zuckerman JD, Vieth RG, Johnson KD, Bach AW, Hansen ST, Solvik S (1987) Treatment of unstable femoral shaft fractures with closed interlocking intramedullary nailing. J Orthop Trauma 1:209–218.
34. Hung LK, Chan KM, Chow YN, Leung PC (1985) Fractured patella: operative treatment using the tension band principle. Injury 16:343–347
35. Rosenberg NJ (1964) Osteochondral fractures of the lateral femoral condyle. J Bone Joint Surg [Am] 46:1013–1026
36. Ahstrom JP (1965) Osteochondral fracture in the knee joint associated with hypermobility and dislocation of the patella – Report of eighteen cases. J Bone Joint Surgery [Am] 47(8):1491–1520
37. Kennedy JC, Grainger RW, McGraw RW (1966) Osteochondral fractures of the femoral condyles. J Bone Joint Surgery [Br] 48(3):436–440
38. Milgram JW, Rogers LF, Miller JW (1978) Osteochondral fractures: Mechanisms of injury and fate of fragments. AJR Am J Roentgenol 130(4):651–658.

39. Leung PC, Mak KH, Lee SY (1983) Percutaneous tension band wiring – a new method of internal fixation for mildly displaced patellar fractures. Trauma 23:62
40. Ma YE, Zhang YF, Qu KF, Yeh YC (1984) Treatment of fractures of the patella with percutaneous suture. Clin Orthop 191:235

14 Fractures Around the Ankles and Foot

K.S. Leung

Advances in the treatment of fractures in the ankle and the foot have been obvious in the past 10 years. The unique features of ankle and foot fractures lie in the frequent involvement of the articular surfaces. The modern concept of treating intra-articular fractures with operation that aims at anatomical reduction, stable fixation and early mobilisation forms the basis of the management of fractures around the ankle and the foot. Further knowledge of the complex biomechanics of the foot also helps to treat these fractures with more predictable outcome. The problems involved in managing the fractures include the frequent association of soft-tissue trauma, the difficulty in restoring the congruity of the articular surface and the early restoration of function as a weight-bearing joint complex.

Fractures of the Ankle

The two common classifications of ankle fractures are those of Lauge and Hansen [1] and of Danis and Weber [2]. The Lauge-Hansen classification [1] is based on cadaveric study and classifies the ankle fractures into four types based on the position of the foot at the time of injury and the direction of the force applied. Each of the categories is further subdivided into stages indicating the severity of the injuries and hence the prognosis. The Danis-Weber schema [2] classifies fractures primarily at the level of the fibular fractures and the association of syndesmotic injuries. The higher the fibular fractures, the more severe are the injuries which involve the syndesmosis. Both classifications are well known and widely used [3,4]. The Lauge-Hansen classification has been criticised for being too comprehensive and difficult in clinical application; it is of greatest value as a basis for conservative treatment since it is intended to provide information about the mechanism of the fracture. The Danis-Weber classification is criticised for being too simple and leaving out significant information. However, it is valuable in deciding the appropriate form of surgical treatment in clinical practice.

Fractures of the ankles are intra-articular fractures. In applying the principles for treating intra-articular fractures, displaced fractures should be treated with anatomical reduction and stable internal fixation to allow early mobilisation [5–9]. Fractures of the ankles are complicated by injuries involving the syndesmosis of the distal tibio-fibular joint. The importance of the syndesmosis is best illustrated by the classification of ankle fractures proposed by Danis-Weber [2]. The higher the fibular fractures, the more severe are the syndesmotic injuries and the displacement of the ankle mortise. Biomechanical study also points out the important role of fibula in the weight-bearing and stability of the ankle mortise [10–12]. The close contact of the articular surface of the ankle mortise in all positions of ankle motion is the principal mechanism for load distribution. Normal syndesmotic function is essential for the maintenance of this mechanism.

For fractures not associated with syndesmotic injuries, open reduction and stable internal fixation with the AO principle is the most accepted method [7,8,13–16]. This method ensures anatomical reduction of the articular surface and early restoration of motion of the ankle joint. The results of treating these fractures are uniformly good. Much of the controversy lies in the treatment of fractures with syndesmotic problems. Syndesmotic injuries may involve either ligamentous disruption or avulsion with a bony attachment, or a combination of these two injuries. The aim of treatment of these injuries is the exact anatomical restoration of the ankle mortise so as to provide perfect congruity with the talus and stability. In this aspect, the exact length of the fibula and the ligamental integrity of the tibio-fibular bond must be reconstructed. The fibular length can be restored in most cases except in those with extensive comminutions, in which the fibular facet of the talus can be used as a guide to the length.

Reconstruction of the syndesmosis depends on the recognition of the pattern of the injury [17]. With the disruption of the syndesmosis of pure ligamental injuries, the fibular fracture is fixed first with the plate and screws: the stability of the syndesmosis is restored with a 4.5-mm cortical screw fixing the fibular to the tibia by purchasing the three cortices. The screw should be fully treaded and inserted as a fixation screw instead of a lag screw (Fig. 1). Biomechanical study shows that the insertion of the syndesmotic screw significantly interferes with ankle motions [18]. The common clinical finding that lucent changes develop around the screw indicates that movement occurs around the screws due to the relative movement of the fibula and the tibia [19]. Screw breakage may occur as metal fatigue sets in if weight-bearing walking is allowed. The recommended regime is to remove the syndesmotic screw at the end of 6 weeks post-operatively, before weight-bearing walking is allowed. The removal of the screw requires another operation; the use of an absorbable implant, such as those made of poly-glycolic acid, may be especially indicated in such circumstances (Fig. 2). In fact, the use of absorbable implants in the form of pins and rods has been advocated in the treatment of fractures around the ankle [20,21]. The need for a prolonged period of immobilisation after the fixation makes this treatment modality less attractive. However, the recent appearance of absorbable implants in the form of screws with better mechanical properties indicates the need for further exploration.

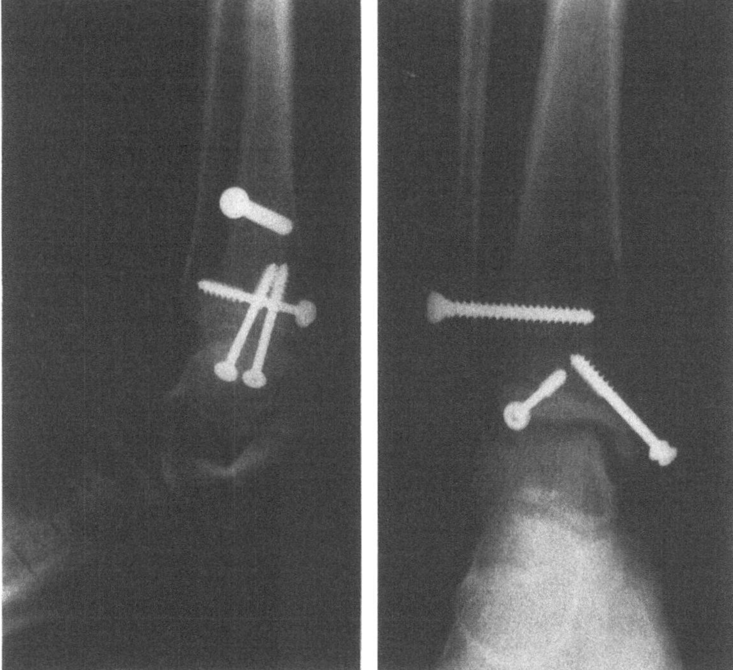

Fig. 1. Fixation of a high fibular fracture together with the medial and posterior malleolar fractures. Stability of the syndesmosis is restored with the screw fixing the fibula to the tibia as well as the fixation of the posterior malleolus

In syndesmotic injuries with avulsion fractures of the anterior and posterior tibio-fibular ligaments, fixation of avulsed fragments with screws also provides excellent results provided that these fragments are large enough for screw fixations (Fig. 3). In those with small fragments, with the reduction and restoration of the correct length of the fibula, most of the fragments are spontaneously reduced and held in the reduced positions by the thick periosteum. Fixation with screws may be unnecessary if not impossible. The restoration of syndesmotic stability is best achieved by the use of the syndesmotic screw. However, if the fragment is sizable, screw fixation has the definite advantage of early stabilisation of the syndesmosis without interfering with ankle movements, as occurs when the syndesmotic screw is used. This certainly facilitates early mobilisation after the operation.

In fractures with a large posterior fragment together with part of the posterior articular surface of the tibial plafond, fixing the fibula and the posterior fragment through a postero-lateral incision is an excellent approach. The use of a 4-mm cancellous screw as the lag screw fixing the posterior fragment is much better mechanically compared with fixation by the anterior route. The other advantage of employing the posterior route is

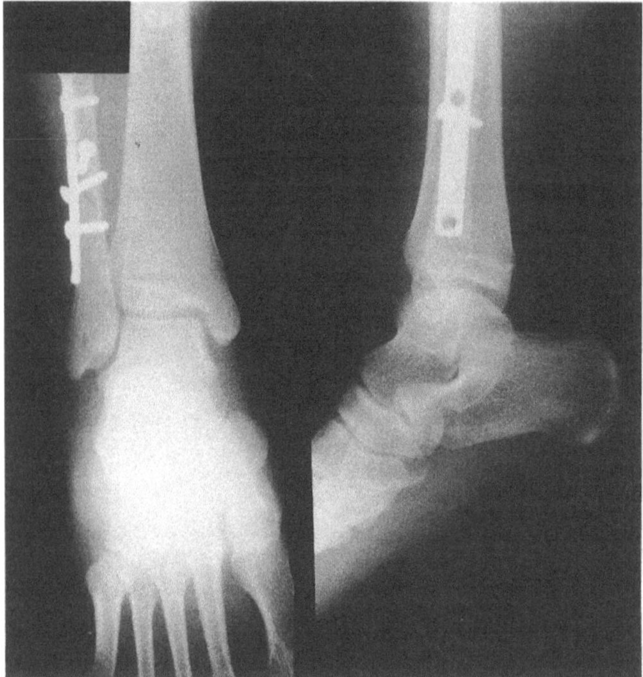

Fig. 2. Use of the absorbable screw as the syndesmotic fixation. Note the apparent empty screw hole in the most distal part of the plate and the screw tread across the fibula to the tibia

better visualisation of the reduction. Long-term study also shows that anatomical stabilisation of the posterior fragment decreases significantly or precludes arthrosis [22].

Fractures of the Talus

Fractures of the talus are uncommon, but the sequelae of the fractures are serious. These sequelae result from the problems of obtaining anatomical reduction of the intra-articular fractures particularly in situations in which major comminution occurs. The restoration of the complex geometric relationship of the three articular surfaces of the talus dictates an absolute anatomical reduction to regain normal motion in the ankle, hindfoot and talonavicular joint. The second problem is the risk of avascular necrosis of the body of the talus after fracture dislocations. As 60% of the surface area is articular surface, and there is no muscular and tendinous attachment, the vascular supply of the talus depends on the blood vessels in the surrounding soft-tissue integrity. As soft-tissue injuries are commonly associated with

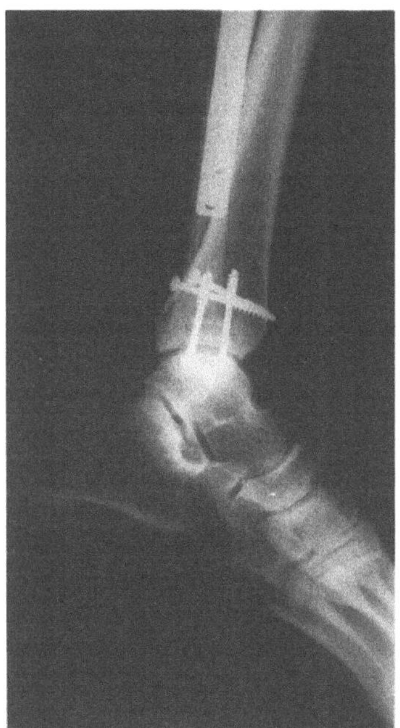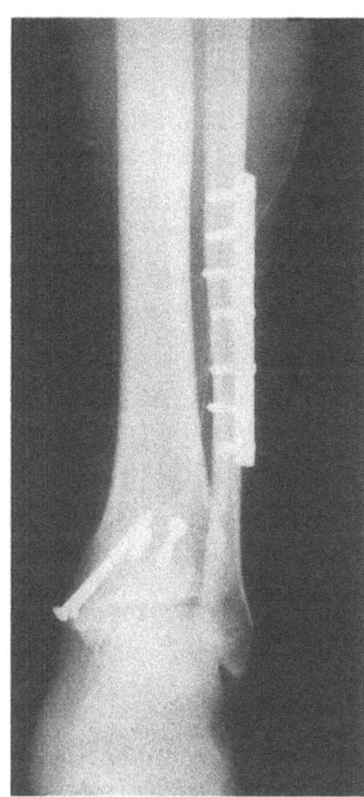

Fig. 3. Stability of the syndesmosis is restored with the screws fixing the posterior malleolus in a Danis-Weber type C fracture. Temporary transfixing the fibula to the tibia is not necessary

fractures and dislocations around this region, the vascular supply of the talus, particularly the body, is thus in danger and could easily be jeopardised during fractures and dislocations. Numerous vascular studies have shown that the major arterial supply of the talus is from the medial side by the branches of the posterior tibial artery [23–25].

There is extensive extra-osseous and intra-osseous anastomosis for the blood supply of the talus. The blood supply of the talus is thus well maintained in isolated fractures unless associated with dislocation which causes soft-tissue damage. The other significant conclusion from these vascular studies is that the preservation of the medial soft-tissue is of the utmost importance during surgical treatment of the fracture dislocations as most injuries of the talus occur with dorsiflexion and inversion, and the medial soft tissues including the artery may remain intact, which ensures the viability of the body of the talus. As the principle of treating intra-articular fractures is anatomical reduction and stable internal fixation, operative treatment is commonly employed for displaced fractures. The conflicting needs of reduction and exposure must be carefully considered, and the preservation of the soft tissue cannot be overemphasised.

Fractures of the talus are classified anatomically into body fractures and neck fractures. Both types may be associated with subtalar dislocations and total dislocation from the ankle mortise. In fractures of the talar body, management of the comminuted dome fractures can be difficult, and primary fusion may be considered. In considering the operative fixation of the fractures the problems lie in anatomical reduction and stable fixation of the articular osteochondral fragments. Bilateral exposure may be required. The use of absorbable implants may be helpful in fixing the osteochondral fragments. Patchy avascular necrosis and late collapse are common. Fortunately, in most cases the symptoms and functional disturbance are far less severe than the radiological findings suggest [26].

Fractures of the neck of the talus are completely different both in management and prognosis from those of the body. Hawkins's classification of fractures of the talar neck is the most widely used [27]:

Type I: non-displaced vertical fracture of the talar neck
Type II: displaced fracture of the talar neck with subluxation or dislocation of the subtalar joint (the ankle joint remains aligned)
Type III: displaced fracture of the talar neck with dislocation of the body of the talus from both the subtalar and ankle joints

The progressive displacement of the fractures, the progressive disruption of blood supply and hence an increasing incidence of avascular necrosis form the basis of this classification. Dislocations of the head fragment with the combination of a type III fracture have been classified as type IV injuries [28]. Diagnosis of type I fracture must be made carefully. There must be no displacement of the fracture, and the anatomical alignment of the subtalar joint is preserved. Treatment consists of a short leg cast and non-weight-bearing walking for 8 weeks. The results of treating this fracture are good. The complication of avascular necrosis is rare. In type II fractures, because of the displacement and subluxation of the body of the talus, anatomical reduction must be achieved. In most cases, open reduction and internal fixation is the preferred method. The use of lag screws to achieve stable fixation should be the standard (Fig. 4).

There are at least three approaches to the exposure of the fractures. Those who advocate the use of the antero-lateral approach claim that the medial soft tissue remains undisturbed, and thus the important vascular blood supply to the body is not further jeopardised. However, there is considerable difficulty in fixation of the fracture as the lateral side of the talar head is wedge shaped, and the lag screws must be inserted through the articular surface of the talonavicular joint to achieve a stable fixation. This would mean another exposure, and the talonavicular joint is affected. Those who advocate the posterior approach (Fig. 5) again face difficulty in controlling the accuracy of the reduction; there is limited exposure through the posterior approach due to the deep seated talo-tibial joint. The medial approach is perhaps the most common. The exposure is simple, and the lag screw fixation through the non-articular surface of the talus ensures a firm grip (Fig. 6). Care must be taken not to disturb the medial soft tissue,

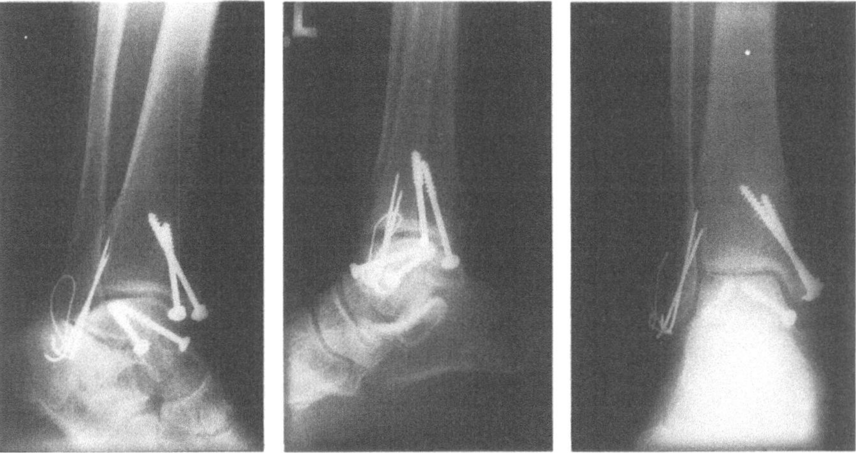

Fig. 4. Fracture of the neck of the talus fixed with medio-lateral screw fixation

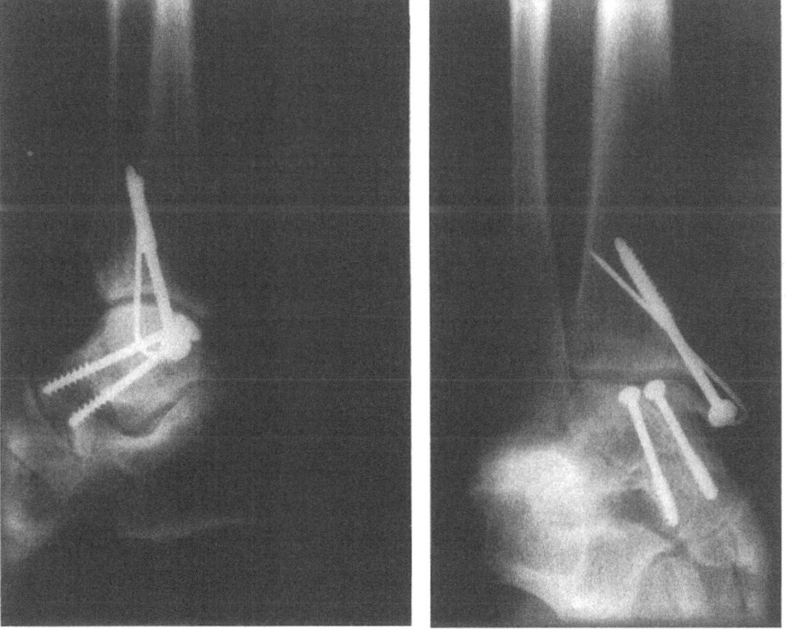

Fig. 5. Fixation of the talar neck fracture with posterior approach

especially the deltoid ligaments, so that the blood supply can be preserved. The exposure can be further improved by osteotomy of the medial malleolus and reflecting it distally. The common association of medial malleolar fracture with talar neck fracture makes this approach even more practical.

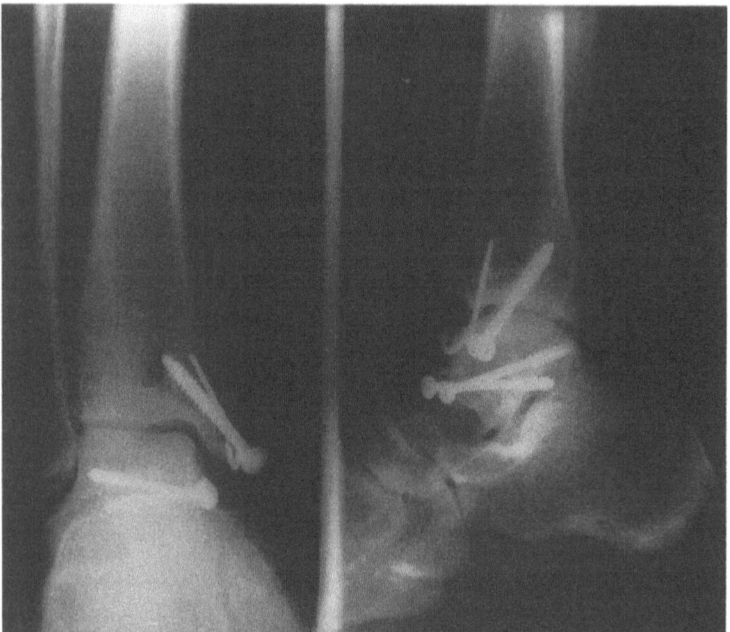

Fig. 6. Fixation of the talar neck fracture with antero-medial approach

The incidence of avascular necrosis after a type II fracture is reported to be around 20%–50%. The diagnosis of avascular necrosis is by radiological means. The appearance of subchondral osteopenic changes on the X-ray film taken 6–8 weeks after the injury (Hawkins's sign) is a reliable indication of the viability of the talar body. The availability of the magnetic resonance imaging is very helpful for the detection of avascular necrosis. Clinical review shows that the majority of type II fractures do not develop significant avascular necrosis leading to collapse. Revascularisation by creeping substitution occurs in most cases. Accurate reduction with stable fixation certainly facilitates this natural revascularisation process. It is therefore not necessary to undertake more radical primary surgical treatments such as primary fusion or talectomy.

For type III fractures, with extensive soft-tissue injury and marked displacement of the talar body after fracture, the treatment becomes a surgical emergency. Speedy relocation of the extruded body of the talus releases the pressure effect on the soft tissue and the neuro-vascular bundle. Open reduction should be carried out after one or two unsuccessful attempts at closed reduction. As more than 50% of these fractures are associated with medial malleolar fractures, the medial approach is chosen most of the time. With accurate reduction, internal fixation can be achieved with lag screws through the talar head. Because of the total detachment of the soft tissue from the talar body the incidence of avascular necrosis approaches 100%,

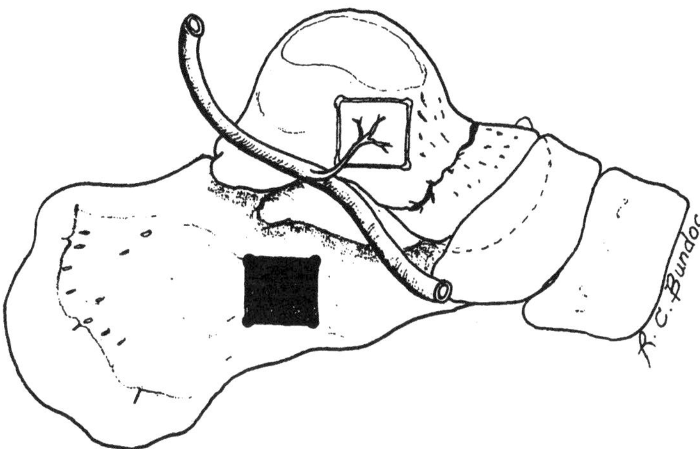

Fig. 7. Schematic drawing of the revacularisation of the talar body with vascularised bone graft isolated from the os calcis

and the outcome is even less predictable. Talo-calcaneal fusion or Blair's fusion is advocated as the salvage operation to reconstruct a stable hindfoot. To prevent or treat avascular necrosis, the microvascular procedure for revascularisation of the talar body has been carried out by transferring a vascularised pedicle bone graft from the medial side of the calcaneum and fixing it into the talus. The fracture is approached through the medial side. After accurate reduction and internal fixation with lag screws the medial calcaneal branch of the medial plantar vessel is isolated and traced to the periosteum of the medial surface of the calcaneum (Fig. 7). The periosteum and the underlying bone is harvested with the pedicle intact. The graft is then turned upwards and fixed across the fracture site by a small Kirschner wire or screw. Preliminary results of treating five cases show good union and revascularisation after a period of months (Fig. 8). Further study must be carried out to confirm this technique for the treatment of type III fractures of the talar neck.

Calcaneal Fractures

The calcaneum is the largest tarsal bone of the foot. It is also the most frequently fractured bone in the foot. Almost all the fractures are produced by axial loading in which the calcaneum is driven upwards against the talus. This results in a primary fracture line that forms posterior to the interosseous ligament of the sinus tarsi and runs obliquely from postero-medially to antero-laterally in the body of the calcaneum (Fig. 9). The sustentaculum tali remains in normal position by the attachment of the interosseous ligament, and this is the key-stone for reduction when operative treatment is

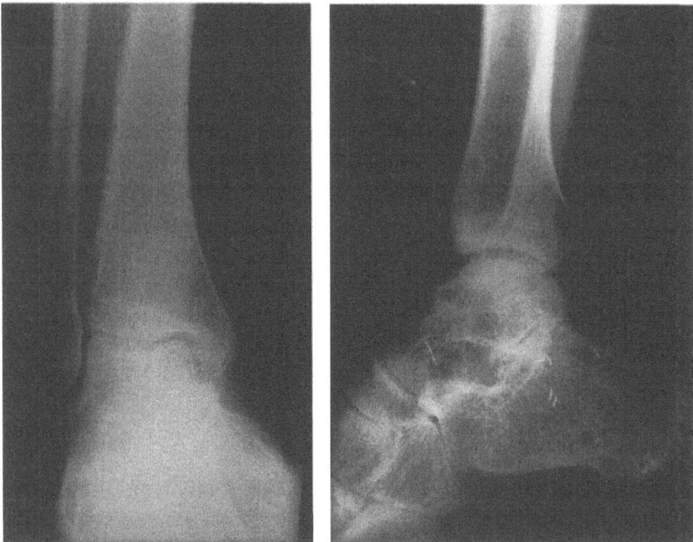

Fig. 8. Hawkin's type III fracture of the talus treated with early revascularisation procedure with the vascularised pedicle bone graft from the os calcis. No signs of avascular necrosis after 1 year follow-up

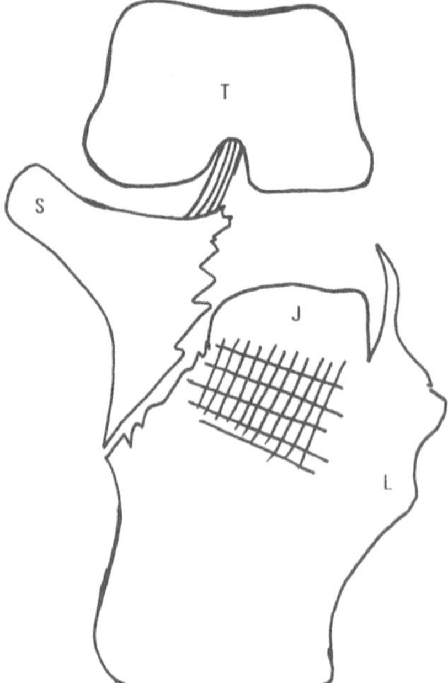

Fig. 9. Schematic drawing of the axial view of the calcaneal fracture. *T*, Talus; *S*, sustentaculum tali; *J*, depressed articular surface; *L*, burst lateral wall of the os calcis

contemplated. With further impaction either the lateral part of the posterior facet of the subtalar joint is fractured and driven into the cancellous part of the body, or the whole articular surface with the subchondral plate is rotated 90° and sinks into the body. To accommodate the osteochondral fragment, the lateral wall of the calcaneum is pushed laterally and fractured. Secondary fracture lines are created. These fracture lines may be vertical, horizontal or oblique and involve substantial compression of the cancellous bone in the calcaneum. The anterior facet and the articular surface of the calcaneocuboid joint may also be fractured. The resultant deformities of the injury are a depressed articular surface in the posterior facet while the osteochondral fragment sinks into the body of the calcaneum, which becomes broader in the transverse diameter and shorter in height. Clinically, there is a loss of congruity of the subtalar joint, a shortened and widened hindfoot with varus deformity and entrapment of the peroneal tendons due to the bulging of the lateral wall of the calcaneum.

The calcaneal fractures can be broadly classified into extra-articular and intra-articular groups. The treatment for extra-articular fractures is mainly conservative and aims at pain relief. The exception to this may be avulsion fracture of the Achilles tendon. Sudden violent contraction of the tricep surae causes this fracture, which is frequently associated with skin problems. The pressure effect of the avulsed fragment calls for special care in operative treatment. Prompt reduction of the fracture decreases the chances of wound ischaema. The use of the tension band wiring principle is well indicated in the treatment of this fracture. The treatment of intra-articular fractures has proven difficult. The availability of a uniform comprehensive classification that allows comparisons of treatment results is perhaps the most vital factor for the recommendation of treatment protocol. Many classifications of the intra-articular fractures have been proposed but none has been widely accepted [29–34]. The use of computed tomography to delineate the fracture patterns may add further information and subsequently a better classification system of these fractures [32,35–38]. Until then, the treatment of the calcaneal fractures should follow the principles for treating intra-articular fractures of the major weight-bearing joint in the lower extremity, that is, anatomical reduction, stable fixation and early mobilisation with weight-bearing.

Conventional X-ray investigation in most circumstances can delineate the fracture pattern adequately. This should include lateral, internal oblique and axial views. The lateral view gives most of the information on the fractures (Fig. 10); it shows readily the displacement of articular fractures, the loss of Bohler's angle and the changes in the crucial angle of Gissane. The oblique view shows particularly the articular displacement of the posterior facet as well as the anterior process. The axial view is the most informative for demonstrating depression of the osteochondral fragment of the posterior facet, the lateral bursting fracture of the lateral wall and the varus deformity of the tuberosity fragment. It also gives important informa-

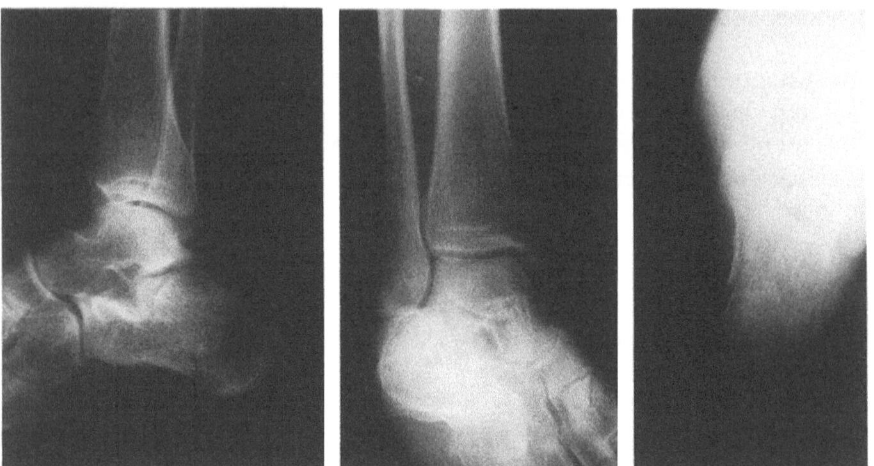

Fig. 10a–c. Three views of the os calcis. (a) lateral view. (b) internal oblique view. (c) axial view

tion on the intact bone fragments into which screws can be inserted for stable internal fixation. Although computed tomography is very helpful if it is readily available, care must be taken to interpret the posterior facet displacement. Rotatory displacement in the transverse axis may not be recognised on the computed tomography scan even then the whole articular surface is rotated 90° in case of the joint depression type by the classification of Essex and Lopresti (Fig. 11).

The treatment of displaced intra-articular fractures of the calcaneum remains controversial [39–44]. We believe that the subtalar joint should be treated according to the same principles as any other weight-bearing joints with displaced intra-articular fractures. During the past five years we have treated displaced intra-articular fractures of the calcaneum by open reduction, internal fixation and primary bone grafting [45]. The operation is performed after the swelling of the foot is well under control. As one of the common complications of operation around the hindfoot is the wound problem, care must be taken in making the incision and exposure of the fracture. The lateral incision is the preferred incision because it gives a direct approach to the pathology of the injury. The incision starts 50 mm above the tip of the lateral malleolus and runs parallel and posterior to its posterior edge until 10 mm inferior to the tip of the lateral malleolus; it runs horizontally for 50–60 mm anteriorly. Anterior extension of the wound may be required when the fracture involves the calcaneocuboid articular surface. Medial exposure is seldom required except when the fracture involves the sustantacular tali. In the lateral approach the sural nerve is identified and retracted inferiorly. The distal skin flap is raised by sharp dissection down to the subperiosteal plane and the proximal flap subfascially. This ensures a

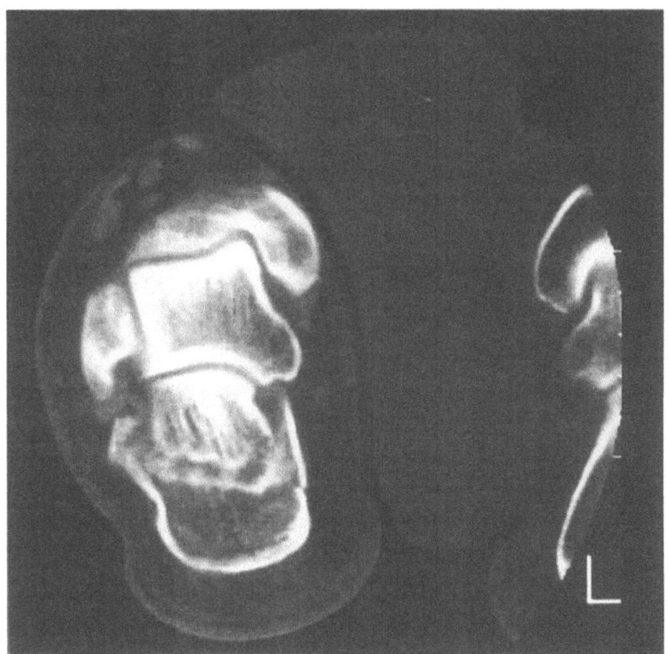

Fig. 11. Computed tomography scan of the os calcis fracture showing apparent congruity of the subtalar joint. Note the loss in height and increase in width of the os calcis

satisfactory blood supply and decrease wound problems. With this approach the subtalar joint is exposed adequately by dislocating the peroneal tendons superiorly and excising the fibulo-calcaneal ligament. Excision of the fibulo-calcaneal ligament does not lead to instability of the subtalar joint since it is common to find stiffness rather than laxity after injury and surgery in the region. The depressed osteochondral fragment can be elevated, and the congruity of the subtalar joint is restored (Fig. 12).

The reduction is secured with lag screws which fix the elevated articular fragment to the antero-medial part of the posterior facet. The subchondral bone of the calcaneum is perhaps the strongest part of the bone and thus ideal for holding the screws. Mechanically it is more stable to lag the lateral mobile fragment to the intact medial part by 4-mm AO cancellous screws. After the elevation and reduction of the osteochondral fragment, a substantial space is created due to the impaction of the cancellous bone of the body of the calcaneum by the osteochondral fragment. This space is packed with cortico-cancellous bone graft from the ipsilateral iliac crest. The major fragments are fixed temporarily with Kirschner wires. The height of the calcaneum is reconstructed by reducing the lateral wall of the calcaneum. Finally, the lateral wall is stabilised with either a cervical plate or a multi-

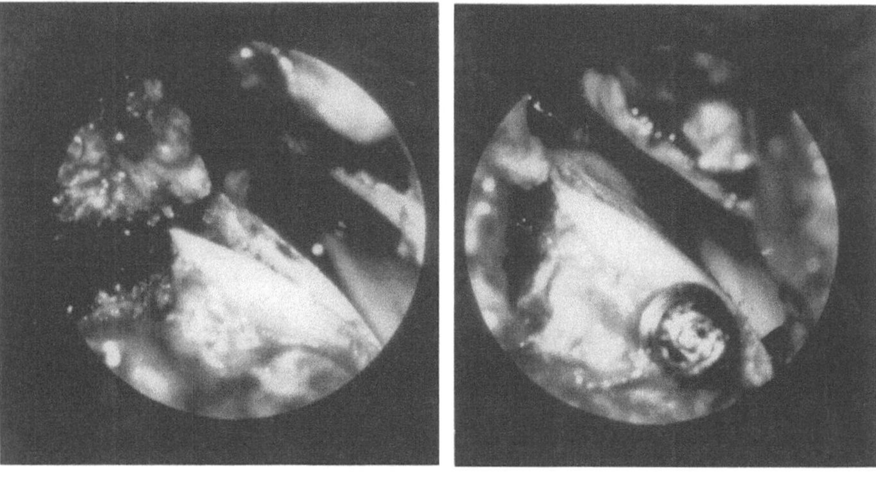

Fig. 12a–b. Reduction of the subtalar joint after elevation of the lateral half of the posterior facet and fixation with lag screw. **a** Pre-reduction. **b** Post-reduction

fragment plate which acts as buttress plate. The plate is fixed to the calcaneum by 3.5- or 4-mm cancellous screws which anchor into the sustentaculum tali and the infero-medial tubicle of the calcaneum. Together with the sub-chondral bone of the posterior facet, the sustantaculum tali and the infero-medial tuberosity of the calcaneum usually remain intact after the injury. The screws from the lateral side should be aimed at these parts of the calcaneum for better anchorage (Fig. 13). This is an additional reason for preferring the lateral approach to the medial approach.

Post-operative management consists of energetic control of swelling and early passive mobilisation of the subtalar joint. A specially designed continuous passive motion machine is most useful in these circumstances. Both the active and passive mobilisation of the ankle and subtalar joints should be carried out energetically. Graduated weight-bearing walking may be started 6 weeks after the operation and full weight bearing at 8–10 weeks post-operatively.

The early results of treating displaced intra-articular fractures with open reduction, internal fixation and primary bone grafting are encouraging [45]. With careful observance of the above regime one can achieve very good reduction of the articular surface and stable fixation. The need for bone grafting in these fractures has been the subject of substantial debate [34,42,44–46]. We have found that there is a huge space after the elevation of the depressed articular surface of the posterior subtalar facet. By packing this space with cortico-cancellous graft the reduced articular osteochondral fragment can be supported, and with the buttressing effect of the lateral side plate the stability of the post-reduction construct is very much enhanced. We believe that this is the reason that our patients can start early passive

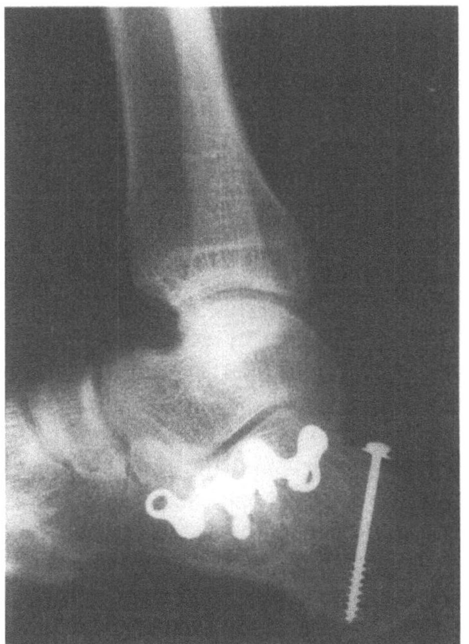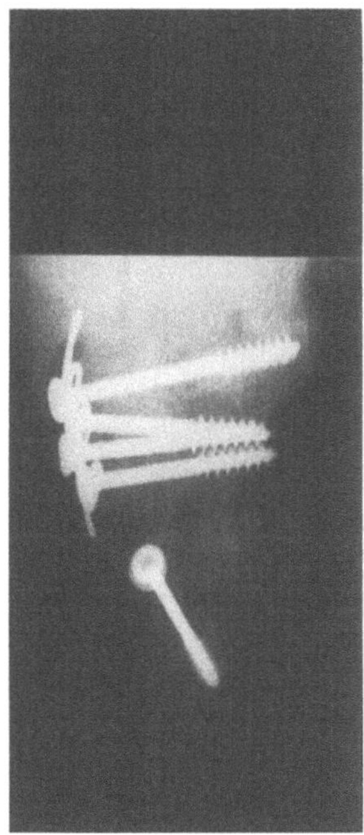

Fig. 13. Fixation of the os calcis fracture with screws fixing the osteochondral fragment. Note the long lag screw anchoring into the sustentaculum tali in the axial view. The posterior screw fixing the tongue fragment anchoring into the postero-medial part of the os calcis

mobilisation and weight-bearing exercise after the operation. Recently, we have started to use the bone substitutes instead of autogenous bone graft. All these contribute to the very good early results of the treatment. At an average follow-up period of 10.6 months, all (64 fractures) had minimal pain, swelling and deformity. An average of 67.8% active and 80.7% passive subtalar joint movements were regained. Over 80% of patients resumed working within 6 months after the injuries. Radiologically, 80% of patients had normal Bohler's angle and 93.5% had normal crucial angle. The latest follow-up of this group of patients confirms the excellent results. At an average follow-up of 3.8 years, 48 patients were assessed clinically with the scoring system proposed by Crosby and Fitzgibbons [32], and the average score was 97.5. The radiological assessment showed minimal changes in the position of the implants, Bohler's angle, crucial angle, height and width. Articular congruity and arthritis grading were assessed as proposed by Knirk and Jupiter [47]; the average articular incongruity grading was 0.75 and that for arthritis 0.89. These results show that the long-term results of operative treatment for displaced intra-articular fractures provides predictably good results [48].

Injuries of Tarsal-Metatarsals

Lisfranc joint dislocations have been reported to be very rare. The fact that this injury is easily missed may account for the low reported incidence. With the increasing incidence of high-energy trauma, it is imperative to diagnose this injury with substantial suspicion as the long-term disability can be significant if treatment is inadequate.

Lisfranc joints is in fact the collective term for the tarso-metatarsal joints. They comprise the osseous, ligamental and the other soft-tissue elements. The five metatarsals, three cuneiforms and cuboid form the osseous elements. The stability of the joints is partly contributed by the arrangement of the osseous elements. The trapezoidal shape of the three cuneiforms with the similar pattern of the base of the medial three meta-tarsals form the so-called "Roman arch" configuration. The second meta-tarsal is recessed into the space between the first and the third cuneiform and thus acts as a keystone in this transverse Roman arch [49,50]. The inherently stable bony configuration together with the dorsal, planter and inter-osseous ligaments form a very stable arch in the midfoot. It therefore requires a violent force to create fracture dislocations, and the commonest mechanism to produce this injury is axial loading of the planter-flexed fixed foot. This is also the culprit in the missed diagnosis since most of the pa-tients are polytraumatised, and the other injuries often divert the attending surgeons' attention until the patient starts to ambulate. Careful examination and radiological evaluation are therefore recommended when there is suspicion of such injury.

Recognition of the constant anatomical relationships on the X-ray exam-ination of the foot is vital to the diagnosis of these uncommon injuries [51,52]. The first metatarsal aligns with the medial cuneiform, the second metatarsal with the middle cuneiform, the third metatarsal with the lateral cuneiform, and the medial border of the fourth metatarsal with the medial border of the cuboid. The fourth and the fifth metatarsals always move as a unit in their relationship with the cuboid. It has been shown that even minimal subluxation or disruption of these normal lines is significant. The association of small fragments around the base of the second metatarsal or along the lateral border of the cuboid is also significant.

The classification proposed by Quenu and Kuss [53] is commonly em-ployed. Homolateral dislocations are those with the five metatarsal displaced in the same direction. The isolated group involves one or two metatarsals being displaced from the others, and the divergent group involves displace-ment of the metatarsals in both the coronal and sagittal planes. The common displacement is that in lateral and dorsal direction.

Concerning treatment, controversies exist over the methods of reduction and fixation, although most agree that the primary aim of the treatment should be the restoration of a painless, stable and plantegrade foot. Those who advocate operative treatment claim that most of the injuries are associated with comminution of the articular surface with resultant entrapment of bony fragments [54–56]. This has been our finding as well. Since the injuries are usually caused by high-energy trauma, soft-tissue trauma is common; the normal anatomical bony configuration is also difficult to reestablish by closed means. Furthermore, post-reduction immobilisation is also difficult without internal fixation. For regaining normal foot mechanics there is a strong indication for operative treatment. During exploration the loose fragments can be removed, the entrapped soft tissue, for example, the anterior tibial tendon, can be released, and the dislocations reduced and stabilised with temporary fixations.

Exposure for these dislocations is by direct longitudinal incisions on the dorsum of the foot. The cutaneous nerves, superficial veins and dorsalis pedis artery are protected. In frank total dislocations, the key to successful reduction is restoration of the second metatarsal to the recess between the medial and the lateral cuneiforms. The reduction is maintained with temporary Kirschner wire. For definitive stabilisation we have found the method suggested by Arntz and Hansen to be very useful [55]. The use of a 4-mm AO cancellous screw as a temporary lag screw across the joint provides a stable fixation (Fig. 14). Similar treatment can be applied to the other

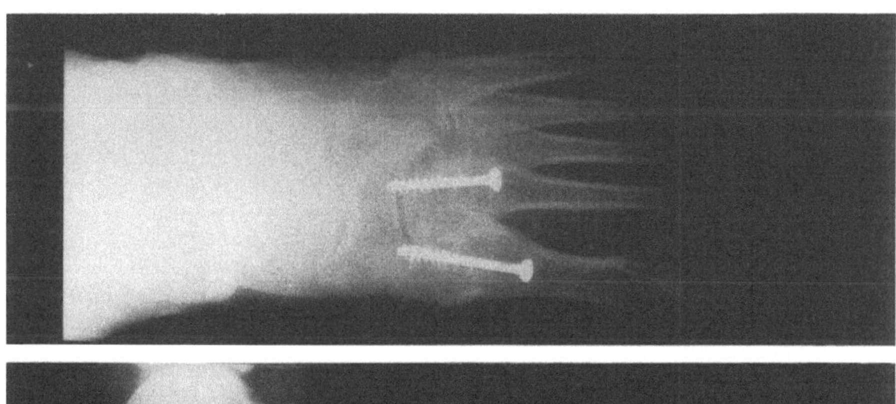

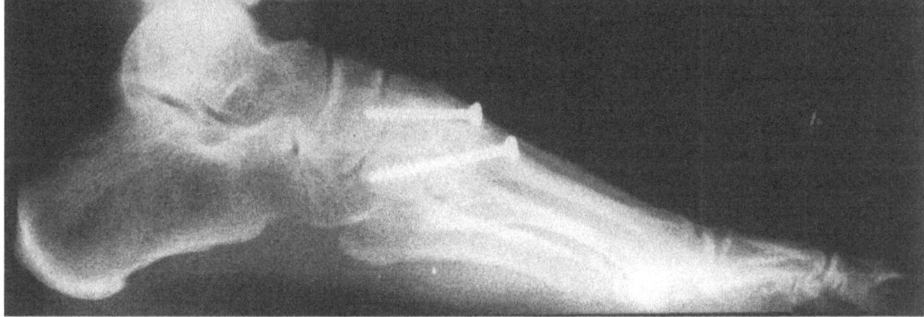

Fig. 14. Temporary fixation of the Lisfranc joints with 4-mm trans-articular lag screws

metatarsotarsal joints. Restoration of the fourth and the fifth metatarsals can be achieved by reducing the fifth metatarsal to the cuboid and maintaining the reduction with a 4-mm AO cancellous screw inserted percutaneously from the fifth metatarsal to the cuboid. The use of the screw for temporary stable fixation seeks to ensure proper healing of the soft tissue around the Lisfranc joints and does not aim at arthrodesis. The removal of the screws at 3 months allows movement around these joints so that a certain degree of subtleness may be regained. The disadvantage of this method is that the patient must undergo another operation to remove the screws after a period of 3 months. The recently available 3.5-mm absorbable screws made of polylactic acids may be a good substitute for the conventional screws (Fig. 15). It is claimed that these absorbable screws can retain their strength for 10–12 weeks after implantation and be absorbed in 1 year [57]. This would be ideal for situations in which temporary rigid fixation is indicated.

Post-operative management consists of high elevation and plaster slab immobilisation. After the stitches are removed, a short leg cast bracing made of fibreglass casting material is applied. The foot is immobilised by a well-moulded cast to maintain the arch. A hinge joint connects the foot cast to the calf plaster so that the ankle can be mobilised. The patient is allowed to walk with graduated weight bearing with the cast bracing for 3 months until the screws are removed.

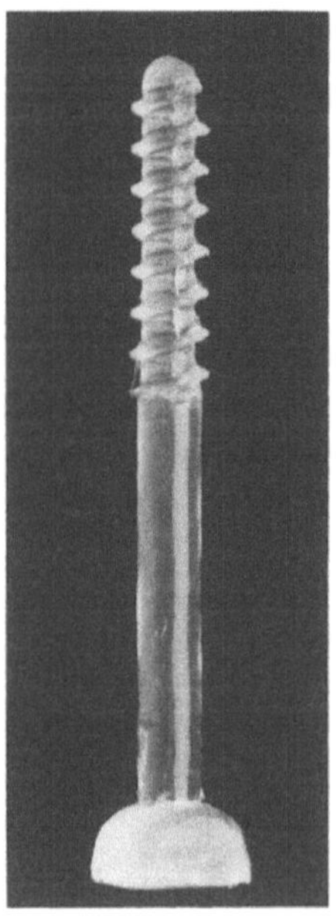

Fig. 15. A 3.5-mm absorbable screw made of poly-L-lactide

Conclusion

The management of fractures around the ankle reflects the principles of treating intra-articular fractures of any weight bearing joint. Restoration of normal anatomy and structure is the primary goal of the treatment. The modern method of operative treatment enables the restoration of early stability and hence early mobilisation and the regaining of function and activities. With the operative treatment the conflicting need for exposure for anatomical fracture reduction and that for soft-tissue preservation are frequently encountered. The delicate status of the soft tissues also makes them particularly susceptible to injury, and hence the complications associated with trauma and fracture management are common. On the other hand, the modern concept of stabilisation of fractures to facilitate post-injury soft-tissue repair calls for careful handling of soft tissues while tackling the fractures around the ankle. In extensive soft- and hard-tissue damage, restoration of the normal articular relationship may not be feassible, and the goal must be directed towards the achievement of a pain-free plantigrade foot. With these points well considered, the results of treating fractures around the ankle can be much improved.

References

1. Lauge-Hansen (1950) Fractures of the ankle. II. Combined experimental-surgical and experimental-roentgenologic investigations. Arch Surg 60:957
2. Müller ME, Allgöwer M, Willenegger H (1970) Manual of internal fixation. Springer, Berlin Heidelberg New York
3. Yde J (1980) The Lauge-Hansen classification of malleolar fractures. Acta Orthop Scand 51:181
4. Lindsjo U (1985) Classification of ankle fractures: the Lauge-Hansen or AO system? Clin Orthop 199:12
5. Olerud C, Molander II (1986) Bi-and trimalleolar ankle fractures operated with nonrigid internal fixation. Clin Orthop 206:253
6. Bauer M, Bergstrom B, Hemborg A, Sandegard J (1985) Malleolar fractures: nonoperative versus operative treatment – a controlled study. Clin Orthop 199:17
7. Yde J, Kristensen KD (1980) Ankle fractures: supination-eversion fractures of stage IV. Acta Orthop Scand 51:981
8. Mak KH, Chan KM, Leung PC (1985) Ankle fracture treated with the AO principle – an experience with 116 cases. Injury 16:265
9. Segal D (1984) Internal fixation of ankle fractures, part I. Instr Course Lect 33:107–117
10. Ramsey PL, Hamilton W (1976) Changes in tibiotalar area of contact caused by lateral talar shift. J Bone Joint Surg [Am] 58:356
11. Gollish JD, Tile M, Begg R (1977) Fractures of the ankle. J Bone Joint Surg [Br] 59:510
12. Lambert K (1971) The weight bearing function of fibula. J Bone Joint Surg [Am] 53:507
13. Cedell CA (1985) Is closed treatment of ankle fractures advisable? Acta Orthop Scand 56:101

14. Devalentine S (1985) Evaluation and treatment of ankle fractures. Clin Podiatry 2(2):325
15. Lindsjo U (1985) Operative treatment of ankle fracture-dislocations – a follow-up study of 306/321 consecutive cases. Clin Orthop 199:28
16. Phillips WA, Schwartz HS, Keller CS, Woodward HR, Rudd WS, Spiegel PG, Laros GS (1985) A prospective, randomized study of the management of severe ankle fractures. J Bone Joint Surg [Am] 67(1):67
17. Sclafani SJA (1985) Ligamentous injury of the lower tibiofibular syndesmosis: radiographic evidence. Radiology 156:21
18. Needleman RL, Skrade DA, Stiehl JB (1989) Effect of the syndesmotic screw on ankle motion. Foot Ankle 10:17
19. Kaye RA (1989) Stabilization of ankle syndesmosis injuries with a syndesmosis screw. Foot Ankle 9:290
20. Rokkanen P, Vainionpaa S, Tormala P, Kilpikari J, Bostman O, Vihtonen K, Laiho J, Tamminmaki M (1985) Biodegradable implants in fracture fixation: early results of treatment of fractures of the ankle. Lancet 2:1422
21. Bostman O, Hirvensalo E, Vainionpaa S, Makela A, Vihtonen K, Tormala P, Rokkanen P (1989) Ankle fractures treated using biodegradable internal fixation. Clin Orthop 238:195
22. Heim UFA (1989) Trimalleolar fractures: late results after fixation of the posterior fragment. Orthopedics 12:1053
23. Haliburton RA, Sullivan CG, Kelly PJ, Peterson LFA (1958) The extra-osseous and intra-osseous blood supply of the talus. J Bone Joint Surg [Am] 40:1115
24. Kelly PJ, Sullivan CR (1963) Blood supply of the talus. Clin Orthop 30:37
25. Mulfinger GL, Trueta J (1970) The blood supply of the talus. J Bone Joint Surg [Br] 52:160
26. Schatzker J, Tile M (1987) The rationale of operative fracture care. Springer, Berlin Heidelberg New York, p 414
27. Hawkins LG (1970) Fractures of the neck of the talus. J Bone Joint Surg [Am] 52:991
28. Pantazopoulos T, Galanos P, Vayanos E et al. (1974) Fractures of the neck of the talus. Acta Orthop Scand 45:296
29. Essex-Lopresti P (1952) The mechanism, reduction technqiue, and results in fractures of the os calcis. Br J Surg 39:395
30. Rowe CR, Sakellarides HT, Freeman PA, Sorbie C (1963) Fractures of the os calcis. A long-term follow-up study of 146 patients. JAMA 184:920
31. Carr JB, Hamilton JJ, Bear LS (1989) Experimental intra-articular calcaneal fractures: anatomic basis for a new classification. Foot Ankle 10(2):81
32. Crosby LA, Fitzgibbons T (1990) Computerized tomography scanning of acute intra-articular fractures of the calcaneus. J Bone Joint Surg [Am] 72(6):852
33. Soeur R, Remy R (1975) Fractures of the calcaneus with displacement of the thalamic portion. J Bone Joint Surg [Br] 57(4):413
34. Burdeaux BD (1987) Calcaneus fractures: rationale for the medial approach technique of reduction. Orthopaedics 10:177
35. Floyd EJ, Ransom RA, Dailey JM (1984) Computed tomography scanning of the subtalar joint. J Am Podiatry Assoc 74(11):533
36. Segal D, Marsh JL, Leiter B (1985) Clinical application of computerized axial tomography (CAT) scanning of calcaneus fractures. Clin Orthop 199:114
37. Solomon MA, Gilula LA, Oloff LM, Oloff J (1986) CT scanning of the foot and ankle. II. Clinical applications and review of the literature. Am J Roentgenol 146:1204
38. Cronier P, Pillet JC, Talha A, Ghestem P, Liebault B, Rieux D, Mercier P, Lescalie F, Pillet J (1988) Scanographic study of the calcaneus: normal anatomy and clinical applications. Surg Radiol Anat 10:303
39. Lance EM, Carey EJ, Wade PA (1963) Fractures of the os calcis: treatment by early mobilization. Clin Orthop 30:76

40. Pennal GF, Yadav MP (1973) Operative treatment of comminuted fractures of the os calcis. Orthop Clin North Am 4(1):197
41. Omoto H, Sakurada K, Sugi M, Nakamura K (1983) A new method of manual reduction for intra-articular fracture of the calcaneus. Clin Orthop 177:104
42. Letournel E (1984) Open reduction and internal fixation of calcaneus fractures. In: Spiegel PG (ed) Techniques in orthopaedics – topics in orthopaedic trauma. University Park Press, Baltimore, pp 173–192
43. Harding D, Waddell JP (1985) Open reduction and depressed fractures of the os calcis. Clin Orthop 199:124
44. Palmer I (1948) The mechanism and treatment of fractures of the calcaneus – open reduction with the use of cancellous grafts. J Bone Joint Surg [Am] 30:2
45. Leung KS, Chan WS, Shen WY, Pak PPL, So WS, Leung PC (1989) Operative treatment of intraarticular fractures of the os calcis – the role of rigid internal fixation and primary bone grafting: preliminary results. J Orthop Trauma 3(3):232
46. Stephenson JR (1987) Treatment of displaced intra-articular fractures of the calcaneus using medial and lateral approaches, internal fixation and early motion. J Bone Joint Surg [Am] 69:115
47. Knirk JL, Jupiter JB (1986) Intra-articular fractures of the distal end of the radius in young adults. J Bone Joint Surg [Am] 68(5):647
48. Leung KS, Yuen KM, Chan WS (1993) Long term results of operative treatment of displaced intra-articular fractures of the os calcis. J Bone Joint Surg [Br] (in press)
49. Lenczner EM, Waddell JP, Graham JD (1974) Tarsal-metatarsal (Lisfranc) dislocation. J Trauma 14:1012
50. Hesp WLEM, Werken C, Goris RJA (1983) Lisfranc dislocations: fractures and/or dislocations through the tarso-metatarsal joints. Injury 15(4):261
51. Stein RE (1983) Radiological aspects of the tarsometatarsal joints. Foot Ankle 3(5):286
52. Foster SC, Foster RR (1976) Lisfranc's trasometatarsal fracture-dislocation. Diagn Radiol 120:79
53. Quenu E, Kuss G (1909) Etude sur les luxations du métatarse (luxations métatarso-tarsiennes) du diastasis entre le 1. et le 2. Metatarsien Rev Chir Paris 39:281, 720, 1093
54. Jeffreys TE (1963) Lisfranc's fracture-dislocation – a clinical and experimental study of tarso-metatarsal dislocations and fracture-dislocations. J Bone Joint Surg [Br] 45(3):546
55. Arntz CT, Hansen ST (1987) Dislocations and fracture dislocations of the traso-metatarsal joints. Orthop Clin North Am 18(1):105
56. DeBenedetti MJ, Evanski PM, Waugh TR (1978) The unreducible Lisfranc fracture. Case report and literature review. Clin Orthop 136:238
57. Partio EK, Böstman O, Vainionpää S, et al. (1988) The treatment of cancellous bone fractures with biodegradable screws. Acta Orthop Scand Suppl 227:18

15 Problems in Spinal Fractures

S.Y. Lee

Rationale for Treatment in Spinal Injuries

Several major goals should be attained in the ideal treatment of any spinal injury. Spinal alignment must be restored by appropriate means of reduction to retain normal spinal biomechanics. This allows early painless mobility, prevents or minimizes neurological deficits, provides stability at the injured site, and prevents progressive late-occurring spinal deformity, pain and possible neural compromise. The treatment should also aim to provide the neural structures with the optimal environment for function, healing and regeneration and minimize non-spinal complications such as deep vein thrombosis, pulmonary embolism, decubitus ulcers, and chest and urinary tract infections.

Treatment for injuries with neither instability nor neural compromise is relatively simple, such as in isolated fractures of the neural arch (e.g. fractured transverse process, spinous process, lamina) and simple wedge compression fractures. These injuries can be treated by early mobilization with appropriate external support. When the injuries are at risk for instability with or without initial neurological deficits, early mobilization without achieving stability can result in neural compromise, at the outset or at later stages. These injuries are best managed by surgical stabilization, and in the absence of surgical expertise the patients should be kept immobilized in bed until healing has been achieved to allow stable ambulation with external support.

Stable and Unstable Injuries

Determining whether the injury is stable or unstable is of prime importance before definite treatment can be planned. A spinal column injury is considered unstable when on stress there is a risk of causing deformity, neurological damage or deterioration in an already existing neurological impairment. A stable spinal injury is a lesion without such a risk, which is thus able to withstand stress without progression in deformity or further neurological damage [1]. Compared to a stable injury, the unstable injury

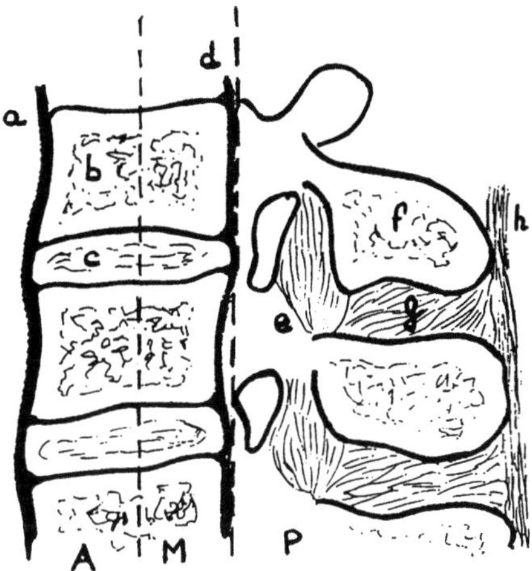

Fig. 1. Denis' three-column concept. The anterior column (*A*) comprises the anterior longitudinal ligament (*a*), anterior halves of vertebral body (*b*) and annulus fibrosis (*c*); the middle column (*M*) comprises the posterior halves of vertebral body and annulus fibrosis, and posterior longitudinal ligament (*d*); the posterior column (*P*) includes the remaining bony parts and the ligamentous complex of ligamentum falvum (*e*), inter-spinous ligaments (*g*) and supra-spinous ligament (*h*)

definitely requires a more restrictive form of immobilization and for a much longer duration to prevent any possible neural tissue damage.

In the neck region the most precise definition of stability is that of White and Panjabi [2], who define cervical spine instability as translatory motion greater than 3 mm or angular deformity of more than 11° difference between the bony segments adjacent to the injured level. This definition is widely used in the evaluation of cervical injuries to assist in determining the most appropriate treatment for a particular injury. Denis' concept of a three-column spine [3,4] (Fig. 1) provides a definition of spinal stability in the thoraco-lumbar spine which is based on the status of the middle column (the posterior half of vertebral body, annulus fibrosus and posterior longitudinal ligament) and not only the posterior ligamentous complex, as understood by earlier authors. The refinement of the classification of spinal injuries by Holdsworth [5] has enhanced our knowledge of mechanisms of injury and led to a better understanding of that which constitutes instability in the thoraco-lumbar spine, the consideration of which dictates the management.

Spinal Cord Injury In Trauma

The hallmark of spinal cord injury after trauma is neck or back pain accompanied by numbness, tingling sensation and weakness of motor power. The presence of any neurological deficit after an injury to the spine indicates the highest likelihood of an unstable vertebral fracture or dislocation. Further injury to the neural tissues is likely to occur if the spinal column is not protected during any moving or transportation of the patient. The level of vertebral injury can often be localized by careful neurological examination. In unconscious or confused patients the physical examination is not reliable for ruling out spinal injuries that could have resulted in incomplete lesions. In such a situation the cervical spine must always be protected by neck collars and sand bags until radiographic examination of the neck can be performed. Occult injuries of the lower cervical and thoracic spine are more difficult to detect by simple radiography and are therefore frequently overlooked in patients with multiple injuries or unconsciousness. Special views of the suspected regions should be sought whenever it is doubtful.

Documented progression of neurological deficits suggests cord compression that should be investigated and treated promptly. Repeated, careful neurological examination, myelography, computed tomography and magnetic resonance imaging can detect the underlying causes and enable prompt intervention. Certain conditions – spinal epidural haematomas, herniated discs, displaced bone fragments from burst fractures of the vertebral body – are well recognized as potential causes of reversible neurological deterioration during the acute phase of management. This early detection and appropriate prompt surgical intervention is one of the primary goals.

Following trauma delayed haemorrhage is common in the central grey matter of the spinal cord. The extent to which this and other mechanisms contribute to the ultimate neurological deficit is far from settled [6]. There are many proposed therapeutic manoeuvres to change the neurological consequences of an inflicted injury, such as steroids, mannitol and urea, localized spinal cord cooling [7], omental transplantation [8], and spinal cord decompression and stabilization in the absence of demonstrated cord compression [9]. However, none of these treatment modalities has ever gained wide acceptance. The primary and immediate clinical goal in spinal cord injury, after instituting the necessary resuscitative measures, still remains to assure stability of the spinal column and relieve any demonstrated cord compression in patients with progressive or incomplete loss of function below the level of injury.

Complete Cord Injury

Below the level of a severe cord injury there is complete loss of all motion and sensory function and absence of all monosynaptic reflexes, resulting in a flaccid paralysis known as spinal shock, which may last from a few days to a number of weeks. Its physiological basis is unknown, although Sherrington [10] thought it could be due to release of segmental reflexes from higher facilitating systems. The earliest signs of recovery from spinal shock are return of the bulbocavernosus reflex, Babinski's reflex and flexion withdrawal.

Rapid early recovery within a few hours or days may be seen rarely in a clinically complete cord injury. For those complete cord injuries in which no change has been detected within the initial 24–48 h there is usually persistent severe motor and sensory paralysis. Autonomic dysreflexia may appear as the recovery from spinal shock continues. This condition, characterized by paroxysms of sweating, hypertension, bradycardia and headache, is a problem which is often overlooked by clinicians unfamiliar with the management of spinal cord injury. Common causes include bladder distension, rectal impaction, urinary tract infections, appendicitis and decubitus ulcer. Initial treatment is directed at removing the underlying stimulus and diminishing the hypertension. Putting the patient in sitting position is the first step in lowering blood pressure. Urinary catheter blockage and impacted, hard faeces are the two most common causes to look for. Various medications have been used to lower blood pressure. Nifedipine (10 mg) sublingually has been found to be very effective in rapidly decreasing dangerously elevated blood pressure.

Surgical intervention in these complete cord injuries with anatomical transection, and obviously no hope of reversing the neurological deficit, is aimed at providing stability and facilitating the early rehabilitation of the patient. Although this procedure is not widely accepted among conservative spinal clinicians, there are several advantages in some cases. A completely dislocated vertebra in the thoraco-lumbar/lumbar region through the disc is grossly unstable and usually results in pseudo-arthrosis, causing girdle pain on movement which could severely affect the patient's wheel-chair ambulatory activities. Reduction of the dislocated spine with implant stabilization and bone grafting at the injured site not only prevents the future disability but also provides easier nursing care and early ambulation training, thus reducing the complications and side effects of prolonged bed rest in the early management.

If using posterior instrumentation, such as Harrington's and Luque's in which several additional levels must be fixed, it is advisable to remove the implants after bone grafting is consolidated, normally at 9–12 months after surgery. In the author's experience in 20 paraplegics receiving posterior instrumentation, each could perform their wheel-chair manoeuvres much better, with obvious recovery of some trunk motion after the implant removal.

Partial Cord Injury

Partial cord injury involves both anatomical and functional preservation of a portion of the spinal cord. In general, such injuries have a much better prognosis for neurological recovery. It is important to rule out the presence of any compression of the cord by bone fragments, extruded disc or haematoma by means of appropriate investigations as early surgical decompression can reverse the neurological deficit in these cases. Several specific syndromes of partial cord injury may occur. Anterior cord syndrome, characterized by paralysis and spino-thalamic sensory deficits below the level of injury, sparing the posterior column [11], is commonly caused by acutely herniated discs and acute flexion fracture dislocations (tear-drop fracture). Although injury/thrombosis to the anterior spinal artery leading to actual neural tissue destruction may be the major cause contributing to permanent neurological deficits, it is not possible to differentiate this clinically from reversible deficits caused by cord compression. Aggressive early investigation and surgical intervention is recommended.

Spinal trauma in children is not as common as in adults and is generally associated with better prognosis, except when spinal cord injury occurs without detectable radiological abnormality. The latter condition occurs more commonly in children under 8 years of age and is attributed to the biomechanical features of the spine in this age group which allows a greater degree of mobility of the spine, thus compressing/stretching the cord in extreme degrees of flexion and extension, or enables the spine to undergo momentary subluxation with spontaneous stable reduction [12]. Children with this injury are also at risk for recurrent spinal cord injury [13]. The neurological deficit may be delayed and is often severe. Hadley et al. [14] in their review of 122 children with spinal cord injury found a similar condition among children under 9 years of age.

Common Problems in Acute Management

Although spinal cord injury is usually associated with vertebral fracture/dislocation, it may not be so in children who have a cartilaginous and elastic spinal column and in elderly individuals with hyperextension force in the presence of marked cervical spondylosis. Every effort should be made to exclude the presence – through radiographic documentation of the spinal column injury if a fracture is not detected in the initial plain film – as this affects the subsequent management of the patient.

It is not uncommon to miss a linear fracture line in a patient with ankylosing spondylitis or one with extensive degenerative changes. Lateral cervical radiographs repeated with head in slight extension and flexion reveal vertebral subluxation or separation of an anterior intervertebral space due to damage of the anterior longitudinal ligament. In general, there is a correlation between the level of the spinal cord injury and that of the vertebral fracture, and the discrepancy between these two levels should not be more than two or three segments, for example, a C5 fracture may be associated clinically with a C6 or C7 cord injury. An odontoid fracture may be missed if it is not clinically associated with a C3 or C4 neurological deficit. Bilateral facet dislocation with vertebral fracture in the region of C6–C7 or C7–T1 is notably very unstable because of extensive damage of the ligaments protecting the facet joints. Reduction of the dislocation in these patients can normally be achieved without much difficulty, but redislocation tends to occur if a relatively rigid immobilization cannot be provided during the transfers, or if skull traction is discontinued prematurely. Early surgical fusion is recommended especially in the presence of neurological impairment. Post-operative immobilization with a halo-body brace is indicated in these cases.

Acute post-traumatic spinal epidural haematoma is uncommon in spinal cord injuries, with an estimated incidence of only 1%–2% [15]. However, this is a treatable cause of neurological deterioration, with early surgical evacuation to relieve the compression on the cord. It occurs most commonly in the region of cervical and cervico-thoracic vertebrae and in patients with ankylosing spondylitis, rheumatoid arthritis, cervical spondylosis, Farestier's disease or bleeding disorders. The diagnosis can be made by computed tomography or magnetic resonance imaging of the spine.

Increased neurological deficits have been noted in patients turned in a Stryker bed, which is no longer used in our service. If continuous traction is needed for a long period, the patient should be turned in a tilting and turning bed (e.g. the Stoke Mandeville Egerton bed), which can better maintain a constant alignment of the traction during the manoeuvres (Fig. 2).

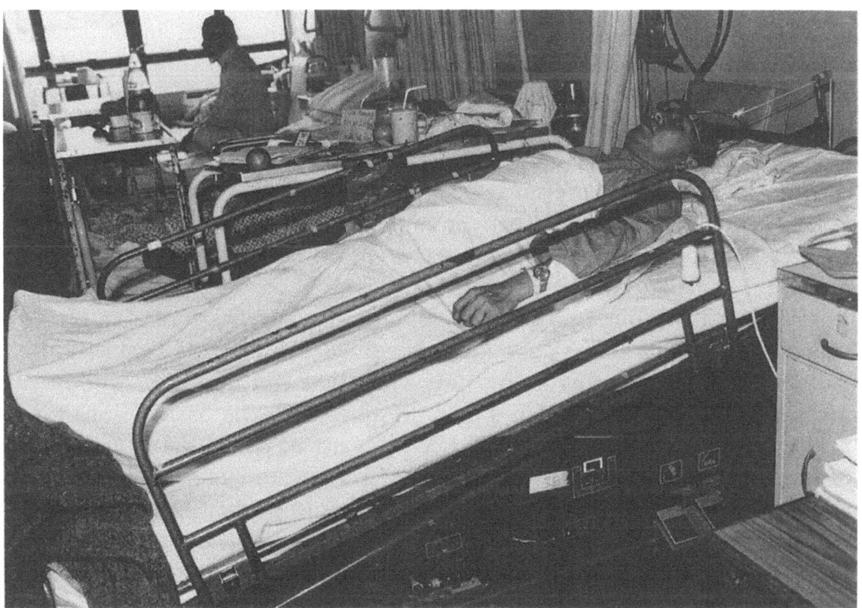

Fig. 2. A more constant and better alignment of the traction can be maintained in a special tilting and turning bed, thus preventing complications during the manoeuvres

Cervical Injuries

Although spinal column injuries are seen less commonly in the cervical region than in the lower thoracic and lumbar vertebrae, they are often more serious. Neck injuries not only have a greater risk of damaging the spinal cord but also have a greater liability to persistent disability in the form of aching pain and stiffness of neck. The incidence of so-called whiplash injury – subluxations and strains in the neck – caused by a sudden recoil of the head in rear-end automobile collisions is increasing in modern society with ever more motor vehicles on the road. In most of these cases the structural effects are relatively minor, but disability may nevertheless be very much prolonged.

Understanding the mechanisms of injury is important in any spinal column trauma before a definite treatment modality can be planned. Because of the coupling actions of the cervical spine, most injury patterns are composed of motion in two or more planes, although one usually predominates [16].

Diagnostic Evaluation

Cervical injuries are often associated with head injuries, the effects of which may mask the spinal lesion and very often cause it to be overlooked. In every case of serious head injury, an unconscious post-traumatic patient, or neck pain and stiffness associated even with only trivial injury, cervical column injury must be suspected until proven otherwise. Clinical evaluation of a patient with suspected cervical injury should begin with adequate immobilization, i.e. sandbags and a hard neck collar (Philadelphia collar) along with the ABC of trauma care (airway, breathing, circulation). Bulbo-cavernosus and anal wink must be tested in the unconscious patient – the absence of which means the patient is in spinal shock. Failure to detect this sign, not uncommon even among experienced surgeons, could result in a disastrous outcome for the patient.

After the thorough physical examination, a lateral cervical spine X-ray which must include C7–T1 should be obtained before other views. With the patient lying supine, this is the only view that can be taken without disturbing or moving the head and neck. It also shows the basic lesions for the majority of neck bone injuries. The X-ray must be evaluated in a systematic fashion, so as not miss any pathology. The overall alignment should be assessed. Pre-vertebral soft-tissue swelling should be measured opposite C4, which normally must not exceed 40% of the antero-posterior diameter of the vertebral body (Fig. 3). Occipito-atlantal disruption can be determined by measuring the distance from the tip of odontoid process of C2 to the basion – the anterior border of the foramen magnum, which should not exceed 5 mm. Disruption of the transverse ligament can be assessed by an increased anterior atlanto-dental interval, which normally should not be

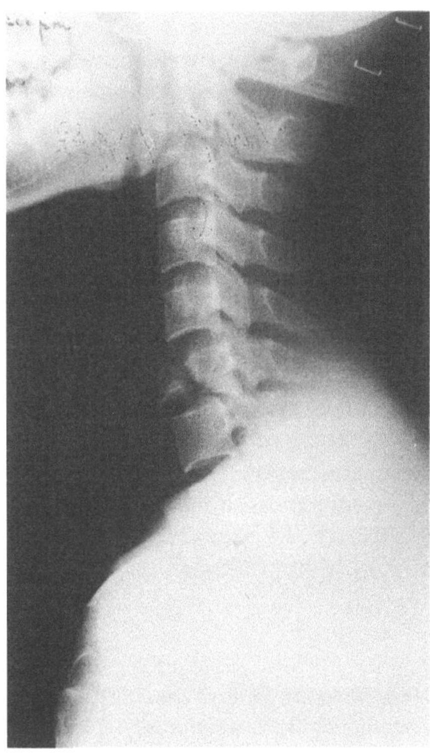

Fig. 3. Careful observation of prevertebral soft-tissue opposite C4 is important. Increased pre-vertebral soft tissue in a 31-year-old man involved in a road traffic accident. A later film (not shown) revealed the subluxation of C6 over C7

more than 3 mm in adults and 4 mm in children. The lateral radiograph may be supplemented as necessary by other views of plain films such as open-mouth view of C1–C2, antero-posterior projection of the cervical spine or oblique views. Many times the lowermost part of the cervical spine (C6–T1) cannot be shown on the lateral radiograph because of the short neck or obstruction by a prominent shoulder. Swimmer's view does not give a clear picture of the region especially in obese persons. Conventional tomography, computed tomography or magnetic resonance imaging is more helpful in such circumstances. Myelography, although still practised as a routine procedure in some European centres, is not the most appropriate investigation in cervical fractures, with a few exceptional situations. It is an invasive procedure and provides little information to affect the definitive treatment in cervical injuries except in cases in which soft-tissue compression on cord is suspected and magnetic resonance imaging is not available.

Once the injury is identified both clinically and radiologically, temporary stabilization of the neck injury is afforded either by a skull tong or Halter's traction. If the attending surgeon can foresee the likelihood of using a halo-body bracing as the definitive treatment to be rendered later, it is obviously advantageous to apply halo ring skull traction from the start instead of using a temporary skull tong. Whenever a skeletal type of traction is necessary for the neck injury, it is advisable to use the halo, if available, because of its flexibility in application of a different line of traction force to induce reduction and the readiness of its conversion into a very stable external fixation system for immobilization with or without surgical treatment for the injury.

Atlanto-Occipital Dislocation

Atlanto-occipital dislocation is a rare and very serious injury, virtually incompatible with life, although survivors have been reported [17]. The injury is caused by a distraction force most commonly associated with high-speed collisions [18]. The diagnosis can be made on the lateral view of the upper cervical spine and applying a simple ratio described by Powers et al. [19] (Fig. 4). The ratio is valid only when there are no other fractures of the atlas [19]. Traction is contraindicated for this injury because it leads to further distraction of the cord. Initial treatment is immobilization with an external support (halo-body brace) followed by intubation. When the patient is stable, an occiput to C2 fusion should be performed.

Odontoid Fracture

Fractures of the odontoid process are classified into three types [20]. Type I fracture is an avulsion of the tip of odontoid at the attachment of the alar ligament. An antero-posterior Water's view radiograph may help to reveal

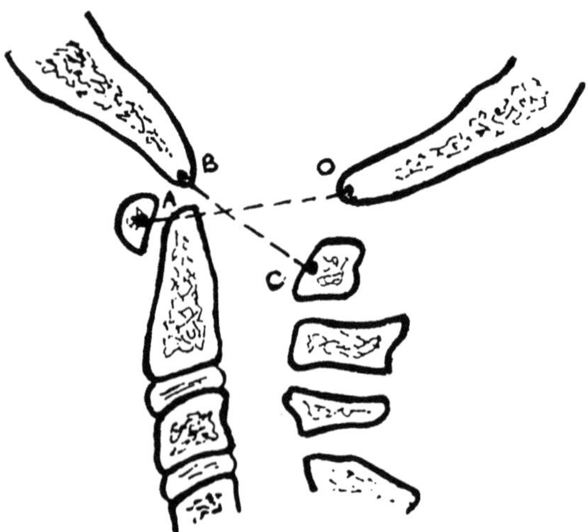

Fig. 4. Powers et al.'s ratio. The distance between the basion (*B*) and the spinolaminar line of C1 (*C*) is divided by the distance between the posterior margin of the foramen magnum (*O*) and the posterior margin of the anterior arch of C1 (*A*). BC/OA ≥ 1 indicates anterior atlanto-occipital dislocation

this injury in some cases. This fracture is considered stable, and patients simply need immobilization with a Philadelphia collar for about 6 weeks. Type II fractures occur through the isthmus (junction of the odontoid process with the body of C2), the region with the poorest blood supply. This is also the most common type of odontoid fracture. It is an unstable fracture and with a non-union rate of up to 60% [21], with the greatest incidence in older individuals with displaced fractures. For patients with angulation of more than 10° the incidence of non-union has been reported to be 29%, whereas fractures with more than 5 mm displacement have a non-union rate of 26%. A logical recommendation for treatment of type II fractures is to immobilize with halo-body brace for those without displacement. If motion at the fractured site is detected at 3 months after immobilization, posterior C1–C2 fusion should be performed. For type II fractures with displacement greater than 5 mm or angulation of more than 10° primary C1–C2 fusion is recommended (Fig. 5). Type III fracture occurs within the body of C2 and has a high incidence of healing with proper immobilization in those without

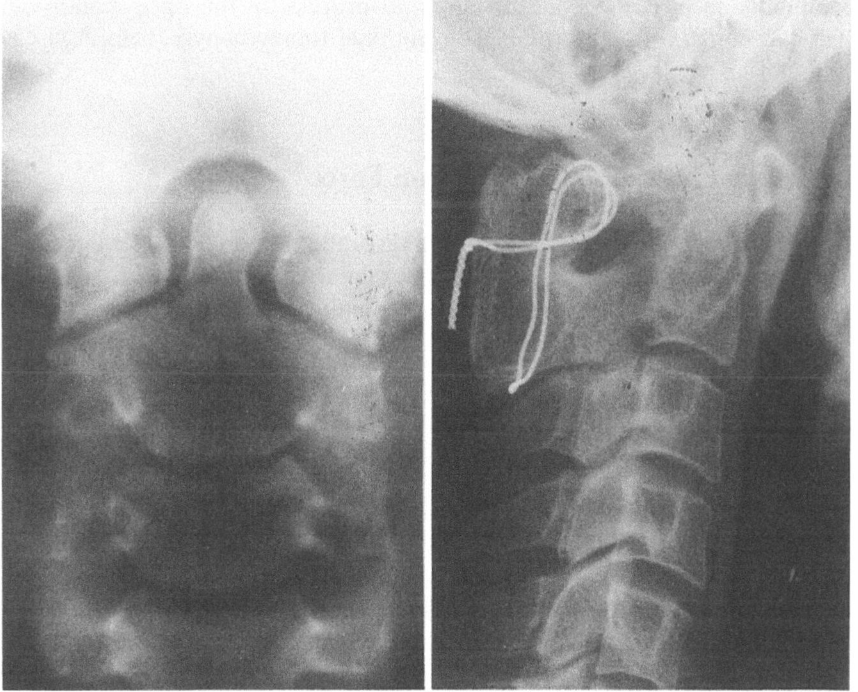

a   b

Fig. 5. a 23-year-old man complained of neck pain after a road traffic accident. Conventional plain X-rays were not conclusive, and a tomogram revealed fracture odontoid. **b** Odontoid fractures after halo-body immobilization still showing signs and symptoms of instability should be surgically fused posteriorly with autogenous bone graft displacement. An initial halo traction to realign any displacement is followed by halo-body bracing for 12 weeks if reduction is satisfactory. Limited immobilization with a Philadelphia collar for a further 3 months after the bracing is recommended. However, fractures with displacement more than 5 mm or angulation greater than 10° do have a higher incidence of non-union, showing 20% and 40%, respectively. Thus, if a satisfactory reduction is not achieved with halo traction, a primary C1–C2 fusion is indicated. Displacement and angulation of the fracture, and blood supply are among the six influencing factors outlined by Southwick [22] that may affect the healing of odontoid fractures. Non-union is uncommon after a proper treatment in these undisplaced type III fractures. If halo-body bracing is not available, a skull-tong traction in bed for 8 weeks followed by a sterno-occipito manubrium immobilization (SOMI) type of bracing to allow ambulation is the alternative treatment. In the author's experience, the compliance with the SOMI brace has been shown to be quite low.

It is important to realize that odontoid fractures can easily be missed on the lateral view radiograph alone. Close inspection of the open-mouth view is important. A common pitfall to be aware of is that of Mach's band commonly seen at the bone of odontoid process on the open-mouth view that can mimic a fracture [23]. Conventional tomography is helpful in case of doubt.

Injuries with Predominant Flexion Force

A flexion-predominate injury results in disruption of the posterior ligaments. The degree of injury ranges from a sprain (hyperflexion) to a significant kyphosis due to subluxation of the facet joints, depending on the extent of ligamental disruption.

Transverse Ligament Rupture

Transverse ligament rupture results from an excessive flexion force. The atlanto-dental interval space on a lateral view showing more than 3 mm in adults and 4 mm in children should suggest the possibility of ligamental rupture. Halo-body immobilization is recommended as the initial treatment in these injuries, as avulsion tears of the lateral mass of C1 may heal with a good immobilization. If the tears are at the mid-substance of the transverse ligament, the healing is unlikely in most instances with immobilization. A dynamic flexion extension view of C1–C2 should be taken after 6 weeks of halo immobilization, and those with no signs of healing require a posterior C1–C2 fusion using either Brooks' or Gallie's technique. The healing of avulsion tears of C1 lateral mass can be identified by the presence of a bony spicule along the lateral aspect of the transverse ligament.

Wedge Compression Fracture

Wedge compression fracture is a hyperflexion injury causing impaction of the anterior portion of the vertebral body resulting in a mild kyphosis. It is usually a stable injury, but if the kyphotic angle exceeds 11° difference with the adjacent bone segments, as described by White and Panjabi [2], it should be treated as an unstable injury and immobilized with halo-body or SOMI brace after reduction by skeletal traction. For stable injuries, a Philadelphia collar worn for 8–12 weeks allows healing at the fractured site.

Clay-Shoveller's Fracture

Clay-shoveller's fracture refers to avulsion fractures of the spinous processes occurring in the lower cervical spine and upper thoracic region (C6–T1) caused by an abrupt involuntary forced flexion against the opposing voluntary action of the inter-spinous and supra-spinous ligaments. Occasionally it is difficult to visualize the spinous process in the cervico-thoracic region in lateral films. An antero-posterior view can be helpful by looking for the double spinous process sign, as described by Cancelmo [24]. It is a stable fracture and requires only a good cervical collar to prevent flexion motions of the neck before the fracture heals.

Flexion Tear-Drop Fracture

Flexion tear-drop fracture involves the complete disruption of posterior ligaments, disc, and facet capsules along with a large triangular fragment of bone avulsed from the anterior aspect of the vertebral body. It is a severely unstable injury and occurs most ommonly at the C5 level [25]. The characteristic of this injury is its frequent association with anterior cord syndrome, which consists of tetraplegia with loss of pain, temperature and touch while posterior column position, motion and vibration are preserved. Some patients may have only partial deficits or be neurologically intact [25,26]. A review of major cervical injuries admitted to Prince of Wales Hospital from 1984 to 1990 found that more than half of flexion tear-drop fractures were neurologically intact. The mechanism of the injury is flexion and axial compression, and common causes are diving accidents, auto accidents and falls from heights [25] (Fig. 6).

Typical radiographic findings are seen on the lateral view and include: fracture of the anterior inferior portion of the vertebral body (usually C5) which maintains alignment with the lower bone segment; posterior displacement of the posterior fracture fragment; kyphotic angulation at the level of injury; widening of the inter-laminar distance, inter-spinous spaces and facet joints; and frequently associated sagittal body and laminar fractures. With complete disruption of all the supporting ligaments at the level of injury, this fracture is the most dangerous injury because it causes neurological

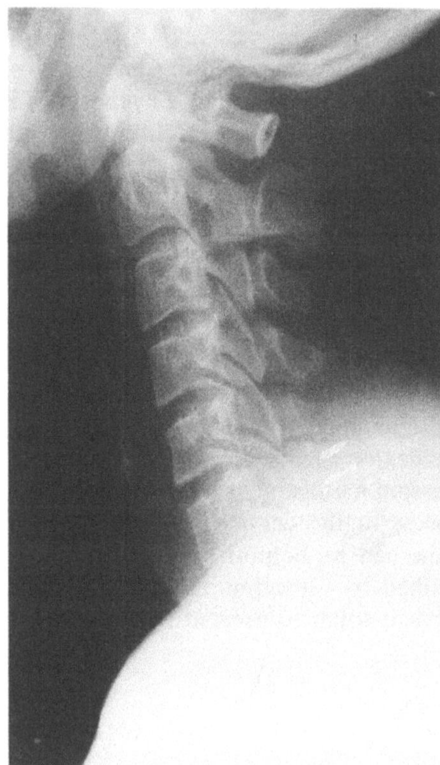

Fig. 6. A 20-year-old man sustaining a flexion tear-drop fracture of C6, resulting in tetraplegia. Notice the anterior inferior portion of the fracture retaining alignment with the lower segment (C7) and the marked posterior displacement of the posterior fracture fragment

damage or further deterioration in cases already having neurological impairment. Halo traction should be applied immediately after the radiological diagnosis, followed by halo-body immobilization. For fractures with persistent neurological impairment after immobilization with the fracture reduced to satisfactory alignment, myelographic computed tomography or magnetic resonance imaging is helpful in determining any mechanical obstructions insulting the cord, where surgical decompression might be indicated. If the injury still shows signs and symptoms of instability after 3 months immobilization, anterior interbody fusion should be performed to prevent futher or any future myelopathy (Fig. 7).

Bilateral Facet Dislocation

Bilateral facet dislocation results from complete disruption of all posterior ligaments at the level of injury, resulting in anterior translation of the affected vertebral body of at least 50% of its antero-posterior diameter in relation to the adjacent distal segment. The inferior facets of the proximal vertebra are displaced and become anterior to the superior facets of the distal vertebra.

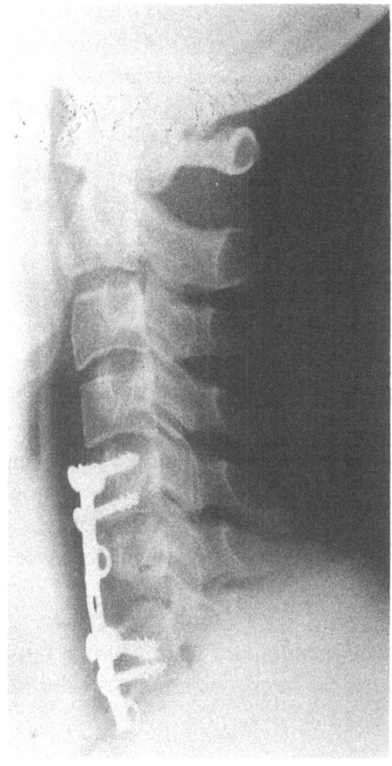

Fig. 7. Conservative traction could not achieve satisfactory alignment in the case show in Fig. 6. Anterior decompression and stabilization with autogenous interbody bony fusion was performed 1 week after the injury. He had some functional recovery. (Note: the length of the plate used was not appropriate)

Reduction should be attempted by skull traction with the neck in a flexed position. Closed supervision is necessary. Any change in neurological impairment in an incomplete lesion, increased intensity of neck pain/radiculopathy are the main criteria in adjusting the amount of weight/force necessary for traction. Once reduction is achieved, the neck should be kept in extension to lock the facets in place. Posterior fusion of the two affected bony segments is then indicated. If closed reduction by traction is unsuccessful, open reduction is required, followed by a posterior fusion. A wiring fixation posteriorly is good enough to hold the reduced facets in place, but an appropriate cervical brace still needs to be added to prevent excessive motion of the injured site, which may result in failure of the fixation before the fusion mass is consolidated. A halo-body vest is indicated for post-surgical immobilization if the patient is uncooperative or uncompliant with the cervical braces.

Unilateral Facet Dislocation

Unilateral facet dislocation occurs with an excessive flexion force combined with rotatory displacement. The facet on the side opposite to that of the rotation is dislocated (i.e. an injury with force of flexion and left lateral rotation results in a right facet dislocation). The disruption is at the unilateral facet capsule and posterior ligaments. The amount of displacement of the affected vertebra does not exceed 25% of the antero-posterior diameter of the inferior vertebra.

The initial treatment should be reduction with skull traction. If successful, the neck is immobilized in a halo-body brace for 8 weeks and a stress view of cervical spine checked for stability. If the finding is not satisfactory, a further 4 weeks of halo immobilization is indicated. If reduction by traction is not successful, a manipulative closed reduction or open reduction must be considered. In such cases conventional myelography, with or without computed tomography, or magnetic resonance imaging is required prior to the reduction. The purpose is to rule out the possibility of disc herniation at the level of injury. Failure to recognize and remove the protruded intervertebral disc may precipitate neurological damage during the course of the closed or open reduction. Unilateral facet dislocations discovered 3–4 weeks after the initial injury cannot be reduced by traction and closed reduction methods because of fibrosis. Open reduction and fusion is indicated in these cases. Late discoveries, diagnosed only after 6–8 weeks and without neurological deficit, should be treated conservatively unless symptoms develop later. Myelography or magnetic resonance imaging is necessary for all these late cases when surgical intervention is considered.

Injuries with Predominant Extension Force

Avulsion of Anterior Arch of C1

Avulsion of anterior arch of C1 is an avulsion of the attachments of the longus colli and anterior longitudinal ligament at the tubercle of the anterior arch and appears as a horizontal fracture on the radiograph. Treatment is by applying a SOMI or similar cervical brace to prevent excessive extension of the neck for 6–8 weeks.

Isolated Posterior Arch Fracture of C1

An isolated posterior arch fracture of C1 should not be mistaken for a Jefferson fracture; the ring of the atlas is not disrupted anteriorly, and the force of injury is different. This injury occurs from compression of the C1 spinous process between the occiput above and the C2 spinous process below in an excessive extension force of the neck. These are stable injuries, and treatment consists merely of a neck collar for symptomatic relief of pain.

Extension Tear-Drop Fracture

Extension tear-drop fracture is characterized by a triangle-shaped fracture fragment at the anterior inferior corner of the vertebral body, resulting from avulsion of the anterior longitudinal ligament or Sharpey's fibres [27]. This fracture is found typically at C2 [26] and is unstable in extension but stable in flexion. Martinez et al. [28] have found that hangman's fracture and locked facet may be associated with extension tear-drop fractures. Lee et al. [29] have also reported an association with thoracic spinal fractures in these C2 injuries. It is important that one be alert to associated thoracic spine fracture, which may be the cause of paraplegia when radiography reveals an obvious C2 injury which alone may not be associated with neurological damage. Extension tear-drop fracture alone should be treated with halo-body immobilization or SOMI with the neck in slight flexion for 8–12 weeks.

Hangman's Fracture

Hangman's fracture is a bilateral fracture of the pars intercularis of C2 occurring between the superior and inferior facet joints [30,31], with or without anterior subluxation of C2 on C3. Classically it is the result of acute hyperextension [28]. Hangman's fractures most commonly occur in motor vehicle accidents and typically are not associated with spinal cord damage [32–34]. Hangman's fracture causes widening of the spinal canal which is significantly different from a fracture through the posterior body of C2, which at first glance may simulate a hangman's fracture. The displacement of the fracture through the C2 body narrows the spinal canal, in contrast to hangman's fracture. The narrowing of the spinal canal predisposes to neurological sequelae. Radiographic findings in cases of hangman's fracture include fracture of the C2 neural arch with or without anterior subluxation of C2 on C3, narrowing of disc space between C2 and C3 and significant pre-vertebral soft-tissue swelling [28]. As with all other cranio-vertebral junction fractures, one should look for any associated fractures in the lower cervical, thoracic and lumbar regions [29]. Hangman's fracture should be treated by traction to reduce the subluxation, if present, and followed by halo-body brace immobilization for 12 weeks.

Hyperextension Dislocation

Hyperextension dislocation occurs with a distraction and hyperextension force to the neck. The anterior longitudinal ligament is disrupted, and in more severe cases the fracture may also rupture the posterior longitudinal ligament. If there is spontaneous reduction of the dislocation, the initial lateral radiograph may not show any obvious signs of the injury, but it is often identified on a forced extension X-ray. Treatment should be rigid immobilization in the reduced alignment for 6–8 weeks. It should then be assessed for its stability by flexion and extension views. Anterior interbody fusion is indicated if it is found to be unstable.

Pillar Fracture

Pillar fracture results from a combination of hyperextension and rotation forces. The pillars represent the lateral masses of the vertebrae, and this fracture usually includes a portion of the articular facet joint. For patients with suspected hyperextension injuries or when there is a question of abnormality on the antero-posterior radiograph, a special pillar view is helpful to visualize these fractures [35]. This radiographic veiw is obtained with the head rotated 45°–50° towards the unaffected side with the central X-ray beam directed at C7 in 30°–40° of caudal angulation [36]. Most lateral mass fractures are stable injuries, and a Philadelphia collar is used. If instability is present with neurological deficit, a halo-body or SOMI type of immobilization is necessary depending upon the level of the injury. For fractures in the lower cervical spine, the amount of immobilization provided by halo-body and SOMI braces shows no significant difference [37]. The halo vest or SOMI is recommended for 3 months.

Injuries with Vertical Compression Force

Burst Fracture of C1

Burst fracture of C1, or Jefferson fracture, by definition indicates an injury that results in fractures through both the anterior and posterior arches of the C1 ring [32]. It occurs with falls, auto accidents or diving accidents [38,39]. The axial loading or vertical compression forces on the skull cause the occipital condyles to compress the lateral masses of C1 against the facets of C2. Owing to the oblique orientation of the articular surfaces of C1 and the occipital condyles, a compression force tends to spread and displace the lateral masses in an outward direction. Normally the displacement increases the spinal canal area, and thus neurological deficit is uncommon in these injuries [38]. However, spread of the lateral masses by more than 6.9 mm indicates disruption of the transverse ligament and may lead to C1–C2 instability and neurological impairment [40,41]. One should be aware that the initial lateral radiograph may appear normal and the fracture not be visible. The open-mouth view reveals the lateral displacement of the C1 lateral masses with or without an avulsion fracture. Most Jefferson fractures represent stable injuries, and treatment with an appropriate cervical collar (Philadelphia) is adequate. For patients with evidence of instability (e.g. rupture of transverse ligament), a halo-body brace should be used for 3 months followed by flexion and extension view X-rays of the neck. If the radiograph then reveals instability, posterior cervical fusion is indicated [42].

Burst Fracture of Cervical Spine

When a uniform vertical compression force is applied to the vertebral bodies, a burst fracture can occur at any level from C3 to C7 in the neck region. The bone or disc fragments resulting from the injury may be retropulsed into the spinal canal, leading to significant neurological compromise. There is no difficulty in diagnosing such fractures radiologically. The treatment is traction, initially with the neck in neutral postion. Computed tomography is helpful in revealing any retropulsion of bone fragments into the canal. Computed tomographic myelography or magnetic resonance imaging shows better any soft-tissue compression on the cord. The conservative treatment is halo-body immobilization for 3 months, whereupon one should check radiographically for any instability. For those patients with obvious bone or soft-tissue compression on the cord revealed by tomography or myelography, anterior decompression and interbody fusion with or without implant fixation is indicated. External immobilization with halo vest or neck collar is necessary depending upon the degree of immediate stability provided by the surgical fixation.

Halo Immobilization

Perry and Nickel [43] introduced the halo fixation device in 1959 for postoperative stabilization of cervical spine fusion in poliomyelitis. The usefulness of the halo in treating cervical spine injuries – when rigid immobilization is desired – is well documented [44–52]. The advantages of halo traction over the earlier skull tongs in the treatment of cervical spine injuries and instabilities resulting from other causes has caused it almost completely to replace the other devices nowadays. Its ease of conversion into halo-body bracing after accomplishing the reduction, allows the patient to be ambulated much earlier, thus shortening the rehabilitation period.

Although initially thought to be relatively free of complications, the halo has been shown by subsequent experience at various centres to result in complications up to 30% of the time [53–56]. The most common complications encountered are pin loosening, pin site infections and pain, disfiguring scars at the pin sites, and less commonly nerve injury, bleeding at the pin sites and dural puncture. In those with halo-body bracing, pressure sores under the vest or cast and dysphagia are reported.

Complications and Preventive Measures

Pin loosening is the most frequent complication encountered by all patients using halo traction. Pain at the pin sites, which was not experienced by the patient in the earlier stages, and an increasing amount of serous discharge at the pin site noticed during daily care should alert the examiner to the possibility of a loosened pin. A loosened pin can be twisted freely without resistance. Pin loosening may lead to many other serious complications, such as complete dislodgement of the halo with subsequent loss of the reduction. Loosened pins also predispose to pin site infections, pain and disfiguring scars after removal of the halo. Pin loosening is not merely a late complication in halo immobilization but is encountered with an equally high incidence of 40%–50% in the first and second months of application. For unclear reasons, the two front pins placed antero-laterally are found to have a slightly higher incidence of loosening than those placed postero-laterally.

Botte et al. [57] have found that the current pins do not completely penetrate the outer cortex of skull bone when inserted at 6 inches – pounds of torque – the usual recommended force to be applied. Thus a margin of solid cortical bone still exists for the pin to be retightened further if loosening occurs.

All pins after the initial application should be routinely retightened after the second or third day, and locked. Failing to lock the pins is a very common oversight among inexperienced and infrequent users of halo immobilization. This no doubt gives rise to an early loosening. A loose pin should be retightened once only. Recurrent loosening of the same pin calls for inserting a new pin in a different suitable location. If on retightening pins, no resistance is encountered after two complete turns, they should not be retightened further but replaced with a new pin at a new location. All new pins should be inserted first before the loosened ones are removed in order to maintain the position of the halo ring and thus the reduction of the cervical fracture or dislocation.

Infection at the pin sites can pose a serious problem for patients who need to be immobilized with a halo device for a relatively lengthy period. Severe infections, such as osteomyelitis, brain abscess, and septicaemia have been reported by several authors [53–56]. Prevention of pin site infection begins with meticulous local pin care. Pin sites should be cleansed once every day or on alternate days. Swabbing with a povidine-iodine or hydrogen peroxide solution is recommended. No cover dressing is necessary for pin sites. Once infection becomes established, the wound discharge should be cultured, and appropriate antibiotics may be necessary for wounds with persistent drainage or cellulitis even when aggressive local treatment has been instituted.

Injuries to the nerves of the scalp are minimized if attention is paid to anatomical detail when applying the halo. Anterior pains placed too far medially (medial one-third of the orbit) are likely to damage the supra-orbital/supra-trochlear nerves. This is manifested by severe pain and para-esthesia radiating superiorly into the frontal region above the pin site. Immediate removal of the pin and reinserting it to a more lateral location (on the middle or lateral one-third of the eye brow) resolves the symptoms.

Pain at the pin sites not due to loosening or infection is uncommon if the pins are inserted properly. Pain during mastication is due to pins inserted behind the hairline in the temporal region. The temporal fossa, where the calvarium is the thinnest, also has the highest risk of dura penetration. Inserting the antero-lateral pins behind the hairline in the hope of achieving cosmetically more acceptable scarring should be avoided in view of all the high risks mentioned.

Excessive bleeding resulting from a misplaced pin lacerating the superficial vessels is not common. However, in patients who are on anti-coagulant therapy, persistent pin site bleeding may be a problem and does not resolve unless the anti-coagulants are tapered.

In injuries requiring immobilization of the head in hyperextension to maintain the reduction of injury, the patient may complain of difficulty in eating or swallowing, due to over-distraction. Careful repositioning of the head and neck without disrupting the original reduction resolves the symptom of dysphagia.

Excessive pin penetration leading to violation of the dura occurs occasionally. This may result from repetitive retightening of the pin or a fall or direct blow to the halo apparatus. Complaints of headache, lethargy, dizziness, visual disturbances, chills and fever should warn the clinician to carry out a detailed investigation. The problem can be identified by skull X-rays demonstrating pin penetration through the inner cortex of skull bone into the brain and presence of cerebrospinal fluid at the pin site after removing a loose pin.

Pressure sores over the bony prominence of the upper trunk, especially over the sternum and scapula are less common in patients wearing the new polyethylene vest with better padding, more uniform pressure and allowing easier skin inspection by nurses. For those using plaster cast, sores are much more common and occasionally result in extensive skin breakdown that requires removal of the cast for wound débridement and skin grafting.

Patients should be asked to close their eyes tightly before insertion of the two antero-lateral pins. Failure to do so may result in the patient's inability to close the eyes completely due to traction on eyelid skin and muscles – a very common mistake made by inexperienced surgeons.

With proper methods of application, following strict guidelines for every step of the procedure in halo immobilization, most of the complications are preventable.

Thoracic, Thoraco-Lumbar and Lumbar Spine Injuries

Injuries in the thoracic and lumbar spine result from abnormal forces in compression, distraction, shear, rotation, or a combination of these. Major injuries to these regions of the spinal column have both similarities and differences. Significant regional anatomic differences in osseous, soft-tissue and neural structures are responsible for varying patterns of injury. The sternum and rib cage add stability to the thoracic spine from T2 to T10, significantly restricting flexion, extension and lateral bending and increasing overall stiffness [58]. This configuration with the articular facets situated in the coronal plane, however, offers minimal resistance to torsional loads [59]. Lumbar vertebrae are the largest and strongest segments in the pre-sacral spine. The facet joints, in addition to the strong ligamental complex, play a crucial role in the stability of the lumbar spine. These facets are oriented mostly in the sagittal plane, in contrast to the thoracic spine, thus permitting significant flexion and extension and limiting only axial rotation. The physiological thoracic kyphosis also predisposes to flexion instability after traumatic or surgical (laminectomy for decompression) disruption of the posterior column [60].

The thoraco-lumbar region is one of transition. The facet orientation changes abruptly from coronal to sagittal between T9 and T12, and the last two thoracic vertebrae (T11 and T12) have characteristics of both the thoracic and lumbar vertebrae. The stability in this region is therefore between being most resistant to antero-posterior translation (in the thoracic spine) and being most resistant to rotational forces (in the lumbar spine).

Neurological injuries have a relatively better outcome in the thoraco-lumbar and lumbar regions than in the thoracic due to the significant differences in the neural structures and their respective environment. For example, although the conus medullaris and cauda equina have a relatively extensive blood supply, the spinal cord between T4 and T9 has relatively sparse segmental arterial anastomotic network and is thus more vulnerable to vascular ischaemia [61].

Classification of spinal fractures based on mechanisms of injury are useful only when they are simple and able to describe the common injury patterns seen in clinical practice. Denis [4], Ferguson and Allen [62] and McAfee et al.'s [63] classifications have all shown significant improvements on previous ones and are most useful in determining the treatment options.

Anterior Compression Fracture

Anterior compression fracture (wedge compression fracture) is generally the result of a pure flexion force delivered to the anterior column of the spine, producing a wedge-shaped deformity of the vertebral body, and most commonly occurs at the thoraco-lumbar region. This is a stable fracture because the posterior osseous and ligamentous structures remain intact. The loss of height of the anterior vertebral body is rarely greater than 50% and is rarely associated with neurological injury. When the injury results from a much greater flexion force, there may be an associated failure of the posterior column in tension, but still with the middle column remaining intact. Any wedge-compression fractures with loss of more than 40% of anterior vertebral body height or with significant kyphosis (30° or more) should warrant further investigation into the status of the posterior elements, which are usually injured [64]. Posterior element disruption may be manifested by widening of the inter-spinous process distance and subluxation of facet joints (Fig. 8).

Treatment of this injury is based upon consideration of the amount of anterior vertebral body wedging and the presence of posterior ligament disruption. Wedge compression fractures with loss of no more than 30% of anterior vertebral body height may be treated with early ambulation as soon as the back pain is allowed. Patients with loss of 30%–50% of anterior vertebral body height should undergo closed reduction with hyperextension immobilization to regain the lost vertebral body height. The author has applied postural reduction with the patient tracted in a Stryker rotation bed tilted to 40°–50° and a pillow underneath the thoraco-lumbar spine to increase the lordosis (Fig. 9). More than 60% of patients have achieved a significant restoration of vertebral body height after 48 h of traction. They are then ambulated in a well-moulded, modified Knight-Taylor brace for 6 months.

Patients with evidence of posterior ligamentous disruption have a propensity to develop progressive kyphosis and should undergo posterior spinal instrumentation and fusion [64]. Such a situtation, however, is not very common in daily practice.

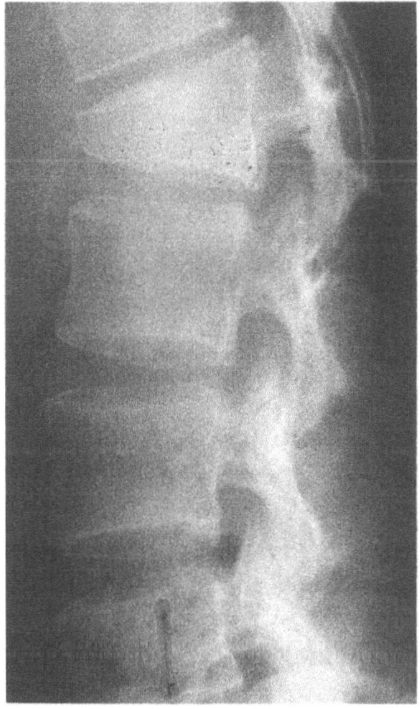

Fig. 8. Posterior element disruption should be suspected in wedge compression fractures with significant kyphosis (30° or more) and widened inter-spinous process distance

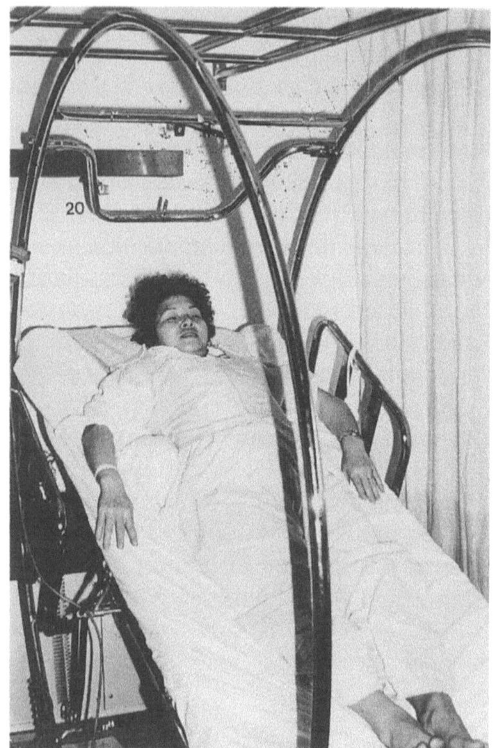

Fig. 9. Postural reduction with the patient tracted in a Stryker rotation bed tilted to 40°–50° with a pillow placed underneath the thoraco-lumbar spine to increase the lordosis

Burst Fracture

Burst fracture represents a failure of the entire vertebral body to resist a vertical axial load. Both the anterior and middle columns are damaged with disc material and/or bone fragments retropulsed into the spine canal (Fig. 10). The posterior column may also fail in compression. A plain radiograph showes fracture of the posterior wall of the vertebral body with a decrease in vertical height. The interpedicular distance is widened due to a sagittal body fracture both anteriorly and posteriorly. These findings are best shown on computed axial tomography. Loss of vertebral body height combined with laxity or disruption of the posterior ligaments may cause the subsequent development of kyphosis.

Neurological status varies widely depending upon the level of injury. Thoracic levels, owing to the high ratio of cord to canal diameter, result in higher rates of neurological deficits, with most of these producing complete spinal cord injuries. Thoraco-lumbar injuries result in a higher relative percentage of incomplete and mixed cord/conus/root lesions. The cauda equina in the lower lumbar spine, on the other hand, does not tolerate chronic compression very well. All these facts are important in relation to

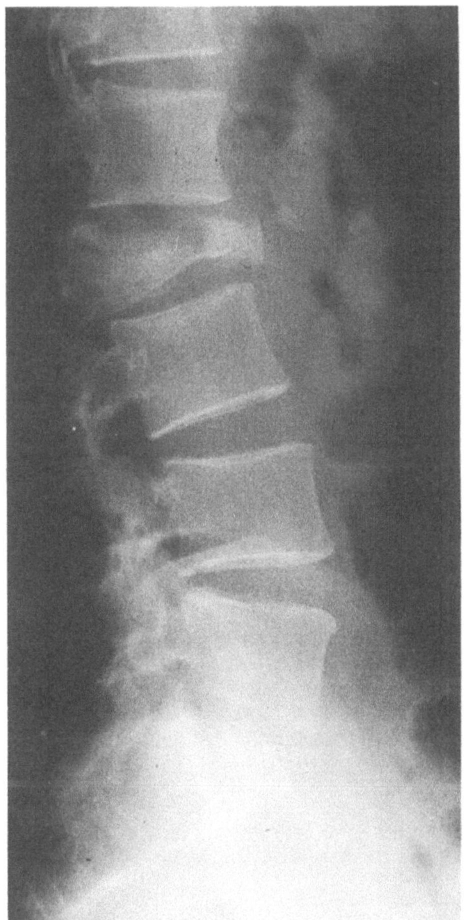

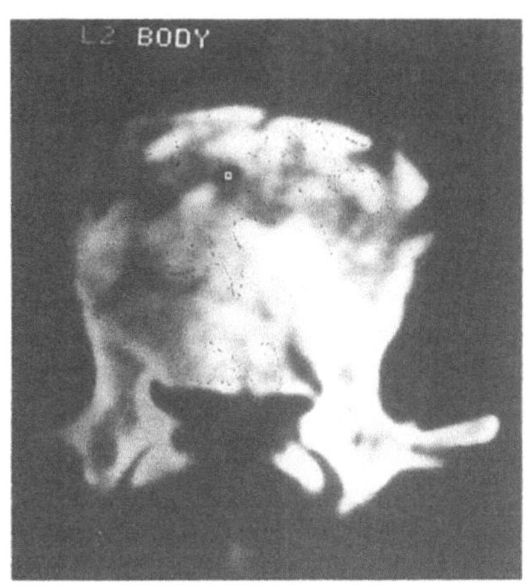

Fig. 10. a Burst fracture of L2 in a 28-year-old man after an industrial accident. Anterior and middle columns are severely damaged, with retropulsion of bone fragments into the spinal canal. **b** Computed tomography shows the damage of vertebral body and bone fragments in the spinal canal

neural relief in the treatment. The presence of neurological deficit and posterior column injury are major factors in determining the treatment of burst fractures. Burst fractures with intact posterior column and neurological function are usually relatively stable and can be treated with 6–8 weeks of bed rest immobilization followed by ambulation in a well-moulded spinal orthosis.

In patients with failure in all three columns, surgical intervention is usually indicated because of the tendency to develop of post-traumatic kyphosis [65,66], by means of posterior spinal distraction instrumentation and fusion with postero-lateral decompression. Classic Harrington's instrumentation and the newer pedicle screw-plate systems have the disadvantage that two levels must be fixed above and below the level of injury. This disadvantage becomes more significant in the lower lumbar spine with a resultant loss of motion segments, especially close to the sacrum. Instrumentation in these high-stress areas of the spine hastens degenerative processes. Pedicle rod systems have the advantage of shortening the length of spine to be instrumented and providing increased stability. Luque's rods with segmental wiring should have no place in the treatment of burst fractures, as the smooth rods provide no distraction force and thus cannot prevent vertebral collapse.

Others [66–68] have advocated an anterior approach in an effort to limit fusion length with or without instrumentation. The anterior approach has the advantage of providing a more direct approach to neural compression in burst fractures. The essence of a good result, whether approached posteriorly or anteriorly, is a thorough decompression of the cord and a successful arthrodesis with autogenous bone grafting. The author's experience has been mostly with the anterior retroperitoneal approach and autogenous iliac bone graft with or without Kaneda's device depending on whether the posterior column is injured, as established by computed tomography (Fig. 11).

Patients with intact neurological function but with spinal canal compromise of more than one-third [69] and thoracic spine injuries with kyphosis of greater than 30° should also be treated surgically.

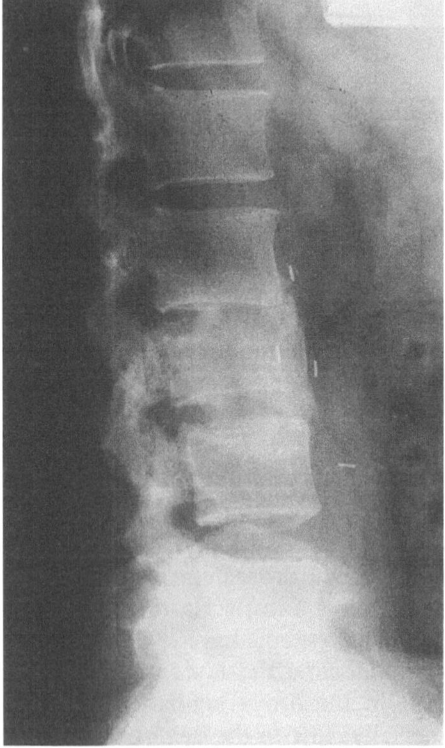

Fig. 11. Anterior retroperitoneal approach provides a more direct approach to neural compression in burst fractures; the autogenous iliac bone graft contributed to a successful arthrodesis

Flexion-Distraction Injuries

Flexion-distraction injuries ("seat-belt" injuries) arise from the failure of both the middle and posterior columns under tension forces and the anterior column failing in compression. The anterior aspect of the vertebral body has a shortened height, while the posterior part does not, causing its failure in tension. Facet fractures and subluxation or dislocation are common, and there is potential for development and progression of neurological deficits and spine deformity [62]. As the anterior longitudinal ligament remains intact in these injuries, translation is unusual.

Neurological status guides the treatment of this injury. In patients with incomplete or no neurological deficit, the treatment should aim at achieving reduction of neural impingement and spinal deformity to prevent progression. Postero-lateral decompression followed by posterior spinal compression instrumentation and bone fusion is indicated. In patients with mid-thoracic injury, postero-lateral decompression may have a high risk of causing undue retraction of the cord, in which cases anterior decompression and fusion should be performed first, followed by posterior instrumentation for stability.

In seat-belt trauma there is a high incidence of associated intra-abdominal injury which one should carefully look for. Flexion-distraction injuries of the lumbar spine may also involve two levels, leading to a greater chance of instability. Unless alert to this possibility, surgeons treating these injuries may render only the obvious injured level stable, thus increasing the stress at the other, unrecognized level of injury. Conventional plane lateral tomography generally displays these injuries, and computed tomography provides little additional information because of the nature of the fracture pattern.

Chance Injuries

Chance injuries result from a significant flexion force applied anterior to the anterior longitudinal ligament [70], leading to all three columns failing in distraction (tension force). The pattern of injury can be all bony involvement in three columns (chance fracture), all soft-tissue injury disrupting the ligaments and disc (chance dislocation), or a combination of bone and soft-tissue elements. The commonest site of these injuries is the thoraco-lumbar junction. As in other types of flexion-distraction injuries, conventional lateral tomography reveals better detail of the pattern than computed tomography, in which the axial views may miss the horizontal injury. Pure soft-tissue injury (chance dislocation) and the combined pattern with translation may lead to progression of deformity and neurological deficit due to poor healing of ligaments [63,71].

Treatment of chance injuries is based upon the presence of neurological status, translation and the anatomy of the injury site (bone versus soft tissue). Posterior spinal compression instrumentation and bone fusion with or without postero-lateral decompression is indicated in patients with significant translation, soft-tissue (ligamentous) disruption, or both. For injuries having significant translation, the instrumentation should be extended one additional level above and below the lesion. Pre-operative scrutiny of imaging studies is mandatory to detect any bone fragments or soft-tissue (disc) materials causing neural impingements. Patients with pure bone injury (chance fracture) and having no translation can be treated conservatively in a moulded hyperextensive spinal orthosis, allowing ambulation. The brace should be worn 3–6 months, with the bone healing monitored.

Fracture-Dislocations

Fracture-dislocations with or without neurological deficit are unstable injuries. They represent failure of all the three columns under a variety or combination of forces in flexion, compression, tension, rotation and shearing. The shear with a translational force entails a significant soft-tissue disruption in ligaments and disc. Anterior translation exceeding 25% of the body usually signifies disruption of the anterior longitudinal ligament [2,63]. Torsional flexion implies a shear and axial rotational force combined with an element of anterior column compression and posterior column tension. The result is the most highly unstable injuries. Facet joints are usually fractured/ dislocated, especially in the thoraco-lumbar spine, where they provide significant resistance to torsion and rotation. The real danger in these types of injuries, in the absence of initial neurological deficit, is unrecognized instability, with a high incidence of delayed neurological injury, deformity (especially in the thoraco-lumbar region) and non-union [5].

Surgical stabilization is imperative in these injuries to deal with both the immediate and potential late problems. Patients with a complete spinal cord injury should undergo posterior spinal distraction or compression instrumentation and bone fusion supplemented by sub-laminar wires. These constructs provide maximum stability for immediate ambulation and rehabilitation. Sub-laminar wires should be avoided in patients with incomplete or no neurological deficits, as the wires add the risk of causing iatrogenic neural injury. Postero-lateral decompression should be performed in cases with neural impingement. Distraction rods may be supplemented with inter-spinous process wires (e.g. Wisconson wires) for additional stability. It is most important to check that the distraction is not exagerated in the case of significant anterior translation, which may indicate a disrupted anterior longitudinal ligament. Intra-operative X-ray monitoring of the vertebral relations is mandatory. For pure translational injuries, Luque's rods alone can be used, but not in compression or tension failure injuries as these rods do not resist compressive or tensile forces.

Summary

The definition as stable or unstable injury is crucial in the management of spinal column injuries. Treatment guidelines should be based upon careful understanding of the mechanism and force of injury, including consideration of regional anatomical differences along the spinal column, neurological status, potential late complications and associated injuries. Detailed radiographic and special imaging studies are crucial to classify the injury for clinical application in the treatment plan. Laminectomy alone aiming to decompress the spinal cord, without appropriate posterior stabilization and bone fusion has no place in the management of any acute spinal injuries [72]. An injury associated with a neurological deficit must be considered unstable, and it is mechanically unsound to allow early ambulation of the patient without internal fixation. When surgical facilities are not available, sufficient time of immobilization in bed should be implemented to allow healing before allowing ambulatory activity.

Recumbency is an adequate treatment for many spinal column injuries. For multiple trauma victims, however, it is totally unsuitable as early mobilization in these cases improves survival chances. Aggressive surgical stabilization is indicated in such situations.

References

1. Whitesides TE (1977) Traumatic kyphosis of the thoracolumbar spine. Clin Orthop 128:78–92
2. White AA, Panjabi MM (1978) Clinical biomechanics of the spine. Lippincott, Philadelphia
3. Denis F (1983) The three column spine and its significance in the classification of acute thoraco-lumbar spinal injuries. Spine 8:817–831
4. Denis F (1984) Spinal instability as defined by the three-column spine concept in acute spinal trauma. Clin Orthop 189:65–76
5. Holdsworth F (1970) Fractures, dislocations and fracture-dislocations of the spine. J Bone Joint Surg [Am] 52:1534–1551
6. Kobrine AI, Bernstein JJ (1985) Experimental spinal cord injury. In: Wilkins RH, Rengachary SS (eds) Neurosurgery, vol 2. McGraw-Hill, New York, pp 1694–1700
7. Bricolo A, Dalle Ore G et al. (1976) Local cooling in spinal cord injury. Surg Neurol 6:101–106
8. Abraham J, Paterson A et al. (1987) Omento-myelo-synangiosis in the management of chronic traumatic parapledia. Paraplegia 25:44–49
9. Yashon D (1988) Surgical management of trauma to the spine. In: Schmidek HH, Sweet WH (eds) Operative neurosurgical techniques, 2nd edn. Grune and Stratton, New York, pp 1449–1469
10. Sherrington CS (1947) The integrative action of the nervous system, 2nd edn. Yale University Press, New Haven
11. Schneider RC (1955) Syndrome of acute anterior spinal cord injury. J Neurosurg 12:95–122
12. Pang D, Wilberger JE Jr (1982) Spinal cord injury without radiographic abnormalities in children. J Neurosurg 57:114–119

13. Pollack IF, Pang D et al. (1988) Recurrent spinal cord injury without radiographic abnormalities in children. J Neurosurg 69:177–182
14. Hadley MN, Zabramski JM et al. (1988) Paediatric spinal trauma: review of 122 cases of spinal cord and vertebral column injuries. J Neurosurg 68:18–24
15. Foo D, Rossier AB (1982) Post-traumatic spinal epidural hematoma. Neurosurgery 11:25–32
16. Berquist TH (1986) Imaging of orthopaedic trauma and surgery. Saunders, Philadelphia
17. Bools JC, Rose BS (1986) Traumatic atlanto-occipital dislocation: two cases with survival. AJNR 7:901–904
18. Bohlman H, Ducker T, Lucas J (1982) Spine and spinal cord injuries. In: Rothman R, Simeone F (eds) The spine, 2nd edn. Saunders, Philadelphia, pp 661–756
19. Powers B, Miller MD et al. (1979) Traumatic anterior atlanto-occipital dislocation. Neurosurgery 4:12–17
20. Anderson LD, D'Alonzo RT (1974) Fractures of the odontoid process of the axis. J Bone Joint Surg [Am] 56:1663–1674
21. Clark C, White A (1985) Fractures of the dens. J Bone Joint Surg [Am] 67:1340–1348
22. Southwick W (1980) Management of fractures of the dens. J Bone Joint Surg [Am] 62:482–486
23. Daffner RH (1977) Pseudo fracture of the dens: Mach bands. Am J Radiol 128:607–612
24. Cancelmo JJ (1972) Clay shoveler's fracture: a helpful diagnostic sign. Am J Radiol 115:540–543
25. Kim KS, Chen HH et al. (1989) Flexion teardrop fracture of the cervical spine: radiographic characteristics. Am J Radiol 152:319–326
26. Harris JH (1978) Acute injuries of the spine. Semin Roentgenol 13:53–68
27. Lee C, Kim KS, Rogers LF (1982) Triangular cervical vertebral body fractures: diagnostic significance. Am J Radiol 138:1123–1132
28. Martinez S, Morgan CL et al. (1979) Unusual fractures and dislocations of the axis vertebra. Skeletal Radiol 3:206–212
29. Lee C, Rogers LF et al. (1984) Fractures of the cranio-vertebral junction associated with other fractures of the spine: overlooked entity? AJNR 5:775–781
30. Mirvis S, Young J et al. (1987) Hangman's fracture: radiologic assessment in 27 cases. Radiology 163:713–717
31. Peppin J, Hawkins R (1981) Traumatic spondylolisthesis of the axis: hangman's fracture. Clin Orthop 157:133–138
32. Effendi B, Roy D et al. (1981) Fractures of the ring of the axis: a classification based on the analysis of 131 cases. J Bone Joint Surg [Br] 63:319–327
33. Elliott JM, Rogers LF et al. (1972) The hangman's fracture: fractures of the neural arch of the axis. Radiology 104:303–307
34. Seljeskog EL, Chou SH (1976) Spectrum of the hangman's fracture. J Neurosurg 45:3–8
35. Miller MD, Gehweiler JA et al. (1978) Significant new observations on cervical spine traumas. Am J Radiol 130:659–663
36. Ballinger PW (ed) (1986) Merrill's atlas of radiographic positions and radiographic procedures, vol 1, 6th edn. Mosby, St Lauis
37. Koch RA, Nickel VL (1978) The halo-vest: an evaluation of motion and forces across the neck. Spine 3:103–107
38. Han SY, Witten DM, Mussleman JP (1976) Jefferson fracture of the atlas. J Neurosurg 44:368–371
39. Sherk HH, Nicholson JT (1970) Fractures of the atlas. J Bone Joint Surg [Am] 52:1017–1024
40. Spence K, Decker S, Sell K (1970) Bursting atlantal fracture associated with rupture of the transverse ligament. J Bone Joint Surg [Am] 52:543–546

41. Zielinski C, Gunther S, Deeb Z (1982) Cranial nerve palsies complicating Jefferson fractures. J Bone Joint Surg [Am] 64:1382–1384
42. Segal LS, Grimm JO, Stauffer ES (1987) Non-union of fractures of the atlas. J Bone Joint Surg [Am] 69:1423–1434
43. Perry J, Nickel VL (1959) Total cervical spine fusion for neck paralysis. J Bone Joint Surg [Am] 41:37–59
44. Anderson LD, D'Alonzo RT (1974) Fractures of the odontoid process of the axis. J Bone Joint Surg [Am] 56:1663–1674
45. Chan RC, Schweigel JF, Thompson GB (1983) Halo-thoracic brace immobilization in 188 patients with acute cervical spine injuries. J Neurosurg 58:508–515
46. Cooper PR, Maravilla KR et al. (1979) Halo immobilization of cervical spine fractures. Indications and results. J Neurosurg 50:603–610
47. Koch RA, Nickel VL (1978) The halo vest. Spine 3:103–107
48. Kostuik JP (1981) Indications for the use of halo immobilization. Clin Orthop 154:46–50
49. Schweigel JF (1979) Halo-thoracic brace management of odontoid fractures. Spine 4:192–194
50. Seljeskig EL (1978) Non-operative management of acute upper cervical injuries. Acta Neurochir (Wien) 41:87–100
51. Zwerling MT, Riggins RS (1974) Use of the halo apparatus in acute injuries of the cervical spine. Surg Gynecol Obstet 138:189–193
52. Zimmerman E, Grant J et al. (1976) Treatment of Jefferson fracture with a halo apparatus. Report of two cases. J Neurosurg 44:372–375
53. Garfin SR, Botte MJ et al. (1986) Complications in the use of the halo fixation device. J Bone Joint Surg [Am] 68:320–325
54. Goodman ML, Nelson PB (1987) Brain abscess complicating the use of a halo orthosis. Neurosurgery 20(1):27–30
55. Humbyrd DE, Latimer FR et al. (1981) Brain abscess as a complication of halo traction. Spine 6:365–368
56. Victor DI, Bresnan MJ, Kellar RB (1973) Brain abscess complicating the use of halo traction. J Bone Joint Surg [Am] 55:635–639
57. Botte MJ, Byrne T, Garfin SR (1987) Application of the halo cervical immobilizer utilizing an increased torque pressure. J Bone Joint Surg [Am] 69:750–753
58. Andriacchi TP, Schultz AB et al. (1974) A model for studies of mechanical interactions between the human spine and rib cage. J Biomech 7:497
59. Markolf KL (1972) Deformation of the thoraco-lumbar intervertebral joints in response to external loads: a biomechanical study using autopsy material. J Bone Joint Surg [Am] 54:511–533
60. White AA, Hirsch C (1971) The significance of the vertebral posterior elements in the mechanics of the thoracic spine. Clin Orthop 81:2–14
61. Dommisse GF (1974) The blood supply of the spinal cord. A critical vascular zone in spinal surgery. J Bone Joint Surg [Br] 56:225–235
62. Ferguson RL, Allen BL (1984) A mechanistic classification of thoraco-lumbar spine fractures. Clin Orthop 189:77–88
63. McAfee PC, Yuan HA et al. (1983) The value of computed tomography in thoraco-lumbar fractures: an analysis of 100 consecutive cases and a new classification. J Bone Joint Surg [Am] 65:461–473
64. Bohlman HH (1985) Current concepts review: treatment of fractures and dislocations of the thoracic and lumbar spine. J Bone Joint Surg [Am] 67:165–169
65. McAfee PC, Yuan HA, Lasda NA (1982) The unstable burst fracture. Spine 7:365–373
66. McAfee PC, Bohlman HH, Yuan HA (1985) Anterior decompression of traumatic thoraco-lumbar fractures with incomplete neurological deficit using a retroperitoneal approach. J Bone Joint Surg [Am] 67:89–104

67. Kaneda K, Abumi K, Fujiya M (1984) Burst fractures with neurologic deficits of the thoracolumbar spine. Results of anterior decompression and stabilization with anterior instrumentation. Spine 9:788–795
68. Kostuik JP (1984) Anterior fixation for fractures of the thoracic and lumbar spine with or without neurologic involvement. Clin Orthop 189:103
69. Edwards CC, Levine AM (1986) Early rod sleeve stabilization of the injured thoracic and lumbar spine. Orthop Clin North Am 17:122–145
70. Chance GQ (1948) Note on a type of flexion fracture of the spine. Br J Radiol 21:452–453
71. Kaufer H, Hayes JT (1966) Lumbar fracture-dislocation – a study of twenty-one cases. J Bone Joint Surg [Am] 48:712–730
72. Morgan TH, Wharton GW, Austin GN (1970) The results of laminectomy in patients with incomplete spinal cord injuries. J Bone Joint Surg [Am] 52:822

Subject Index

Absorbable implant   420
   Screw   378, 436
   Pins   287
Acupuncture   2
Adjunctive internal fixation   69
Aerobe/anaerobe cultures   182
Agee   281
Aligment index of Garden   381
Ambulatory brace   241
Amputation   169
Angiogenesis   16
Ankle mortise   420
Anterior compression fracture   460
AO classification 168, 340
   School   302
Arthrodesis   252
Arthroscopically assisted procedures
   404
Articular cartilage   416
Artificial skin   171
Aseptic technique   4
Atlanto-occipital dislocation   448
Atraumatic techniques   6
Atrophic nonunion   151
Avascular necrosis   366
Avulsion of anterior arch of C1   454
Axial dynamization   31
Axial force transmission 71
Axial readjustment   44
Axillary artery damage   367

Barton   101
Base metacarpals   289
Baumann's angle 327
Benjamin Hobson   4
Bennett   108, 289
Bilateral facet dislocation   452
Bioelectric potentials   46
Biomaterial   9
Biomechanics   6, 10
Biplanar raduigraphy   348
Bohler   310
   Angle   429
Bolt   284

Bone-external fixator system   29
Bone-pin interface   62
Bone-plate system   29
Bone-to-bone union   379
Bone cysts   213
Bone grafting   206
Bone loss   169
Bone marrow   46
Bone setters   2
Bone stabilization   171
Bone transplantation   212
Bone transport   206, 212
Boxing glove   297
Brachial plexus injury   367
Brinell's hardness   18
Buckling fractures   229
Burst fracture   462
   C1   456
   Cervical spine   457

Calcium content   18
Callus   6, 17
   Cartilaginous   16
   External   24
Capitellum fractures   263
Carpal
   Injuries   293
   Osteotomy   189
Cast   5, 295
Cellular mediator mechanisms   52
Cervical injuries   446
Chance injuries   465
Charnley 82
Chemical messengers   15
Chin dynasty   1
Chinese   1
Ching dynasty   4
Chondral fractures   407
Chronic osteomyelitis   211
Circular external fixators   85
Circulation   8
Circumferential frame   98
Civilization   1
Clay-shoveller's fracture   451

Closed intramedullary nailing   134
Closed osteotomy   153
Closed reduction   224, 328
Clyburn external fixator   310
Comminuted fractures   7, 251, 348
Comparative doppler   175
Compartment syndrome   76, 141
Complete cord injury   442
Complete fractures   229
Complication hand fractures   297
Compression arthrodesis   59
Compression mode   69
Compression plate   10, 342
Computed tomography   359
Congenital pseudarthrosis   212
Continuous passive mobilisation   265
Contracture   83, 210
Controversy fracture management   253
Coral   314
Corticosteroid   297
Crack propagation   14
Crucial angle of Gissane   429
Cyclical loading   70

Danis-Weber classification   419
Debridement   198
Deep circumflex iliac artery   204, 382
Deformities   297
Delta frame   80
Diagnosis   219, 327
Diaphyseal fractures   11
Diepunch fragments   101, 310
Digital nerve   270
Distal radio-ulnar joint   100, 320
Distal targeting device   130
Distraction-fixation   109
Distraction   285
Dorsal angulation   309
Double-cluster   98
Dowel bolt   131
Dynamic axial fixator   88
Dynamic compression   24
Dynamisation   7, 47, 71, 81, 121

Early mobilisation   254
Electrical potentials   46
Electromagnetic   45
Energy-absorbing   12
England   4
Epidemiology   354
Epiphyseal fractures   337
   Lines   356
   Plates   295
Epiphysis   222
Eponychium   273
Exchange nailing   153

Extension tear-drop fracture   455
Extensor digitorum longus   206
Extensor tendon   287
External fixation   28
   Fixator   7, 198, 259, 263
External splintage   249, 250

Fabricius Hildanus   4
Far east   1
Fat-pad sign   222
Fatigue fractures   157
Fatigue load   14
Femoral-condylar fractures   408
Femoralbrace241
Femoral neck fracture   137
Femoral shaft fractures   240
Femur   88
Fibula   196, 204, 212, 420
Fibular pro-tibia   206
Fibulectomy fasciotomy   178
Fixation   249
   Device   255
Fixed pelvic volume   94
Flexion-distraction injuries   465
Flexion tear-drop fracture   451
Flexor retinaculum   291
Forearm brace   313
Forearm shaft fractures   230
Transverse compression   69
Fracture-dislocations   466
Fracture alignment   81
Fracture closed treatment   252
Fracture fixation   1
Fracture management   1, 249
Fracture mechanics   224
Fracture open treatment   252
Fractures   295
Fractures avulsion   278
Fractures comminuted   249
Fractures metacarpals   284
Fractures middle proximal phalanges
   277
Fractures of the distal humerus   340
Fractures of the radial head   348
Fractures of the radial neck   351
Fracture stabilisation   80
Fractures terminal phalanx   273
Frame assembly   80
Framis Glisson   4
Free-flap   196, 197
Frykman   309
Functional brace   5, 311
Functional recovery   6

Gamma nail   389
Gap healing   24

Garden's classification   380
Gastrocnemius muscle   196
Gracilis   202, 208
Grafting bone   204
Green-stick fractures   224, 229
Gue-hung   1
Gustilo's classification   75

Half pins   62
Halo immobilization   457
Halter's traction   447
Hand   187
Hangman's fracture   455
Hanover fracture scale   169, 170
Hawkin's classification   424
Hemi-arthroplasty replacement shoulder
   363
Herbert   293
   Screw   319
Heterotopic ossification   367
High-energy injuries   13
Hip brace   376
History   1
Hoffmann external fixator   272, 312
Humeral-ulnar angle   327
Humoral factors   8
Hydroxyapatite   314
Hyperextension dislocation   455
Hypertrophy   212

Iliac crest   204, 212
Ilizarov's   85
Immobilization   224, 227
Impingement syndrome   365
Indications digital replantation   189
Infection   270, 297
Inflammation phase   15
Inter-condylar fractures   340
   Eminence fractures   404
Interfragmental contact   69
Interfragmentary motion   15
   Strain   21
Internal fixation   251, 341
Interphalangeal joint   267
Interstitial fluid pressure   177
Intra-articular   346
   Fracture   7, 263, 340
Intra-operative films   327
Intra-cortical bone formation   39
Intramedullary fixator   121
Intramedullary implants   258
Intramedullary nailing   10, 31, 88
   Interlocking   34, 82
Intramedullary saw   153
Intramedullary splinting   237
Intraosseous wiring   107

Intrinsic stability   69
Irreducible fractures   329
Ischaemic time   190
Isolated posterior arch fracture of C1
   454
Isotropic material   12

Jet lavage   171
John Hunter   4
Joint degeneration   286
Joint movement   81
Journal of bone and joint surgery   4
Juxta-articular fracture   251, 400

K-wire   263, 272, 273, 275, 259, 295
Klinert   272

Lateral condylar fractures   337
Latissimus dorsi   202, 208
Lauge-Hansen classification   419
Leprosy 193
Li Chong-nam 3
Ligamentotaxis   73, 102, 301
Lisfranc joint   434
Lister   4
Little   4
Li Xi-chun   3
Long gamma nail   158, 383
Loss of tamponade   95
Lower limb replantations   191
Lumbar spine injuries   459

Malunion   228, 366
Material properties   9
Mechanical stimulations   36, 45
Medial epicondyle   340
Meiji   4
Metallurgy   6
Metaphyseal-diaphyseal angle   327
Metatarsophalangeal joint   206
Micro motion   31, 47, 67
Microsurgical techniques   187
   Children   210
   Pathological fractures   212
Ming dynasty   3
Mini-external fixator   107, 202
Mini-pin   284
Mini-plate   255, 270
Mobilisation   249, 272
Modular frame   60
Modularity   67
Modulation   9
Molecular stimulus   9
Monteggia's   237
Moulding   234
mRNA   16

Multiplanar frame   59, 68
Multiple toes   208
Multitrauma   9
Musculocutaneous flap   201
Mutilated hand   206
Myoelectric hands   269
Myoelectric prosthesis   191

Nerve
  Injuries   328
  Palsies   332
Neutralisation   88
  Mode   71
Non-telescoping implants   387
Nonunion   147, 211, 228, 273, 366
Nutrient artery   122

Oblique locking screw   128
Odontoid fracture   448
Olecranon
  Fractures   346
  Osteotomy   343
Open fracture   196, 268
Open reduction   227, 328
Operative treatment   5
Orthofix   43
Ossification   17
  Centres   222
Osteo   284
Osteoblastic activity   17
Osteochondral
  Fractures   263, 413
  Grafts   285
Osteocutaneous flap   204
Osteogenesis   17, 73
  Cells   45
Osteopenia   8, 31
Osteoporosis   373
Over diagnosis   222
Over growth   241
Over reaming   143

Palmar tilt   310
Partial cord injury   443
Patella-femoral joint   400
Patellar fractures   413
Pathological fractures   135
Pedicle vascularised bone graft   381
Penning fixator   310
Percutaneous fixation   227, 333, 328,
  404
Perforators   202
Periosteal blood supply   122
Periosteal callus   14
Periosteal stripping   168
Phemister's technique   211

Piezoelectric properties   46
Pillar fracture   456
Pin-bone interface   29
Pin care   81
Pipkin's classification   375
Piriform fossa   125
Plastering technique   225
Plastic deformation   232
Pohl   387
Polylactic acids   436
Polytrauma   83
Post-traumatic osteitis   180
Posterior instability   94
Preloading   64
Presacral venous plexus   95
Pressure glove   297
Primary bone grafting   311
Primary bone healing   6, 23
Primary callus response   15
Primary fusion   267
Primary operation   252
Prosthetic compliance   190
Proximal femoral fractures   123
Proximal humeral fracture   354
Proximal locking 128
Proximal phalanx   278
Prussia   4
Pull-out strengths   64
Pulled elbow   238

Quantitative magnetic resonance   49

Radial displacement   309
Radial inclination   99
Radial length   99
Radical débridement   171
Radiograph   219, 327
Re-displacement   228
Reamer products   121
Reaming   33
Reconstruction   187
Rectus abdominis   202
Reduction   3, 224, 249, 327
Regeneration   15, 191, 297, 366
Re-implantation   187
Remodelling   230
  Potential   241
Replantation   187, 188
  Arm   189
  Forearm   189
  Salvage   196
Retroperitoneal haemorrhage   99
Revascularisation   7, 187, 376, 427
Reverse Barton's   101
Rigid compression plating   30
Rigid fixation   6, 73

Ring avulsion amputation   187
Röntgen   5
Rotational deformity   230, 241
Royal orthopaedic hospital   4

Sacroiliac instability   95
Salter-Harris   337
Saucerisation   211
Scaphoid fracture   293
Scapular fracture   368
Secondary bone healing   23
Secondary osteons   20
Secondary reamed intramedullary
        nailing   90
Shaft metacarpal   287
Shanghai   4
Shear stress   11
Skeletal traction   241
Skin flap   201
Skin traction   241
Soft-tissue   169
    Coverage   196, 198
    Injury   168
    Score   179
Spica cast   241
Spinal cord injury   440, 441
Spiral fracture   249
Splint   4, 279
Stability   253, 400
Static compression   24, 41
Static interlocking   35
Stiffness   297, 366
Stimulating factor   5
Stress   8
    Concentration   62
    Planes   12
    Protection   32
    Shielding   71
    Tensile   64
Stress x-ray   403
Strickland   269
Structural rigidity   26
Subcapital transverse fractures   351
Subtotal amputations   169
Subtrochanteric   35
Sudek's dystrophy   310
Sukhtian-Hughes   39
Supracondylar dilemma   328
Supracondylar fractures   328
Sural nerve   208
Surgeons physicians   302
Sustentaculum tali   427
Syndesmotic injuries   420

Tang dynasty   3
Taoist   1, 2

Tendocutaneous flap   206
Tendon avulsion   275
Tendon
    Grafts   206
    Injuries   272
Tension band   107, 343, 414
Tension failure   12
Thenar muscles   208
Thermal crush   207
Thermal necrosis   64
Thoracic   459
Thoraco-lumbar   459
Three-point principle   231
Tibial blood supply   122
Tibial plateau and plafond   83
Tibial plateau fractures   401
Tibial shaft   241
Toe joint transplantation   268
Tomography   403
Torsional strength   64
Torsion injury   12
Traction   3
Trans-capitellar kirschner wire   351
Transfixion pins   61
Transforming growth g factors   46
Transiliac insertion   97
Transposition of the ulnar nerve   345
Transverse ligament rupture   450
Trapezoidal frame   95
Trauma energy   11
Triangular fibro-cartilage   309, 320
Tricalcium phosphates   314
Tscherne's classification   77, 168

Ulnar collateral ligament   320
Ulnar nerve   292
Ulnar styloid   320
Ulnar wrist complex   316
Unilateral facet dislocation   453
Unilateral frame   59
Unreamed nails   122
    Interlocking   82

Valgus deformity   245
Varus deformities   336
Vascular injuries   328
Vascular integrity   168
Vascularised bone grafts   204
Vascularised joint transplantation   286
Vascularity   7
Venous anastomosis   198
Vibration methods   49
Viscoelastic properties   14
Volar Barton's   318
Volar plate   279

Volkmann's ischaemic contracture 177, 210

Wedge compression fracture 451
Western approach 5

Wiring 258
Wolff's law 46

Yüan dynasty 3